INNOVATIONS IN CLINICAL PRACTICE: A SOURCE BOOK

Volume 18

Edited by
LEON VANDECREEK
THOMAS L. JACKSON

PROFESSIONAL RESOURCE PRESS
P.O. Box 15560
Sarasota, FL 34277-1560

Published by Professional Resource Press
(An imprint of Professional Resource Exchange, Inc.)
Post Office Box 15560
Sarasota, FL 34277-1560

Printed in the United States of America

Looseleaf Edition ISBN: 1-56887-059-0
Hardbound Edition ISBN: 1-56887-060-4
Library of Congress Catalog Card Number: 82-7614
ISSN 0737-125x

The copyeditor for this book was Patricia Rockwood, the managing editor was Debbie Fink, and the production coordinator was Laurie Girsch.

Preface

This is the eighteenth yearly volume of the *Innovations in Clinical Practice: A Source Book* series. Over 775 authors have now contributed to making the *Innovations* series a valued resource for practicing mental health clinicians. All volumes in the series follow the same basic format with five separate sections. No single volume is comprehensive or built around a particular theme. *Innovations* is a wide-ranging clinical resource series that contains topics either selected by the editors, suggested by readers, or, in some cases, based on manuscripts that have been submitted for review. We continue to receive very positive feedback from clinicians who have purchased the volumes, and are pleased that we have apparently played an important role in disseminating information to practicing clinicians.

Peter A. Keller was the senior editor of the series from its inception in 1981 through Volume 10 in 1991. We are all deeply indebted to him for his hard work, outstanding editorial judgment, and insights regarding the types of contributions that mental health practitioners need and want. Lawrence G. Ritt served as co-editor of the first five volumes and continues to consult about the development of subsequent volumes. Steven R. Heyman was co-editor for Volumes 6 through 10.

Beginning with the eleventh volume, Leon VandeCreek assumed the position of senior editor. Samuel Knapp served as an associate editor for Volumes 11 through 16. Thomas L. Jackson has served as an associate editor since Volume 11.

There are two other individuals who have made important contributions to the production of the eighteen *Innovations* volume. From the onset of this series, Debra Fink has supervised the final production of each volume and insured careful attention to details that others might have missed. Laurie Girsch has ably assisted her since Volume 8. We appreciate their thoroughness and cooperative spirit. Each year they have become more important to the success of the series.

Other contributors to the preparation of this volume include Patricia Rockwood and Judy Warinner, who have worked many hours copyediting and proofreading the manuscripts. Without their skilled assistance, this volume would not be a reality. We would also like to thank Susan Bach, Shelley Holland, and Josh Wilhelm for their help in preparing this volume for distribution.

Responsive to feedback from our customers, we have made a few changes to modernize this and future volumes in the *Innovations* series. To improve readability, we have narrowed the margins and decreased the type size very slightly. This allows us to include the same amount of content as prior volumes in a significantly easier-to-read format. We have also upgraded the binder used in the deluxe binder edition. Although the new D-ring style binder used in this edition is more expensive to manufacture than the standard binder used in previous volumes, it has a number of advantages: the new D-ring bind is 1/2" thinner and requires less bookshelf space; it holds the same number of pages as the standard binder; and pages are easier to turn, lay flatter for easier reading, and are less prone to tear.

We believe that the *Innovations in Clinical Practice* series is successful because of its highly applied focus. Our primary audience is mental health practitioners. To insure the continuing value of the series, we need the help of readers, and we invite your ideas and feedback on this volume. We also encourage you to consider the possibility of submitting a contribution.

An Invitation to Submit a Contribution

The editors are currently soliciting contributions for future volumes in the *Innovations* series. If you are doing something innovative in your work, please let us hear from you. Contact Dr. Leon VandeCreek, Senior Editor, School of Professional Psychology, 3640 Colonel Glenn Highway, Wright State University, Dayton, OH 45435, if you would like more detailed information on becoming a contributor.

Continuing Education

The Professional Resource Exchange is approved as a continuing education (CE) sponsor by both the American Psychological Association and the National Board for Certified Counselors, and credits may be obtained by readers who are required to participate in CE programs, as well as by those who simply wish to validate their learning. Interested readers are referred to the material at the back of this volume to learn how to obtain home study continuing education credits through the *Innovations in Clinical Practice* series. These programs provide an economical means of obtaining continuing education credits while acquiring relevant clinical knowledge. Readers have been consistently positive about the experience of obtaining CE credits through this series.

Copyright Policies

Most of the material in this volume may be duplicated. You may photocopy materials (such as office forms and instruments) or reproduce them for use in your practice or share contributions with your students in the classroom. For materials on which the Professional Resource Exchange holds the copyright, no further permission is required for noncommercial, professional, or educational uses. However, unauthorized duplication or publication for resale or large-scale distribution of any material in this volume is expressly prohibited.

Any material that you duplicate from this volume (with the exceptions mentioned below) must be acknowledged as having been reprinted from this volume and must note that copyright is held by the Professional Resource Exchange, Inc. The format and exact wording required in the acknowledgment are shown on the copyright page of this volume. The only exception to this policy is that clinical and office forms (not instruments) for use with clients in your own office may be reprinted without including the acknowledgment mentioned above.

There are exceptions to our liberal copyright policy. We do not hold copyright on some of the materials included in this volume and, therefore, cannot grant permission to freely duplicate those materials. When copyright is held by another publisher or author, such copyright is noted on the appropriate page of the contribution. Unless otherwise noted in the credit and copyright citation, any reproduction or duplication of these materials is strictly and expressly forbidden without the consent of the copyright holder.

Leon VandeCreek
Wright State University

Thomas L. Jackson
University of Arkansas

Biographies

Leon VandeCreek, PhD, Senior Editor, is Dean of the School of Professional Psychology at Wright State University. He was awarded the Diplomate in Clinical Psychology from the American Board of Professional Psychologists in 1989, and he is a Fellow of Divisions 12 (Clinical), 29 (Psychotherapy), and 42 (Independent Practice) of the American Psychological Association (APA). He is the author or coauthor of approximately 50 articles, books, and chapters in psychology. He is a contributing editor for *The Psychotherapy Bulletin* and a member of the editorial board for *Psychotherapy*, both publications of Division 29 of the APA. His interests include professional training, law and psychology, and ethics. Dr. VandeCreek may be contacted at School of Professional Psychology, 3640 Colonel Glenn Highway, Wright State University, Dayton, OH 45435.

Thomas L. Jackson, PhD, Associate Editor, is Professor and Director of Clinical Training in the Department of Psychology at the University of Arkansas. His research and clinical interests include the areas of sexual assault and violence and have resulted in over 50 articles, chapters, and books, as well as consultation and paper presentations to over 70 regional, national, and international groups. He has directed two American Psychological Association-accredited clinical psychology doctoral training programs, and has chaired the Boards of Examiners in Psychology in two different states. Dr. Jackson is a Fellow in Division 12 (Clinical) of the American Psychological Association as well as in the American Association of Applied and Preventive Psychology, the Association of State and Provincial Psychology Boards, and is Past Chair of the Committee of Accreditation of the American Psychological Association. Dr. Jackson may be contacted at the Psychology Department, 216 Memorial Hall, University of Arkansas, Fayetteville, AR 72701.

Table of Contents

Preface *iii*

Biographies *v*

Introduction to the Volume 1

SECTION I: CLINICAL ISSUES AND APPLICATIONS

Introduction to Section I 3

Time-Limited Dynamic Psychotherapy for Difficult Patients
Hanna Levenson 5

Interpersonal Psychotherapy for
Treating Late Life Depression
Gregory A. Hinrichsen 21

Chronic Medical Conditions:
Working With Patients and Their Families
Janet R. Schultz and Melissa Foti 33

Solution Focused Family of Origin Therapy
Terry D. Hargrave and Linda Metcalf 47

The Assessment and Treatment of Erection Dysfunction
Frederick L. Peterson, Jr. 57

Integration of Psychotherapy and Medication in the
Treatment of Severe Personality Disorders
Paulette Marie Gillig 73

A Cognitive-Experiential Model of
Dream Interpretation for Couples
Misty R. Kolchakian and Clara E. Hill 85

Parent-Child Interaction Therapy
Amy D. Herschell, Vicki A. Lumley, and Cheryl B. McNeil 103

Assessment and Treatment of Chronic Headaches
In Adolescents
Vanessa K. Jensen and Dunya T. Yaldoo 121

Assessment and Treatment of PTSD
In Motor Vehicle Accident Survivors
Jillian C. Shipherd, J. Gayle Beck, Jessica L. Hamblen, and Jennifer B. Freeman 135

Directed Family Therapy: Treatment for
Divorcing Families in Conflict
Kevin D. Arnold and Jeff D. Sherrill 153

Collaborative Divorce: An Interdisciplinary
Approach for Resolving Divorce Conflicts
A. Rodney Nurse and Peggy Thompson 169

Evaluation and Treatment of Sexual Disorders: Frottage
Richard B. Krueger and Meg S. Kaplan 185

Assessment of Dementia
Martin D. Zehr 199

SECTION II: PRACTICE MANAGEMENT AND PROFESSIONAL DEVELOPMENT

Introduction to Section II 211

What to Do When You Receive an Ethics,
Legal (Malpractice), or Licensing Complaint
Robert Henley Woody 213

Risk Management and Ethical Issues Regarding
Termination and Abandonment
Jeffrey E. Barnett, Sherry G. MacGlashan, and Alicia J. Clarke 231

Ethical Dilemmas in Interactions With the Media
Leonard A. Jason, Susan C. Jahn, and Meredith S. Miller 247

Maintaining Professional Competence for Working
With Culturally Diverse and Aging Clients
Jeffrey E. Barnett and Nicole Polakoff 257

Using Quality of Care Indicators as a Marketing Tool
John Rudisill 273

SECTION III: INSTRUMENTS AND OFFICE FORMS

Introduction to Section III 279

Psychotherapist-Patient Contract
Eric A. Harris, Bruce E. Bennett, and APA Insurance Trust 281

The Emotional, Sexual, and Spiritual Intimacy Scale (ESSI)
Joanne L. Davis, Rachel J. Pallen,
Christine M. DeMaio, and Thomas L. Jackson 289

Pre-Authorization Forms and Policies for
Increasing Fee Collections
Lawrence G. Ritt 297

A Clinical Supervision Documentation Form
Astra P. Brantley 301

SECTION IV: COMMUNITY INTERVENTIONS

Introduction to Section IV 309

Psychoeducational Groups for Adolescent Sex Offenders
Garry P. Perry, Stan Dimnik, Phyllis Ohm, and Brenda L. Wilks 311

Psychological Interventions for Surgery Patients
William W. Deardorff 323

Adventure Therapy With Adolescents
Jennifer Davis-Berman and Dene S. Berman 335

Improving Athletic Performance and Motivating Athletes
Bobby L. Stinson, II, Robert D. Friedberg,
Richard A. Page, and Michael J. Cusack 349

Providing Mental Health Services to the Deaf Community
Robert N. Basil 369

SECTION V: SELECTED TOPICS

Introduction to Section V 383

Integrating Telehealth Into Mental Health Care
B. Hudnall Stamm 385

Alternative Medicine's Contribution
To Mental Health Treatment
Kathryn P. White 401

Dyslexia: Overview and Treatment
George S. Grosser and Carol S. Spafford 417

Compassion Fatigue: When Caregiving Begins to Hurt
Jackson P. Rainer 441

A Simple Technique to Aid in the
Assessment of Resistant Children
Susan K. Skinner and Paul C. Guthrie 455

Marital and Sexuality Issues in
Clients With Disabilities
Martin G. Brodwin and Roy K. Chen 459

Working With Marital Affairs: Learning From the Clinton Triangles
Emily M. Brown 471

Introduction to the Client Handouts 479

Managing Traumatic Stress: Tips for Recovering
From Disasters and Other Traumatic Events
American Psychological Association Practice Directorate 481

Breast Cancer: How Your Mind Can Help Your Body
Alice F. Chang and Sandra B. Haber 485

Subject Index to Volume 18 487

Information for Contributors 491

Continuing Education 493

Introduction To the Volume

As in previous volumes, *Innovations in Clinical Practice: A Source Book* (Volume 18) is organized into five sections that reflect the diversity of contributions to the series. The subject index for this volume is contained on pages 487 to 490. A cumulative index to all 18 volumes is also available from the publisher.

The first section, CLINICAL ISSUES AND APPLICATIONS, deals primarily with therapeutic concerns. The various contributions, however, go beyond traditional therapeutic issues and also address important questions of assessment, as well as treatment. Issues that relate to a number of different types of clients and situations are covered.

The second section addresses PRACTICE MANAGEMENT AND PROFESSIONAL DEVELOPMENT. This section is included because of the increasing number of clinicians who work independently and require a source of information on practice management and professional development issues. We remain in a period of dramatic changes that affect the nature of our practices. New risks as well as opportunities are constantly emerging in this era of health care reform. In this section, we try to address relevant issues that we believe will be of interest to our readers. Some of our discussions here also should be of interest to students and clinicians who practice in organizations or agencies.

The third section includes assessment INSTRUMENTS AND OFFICE FORMS. The assessment instruments are primarily informal and designed to assist clinicians in collecting information about clients. Our goal is to publish screening instruments and forms that aid in the organization of data, rather than the making of formal inferences. There are some exceptions to this rule; however, we believe all fall within the bounds of accepted professional practice in the format in which they are presented. The materials presented here should be useful to psychologists and other professionals, with minimal potential for misuse. We assume that readers will be thoroughly familiar with any disorders or processes that they attempt to evaluate, and readers are advised to carefully review the introductory materials that accompany contributions to this section.

The fourth section on COMMUNITY INTERVENTIONS reflects our view that mental health practitioners have much to offer in the community beyond traditional clinical services. We trust that the material in this section will be of assistance to those who are interested in mental health consultation, education, prevention, and expanding their services to reach new and broader populations.

The fifth section, SELECTED TOPICS, includes a variety of contributions that do not fit neatly into one of the other sections. We also have included two handouts for use with your clients in this section.

Introduction to Section I: Clinical Issues and Applications

The CLINICAL ISSUES AND APPLICATIONS section includes contributions that are primarily related to new developments in assessment and treatment. No unifying themes are intended, and the range of topics is quite broad. This section provides a means for practitioners to access current information about new clinical techniques that might be incorporated into their practices, or to learn of new developments in specialized areas.

In the first contribution, Hanna Levenson describes a model of Time-Limited Dynamic Psychotherapy (TLDP) for Difficult Patients. TLDP is an interpersonal treatment approach for patients with chronic, pervasive, dysfunctional ways of interacting with others. The focus is on changing ingrained patterns of personality style. While the theoretical framework is psychodynamic, TLDP incorporates current developments in interpersonal, object-relations, and self-psychology theories, as well as cognitive-behavioral and systems approaches.

In the next contribution, Gregory Hinrichsen presents a framework for working with depression in older adults. He examines how interpersonal relationships are important in depression and describes the application of Interpersonal Psychotherapy to depressed older adults.

Almost every therapist will work with a patient who lives with chronic illness. In the third contribution, Janet Schultz and Melissa Foti describe the biopsychosocial model of working with patients with chronic illness. In addition to the familiar notion that the development and experience of illness is influenced by biological, psychological, and social factors, the model also posits that there are many nested levels to the system which influence health and illness. The model also shows that there are a variety of levels on which physicians, psychotherapists, and other health care professionals can intervene to alter the experience and course of the illness.

In the fourth contribution, Terry Hargrave and Linda Metcalf present a picture of Solution Focused and Family of Origin therapies and how they have merged the two models. They show how to make the Family of Origin model more efficient and action oriented while making the Solution Focused approach able to integrate and use information about the past.

Frederick Peterson, Jr., introduces mental health professionals to the latest thinking about treatment for erection dysfunction (ED). The objective of the contribution is for mental health professionals to develop a general understanding of how to respond with clients complaining of ED from the context of the multidisciplinary field of sex therapy. Assessment and treatment options are presented, including behavioral, mechanical, and pharmacological.

Medication is sometimes helpful in the treatment of severe personality disorders because biological factors, such as temperament, likely play an important role in the emotional and cognitive coping styles that shape a personality. Paulette Marie Gillig describes how to integrate psychotherapy and medication in the treatment of severe personality disorders.

Misty Kolchakian and Clara Hill present a cognitive-experiential model of dream interpretation for couples. They support the notion that dream interpretation is one useful way for couples to learn about themselves, their partners, and their relationship. Although the use of dreams is not new, few models have been described to ensure that therapists are employing the methods as recommended. The authors modified the Hill cognitive-experiential model of working with dreams with individuals to working with couples.

In the next contribution, Amy Herschell, Vicki Lumley, and Cheryl McNeil describe the Parent-Child Interaction Therapy (PCIT) for working with families with children between the ages of 2 and 7 who are experiencing a broad range of behavior problems. PCIT is a short-term, empirically investigated intervention that focuses on the parent-child relationship and on establishing a structured, consistent discipline program.

An occasional headache is common among individuals of all ages. Severe headaches, on the other hand, often interfere with daily activities. Vanessa Jensen and Dunya Yaldoo present a summary of research into assessment and treatment of chronic headaches in adolescents. The research has demonstrated the effectiveness of biobehavioral interventions.

Within the last decade, an increasing number of patients have presented for assistance for posttraumatic stress disorder (PTSD). In the next contribution, Jillian Shipherd, J. Gayle Beck, Jessica Hamblen, and Jennifer Freeman outline a cognitive-behavioral treatment approach that is targeted at individuals who are experiencing PTSD following a serious motor vehicle accident. The approach can be used in either an individual or a small group format.

Most clinicians have worked with clients with problems with divorce and its aftermath. The next two contributions focus on how to work with the most difficult divorcing families. Kevin Arnold and Jeff Sherrill describe Directed Family Therapy, which is a structured treatment protocol. Their model was developed in response to the ongoing litigation in which many families find themselves after divorce and under a shared parenting agreement. It is designed for couples at the more serious levels of conflict where there are threats to litigate or threats of violence with displays of intimidating behaviors. The contribution by A. Rodney Nurse and Peggy Thompson describes Collaborative Divorce, which is an interdisciplinary team approach for solving problems that arise in divorce. The team typically consists of a male/female coaching team comprised of two mental health professionals, a child specialist, a financial counselor who works with both parties, and lawyers who are trained in this approach.

Richard Krueger and Meg Kaplan present a discussion about the evaluation and treatment of a sexual disorder called frottage. Frottage is a sexual disorder that entails sexually arousing fantasies, sexual urges, or behaviors involving touching and rubbing against a nonconsenting person. Their contribution includes a discussion about assessment, treatment options, and several case studies.

In the final contribution of Section I, Martin Zehr describes the assessment of dementia in older patients. He provides clinicians with guidelines for conducting an initial evaluation of dementia that may be relied upon when deciding to advise a patient to pursue a more intensive assessment or to consider practical issues such as possible changes in living arrangements and needs for assistance.

Time-Limited Dynamic Psychotherapy for Difficult Patients*

Hanna Levenson

A now-classic series of studies on good and poor outcome cases treated in brief therapy reveals that patients who were hostile, negativistic, inflexible, mistrusting, or otherwise highly resistant uniformly had poor outcomes (Strupp, 1980a, 1980b, l980c, 1980d). Apparently their therapists became entrapped into reacting angrily; in general, they responded antitherapeutically to these patients' pervasive negativism and hostility.

Strupp observed that these difficult patients had characterological styles that made it very hard for them to negotiate good working relationships with their therapists. In such cases the therapists' skill in managing the interpersonal therapeutic climate was severely taxed. Because the therapies were brief, this inability to form a therapeutic alliance quickly had deleterious effects on the entire therapy. Based on such studies and clinical experience, Strupp, Binder, and their colleagues developed Time-Limited Dynamic Psychotherapy (TLDP) to help therapists deal more effectively with such difficult patients.

TLDP is an interpersonal, time-sensitive approach for patients with chronic, pervasive, dysfunctional ways of relating to others. The focus is not on the reduction of symptoms per se (although such improvements are expected to occur) but rather on changing ingrained patterns of interpersonal relatedness or personality style. Although the framework of TLDP is psychodynamic, it incorporates current developments in interpersonal, object-relations, and self-psychology theories as well as cognitive-behavioral and system approaches.

TLDP makes use of the relationship that develops between therapist and patient to kindle fundamental changes in the way a person interacts with others and himself or herself. Its premises and techniques are broadly applicable regardless of time limits. However, its method of formulating and intervening makes it particularly well suited for the so-called difficult patient seen in a brief or time-limited therapy. Its particular strengths include (a) applicability to the treatment of difficult patients (broad selection criteria), (b) relevance and accessibility for psychodynamically trained clinicians who want to work more effectively and more efficiently, (c) empirical scrutiny of the model, (d) a flexible framework that allows therapists to adapt it to their own unique therapeutic styles, and (e) avoidance of complex metatheoretical constructs by staying close to observable data where possible.

A TLDP treatment manual was constructed for a research program designed to assess the degree to which clinicians could learn briefer ways of intervening with challenging patients. This manual eventually was reproduced in book form as *Psychotherapy in a New Key: A Guide to Time-Limited Dynamic Psychotherapy* (Strupp & Binder, 1984). A more recently published clinical casebook, *Time-Limited Dynamic Psychotherapy: A Guide to Clinical Practice* (Levenson, 1995), translates TLDP principles and strategies into pragmatically useful ways of thinking and intervening for the practitioner.

---

*Portions of this contribution are taken from *Time-Limited Dynamic Psychotherapy: A Guide to Clinical Practice* (copyright © 1995 by Hanna Levenson), reprinted by permission of Basic Books, a member of Perseus Books, LLC.

TLDP: THE MODEL

An Interpersonal Approach

Historically, TLDP is rooted in an object-relations framework. Because it embraces an interpersonal perspective, the search for and maintenance of human relatedness is considered to be a major motivating force within all human beings. This relational view is in sharp contrast to that of classical psychoanalysis which emphasizes predetermined mental structures to deal with conflicts between gratification of instinctual impulses and societal constraints.

The relational view focuses on transactional patterns where the therapist is embedded in the therapeutic relationship as a participant observer. Transference is not considered a distortion, but rather the patient's plausible perceptions of the therapist's behavior and intent, and countertransference does not indicate a failure on the part of the therapist, but rather represents his or her natural reactions to the pushes and pulls from interacting with the patient.

In TLDP, psychological symptoms and problems are usually seen as arising from interpersonal difficulties. Often when people enter therapy, the presenting complaint involves some symptom (e.g., anxiety, depression) that forms the basis for an Axis I diagnosis (*DSM-IV*; American Psychiatric Association, 1994). Only after tracking the origin of such dysphoric feelings does it often become apparent that its source is interpersonal.

Assumptions Essential to TLDP Treatment

The TLDP model makes five basic assumptions that greatly affect treatment.

Maladaptive Relationship Patterns Are Learned in the Past

Disturbances in adult interpersonal relatedness typically stem from faulty relationships with early caregivers - usually in the parental home. Bowlby (1973) elaborated that early experiences with parental figures result in mental representations of these relationships or working models of one's interpersonal world. The child learns that in order to maintain connections with others and feel secure, he or she must behave in certain ways. These "certain ways" form the building blocks of what will become organized, encoded experiential, affective, and cognitive data (interpersonal schemas) informing one about the nature of human relatedness and what is generally necessary to sustain and maintain emotional connectedness to others.

Such Maladaptive Patterns Are Maintained in the Present

This emphasis on early childhood experiences is consistent with the basis for much of psychoanalytic thinking. From a TLDP framework, however, the individual's personality is not seen as fixed at a certain point, but rather as continually changing as it interacts with others. Although one's dysfunctional interactive style is learned early in life, this style must be supported in the person's present adult life for the interpersonal difficulties to continue. For example, if children have learned to be placating and deferential because they grew up in a home with authoritarian parents, they will unwittingly and inadvertently attempt to maintain this role as an adult by pulling for others to act harshly toward them.

Thus, dysfunctional interactions tend to be sustained in the present, including the current patient-therapist relationship. Accordingly, one can concentrate on the present to alter the patient's dysfunctional interactive style. Focusing in the present allows change to happen more quickly; the majority of the sessions are not spent working through childhood conflicts and discovering historical truths.

Dysfunctional Relationship Patterns Are Reenacted In Vivo in the Therapy

A third assumption is that the patient interacts with the therapist in the same dysfunctional way that characterizes his or her interactions with significant others (i.e., transference), and tries to enlist the therapist into playing a complementary role. From an interpersonal therapy perspective this reenactment is an ideal situation, because it provides the therapist with the very situation that gets the patient into difficulties in the outside world. The therapist is given the opportunity to observe the playing out of the maladaptive interactional pattern, and to experience what it is like to try to relate to that individual. The patient's perceptions of the therapist's behaviors are not considered as static re-creations of previous relationships (i.e., distortions), but as plausible possibilities given the patient's frame of reference.

The Therapeutic Relationship Has a Dyadic Quality

A corollary assumption to the TLDP concept of transference is that the therapist also enters into the relationship and becomes a part of the reenactment of the dysfunctional interpersonal interaction. In Sullivan's terms (1953), the therapist becomes a *participant observer*. The therapist cannot help but react to the patient; that is, the therapist inevitably will be pushed and pulled by the patient's dysfunctional style and will respond accordingly. This transactional type of reciprocity and complementarity (i.e., interpersonal countertransference) does not indicate a failure on the part of the therapist, but rather represents his or her "role responsiveness" (Sandler, 1976) or "interpersonal empathy" (Strupp & Binder, 1984). The therapist inevitably becomes "hooked" into acting out the corresponding response to the patient's inflexible, maladaptive pattern (Kiesler, 1988).

To get oneself unhooked, it is essential that the therapist realize how he or she is fostering a replication of the dysfunctional pattern, use this information to change the nature of the interaction in a more positive way, and collaboratively invite the patient to look at what is happening between them. Importantly, too, the patient can come to appreciate how he or she manages to get the therapist involved in a maladaptive pattern.

The TLDP Focus Is on the Chief Problematic Relationship Pattern

Although patients may have a repertoire of different interpersonal patterns depending upon their states of mind and the particulars of the situation, the emphasis in TLDP is on discerning what is a patient's most pervasive and problematic style of relating (which may need to incorporate several divergent views of self and other). This is not to say that other relationship patterns may not be important. However, focusing on the most frequently troublesome type of interaction should have ramifications for other less central interpersonal schemas and is pragmatically essential when time is of the essence.

Goals

The TLDP therapist seeks to provide a *new experience* and a *new understanding* for the patient.

*New Experience**

The first and major goal in conducting TLDP is for the patient to have a new experience. "New" is meant in the sense of being different and more functional (i.e., healthier) than the maladaptive pattern to which the person has become accustomed. And "experience" emphasizes the affective-action component of change: behaving differently and emotionally appreciating behaving differently. From a TLDP perspective, behaviors are encouraged that signify a new manner of interacting (e.g., more flexibly and independently) rather than specific, content-based behaviors (e.g., being able to go to a movie alone).

The new experience is actually composed of a set of experiences throughout the therapy in which the patient has a different appreciation of self, of therapist, and of their interaction. These new experiences provide the patient with experiential learning so that old patterns may be relinquished and new patterns may evolve.

The therapist determines the type of new experiences that are particularly helpful to a particular patient based on the therapist's formulation of the case (see below). The therapist identifies what he or she could say or do (within the therapeutic role) that would most likely subvert or interrupt the patient's maladaptive interactive style. The therapist's behavior gives the patient the opportunity to disconfirm his or her interpersonal schemata. The patient can

---

*The goal of a new experience presented here is somewhat of a modification of that originally presented by Strupp and Binder (1984).

actively try out new behaviors in the therapy, see how they feel, and notice how the therapist responds. This information then informs the patient's interpersonal schemata of what can be expected from self and others. This in vivo learning is a critical component in the practice of TLDP.

These experiential forays into frightening territory (from the patient's point of view) make for heightened affective learning. A tension is created when the familiar (though detrimental) responses to the patient's presentation are not provided. Out of this tension new learning takes place. Such an emotionally intense process is what "heats up" the therapeutic process and permits progress to be made more quickly than in therapies that depend solely upon more abstract learning (usually through interpretation and clarification). As Frieda Fromm-Reichmann is credited with saying, what the patient needs is an experience, not an explanation.

There are parallels between the goal of a new experience and procedures used in some behavioral techniques (e.g., exposure therapy) where clients are exposed to feared stimuli without negative consequences. Modern cognitive theorists voice analogous perspectives (e.g., Safran & Segal, 1990) when they talk about interpersonal processes that lead to *experiential disconfirmation*. Similarities can also be found in the Plan Formulation Method (Sampson & Weiss, 1986; Weiss, 1993) in which change occurs when therapists pass their patients' "tests."

The concept of a *corrective emotional experience* described more than 50 years ago is also applicable (Alexander & French, 1946). In their classic book *Psychoanalytic Therapy: Principles and Applications,* Alexander and French challenged the then-prevalent assumption concerning the therapeutic importance of exposing repressed memories and providing a genetic reconstruction. Their concept of the corrective emotional experience has been criticized for promoting manipulation of the transference by suggesting that the therapist should respond in a way diametrically opposite to that expected by the patient. For example, if the child had been raised by an intrusive mother, then the therapist should maintain a more restrained stance.

The TLDP concept of the new experience does not involve a direct manipulation of the transference, nor is it solely accomplished by the offering of a "good enough" therapeutic relationship. Specifically, a therapist can help provide a new experience by selectively choosing from all of the helpful, mature, and respectful ways of being in a session those particular aspects that would most effectively undermine a specific patient's dysfunctional style.

With sufficient quality or quantity of these experiences, patients can develop different internalized working models of relationships. In this way TLDP promotes change by altering the basic infrastructure of the patient's transactional world, which then reverberates to influence the concept of self. This emphasis on *experiential learning* allows TLDP to benefit a wider range of patients (broader selection criteria) than many other types of psychodynamic brief therapies that emphasize understanding through interpretation.

New Understanding

The second goal of providing a new understanding focuses more specifically on cognitive changes than the first goal just discussed, which emphasizes the affective-behavioral arena. The patient's new understanding usually involves an identification and comprehension of his or her dysfunctional patterns. To facilitate a new understanding, the TLDP therapist can point out repetitive patterns that have originated in experiences with past significant others, with present significant others, and in the here-and-now with the therapist. Therapists' disclosing their own reactions to the patients' behaviors can also be beneficial. Patients begin to recognize how they have similar relationship patterns with different people in their lives, and this new perspective enables them to examine their active role in perpetuating dysfunctional interactions.

Although the two foregoing TLDP goals have been presented as separate entities, in actuality the new experience and the new understanding are part of the same picture. Both perspectives are always available, but at any one time one becomes figure and the other ground.

New experiences, if they are to be more than fleeting events, have elements of representations (understandings) of self and others. Similarly, new understandings, if they are to be more than mere intellectualizations, have experiential and affective components.

However, in teaching TLDP a conceptual division is made between the idea of a new experience and a new understanding for heuristic reasons; this helps the trainees attend to aspects of the change process that are helpful in formulating and intervening quickly. In addition, because psychodynamically trained therapists are so ready to intervene with an interpretation, placing the new experience in the foreground helps them grasp and focus on the "big picture" - how not to reenact a dysfunctional scenario with the patient.

Inclusion/Exclusion Criteria

TLDP is seen as most suitable for people who have lifelong dysfunctional interpersonal difficulties. The first session is presented to patients as an evaluation session - an assessment of the appropriateness of TLDP treatment for them. However, the evaluation actually begins with the very first contact with the patient - whether directly (e.g., by phone) or indirectly (e.g., through a referral). How a patient handles the first contact with the therapist can be very telling about the patient's hopes, expectations, fears, attitudes, and overall style. For example, the patient who responds in a deferential and obsequious manner to the first phone call from the therapist ("Oh, doctor, I so much appreciate your willingness to see me. I have heard what a marvelous therapist you are and I am so much looking forward to meeting you and am so glad you will be able to see me although you are so busy with more important things") is already affecting the therapist differently than the patient who replies in a challenging, argumentative way ("I can only come in for appointments on Thursday afternoons and I cannot work with anyone who is going to be late. Are you late for sessions?"). And in the face-to-face meeting, much can be learned about dysfunctional patterns of relating to others by observing the nonverbal and paralingual behavior of patients right from the outset.

Table 1 (below) contains the five major selection criteria for determining a patient's appropriateness for TLDP: First, patients must be in *emotional discomfort* so they are motivated to endure the often challenging and painful change process and to make sacrifices of time, effort, and money as required by therapy. Most therapists have confronted the enormous (and frequently insurmountable) problem of trying to treat people who are court-referred or "dragged" into the consultation room by an exasperated family member.

TABLE 1: Selection Criteria for Time-Limited Dynamic Psychotherapy*

Inclusionary
1. Patient is sufficiently uncomfortable with his or her feelings and/or behavior to seek help via psychotherapy.
2. Patient is willing and able to come regularly for appointments and talk about his or her life.
3. Patient is willing to consider the possibility that his or her problems reflect difficulties in relating to others.
4. Patient is open to considering the possibly important role that his or her emotional life plays in interpersonal difficulties.
5. Patient evidences sufficient capacity for relating to others as separate individuals so that identifiable relationship predispositions can be enacted in the therapeutic relationship and then collaboratively examined.

Exclusionary
1. Patient is not able to attend to the process of a verbal give-and-take with the therapist (e.g., patient has delirium, dementia, psychosis, or diminished intellectual status).
2. Patient's problems can be treated more effectively by other means (e.g., patient has specific phobia or manic-depressive illness).
3. Patient cannot tolerate the active, interpretative, interactive therapy process, which often heightens anxiety (e.g., patient has impulse control problems, abuses alcohol and/or substances, or has a history of repeated suicide attempts).

***Note.** Adapted from Strupp and Binder (1984); MacKenzie (1988).

Second, patients must *come for appointments and engage with the therapist* - or at least talk. Initially such an attitude may be fostered by hope or faith in a positive outcome. Later it might stem from actual experiences of the therapist as a helpful partner.

Third, patients must be *willing to consider how their relationships have contributed* to distressing symptoms, negative attitudes, and/or behavioral difficulties. The operative word here is willing. Suitable patients do not actually have to walk in the door indicating that they have difficulties in relating to others. Rather, in the give-and-take of the therapeutic encounter, they must evidence signs of being willing to entertain the possibility that they have problems relating to others.

Fourth, patients need to be *willing to examine feelings* that may hinder more successful relationships and may foster more dysfunctional ones. Also, Strupp and Binder (1984) elaborate that the patient needs to possess "sufficient capacity to emotionally distance from these feelings so that the patient and therapist can jointly examine them" (p. 57).

And fifth, patients should be capable of having a *meaningful relationship* with the therapist. Again, it is not expected that the patient initially relates in a collaborative manner. But the potential for establishing such a relationship should exist. Patients cannot be out of touch with reality or so impaired that they have difficulty appreciating that their therapists are separate people. It would be impossible to conduct an interpersonal therapy if the patient did not know where he or she ended and the therapist began.

The exclusionary criteria for TLDP are very similar to criteria for red-flagging patients in other brief dynamic approaches (MacKenzie, 1988).

TLDP FORMULATION

The Cyclical Maladaptive Pattern

In the past, psychodynamic brief therapists used their intuition, insight, and clinical savvy to devise formulations of cases. Although these methods may work wonderfully for the gifted or experienced therapist, they are impossible to teach explicitly. One remedy for this situation was the development of a procedure for deriving a dynamic, interpersonal focus - the Cyclical Maladaptive Pattern (CMP; Schacht, Binder, & Strupp, 1984).

Briefly, the CMP outlines the idiosyncratic "vicious cycle" of maladaptive interactions that a particular patient gets into when he or she relates to others. These cycles or patterns involve inflexible, self-perpetuating behaviors, self-defeating expectations, and negative self-appraisals that lead to dysfunctional and maladaptive interactions with others (Butler & Binder, 1987; Butler, Strupp, & Binder, 1992).

Development and use of the CMP in treatment is central to TLDP. It plays a key role in guiding the clinician in formulating a treatment plan. It provides an organizational framework which makes a large mass of data comprehensible and leads to fruitful hypotheses. A CMP should not be seen as an encapsulated version of Truth, but rather as a plausible narrative, incorporating major components of a person's current and historical interactive world. It is a map of the territory - not the territory itself (Strupp & Binder, 1984). A successful TLDP formulation should provide a blueprint for the entire therapy. It describes the nature of the problem, leads to the delineation of the goals, serves as a guide for interventions, enables the therapist to anticipate reenactments within the context of the therapeutic interaction, and provides a way to assess whether the therapy is on the right track - in terms of outcome at termination as well as in-session mini-outcomes. The focus provided by the CMP permits the therapist to intervene in ways that have the greatest likelihood of being therapeutic. Thus the therapy can be briefer *and* more effective at the same time.

The TLDP formulation process is described, step by step, in Table 2 (p. 11). However, these steps should not be thought of as separate techniques applied in a linear, rigid fashion, but rather as guidelines for the therapist to use in a fluid and interactive manner.

TABLE 2: Steps in TLDP Case Formulation

1. Let patients tell their stories in their own words.
2. Explore the interpersonal context related to symptoms or problems.
3. Obtain data for the CMP.
4. Listen for themes in the patient's content and manner of interacting (in past and present relationships as well as with the therapist).
5. Be aware of reciprocal reactions (countertransferential pushes and pulls).
6. Develop a CMP narrative describing the patient's predominant dysfunctional interactive pattern.
7. Use the CMP to formulate what new experience might lead to more adaptive relating within the therapeutic relationship (Goal 1).
8. Use the CMP to formulate what new understanding might lead to the patient's increased awareness of dysfunctional patterns as they occur with the therapist and others (Goal 2).
9. Revise and refine the CMP throughout therapy.

Constructing the CMP

In the initial sessions, the therapist lets the patient tell his or her own story (Step 1) rather than relying on the traditional psychiatric interview that structures the patient's responses into categories of information (e.g., developmental history, education). By listening to *how* the patient tells his or her story (e.g., deferentially, cautiously, dramatically) as well as to the content, the therapist can learn much about the patient's interpersonal style. The therapist then explores the interpersonal context of the patient's symptoms or problems (Step 2). When did the problems begin? What else was going on in the patient's life at that time, especially of an interpersonal nature?

The clinician obtains data that will be used to construct a CMP (Step 3). This process is facilitated by using four categories to organize the clinical information.

Acts of the Self

These acts include the thoughts, feelings, motives, perceptions, and behaviors of the patient that have an interpersonal nature. For example: "When I meet strangers, I think they wouldn't want to have anything to do with me" (thought). "I am afraid to take the promotion" (feeling). "I wish I were the life of the party" (motive). "It seemed she was on my side" (perception). "I start crying when I get angry with my husband" (behavior). Sometimes these acts are conscious as those above, and sometimes they are outside awareness, as in the case of the woman who does not realize how jealous she is of her sister's accomplishments.

Expectations of Others' Reactions

This category pertains to all the statements having to do with how the patient imagines others will react to him or her in response to some interpersonal behavior (Act of the Self). "My boss will fire me if I make a mistake." "If I go to the dance, no one will ask me to dance."

Acts of Others Toward the Self

This third grouping consists of the actual behaviors of other people, as observed (or assumed) and interpreted by the patient. "When I made a mistake at work, my boss shunned me for the rest of the day." "When I went to the dance, guys asked me to dance, but only because they felt sorry for me."

Acts of the Self Toward the Self (Introject)

In this section belong all of the patient's behaviors or attitudes toward himself or herself - when the self is the object of the interpersonal pattern. How does the patient treat himself or herself? "When I made the mistake, I berated myself so much I had difficulty sleeping that night." "When no one asked me to dance, I told myself it's because I'm fat, ugly, and unlovable."

For the next step (Step 4), the therapist listens for themes in the emerging material by being sensitive to commonalities and redundancies in the patient's transactional patterns over person, time, and place. The patient's references to past and present relationships outside of therapy, seemingly innocuous comments, associations, and so on, may contain subtle clues as to how the patient is viewing the therapist (i.e., allusions to the transference).

As part of interacting with the patient, the therapist will be pulled into responding in a complementary fashion, recreating a dysfunctional dance with the patient. By examining the patterns of the here-and-now interaction, and by using the Expectations of Others' Reactions and the Acts of Others Toward the Self components of the CMP, the therapist becomes aware of his or her countertransferential reenactments (Step 5). Questions that practitioners may want to ask themselves include: How are you feeling being in the room with this patient? What are you pulled to do or not do? The therapist's internal and external responses to the patient provide important sources of information for understanding the patient's lifelong dysfunctional interactive pattern.

One's reactions to the patient should make sense given the patient's interpersonal pattern. Of course, each therapist has a unique personality that might contribute to the particular shading of the reaction that is elicited by the patient, but the TLDP perspective is that the therapist's behavior is *predominantly* shaped by the patient's evoking patterns (i.e., the influence of the therapist's personal conflicts is not so paramount as to undermine the therapy).

By using the four categories of the CMP and the therapist's own reactions to the developing transactional relationship with the client, a CMP narrative is developed describing the patient's predominant dysfunctional interactive pattern (Step 6). The CMP can be used to foresee likely transference-countertransference reenactments that might inhibit treatment progress. By anticipating patient resistances, ruptures in the therapeutic alliance, and so on, the therapist is able to plan appropriately. Thus when therapeutic impasses occur, the therapist is not caught off guard, but rather is prepared to capitalize on the situation and maximize its clinical impact - a necessity when time is of the essence.

From the CMP formulation, the therapist then discerns the goals for treatment. The first goal involves determining the nature of the new experience (Step 7). This new experience should contain *specific,* possibly mutative, transference-countertransference interactions (Gill, 1993). The therapist-patient "interaction has to be about the right content - a content that we would call insight if it became explicit" (p. 115).

After determining the nature of the new experience, the therapist can use the CMP formulation to determine the second goal for treatment, the new understanding (Step 8) of the client's dysfunctional pattern as it occurs in interpersonal relationships.

The last step (Step 9) in the formulation process involves the continuous refinement of the CMP throughout the therapy. In a brief therapy, the therapist cannot wait to have all the "facts" before formulating the case and intervening. As the therapy proceeds, new content and interactional data become available that might strengthen, modify, or negate the working formulation.

TLDP STRATEGIES

Implementation of TLDP does not rely on a set of techniques. Rather it depends on therapeutic *strategies* that are useful only to the extent that they are *embedded in a larger interpersonal relationship.* The Vanderbilt Therapeutic Strategies Scale (VTSS) was designed by members of the Center for Psychotherapy Research Team at Vanderbilt University (Butler, Henry, & Strupp, 1995) as a measure of how much therapists adhere to TLDP principles. Research indicates that the VTSS is able to reflect changes in therapists' behaviors following training in TLDP (Butler, Lane, & Strupp, 1988; Butler & Strupp, 1989; Butler, Strupp, & Lane, 1987; Henry, Strupp, et al., 1993). The VTSS is divided into two sections: The first is concerned with a general approach to psychodynamic interviewing; the second with therapist actions specific to TLDP. Table 3 (p. 13) contains the 10 TLDP specific strategies from the VTSS.

TABLE 3: Vanderbilt Therapeutic Strategies Scale*

TLDP Specific Strategies

1. Therapist specifically addresses transactions in the patient-therapist relationship.
2. Therapist encourages the patient to explore feelings and thoughts about the therapist or the therapeutic relationship.
3. Therapist encourages the patient to discuss how the therapist might feel or think about the patient.
4. Therapist discusses own reactions to some aspect of the patient's behavior in relation to the therapist.
5. Therapist attempts to explore patterns that might constitute a cyclical maladaptive pattern in the patient's interpersonal relationships.
6. Therapist asks about the patient's introject (how the patient feels about and treats himself or herself).
7. Therapist links a recurrent pattern of behavior or interpersonal conflict to transactions between the patient and therapist.
8. Therapist addresses obstacles (e.g., silences, coming late, avoidance of meaningful topics) that might influence the therapeutic process.
9. Therapist provides the opportunity for the patient to have a new experience of himself or herself and/or the therapist relevant to the patient's particular cyclical maladaptive pattern.**
10. Therapist discusses an aspect of the time-limited nature of TLDP or termination.

***Note.** From *Working Manual for the Vanderbilt Therapeutic Strategies Scale* by S. F. Butler and The Center for Psychotherapy Research Team, 1986. Reprinted with permission.

**Item written by H. Levenson

In TLDP, the therapist specifically addresses transactions in the patient-therapist relationship (Strategy 1). This focus on the here-and-now provides the building blocks for understanding how the interaction may be a microcosm of interpersonal difficulties. The therapist actively encourages the patient to explore thoughts and feelings about the therapist (Strategy 2) and conversely to discuss how the patient imagines the therapist might think or feel about the patient (Strategy 3). It can often be helpful for the therapist actually to self-disclose his or her countertransferential pull to the patient's specific behaviors (Strategy 4). In this way the therapist can guide exploration of possible distortions in the patient's perceptions of others or help the patient appreciate his or her impact on others ("When you did X just now, I felt like doing Y. Can we take a look at this situation?").

Throughout the therapy, the therapist attempts to discover and discuss with the patient any themes emerging in the content and process of the patient's relationships (Strategy 5). These explorations enable the patient to become more aware of problematic patterns of behavior (CMP). Asking about how the patient treats himself or herself (Strategy 6) can further be used to understand how interpersonal processes affect self-structures and vice versa.

The therapist can help depathologize the patient's CMP by guiding him or her in understanding its historical development. From the TLDP point of view, symptoms and dysfunctional behaviors are the individual's attempt to adapt to situations threatening interpersonal relatedness. For example, in therapy a passive, anxious client began to understand that as a child he had to be subservient and hypervigilant in order to avoid beatings. This realization enabled him to view his present interpersonal style from a different perspective and allowed him to have some empathy for his childhood plight.

In TLDP the most potent intervention capable of providing a new understanding is thought to be the therapist's linking the patient's recurrent patterns of behavior to transactions between the therapist and patient (Strategy 7). Although most of the therapy will be devoted to examining the patient's problems in relationships *outside the therapy* (as discussed previously), it is chiefly through the therapist's observations and interpretations about the reenactment of the cyclical maladaptive pattern *in the sessions* that patients begin to have an in vivo understanding of their behaviors and stimulus value. By ascertaining how an interpersonal pattern has emerged in the therapeutic relationship, the patient has, perhaps for the first time, the opportunity to examine the nature of such behaviors in a safe environment.

An oft-asked question is how early in the therapy the therapist can make observations having to do with transactions in the patient-therapist relationship as manifestations of the

CMP (e.g., transference-countertransference reenactments). The rule of thumb is that the therapist needs to allow ample time for the therapeutic relationship to evolve. That is, the therapist *and* patient need to have sufficient experiences in which particular dynamic interactions have played out repeatedly. In this way the interactive pattern is recognized not only by the therapist, but also by the patient.

A quite common error in technique is for the therapist, who is alert to discerning relationship themes, to point out such patterns to the patient long before the patient has had the opportunity to experience such redundancies in interacting with the therapist. These types of premature interpretations are usually met with surprise, hostility, and/or confusion on the part of the patient and can lead to gross ruptures in the working alliance. If the therapist has decided it is the apt time to link a recurrent pattern of behavior with others to transactions between the patient and himself or herself, he or she should make them as detailed and concrete as possible. Such specificity helps the patient experientially recognize himself or herself in the situation.

In Strategy 8 the therapist addresses obstacles (e.g., coming late) that might influence the therapeutic process. In TLDP these obstacles often are the meat surrounding the CMP skeletal structure. That is, such defensive maneuvers help the therapist discover the manner in which the patient tries to maintain a familiar, albeit dysfunctional, pattern. Resistance from the perspective of TLDP is viewed within the interpersonal sphere - as one of a number of transactions between therapist and patient. The assumption is that the patient is attempting to retain personal integrity and ingrained perceptions of himself or herself and others. The patient's perceptions support his or her understanding of what is required to maintain interpersonal connectedness. Resistance in this light is the patient's attempt to do the best he or she can with how he or she construes the world.

Therefore, the manner in which the patient "resists" will be informative regarding the patient's interactive style. The therapist often has the experience of "hitting a wall" when confronted with the patient's resistance. This wall often demarcates the boundaries of the patient's CMP. Rather than continue to hit the wall in an attempt to break through it, the TLDP therapist can stand back, appreciate the wall, and invite the patient to look at the wall also. Such an approach often avoids power plays with hostile patients and helps to promote empathy and collaboration. Because the focus in TLDP is on the interpersonal interaction, the therapist always has the process (between therapist and patient) to talk about when a therapeutic impasse has occurred. It is this focus on the interactive process that is the sine qua non of TLDP.

One of the most important treatment strategies is providing the opportunity for the patient to have a new experience of himself or herself and/or the therapist that helps undermine the patient's CMP (Strategy 9). The following examples illustrate how to intervene with two patients with seemingly similar behaviors but differing experiential goals.

Marjorie's maladaptive interpersonal pattern suggested she had deeply ingrained beliefs that she could not be appreciated unless she were the charming, effervescent ingenue. When she attempted to joke throughout most of the fifth session, her therapist directed her attention to the contrast between her joking and her anxiously twisting her handkerchief. (New experience: The therapist invites the possibility that he can be interested in her even if she were anxious and not entertaining.)

Susan's lifelong dysfunctional pattern, on the other hand, revealed a meek stance fostered by repeated ridicule from her alcoholic father. She also attempted to joke in the fifth session, nervously twisting her handkerchief. Susan's therapist listened with engaged interest to the jokes and did not interrupt. (New experience: The therapist can appreciate her taking center stage and not humiliate her when she is so vulnerable.) In both cases the therapist's interventions (observing nonverbal behavior; listening) were well within the psychodynamic therapist's acceptable repertoire. There was no need to do anything feigned (e.g., laugh uproariously at Susan's joke), nor was there a demand to respond with a similar therapeutic stance to both presentations.

In these cases the therapists' behavior gave the patients a new interpersonal experience - an opportunity to disconfirm their own interpersonal schemata. With sufficient quality and/or quantity of these experiences, patients can develop different internalized working models of relationships. In this way TLDP promotes change by altering the basic infrastructure of the patient's transactional world, which then reverberates to influence the concept of self.

The last strategy is designed to support exploration of the patient's reactions to the time-limited nature of TLDP and termination (Strategy 10). Because TLDP is based on an interpersonal model with roots in attachment theory and object relations, issues of loss are interwoven throughout the therapy and do not just appear in the termination phase. As termination approaches, one can expect to see the patient's anxiety handled in ways characteristic for that particular patient's CMP. The best advice for the TLDP therapist is to stay with the dynamic focus and the goals for treatment while examining how these patterns are evidenced when loss and separation issues are most salient.

Termination can be an emotionally difficult part of the treatment. It may involve leaving a therapist who has been empathic, respectful, and helpful. The process might rekindle memories of other losses and separations the patient has endured. It is no wonder that some patients have a return of symptoms, or express disappointment or anger about the "inadequate treatment." On occasion they might introduce new problems as a way of trying to maintain the relationship.

Clinicians who are inexperienced in the use of brief dynamic approaches can act out their own conflicts with termination. Such therapists may find patients' direct and indirect pleas for continued therapy difficult to handle. Ending a therapy earlier than one is accustomed to usually creates psychological dilemmas; the therapist can avoid or postpone these dilemmas by finding "good reasons" for extending the length of the therapy. Because patients readily provide such reasons, terminations in time-limited dynamic therapy are in jeopardy of being truncated or diluted. The beginning brief therapist can profit from becoming aware of his or her resistances to termination.* See Table 4 (below) for some common resistances to ending therapy.

TABLE 4: Possible Therapist Resistances to Termination**

1. Dependency issues - obtaining vicarious nurturance while offering help
2. The need to be needed
3. Conflicts around separation and loss (saying good-bye)
4. Conflicts around attachment and intimacy (saying hello to new patients)
5. Loss of an intimate and meaningful relationship
6. Therapeutic "perfectionism" - overinvestment in therapeutic results
7. Fear of being seen as sadistic, withholding, and/or rejecting
8. Difficulties accepting the limits of therapeutic intervention
9. Insecurities regarding one's own skill
10. Economic pressures to hold on to that which is profitable and dependable
11. Anxiety over loss of one's professional role
12. Guilt over failing the patient
13. Overconcern for the "successful" termination

****Note:** Includes some material from Bauer and Kobos (1987), Hoyt (1985), and Martin and Schurtman, 1985.

How does the TLDP therapist know when the patient has had "enough" therapy? In doing TLDP, I use five questions to help the therapist judge when termination is appropriate. Table 5 (p. 16) contains these questions presented in approximate order of reassurance to the therapist. If the answer is "no" to more than one of these questions, then I do not consider that the patient has had an adequate course of TLDP. The therapist should consider why this has been the case and weigh the possible benefits of alternative therapies, another course of TLDP, a different therapist, nonprofessional alternatives, and so on.

*I suggest that clinicians or trainees who are learning how to do brief therapy employ a time-limited approach with a definite ending date (as opposed to a specific number of sessions or a focused therapy approach). By having an explicit ending date, therapists are compelled to confront their resistances to terminating in a timely fashion; this can be a very important part of the learning experience.

TABLE 5: Guidelines for Termination in TLDP

1. Has the patient evidenced interactional changes with significant others in his or her life? Does the patient report more rewarding transactions?
2. Has the patient had a new experience (or a series of new experiences) of himself or herself and the therapist within the therapy?
3. Has there been a change in the level on which the therapist and patient are relating (from parent-child to adult-adult)?
4. Has the therapist's countertransferential reaction to the patient shifted (usually from negative to positive)?
5. Does the patient manifest some understanding about his or her dynamics and the role he or she was playing to maintain them?

As with most brief therapies, TLDP is not considered to be the final or definitive intervention. At some point in the future, the patient may feel the need to obtain more therapy for similar or different issues. Such additional therapy would not be viewed as evidence of a TLDP treatment failure. In fact it is hoped that patients will view their TLDP therapies as helpful and as a resource to which they could return over time. This view of the availability of multiple, short-term therapies over the individual's life span is consistent with the position of the therapist as family practitioner, a role consistent with the tenets of managed health care (Cummings, 1995).

Readers may wish to assess the degree to which they use these 10 strategies in their practices (before and/or after learning about TLDP) or they may use the VTSS to keep on track as they try to implement TLDP with a patient. A manual providing rating guidelines for each item with specific examples and rules to assist in making the ratings is contained in *Time-Limited Dynamic Psychotherapy: A Guide to Clinical Practice* (Levenson, 1995).

TRAINING

Therapist Resistances to Learning Brief Dynamic Approaches

Despite advances in the theory and technique of brief dynamic psychotherapy, as well as a number of research studies demonstrating its overall effectiveness, many therapists are still reluctant to learn these methods. Therapists' values and assumptions regarding the nature and practice of brief psychotherapy contribute to this reluctance. The area of negative attitudes toward briefer modes of intervention is extremely important, because such beliefs could adversely affect therapists' willingness and ability to use brief therapy methods effectively. Brief therapists and researchers have warned that a brief therapy could be undermined if the therapist does not feel optimistic and confident about the process. Thus psychodynamically trained therapists learning TLDP may need to work through their own conflicts regarding the approach.

There is evidence that TLDP training can alter the therapeutic values and attitudes of practicing clinicians (Neff et al., 1996) and trainees (Levenson & Bolter, 1988). Specifically, posttraining, therapists were (a) more willing to consider using brief therapy for other than minor disorders, (b) more positive about achieving significant insight, (c) more expectant that the benefits would be long-lasting, and (d) less likely to think that an extended period of "working through" was necessary. Also they were more willing to be active, more likely to see that a time limit was helpful, and more prepared to believe that patients would change significantly after the therapy was over. It is my opinion that dealing with attitudes and values associated with short-term therapy is a necessary component for the success of TLDP as well as any teaching or training program in brief psychotherapy.

Suggestions for Continued TLDP Training

Strupp and his research group undertook a direct investigation into the effects of training on therapist performance (Henry, Schact, et al., 1993; Henry, Strupp, et al., 1993; Strupp,

1993). The findings indicate that their intensive training program was successful in changing experienced therapists' interventions congruent with TLDP strategies (Henry, Strupp, et al., 1993), and that these changes held even with the more difficult patients (Henry, Schact, et al., 1993). However, their study also revealed some unintended and potentially untoward training effects. Although there were positive changes in therapists' skills following training, there were also indications of negative changes. The investigators speculated that there may be a posttraining phase in which therapists' performance declines as they grapple with integrating new techniques into their existing therapeutic mode.

For the reader who wants to learn more about TLDP case formulation and intervention, I recommend a multifaceted approach including reading, supervision (expert or peer), consultation, instructional videotapes, and workshops. There are presently two TLDP manuals available: *Psychotherapy in a New Key: A Guide to Time-Limited Dynamic Psychotherapy* (Strupp & Binder, 1984) describes the basic principles and strategies of TLDP; *Time-Limited Dynamic Psychotherapy: A Guide to Clinical Practice* (Levenson, 1995) provides a practical and pragmatic casebook approach. Several instructional videotapes are also available, illustrating TLDP formulation, intervention strategies, and termination issues.*

After reading/watching videotapes about TLDP, I advise becoming familiar with the steps in TLDP formulation (see Table 2, p. 11) and reviewing the TLDP relevant intervention strategies (see Table 3, p. 13). Next, therapists can practice devising CMP formulations and TLDP goals for their problematic patients (e.g., those with poor therapeutic alliances). Going through this exercise even for ongoing patients in open-ended therapies can be quite informative for therapists, helping them see more clearly where they might be unintentionally colluding with patients in some dysfunctional dynamic.

For those therapists who wish to try out a TLDP therapy, I suggest video- or audiotaping sessions and then reviewing these sessions using the VTSS to assess adherence and deficient areas needing further attention and/or guidance. Peer (or, if possible, expert) consultation is invaluable in becoming aware of nuances in the therapeutic interchange that inform the CMP. In addition, workshops on TLDP occur nationally and regionally sponsored by service-oriented agencies and professional associations. In San Francisco, I have established a training institute - the Levenson Institute for Training (LIFT) - to provide professionals with in-depth training in TLDP.

EMPIRICAL FINDINGS RELEVANT TO TLDP

My own research program has examined TLDP process and outcome with a personality-disordered population. As part of that endeavor, Overstreet (1993) examined the outcomes of 89 male patients with chronic, rigid, and pervasive interpersonal difficulties receiving treatment through two Veterans Affairs Medical Centers. He found that approximately 60% of them achieved positive interpersonal or symptomatic outcomes following an average of 14 sessions with therapists in training. By termination, over 70% of patients felt their problems had lessened.

In a long-term follow-up of these patients (Bein, Levenson, & Overstreet, 1994; Levenson & Bein, 1993), findings reveal that patient gains from treatment (measured by self-reported changes in symptoms and interpersonal problems) were maintained and slightly bolstered. In addition, at the time of follow-up, 80% of the patients thought their therapies had helped them deal more effectively with their problems. Other analyses indicate that patients felt they benefited more from their therapies the more they perceived that sessions focused on TLDP-congruent strategies (i.e., trying to understand their typical patterns of relating to people, exploring childhood relationships, and trying to relate in a new and better way with their therapists). Interventions incongruent or at variance with TLDP (e.g., therapists' giving advice, focusing on symptoms, assigning homework) were unrelated to patients' judgments of benefit.

---

*To obtain instructional videotapes, contact: Hanna Levenson, LIFT, 2323 Sacramento Street, Second Floor, San Francisco, CA 94115 or LiftCenter@aol.com; American Psychological Association, 750 First Street NE, Washington, DC 20002; Psychological and Educational Films, 3334 E. Coast Highway, #252, Corono del Mar, CA 92625.

Another study using these data is relevant for the meaningfulness of TLDP case formulation in a real clinical situation (Hartmann & Levenson, 1995). CMP case formulations written by the treating therapists (after the first one or two sessions with their patients) were read by five clinicians who did not know anything about the patients or their therapies. These raters were able to agree on the patients' interpersonal problems solely based on the information contained in the CMP narratives. Perhaps most meaningful is the finding that better outcomes were achieved the more these therapies stayed focused on topics relevant to the patients' CMPs. Thus, these preliminary findings indicate that the TLDP case formulations convey reliable interpersonal information to clinicians otherwise unfamiliar with the case and lead to better outcomes the more therapists can adhere to them.

CONTRIBUTOR

Hanna Levenson, PhD, has been specializing in the area of brief psychotherapy - as a clinician, teacher, and researcher - for over 20 years. She is Clinical Professor of Psychiatry at the University of California School of Medicine, founder of the Levenson Institute for Training (LIFT), and Director of the Brief Psychotherapy Program at California-Pacific Medical Center in San Francisco. She has published over 60 professional articles, two books - *Time-Limited Dynamic Psychotherapy: A Guide to Clinical Practice* (1995; Spanish ed., 1997), and the *Concise Guide to Brief Dynamic Psychotherapy* (1997) - and a professional videotape, *Time-Limited Dynamic Psychotherapy: Making Every Session Count* (1998). Dr. Levenson may be contacted at 2323 Sacramento Street, Second Floor, San Francisco, CA 94115. E-mail: LiftCenter@aol.com

RESOURCES

Alexander, F., & French, T. M. (1946). *Psychoanalytic Therapy: Principles and Applications.* New York: Ronald Press.

American Psychiatric Association. (1994). *Diagnostic and Statistical Manual of Mental Disorders* (4th ed). Washington, DC: Author.

Bauer, G. P., & Kobos, J. C. (1987). *Brief Therapy: Short-Term Psychodynamic Intervention.* Northdale, NJ: Jason Aronson.

Bein, E., Levenson, H., & Overstreet, D. (1994, June). Outcome and follow-up data from the VAST project. In H. Levenson (Chair), *Outcome and Follow-Up Data in Brief Dynamic Therapy: Caveat Emptor, Caveat Vendor.* Symposium conducted at the annual international meeting of the Society for Psychotherapy Research, York, England.

Bennett, M. J. (1983). Focal psychotherapy: Terminable and interminable. *American Journal of Psychotherapy, 37,* 365-375.

Bowlby, J. (1973). *Attachment and Loss. Vol. 2: Separation, Anxiety, and Anger.* New York:Basic Books.

Budman, A. H., & Gurman, A. S. (1988). *Theory and Practice of Brief Psychotherapy.* New York: Guilford.

Butler, S. F., & Binder, J. L. (1987). Cyclical psychodynamics and the triangle of insight: An integration. *Psychiatry, 50,* 218-231.

Butler, S. F., & The Center for Psychotherapy Research Team. (1986). *Working Manual for the Vanderbilt Therapeutic Strategies Scale.* Unpublished manuscript.

Butler, S. F., Henry, W. P., & Strupp, H. H. (1995). Measuring adherence in time-limited dynamic psychotherapy. *Psychotherapy, 32,* 629-638.

Butler, S. F., Lane, T. W., & Strupp, H. H. (1988, June). *Patterns of Therapeutic Skill Acquisition as a Result of Training in Time-Limited Dynamic Psychotherapy.* Paper presented at the annual meeting of the Society for Psychotherapy Research, Santa Fe, NM.

Butler, S. F., & Strupp, H. H. (1989, June). *Issues in Training Therapists to Competency: The Vanderbilt Experience.* Paper presented at the annual meeting of the Society of Psychotherapy Research, Toronto, Canada.

Butler, S. F., Strupp, H. H., & Binder, J. L. (1992). Time-limited dynamic psychotherapy. In S. H. Budman, M. F. Hoyt, & S. Friedman (Eds.), *The First Session in Brief Therapy,* (pp. 87-110). New York: Guilford.

Butler, S. F., Strupp, H. H., & Lane, T. W. (1987, June). *The Time-Limited Dynamic Psychotherapy Therapeutic Strategies Scale: Development of an Adherence Measure.* Paper presented to the international meeting of the Society for Psychotherapy Research, Ulm, West Germany.

Cummings, N. A. (1995). Unconscious fiscal convenience. *Psychotherapy in Private Practice, 14,* 23-28.

Frank, J. D. (1974). *Persuasion and Healing.* New York: Schocken.

Gill, M. M. (1993). Interaction and interpretation. *Psychoanalytic Dialogues, 3,* 111-122.

Hartmann, K., & Levenson, H. (1995, June). *Case Formulation in TLDP.* Presentation at the Society for Psychotherapy Research meeting, Vancouver, Canada.

Henry, W. P., Schacht, T. E., Strupp, H. H., Butler, S. F., & Binder, J. L. (1993). Effects of training in time-limited dynamic psychotherapy: Mediators of therapists' responses to training. *Journal of Consulting and Clinical Psychology, 61,* 441-447.

Henry, W. P., Strupp, H. H., Butler, S. F., Schacht, T. E., & Binder, J. L. (1993). Effects of training in time-limited dynamic psychotherapy: Changes in therapist behavior. *Journal of Counseling and Clinical Psychology, 61,* 434-440.

Hoyt, M. F. (1985). Therapist resistances to short-term dynamic psychotherapy. *Journal of the American Academy of Psychoanalysis, 13,* 93-112.

Kiesler, D. J. (1982). Confronting the client-therapist relationship in psychotherapy. In J. C. Anchin & D. J. Kiesler (Eds.), *Handbook of Interpersonal Psychotherapy* (pp. 291-312). New York: Pergamon Press.

Kiesler, D. J. (1988). *Therapeutic Metacommunication: Therapist Impact Disclosure as Feedback in Psychotherapy.* Palo Alto, CA: Consulting Psychologists Press.

Lebow, J. (1996). Do-it-yourself research. *Family Therapy Networker, 20,* 61-63.

Levenson, H. (1995). *Time-Limited Dynamic Psychotherapy: A Guide to Clinical Practice.* New York: Basic Books.

Levenson, H., & Bein, E. (1993, June). VA Short-term psychotherapy research project: Outcome. In D. A. Shapiro (Chair), *Long-Term Outcome of Brief Dynamic Psychotherapy.* Symposium conducted at the annual international meeting of the Society for Psychotherapy Research, Pittsburgh, PA.

Levenson, H., & Bolter, K. (1988, August). Short-term psychotherapy values and attitudes: Changes with training. In H. Levenson (Chair), *Issues in Training and Teaching Brief Therapy.* Symposium conducted at the annual convention of the American Psychological Association, Atlanta, GA.

Levenson, H., & Butler, S. F. (1999). Brief dynamic individual psychotherapy. In R. E. Hales, S. C. Yudofsky, & J. A. Talbott (Eds.), *The American Psychiatric Press Textbook of Psychiatry* (3rd ed., pp. 1133-1156). Washington, DC: American Psychiatric Press.

Levenson, H., Butler, S. F., & Beitman, B. D. (1997). *Concise Guide to Brief Dynamic Psychotherapy.* Washington, DC: American Psychiatric Press.

Levenson, H., & Davidovitz, D. (1995, August). *Prevalence of and Training in Brief Therapy: Results of a National Survey of Psychiatrists, Psychologists, and Social Workers.* Presentation at the annual convention of the American Psychological Association, New York, NY.

Levenson, H., & Hales, R. E. (1993). Brief psychodynamically informed therapy for medically ill patients. In A. Stoudemire & B. S. Fogel (Eds.), *Medical-Psychiatric Practice* (Vol. 2; pp. 3-38). Washington, DC: American Psychiatric Press.

Levenson, H., Speed, J., & Budman, S. H. (1994). Therapists' experience, training, and skill in brief therapy: A bicoastal survey. *American Journal of Psychotherapy, 49,* 95-117.

Levenson Institute for Training (LIFT) (Producer), & Holland, J. (Director). (1998). *Time-Limited Dynamic Psychotherapy: Making Every Session Count* [Videotape]. (Available from Hanna Levenson, PhD, LIFT, 2323 Sacramento Street, Second Floor, San Francisco, CA 94115)

MacKenzie, K. R. (1988). Recent developments in brief psychotherapy. *Hospital and Community Psychiatry, 39,* 742-752.

Martin, E. S., & Schurtman, R. (1985). Termination anxiety as it affects the therapist. *Psychotherapy, 22,* 92-96.

Neff, W. L., Lambert, M. J., Kirk, M. L., Budman, S. H., & Levenson, H. (1996). Therapists' attitudes toward short-term therapy: Changes with training. *Employee Assistance Quarterly, 11,* 67-77.

Overstreet, D. L. (1993). *Patient Contribution to Differential Outcome in Time-Limited Dynamic Psychotherapy: An Empirical Analysis.* Unpublished doctoral dissertation, Wright Institute, Berkeley, CA.

Safran, J. D., & Greenberg, L. S. (1991). Affective change processes: Synthesis and critical analysis. In J. D. Safran & L. S. Greenberg (Eds.), *Emotion, Psychotherapy, and Change* (pp. 339-362). New York: Guilford.

Safran, J. D., & Segal, Z. V. (1990). *Interpersonal Process in Cognitive Therapy.* New York: Basic Books.

Sampson, H. (1994). Repeating pathological relationships to disconfirm pathogenic beliefs: Commentary on Steven Stern's "needed relationships." *Psychoanalytic Dialogues, 4,* 357-361.

Sampson, H., & Weiss, J. (1986). Testing hypotheses: The approach of the Mount Zion Psychotherapy Research Group. In L. S. Greenberg & W. M. Pinsof (Eds.), *The Psychotherapeutic Process: A Research Handbook* (pp. 591-614). New York: Guilford.

Sandler, J. (1976). Countertransference and role-responsiveness. *International Review of Psycho-Analysis, 3,* 43-47.

Schacht, T. E., Binder, J. L., & Strupp, H. H. (1984). The dynamic focus. In H. H. Strupp & J. L. Binder, *Psychotherapy in a New Key: A Guide to Time-Limited Dynamic Psychotherapy* (pp. 65-109). New York: Basic Books.

Strupp, H. H. (1980a). Success and failure in time-limited psychotherapy: A systematic comparison of two cases (Comparison 1). *Archives of General Psychiatry, 37,* 595-603.

Strupp, H. H. (1980b). Success and failure in time-limited psychotherapy: A systematic comparison of two cases (Comparison 2). *Archives of General Psychiatry, 37,* 708-716.

Strupp, H. H. (1980c). Success and failure in time-limited psychotherapy: With special reference to the performance of a lay counselor (Comparison 3). *Archives of General Psychiatry, 37,* 831-841.

Strupp, H. H. (1980d). Success and failure in time-limited psychotherapy: Further evidence (Comparison 4). *Archives of General Psychiatry, 37,* 947-954.

Strupp, H. H. (1993). The Vanderbilt psychotherapy studies: Synopsis. *Journal of Consulting and Clinical Psychology, 61,* 431-433.

Strupp, H. H., & Binder, J. L. (1984). *Psychotherapy in a New Key: A Guide to Time-Limited Dynamic Psychotherapy.* New York: Basic Books.

Strupp, H. H., & Hadley, S. W. (1979). Specific versus nonspecific factors in psychotherapy: A controlled study of outcome. *Archives of General Psychiatry, 36,* 1125-1136.

Sullivan, H. S. (1953). *The Interpersonal Theory of Psychiatry.* New York: W. W. Norton.

Weiss, J. (1993). *How Psychotherapy Works.* New York: Guilford.

Interpersonal Psychotherapy for Treating Late Life Depression

Gregory A. Hinrichsen

Late life is a time of considerable change. Friends and family die, health problems develop, social and occupational roles that previously shaped daily life are lost or change, the character of interpersonal relationships may be altered, and the financial security of earlier years may be threatened. Despite these challenges, most older people evidence a remarkable ability to contend with these issues. For some older people, however, the stress of these changes results in major depressive disorder (MDD), adjustment disorder, or dysthymia. Although the rates of diagnosable depressive disorders are lower in this cohort of older people compared with younger individuals, for those with these disorders, the suffering is enormous (Weissman et al., 1991).

What is the most effective way to treat late life depression? Solid evidence attests to the considerable usefulness of antidepressant medication (Salzman, 1994). Some older adults, however, may have medical conditions that make prescribing medications difficult. Often antidepressant medications have side effects. Some older people are reluctant to take psychiatric medications or resist the addition of another prescription to an already complicated regimen of medications for health problems. And although antidepressant medications are often very useful in treating psychiatric symptoms, many older people seeking treatment for depression need guidance to more successfully contend with the difficulties that precipitated the depression or co-exist with it. What is the most effective way to psychotherapeutically treat late life depression? Studies have found that psychodynamic, cognitive-behavioral, and an array of psychosocial interventions are effective in reducing depressive symptoms. Psychotherapy with older adults appears to be as effective as with younger adults (Scogin & McElreath, 1994).

In recent years there has been increasing emphasis on the application of empirically supported treatments. Empirically supported treatments are psychotherapeutic interventions for which there is solid evidence of usefulness. The American Psychological Association's Division of Clinical Psychology (Division 12) Task Force on Promotion and Dissemination of Psychological Procedures (1995) carefully evaluated existing treatments and identified psychotherapies for which there was convincing evidence of efficacy. Interpersonal Psychotherapy of Depression (IPT) was identified as one of several psychotherapies that demonstrated efficacy in the treatment of MDD in younger adults. Increasingly there is evidence that IPT is also useful in the treatment of depression in older adults.

In this contribution I will examine how interpersonal relationships are important in depression, the framework for conducting IPT, and the application of IPT to depressed older adults. The contribution will conclude with a case example that illustrates the use of IPT with a depressed older woman.

WHY INTERPERSONAL RELATIONSHIPS ARE IMPORTANT IN DEPRESSION

Stressful life events, marital disruptions, and other life difficulties have been tied to increased risk for depression and other mental health problems. In studies of older adults, problems in social integration, social support, social stress, and social-psychological resources have been associated with a variety of indicators of poorer emotional well-being, including depression (George, 1994).

In an interesting theoretical paper, James Coyne (1976) posited a downward interpersonal spiral in the context of depression. Coyne argued that when a person becomes depressed, especially problematic interpersonal dynamics develop between the depressed individual and a significant other, typically a spouse. At the onset of depression, the spouse responds with numerous efforts to help reduce the distress of the depressed person. Efforts to help are rejected or seem ineffective. Efforts are often redoubled, but they do not have the desired effect. The spouse becomes increasingly frustrated and may become angry or upset. For the depressed person, the spouse's frustration only confirms the depressed person's feelings of hopelessness. The spouse may feel guilty and try harder to help the depressed person. Eventually the spouse begins to disengage from the depressed relative, further reinforcing the depressed person's sense of worthlessness and hopelessness.

Research has confirmed the troubled interpersonal dynamics that develop in depressive illness. Work from the National Institute of Mental Health Collaborative Treatment of Depression Research Program found that, over 5 years, the psychosocial consequences of affective illness were "surprisingly severe, enduring, and pervasive" (Coryell et al., 1993, p. 723). Coyne's (1976) framework provides suggestive evidence of why this might be. Work by Weissman and Paykel (1974) similarly found that depression negatively affected women's ability to function in the interpersonal sphere in roles as wife, mother, homemaker, and worker. Most troubling was their finding that even after depressive symptoms improved considerably, women continued to have interpersonal problems with significant others, notably spouses.

The sobering reality is that depressed people particularly need significant others at an extremely difficult time in their lives; it has been demonstrated consistently that the quality of relations between a depressed person and significant others affects the course of the depressive episode. The best evidence in this regard comes from studies of expressed emotion (EE) in families. Research on EE has examined the expression of criticism, hostility, and emotional overinvolvement of family members toward persons with psychiatric disorders. Twenty-five years of research has consistently demonstrated that persons with psychiatric problems (most studies involve individuals with schizophrenia) with relatives characterized as "high EE" have a much poorer course of psychiatric illness (Koenigsberg & Handley, 1986). It is important to emphasize that EE is not the expression of emotion per se but chiefly negative emotions. Studies of EE have also included depressed persons and their significant others. These studies have demonstrated that depressed persons may be even more vulnerable to the negative effect of EE in family members than persons with psychotic disorders (Hooley, Orley, & Teasdale, 1986). Interestingly, Hooley and Teasdale (1989) found that simply asking depressed persons how critical they felt their spouse acted toward them was tied to much higher rates of relapse in depression.

The same appears to be true with older adults. My colleagues and I conducted a study of 150 older adults hospitalized for an episode of MDD and the adult children or spouses who provided care to them during the depressive episode. Among several areas in which family members identified problems in the care of the depressed older person, interpersonal difficulties were the most frequently noted (Hinrichsen, Hernandez, & Pollack, 1992). We followed older adults for 1 year to determine which factors were most strongly tied to whether they recovered from the depressive episode or, if they recovered, whether they relapsed. We examined whether demographic characteristics of the patient or family member or indicators of the patient's psychiatric condition (e.g., current and past psychiatric problems) were tied to how the older patient fared clinically over the year. Interestingly, a poorer course of illness in the patient was tied to problems in interpersonally relevant issues between the older patient and the family member who provided care during the depressive episode (Hinrichsen & Hernandez, 1993). With a subset of study participants we examined the influence of EE on the course of depressive illness. There was an interaction between high EE and the identity of the family member. Patients cared for by adult children with high EE had a poorer course of illness over 1 year than those cared for by children with low EE. In contrast, patients cared for by a high EE spouse fared better clinically than those with low EE spouses (Hinrichsen & Pollack, 1997). Results suggest that in older adults the meaning of high EE for the patient depends on the identity of the caregiver.

FRAMEWORK FOR INTERPERSONAL PSYCHOTHERAPY OF DEPRESSION

IPT is a time-limited, manualized psychotherapy originally developed for the treatment of MDD. More broadly, IPT is influenced by the work of the Interpersonal School of Psychiatry of which Harry Stack Sullivan was its best known theoretician and practitioner (Sullivan, 1953). IPT is based on the assumption that interpersonally relevant events influence the development and course of depression. As noted, research supports this proposition. IPT does not assume, however, that for all people interpersonal difficulties are the cause of depression. There are many factors that may precipitate depression, including significant biological vulnerability for some individuals. However, given evidence that interpersonal factors play a very important role in depression, the developers of IPT chose interpersonal issues as the focus of the psychotherapy. IPT has been found effective in the treatment of MDD in acute and longer term studies of depression in younger individuals (see Frank & Spanier, 1995, for a review of studies). IPT has also been adapted for the treatment of other difficulties including dysthymia, bulimia, and bipolar disorders and for the treatment of depressed adolescents and persons with HIV infection who are depressed (Klerman & Weissman, 1993). IPT is listed as a treatment for MDD in adults by the American Psychiatric Association *Practice Guideline* (Karasu et al., 1993), the U.S. Department of Health and Human Services's *Clinical Practice Guidelines* for the treatment of depression in primary care settings (Depression Guidelines Panel, 1993), and, as noted, the American Psychological Association's Task Force on Promotion and Dissemination of Psychological Procedures (1995).

Because IPT is manualized, the rationale, focus, goals, and structure of therapeutic sessions are outlined (Klerman et al., 1984). IPT for depression is typically conducted in 16 sessions in three phases of treatment. In the initial phase (Sessions 1-3) several issues are reviewed. First, patient symptoms are assessed using the *DSM-IV* (American Psychiatric Association, 1994) system to characterize the psychiatric condition. The patient is told the name of the condition. The patient is educated about the nature of MDD and its treatment. MDD is characterized as a medical illness, and it is emphasized that MDD impairs an individual's ability to function. Often individuals blame themselves because of difficulty in performing occupational or social obligations. By characterizing MDD as an illness, temporary reduction in daily obligations is sanctioned until the patient is feeling better. An evaluation is made whether the patient should be referred for antidepressant medications. Although in research studies IPT alone has been found to be effective in the treatment of MDD, in clinical practice both psychotherapy and antidepressant medication may be optimal companion treatments.

Next, current and past interpersonal relationships are reviewed in what Klerman and colleagues (1984) call an "interpersonal inventory." What are satisfying and unsatisfying aspects of the relationship? Are there differences in expectations in the relationship? What changes does the patient wish to make in the relationship?

An interpersonal problem area is then identified from one or two of the four problem areas that are a focus of IPT: *Grief, Interpersonal Disputes, Role Transitions,* and *Interpersonal Deficits.* Finally, the therapist recaps his or her understanding of the problem, and treatment goals are established in conjunction with the patient. Then the specifics of IPT are explained to the patient (e.g., the focus of IPT on the here-and-now, the need for the patient to discuss important issues of concern, the duration of treatment sessions, and the 16-week length of the treatment).

The majority of treatment sessions are within Phase 2 (Sessions 4-13). In this phase, therapeutic strategies are implemented in one or two of IPTs four interpersonal problem areas. Persons with *Role Transitions* experience a major life change. Goals of treatment include helping the patient to mourn and accept the loss associated with the change and to see the new role or roles as more positive by restoring patient self-esteem and developing a more solid sense of mastery of the new role. IPT outlines specific strategies that the therapist uses to achieve goals in this and the other three possible treatment foci.

Persons for whom the therapeutic focus is *Grief* are essentially experiencing a complicated bereavement. Treatment goals include facilitating the mourning process and then helping the patient to reestablish relationships with significant others. Individuals with *Interpersonal Disputes* confront substantive problems in an important relationship, often with a spouse, but also with others, including, for example, a friend, co-worker, employer, or adult child. Some persons may evidence *Interpersonal Deficits*; that is, they may lack the requisite skills to establish satisfying relationships with others or, if established, are unable to sustain those relationships. Goals of treatment are to reduce the patient's social isolation and encourage the development of new relationships.

In the third and final phase of treatment, termination issues are addressed (Sessions 14-16). In this phase there is discussion about the end of treatment, an acknowledgment that ending therapy can be difficult for some, and encouragement of the patient's independent functioning once the therapy has ended.

A variety of treatment techniques may be used in IPT. These include exploration of options, encouragement of affect, clarification, communication analysis, use of the therapeutic relationship, behavioral change techniques, directive strategies (i.e., psychoeducation, direct suggestions, modeling), and role playing.

THE APPLICATION OF INTERPERSONAL PSYCHOTHERAPY TO DEPRESSED OLDER ADULTS

IPT appears particularly relevant to the problems of late life. Many older adults experience a variety of transitions in their roles as worker, spouse, and parent. Numerous studies in gerontology about the nature and impact of late life role changes attest to this (Antonucci, 1990). Although most older people evidence reasonably satisfying relationships with spouse, adult children, and friends, the later years may bring problems in one or more of these relationships. For example, a husband's retirement often increases the amount of time that the older woman spends with him. Many more hours in face-to-face contact may increase the likelihood that existing problems in the marital relationship are sharpened, resulting in heightened conflict. Increasing loss of relatives and friends typically seen in the later years may result in complicated grief. Although most older people adapt to interpersonal losses, notably the death of a spouse, others do not fare as well. The reasons why people experience complicated *Grief* are many but may include overreliance on the deceased spouse for emotional or practical support to the exclusion of other relationships, an ambivalent and psychologically complicated relationship with the deceased, or an extended period of caregiving to the deceased prior to death. Some older people may have evidenced *Interpersonal Deficits* throughout their lives, but the emotional consequences associated with them do not become acute until the later years when they experience life changes. Others may have relied exclusively on established family relationships for support in younger years. With the loss of these relationships they do not possess the skills to rebuild or sustain a social network.

There is growing evidence that IPT is useful in the treatment of depression in older adults. One study found that IPT was as effective as the antidepressant nortriptyline in the treatment of acute depression (Schneider et al., 1986; Sloane, Staples, & Schneider, 1985). In another study, Interpersonal Counseling, a brief form of IPT, was found to reduce depressive symptoms in older adults who were hospitalized with medical problems and who evidenced nondiagnosable yet clinical significant depressive symptoms (Mossey et al., 1996). The largest study of IPT (Reynolds et al., 1999) examined whether nortriptyline, IPT, or the combination was effective in preventing the recurrence of MDD in older adults. In the study, after initial treatment with IPT and nortriptyline, older patients were randomized to several treatments or treatment combinations. After randomization, IPT patients received monthly IPT. The researchers found that over a 3-year study period, both nortriptyline and IPT reduced the recurrence rates of MDD and that the combination of IPT and nortriptyline appeared optimal in reducing recurrence. The researchers felt that it was notable that, after initial treatment, even monthly IPT significantly reduced recurrence of MDD.

My colleagues and I have used IPT to treat MDD, adjustment disorder with depressed mood, or dysthymia in an outpatient geriatric psychiatry clinic at our institution. Some older patients have been treated with IPT alone or in combination with antidepressant medication. In the 20 or so patients whom I have treated or who have been treated by persons under my supervision, about 80% have evidenced significant reductions in depressive symptoms and many of them no longer meet criteria for a *DSM-IV*-defined depressive disorder (Hinrichsen, 1997). Clinically IPT appears especially well suited to treating late life depression and is consistent with general recommendations in doing psychotherapy with older people (Knight, 1996). We have found that IPT requires little or no adaptation when used with older adults. The most frequent problem areas are *Role Transitions* and *Interpersonal Disputes.* We have had few older adults leave treatment and have observed that many older people find the format of IPT appealing: Treatment goals are outlined, depression is treated as an illness (albeit one interwoven with interpersonal problems), the treatment is time-limited and problem-focused, and the therapist is an active participant in the therapeutic process.

We have found, however, that IPT may be less successful with older adults who evidence significant cognitive impairment. For example, one older woman with a severe MDD had cognitive deficits that were more severe than it appeared at the beginning of treatment. As treatment progressed, she evidenced substantive problems in remembering what had been discussed in the previous week's therapy and often failed to implement agreed-upon strategies for change in her daily life. Her son reported that she was less depressed in the 2 or 3 days following psychotherapy but she did not evidence a substantial reduction in depressive symptoms at the end of treatment. It is important to emphasize, however, that mild cognitive loss should not prohibit treating older adults with IPT or other forms of psychotherapy. Yet there may be limits to what one can achieve with IPT with older adults with substantive cognitive impairment.

As an IPT supervisor I have found that some therapists have initial problems in implementing IPT. Particularly for therapists with a predominantly psychodynamic orientation, the active role of the therapist may seem alien. There is much more back-and-forth, give-and-take between therapist and patient than typically occurs in psychodynamic therapy. In IPT the therapist plays the role of coach, supporter, and collaborator and, at times, cheers the patient on when successes are evident. The therapist may offer suggestions and recommendations when the patient has difficulty identifying possible options to deal with specific problems. Some psychodynamic therapists may feel uncomfortable with the IPT focus on current problems rather than presumed historical antecedents of current problems. And although a discussion of early life issues may be appropriate, the discussion ultimately needs to be tied to current problems.

Other therapists find it difficult to circumscribe psychotherapy to 16 weeks and wonder whether substantive change can be made in only 4 months. The characterization of MDD as a "medical illness" may feel uncomfortable to some nonmedically trained mental health care professionals despite the fact that biological changes associated with MDD have been well established. Although there is considerable latitude in IPT for the discussion of a wide range of issues, some therapists find it difficult to maintain a focus on treatment goals and, at times, will permit the patient to discuss issues that are at best tangential to the problems that brought the patient into psychotherapy. Particularly for those with little experience in doing psychotherapy with older adults, there may be a sense that older adults are unlikely to change or that it is doubtful that patients with numerous and complicated life problems can evidence substantive change. Nonetheless, for most therapists these concerns are surmountable. The most convincing evidence for novice IPT therapists is the fact that, consistent with research studies, most of their patients demonstrate significant reductions in depressive symptoms by the end of treatment.

A CASE EXAMPLE*

Phase One of IPT

"I just want to let you know, Doctor, I *hate* being here."

And so began the first session of IPT with Gladys. She continued with a defiant look on her face. "I hate doctors, I hate medication, and I hate the idea that at my age I have to see a shrink."

Gladys, a 70-year-old woman, had come to psychotherapy only after her daughter exerted considerable pressure on her. In the last 4 months Gladys had grown increasingly depressed, had problems with sleeping, had lost weight, had mild suicidal ideation, was hopeless, and was preoccupied with thoughts of her husband. It had become more difficult to accomplish everyday tasks like cooking and cleaning. And, of course, she was very irritable. Gladys told a harrowing story of her husband's stroke. She and her husband were avid hikers. In the middle of a hiking trip to a remote area, he complained of dizziness and then right-sided weakness. He fell to the ground and was unable to move. He had had a severe stroke. For hours she sat by her husband, helpless to do anything. Eventually, other hikers came by and notified authorities. A helicopter took her husband to a hospital far from their home where he remained for months. She made the decision that he would be best cared for in a nursing home where he had remained for the last 2 years.

Gladys returned to work as a real estate salesperson. Often after work she would visit her husband in the nursing home where he remained significantly physically disabled. About 6 months prior to beginning IPT she decided that her work was too demanding and retired. She now made daily visits to the nursing home where she often remained for hours. Within a few months she became depressed.

In the initial phase of treatment Gladys' depressive symptoms were reviewed and she was told that she had an episode of MDD. I administered the Hamilton Depression Rating Scale of Depression (HAM-D; Hamilton, 1960), a measure of depression severity. She had a score of 19 indicating moderately severe depression. She was surprised that there was a name that described how she felt.

"People suffering from MDD can also experience considerable irritability as you are," said the therapist.

With a small smile on her face she said, "I'm glad that somebody knows what's going on around here."

Current and past relationships were also reviewed. She had a reasonably good relationship with her daughter, although she complained about the man her daughter married. Notably, since her husband's stroke she saw little of the couples with whom she and her husband had socialized in the past.

"As far as they are concerned, I'm a widow. They don't want to hear about my husband's problems. And how many times have they visited him in the nursing home? Once? Twice? Some friends, huh?"

She spoke more lovingly of her friends at the real estate office. She had a special friend with whom she would have lunch everyday. She enjoyed the camaraderie with her fellow workers and her contact with real estate clients. Since her retirement she had seen little of her former co-workers, especially since she had become depressed. She said that she and her husband had a good relationship throughout their lives. She spoke admiringly of his many achievements in business and said that she and her husband had been well off financially. Although she said that her husband was very loving toward her during her visits to the nursing home, she confided that she hated the visits. "All that sickness really gets to you." I asked her why she spent so many hours at the nursing home if it was so difficult for her. She replied, "That's a good question." In a discussion of past relationships, Gladys mentioned that when she was a teenager her mother had a serious and ultimately fatal illness. She was required to care for her mother, which she said was difficult. "I was just a teenager. I wanted to

---

*Names and identifying characteristics in this case example have been changed to protect confidentiality.

do things that teenagers did but I couldn't. I had to come home from school and care for mother."

At the end of the third session I shared my understanding of her problems, the goals for treatment, and the plan for psychotherapy.

"As we have discussed, you have a major depression. On a scale that has been used in many studies of depression, you have a score of 19, which indicates moderately severe depression. This has made it much more difficult for you to do the things you normally do and has resulted in many of the symptoms of depression that you are now experiencing. I think it is interesting that your depression began shortly after you stopped working. You have what I call a *Role Transition.* You are transitioning from your role as a full-time worker to that of someone who is not. One result of retirement is that you don't see the friends at work. In fact, there seem to be few people except your husband with whom you have contact. You have also made a transition in your role as caregiver to your husband. While in the past you made visits to the nursing home several times a week, you are now there every day. This is different from the way that things were and it has been more difficult for you in recent months. I also think that because early in life you also cared for a sick mother, this experience has made it more emotionally complicated for you than for other caregivers to infirm spouses.

"MDD is a treatable illness, and I think we can be reasonably sure that you will be better by the end of psychotherapy. Research has shown that this type of psychotherapy is effective with about 80% of people. We also know that antidepressant medication can be effective. I think you can benefit by medication also, and I want you to have an appointment with the psychiatrist for a medication evaluation."

"I really don't want to take medication, but I will make the appointment anyway."

"I understand your concern. And although Interpersonal Psychotherapy has been shown to be effective without medication, I think that antidepressant medication will also help. Of course, this is your decision. There are several goals of our treatment. The first goal is that by the end of treatment you will be out of the episode of major depression. The second goal is that you will better come to terms with the end of your work life and the change in your role in providing care to your husband. The third goal is that you find a way of living your life now that is more satisfying and enjoyable to you. I think it is notable that you have little focus in your life now other than making visits to your husband at the nursing home."

She raised an eyebrow. "You mean this is all going to be accomplished in 16 sessions?" She stopped herself. "Well, that sounds OK with me because, as I told you, I don't want to be here anyway."

"As I mentioned before, for most people this type of psychotherapy has been shown to be effective in 16 weeks. We will meet every week. The focus of our discussion will primarily be on problems that you are confronting in your life now. If there are problems or concerns that you have about the way things are going in the therapy or in your relationship with me I want you to tell me."

"I guess I pretty much told you what I thought from the beginning."

"Yes, you did. I know you were reluctant to come for psychotherapy but I think it will be worth your time."

Phase Two of IPT

In early sessions Gladys said she continued to feel irritable and was prone to disputes with others. She so exasperated her dentist because of her complaints about his staff that he told her she should find another dentist. On the road she frequently honked her horn at other drivers whom she felt were driving too quickly or too slowly. She complained that my office was too bright or too warm, and that despite her long history of hiking, couldn't stand the one flight of stairs she climbed to reach my office. The psychiatrist who evaluated her prescribed antidepressant medication which she hesitated to take. When she did take it she complained of side effects barely after taking the first capsule.

In the early sessions of the middle phase, I urged her to discuss the circumstances surrounding her husband's stroke. She conveyed the story in an almost verbatim way as it had been told in my first meeting with her and without much emotion. Eventually with some reluctance she spoke of her own sense of helplessness and despair waiting for hours for help to come and blamed herself for being so foolish as to hike to a remote area at such an advanced age. "If only, if only I hadn't suggested that we take that hiking trip, things would be alright now." Self-blame was evident also in a discussion of her husband. She said that she should not have placed her husband in a nursing home and that she should care for him at home. In these sessions we focused on a more realistic understanding of how she could not have anticipated that a hiking trip would end in a stroke. We further reviewed the practical problems that would be involved in home care for someone as physically debilitated as her husband.

She continued her daily visits to the nursing home where she would often spend a good part of the day. During these visits she said how sorry she felt for her husband and, not unexpectedly, described conflicts with nursing home staff about the quality of care her husband was receiving. Because the nursing home visits were so distressing to her, we explored other options for visiting: fewer hours, fewer days, or a different structure to the visits. She said that she felt "compelled" to visit her husband and would feel guilty if she were not at the nursing home.

At this point, the therapy shifted to a discussion of her relationship with her husband. She described a happy marriage to an entrepreneurial man whose business success offered a very comfortable lifestyle. I asked whether his extended nursing home stay had put a strain on finances. Her face tightened at mention of finances. "Things are very bad now." She began to talk about the aftermath of her husband's stroke. "I had to take charge of the finances - what a disaster." Unbeknownst to Gladys, her husband had taken their considerable resources and made bad investments in the stock market. To cover his losses, he had taken a second mortgage on their home. Because of this, at the time her husband entered the nursing home, she was forced to sell their home to cover losses and rent an apartment. "This apartment is not a home. It's a place to sleep."

In the next session there was further discussion of options with regard to the frequency of visiting her husband in the nursing home. She said that "it made sense" that she should spend less time at the nursing home and cultivate other activities and friendships. She wondered why it was so difficult. "Do you think that I visit him so often because I am so mad at him?" I encouraged her to discuss this. In this session and the next she spoke of how betrayed she felt by her husband's mishandling of the finances. "He didn't even tell me. But then, after all, I never asked." She spoke of her resentment that his stroke had so dramatically changed her life but said she felt confused by her feelings. "How can you be so angry at someone who is so helpless?" This discussion blended into some recollections of difficulties in the care of her mother when she was a teenager. I pointed out the parallels, which were evident to her at this point, and underscored that in view of her responsibilities for care of her mother during her teenage years, care for a disabled husband was more emotionally complicated for her.

"That makes a lot of sense."

By the 10th session Gladys' depressive symptoms began to improve. She was less depressed and less irritable. She was sleeping better and had more energy. She irregularly took the antidepressant because of perceived side effects. However, I continued to encourage her to have an active dialogue with the psychiatrist about medication. With a sense of pride, she told me that she had joined a Yoga class and a book club at the local library. Although she still felt some guilt about taking time from her nursing home visits, she said that these activities were important to do. She discussed her past work as a real estate salesperson which she appraised as a mixture of "good and bad." She liked contact with clients and co-workers, but the hours were long and there were many aggravations. She mused that perhaps one reason she had worked was because it was a good excuse not to visit her husband every day at the nursing home.

In the remaining sessions of this Second Phase of IPT we continued to examine her nursing home visiting schedule and additional options to enhance her social and recreational life. I pointed out the fact that after the Yoga class and book club meetings she felt better emotionally and felt better about herself. During this time she rekindled a friendship with a former co-worker who seemed delighted that she wanted to reestablish a relationship. By the 13th session Gladys had cut in half the number of hours she spent at the nursing home, continued the social activities she had initiated, and had planned a vacation with her daughter.

Phase Three of IPT

Throughout the psychotherapy I reminded Gladys of remaining sessions. At the 14th session I told her that we had two remaining sessions. She seemed surprised and asked why the psychotherapy needed to end. I reviewed our initial plan of treatment and pointed out that she was doing much better, which she acknowledged. In the remaining sessions we discussed her feelings about termination and ways in which she could build upon the changes that she had made during the psychotherapy.

In the final session I readministered the HAM-D.

"Gladys, in this remaining session I want to review how things have gone during the psychotherapy. As you may recall, at the beginning of psychotherapy, one of our goals was that you would be out of the episode of major depression. The score on the depression rating scale that we did at the beginning of therapy was 19, indicating moderately severe depression. Your score now is 2, indicating a virtual absence of depression. Further, you are out of an episode of major depression."

"It does seem that way," Gladys said.

"The second goal was that you would better come to terms with the end of your work life and change in your role in providing care to your husband. I believe that our talks together underscored why this has been so hard for you. You were angry at your husband because his stroke dramatically changed your life and also angry because your husband had mishandled the finances. This was emotionally confusing for you because you also felt very sad to see how debilitated your husband was. It was further complicated by the fact that early in your life you had to provide care to a sickly mother, a situation about which you held feelings of resentment and pity toward her. Work in real estate provided a good reason for not spending so much time at the nursing home. Without work, however, you felt compelled to spend much more time at the nursing home than you were comfortable with. Because you spent so much time at the nursing home, you cut yourself off from things that were potentially enjoyable and pleasurable to you. The result was the episode of major depression."

"The third goal of the therapy was to find a way of living your life now that was more satisfying and enjoyable to you. I think you've made very good headway here. You have now made time for your Yoga class, the book club, some friendships, and even the trip with your daughter. All these things are related to feeling better and feeling better about yourself."

"This was more helpful than I thought it was going to be," said Gladys.

"Gladys, it is you who has helped yourself. You were the one who came here every week despite feeling very skeptical about psychotherapy. You were the one who struggled with a confusing set of feelings about your husband and yourself. You were the one who has begun to reshape your daily life."

Gladys indicated that in recent weeks she had begun to take the antidepressant on a regular basis. I encouraged her to have an ongoing discussion with the psychiatrist about this. After reviewing different options, Gladys agreed to join a support group for older people caring for debilitated spouses.

RESOURCES FOR CONDUCTING INTERPERSONAL PSYCHOTHERAPY

For those interested in learning IPT the best starting place is Klerman and colleagues' original treatment manual published as *Interpersonal Psychotherapy of Depression* (Klerman et al., 1984). There is also a patient companion guide: *Mastering Depression: A Patient's Guide to Interpersonal Psychotherapy* (Weissman, 1995). Continuing education seminars on IPT are often available at major professional meetings including the American Psychological Association and American Psychiatric Association. Individual supervision of IPT can be arranged sometimes with professionals who have been formally trained in IPT. John Markowitz, MD (1998a, 1998b), in the Department of Psychiatry at the New York Presbyterian Hospital (New York Presbyterian Hospital, 525 E. 68th Street, #1322, New York, NY 10021)) has compiled a list of mental health professionals with IPT expertise. The interested reader may also contact this author to locate IPT supervision. Sometimes supervision of audio- or videotaped IPT sessions can be conducted by telephone.

As the clinical case illustrates, IPT can be used flexibly and effectively in the treatment of MDD in the elderly. Results of this treatment are generally consistent with outcomes with other older individuals with depressive disorders who have been treated by me or those under my supervision. Further, these results are also consistent with those found in studies of younger and older depressed persons treated with IPT.

CONTRIBUTOR

Gregory A. Hinrichsen, PhD, is Director of Psychology Training and the Director of the Geropsychology Fellowship at Hillside Hospital, North Shore - Long Island Jewish Health System. He is also Associate Professor of Psychiatry at the Albert Einstein College of Medicine. Dr. Hinrichsen has been in the gerontology field since 1976 and is President of the American Psychological Association's Division 12, Section II - Clinical Geropsychology. His research interests include family issues in late life depression and dementia. Dr. Hinrichsen may be reached at Research Building, Hillside Hospital, 75-59 263 Street, Glen Oaks, NY 11001. E-mail: hinrichs@lij.edu

RESOURCES

American Psychiatric Association. (1994). *Diagnostic and Statistical Manual of Mental Disorders* (4th ed.). Washington, DC: Author.

Antonucci, T. C. (1990). Social supports and social relationships. In R. Binstock & L. George (Eds.), *Handbook of Aging and the Social Sciences* (3rd ed., pp. 205-226). San Diego, CA: Academic Press.

Coryell, W., Scheftner, W., Keller, M., Endicott, J., Maser, J., & Klerman, G. (1993). The enduring psychosocial consequences of mania and depression. *American Journal of Psychiatry, 150,* 720-727.

Coyne, J. C. (1976). Depression and the response of others. *Journal of Abnormal Psychology, 85,* 186-193.

Depression Guidelines Panel. (1993). *Clinical Practice Guideline: Depression in Primary Care: Treatment of Major Depression* (Agency for Health Care Policy and Research Publication 93-0551). Rockville, MD: U.S. Department of Health and Human Services, Agency for Health Care Policy and Research.

Frank, E., & Spanier, C. (1995). Interpersonal psychotherapy for depression: Overview, clinical efficacy, and future directions. *Clinical Psychology: Science and Practice, 2,* 349-369.

George, L. K. (1994). Social factors and depression in late life. In L. S. Schneider, C. F. Reynolds, B. D. Lebowitz, & A. J. Friedhoff (Eds.), *Diagnosis and Treatment of Depression in Late Life* (pp. 131-153). Washington, DC: American Psychiatric Press.

Hamilton, M. (1960). A rating scale for depression. *Journal of Neurology, Neurosurgery and Psychiatry, 23,* 56-62.

Hinrichsen, G. A. (1997). Interpersonal psychotherapy for depressed older adults. *Journal of Geriatric Psychiatry, 30,* 239-257.

Hinrichsen, G. A., & Hernandez, N. A. (1993). Factors associated with recovery from and relapse into major depressive disorder in the elderly. *American Journal of Psychiatry, 150,* 1820-1825.

Hinrichsen, G. A., Hernandez, N. A., & Pollack, S. (1992). Difficulties and rewards in family care of the depressed older adults. *Gerontologist, 32,* 486-492.

Hinrichsen, G. A., & Pollack, S. (1997). Expressed emotion and the course of late life depression. *Journal of Abnormal Psychology, 106,* 336-340.

Hooley, J. M., Orley, J., & Teasdale, D. J. (1986). Levels of expressed emotion and relapse in depressed patients. *British Journal of Psychiatry, 148,* 642-647.

Hooley, J. M., & Teasdale, J. D. (1989). Predictors of relapse in unipolar depressives: Expressed emotion, marital distress, and perceived criticism. *Journal of Abnormal Psychology, 98,* 229-235.

Karasu, T. B., Docherty, J. P., Gelenberg, A., Kupfer, D. J., Merriam, A. E., & Shodoan, R. (1993). Practice guideline for major depressive disorder in adults. *American Journal of Psychiatry, 150,* 1-26.

Klerman, G. L., & Weissman, M. M. (1993). *New Applications of Interpersonal Psychotherapy.* Washington, DC: American Psychiatric Press.

Klerman, G. L., Weissman, M. M., Rounsaville, B. J., & Chevron, E. S. (1984). *Interpersonal Psychotherapy of Depression.* New York: Basic Books.

Knight, B. G. (1996). *Psychotherapy With Older Adults* (2nd ed.). Thousand Oaks, CA: Sage.

Koenigsberg, H. W., & Handley, R. (1986). Expressed emotion: From predictive index to clinical construct. *American Journal of Psychiatry, 143,* 1361-1373.

Markowitz, J. C. (Ed.). (1998a). *Interpersonal Psychotherapy* [Review of Psychiatry Series]. Washington, DC: American Psychiatric Press.

Markowitz, J. C. (1998b). *Interpersonal Psychotherapy for Dysthymic Disorder.* Washington, DC: American Psychiatric Press.

Mossey, J. M., Nott, K. A., Higgins, M., & Talerico, K. (1996). Effectiveness of a psychosocial intervention, interpersonal counseling, for subdysthymic depression in medically ill elderly. *Journals of Gerontology: Medical Sciences, 51A,* M172-178.

Reynolds, C. F., Frank, E., Perel, J. M., Imber, S. D., Cornes, C., Miller, M. D., Mazumdar, S., Houck, P. R., Dew, M. A., Stack, J. A., Pollock, B. G., & Kupfer, D. J. (1999). Nortriptyline and interpersonal psychotherapy as maintenance therapies for recurrent major depression: A randomized controlled trial in patients older than 59 years. *Journal of the American Medical Association, 281,* 39-45.

Salzman, C. (1994). Pharmacological treatment of depression in elderly patients. In L. S. Schneider, C. F. Reynolds, B. D. Lebowitz, & A. J. Friedhoff (Eds.), *Diagnosis and Treatment of Depression in Late Life* (pp. 181-244). Washington, DC: American Psychiatric Press.

Schneider, L. S., Sloane, R. B., Staples, F. R., & Bender, M. (1986). Pretreatment orthostatic hypotension as a predictor of response to nortriptyline in geriatric depression. *Journal of Clinical Psychopharmacology, 6,* 172-176.

Scogin, F., & McElreath, L. (1994). Efficacy of psychosocial treatment for geriatric depression: A quantitative review. *Journal of Consulting and Clinical Psychology, 62,* 69-73.

Sloane, R. B., Staples, F. R., & Schneider, L. S. (1985). Interpersonal psychotherapy versus nortriptyline for depression in the elderly. In T. R. Norman & L. Dennerstein (Eds.), *Clinical and Pharmacological Studies in Psychiatric Disorders* (pp. 344-346). London: John Libbey.

Sullivan, H. S. (1953). *The Interpersonal Theory of Psychiatry.* New York: Norton.

Task Force on Promotion and Dissemination of Psychological Procedures. (1995). Training in and dissemination of empirically-validated psychological treatments: Report and recommendations. *Clinical Psychologist, 48,* 3-23.

Weissman, M. M. (1995). *Mastering Depression: A Patient's Guide to Interpersonal Psychotherapy.* Albany, NY: Graywind Publications.

Weissman, M. M., Bruce, M. L., Leaf, P. J., Florio, L. P., & Holzer, C. (1991). Affective disorders. In L. N. Robins & D. A. Regier (Eds.), *Psychiatric Disorders in America: The Epidemiologic Catchment Area Study* (pp. 53-80). New York: Free Press.

Weissman, M. M., & Paykel, E. (1974). *The Depressed Woman.* Chicago: University of Chicago Press.

Chronic Medical Conditions: Working With Patients And Their Families

Janet R. Schultz and Melissa Foti

Therapists often think of professionals who work with chronically ill people as specialists whose work is very distant from their own. The fact is, however, that almost every therapist with even a medium-sized caseload is probably working with someone who lives with chronic illness, even if that is not the patient's presenting problem.

One reason for this statistical probability is that chronic illness is more common in Western societies than ever before. First, the population is aging. Life expectancy is now past 72 for both men and women, and a larger proportion of the population than ever before is over 50. With aging comes increasing risk of chronic illness. Second, many conditions that were fatal in the past are now better thought of as chronic in nature. For example, leukemia, which years ago was considered to carry a death sentence, now often brings years of survival during which treatment may be ongoing. More than half of all people with cancer live more than 5 years past diagnosis (National Cancer Institute, 1996). Third, many babies that would have died in the past are surviving into childhood and even adulthood. This includes micropremies, who are at greater risk of having chronic conditions, and children with certain diseases such as cystic fibrosis (CF) and hemophilia, for whom life expectancies have made tremendous gains over the past few decades as new treatments became available. Fourth, some chronic conditions are occurring with higher prevalence than in the past. Asthma is the most outstanding example of this category.

According to 1995 statistics (National Center for Health Statistics, 1993), just under 100 million noninstitutionalized persons live with chronic conditions, of whom about 40% have limitations in function. The magnitude of the number of persons with medical conditions is such that caring for a family member with a chronic illness can now be considered a normative role in adulthood (Monahan & Hooker, 1997). By 2020, it is projected that 134 million will have chronic conditions and almost one-third of them will have limitations in a major activity. Therapists in both private and public sector work will see the increase, but because poverty is associated with higher prevalence of chronic medical conditions (National Center for Health Statistics, 1993), those in the public sector may experience it more.

WHO HAS CHRONIC MEDICAL CONDITIONS?

Although older age is associated with chronic conditions, only about a third of those who have such medical problems are elderly (over 65 years old) (National Center for Health Statistics, 1993). Of the group considered to be "working-age adults" (18-64 years of age), in 1994 almost 22 million were significantly limited in their activities by chronic, nonpsychiatric conditions. To make this large number more meaningful, the number of working-age adults in

1994 who could not work because of a chronic condition could populate either Virginia or Massachusetts. A quarter of the 45- to 64-year-old subgroup were limited by a chronic condition, and more than 40% of those were unable to carry on their major activity, whether paid employment or housework. Of the younger workers, 10% had an activity-limiting condition, with back or spine conditions being disproportionately represented. Similarly, 10% to 20% of children have chronic medical conditions, although only 1% to 2% are categorized as suffering severe disorders. Those figures still translate to over 1 million children with severe conditions and millions more with less severe, but often life-altering, medical conditions.

No age or ethnic group is immune to chronic conditions. Certain diseases such as sickle-cell anemia or cystic fibrosis are well known to differentially affect people of varying racial and ethnic backgrounds, but there are other less well known differences in prevalence rates. For example, diabetes affects African-Americans 70% more often than white Americans, while Hispanics are affected almost twice as much as their white counterparts. Similarly, the prevalence of diabetes among Native Americans is more than twice that for the total population. Five-year survival rates from cancer are also lower for African-Americans than for Caucasians, largely due to later diagnosis. Asian-Americans are more likely to have cleft lip and/or palate than other groups. Despite their longer life expectancies, women account for more than half of all the deaths from cardiovascular disease each year (National Center for Chronic Disease Prevention and Health Promotion, 1999).

Of the nearly 100 million noninstitutionalized people with chronic conditions, more than 40% have more than one medical problem (Hoffman & Rice, 1995). Having more than one chronic condition increases the likelihood of significant limitation of function. People in nursing homes or other institutions have a much higher probability of having two or more chronic diagnoses.

CONTEXT OF THE ILLNESS

Historically, using the biomedical model, disease was considered to be "in the patient," that is, an individual's functioning was impaired, usually in direct proportion to the organic damage present. The disorder was literally viewed as inside the skin of the patient; anything else that affected medical outcome was subsumed under "psychosocial overlay." Over time, however, alternative models have evolved, with one of the most notable being George Engel's (1977, 1980) biopsychosocial model. Besides the now-familiar notion that the development and experience of illness is influenced by biological, psychological, and social factors, the model also posits that there are many nested levels to the system which influence health and illness. These levels, which both affect and are affected by each other, range from the cellular or even molecular to the societal and natural environmental levels. In addition to acknowledging a variety of influences on health outcomes, this model points out that there are also a variety of levels on which physicians, therapists, and other health care professionals can intervene to alter the experience and course of the disease or condition. A visual representation of a modified Engel model in presented in Figure 1 (p. 35).

Engel's approach is based on systems theory, which highlights both organization and interrelatedness. An important implication of this model is that because systems are comprised of interrelated parts, a change in one part is associated with the change in all others. A chronic illness is not just inside the patient, but affects the whole family system. And because systems work to maintain a regular state of balance, familiar homeostatic processes become more noticeable during times of challenge. These processes or patterns (which may look either adaptive or maladaptive) help to provide the members of the family with a sense of stability and continuity. A systems view also takes into account that processes change over time and that both individuals and families have somewhat predictable developmental courses and crises. Although certainly all levels are relevant, this contribution will confine itself to the family level issues involved in chronic illness.

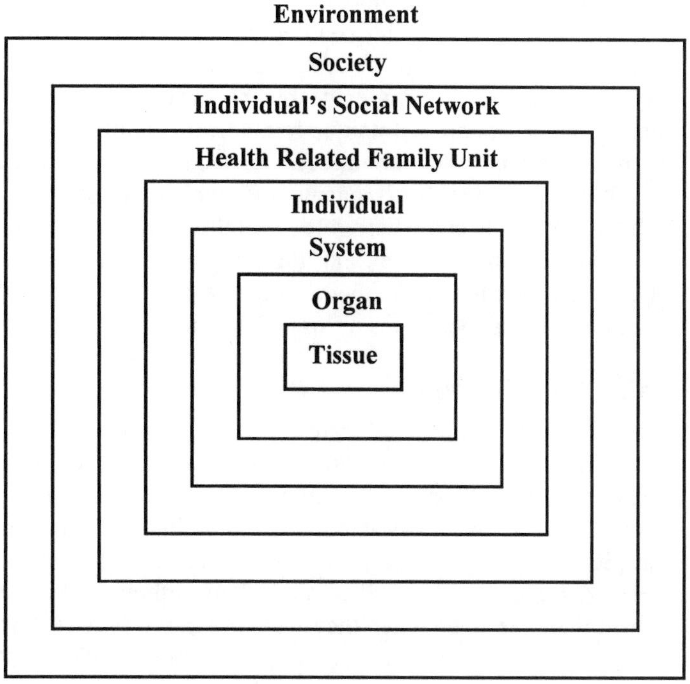

Environment

Society

Individual's Social Network

Health Related Family Unit

Individual

System

Organ

Tissue

Figure 1. Levels in a Biopsychosocial Model.

The Health Related Family Unit

Ransom (1983) emphasized the importance of family in caregiving and used the term "health related family unit" to describe the context in which illness occurs. This unit is not defined by biological or legal status, but rather focuses on relationships and function. Additionally, this concept includes the notion of the family as the primary unit to be addressed when a member is ill. The family is seen as both influencing and being in turn influenced by the illness experience. One of the most important and inevitable functions the family plays is assigning meaning to the illness and events surrounding it. McCubbin and Patterson (1982) argued that the meaning families ascribe is a critical mediating factor in determining family adjustment and adaptation.

This meaning-making activity is one place where therapists can have influence, understanding that the process is based on family legacy, cultural/subcultural influences, and beliefs about health and illness. Family legacy involves the multigenerational contributions to the stories of what members of this family do when faced with major challenges and/or illness, shaping the myths, expectations, and beliefs that influence the kinds of coping that occur. Cultural influences may define the power structure for the family, the roster of persons considered as family, and how one behaves when someone is ill. Health beliefs, often culturally influenced, similarly shape family responses by helping to define the medical challenges. For example, a family that is convinced that the patriarch's prostate cancer is not life-threatening will mobilize differently than one that is convinced that death will be rapid and inevitable, perhaps requiring the selection of an heir to the leadership role. Sometimes competing systems of beliefs impede the family's reaching the goal of constructing a meaning for the chronic condition that preserves its sense of competency and value. Gonzalez, Steinglass, and Reiss (1989) have defined the task in terms of a balance, finding a place for the illness, but keeping the illness in its place.

Certainly all of the characteristics and processes of the family that have been important for any other work are important here. Cohesion and adaptability appear often in the literature on families with chronic illness. As with many aspects of family function, either can be problematic or helpful depending on the extent, the point of development, and the situation under consideration. The same closeness that has been found to be helpful for families with ill children can also result in enmeshment, overprotectiveness, and lack of conflict resolution. Family processes are not unique to medical conditions, but some of the challenges faced by members of this system are directly related to the illness at hand.

A particular family arrangement for which families with a chronically ill member are particularly at risk is one where role flexibility is diminished so that people become locked into roles such as "the sick one" and "the caregiver." Other times, even without the loss of flexibility, family members as individuals or the family as a whole may inadvertently promote or support physical symptoms or loss of function.

The Health Care System

Dealing with the health care system is stressful and challenging for most families, especially when the medical condition is intrusive enough to require multiple contacts with physicians, clinics, and hospitals. Although often close relationships with medical professionals are forged, the health care system may be intimidating. One teen described his experience in the hospital as feeling as if he were captive on another planet: Residents of this planet looked and dressed strangely. They talked about him without looking at him. They used language that was unfamiliar, even when they were talking to him. Instead of saying hello, the citizens of the planet greeted him by removing a ceremonial object that was normally slung around the back of their necks and touching his chest with it. They made him give up his clothes, dressed him in odd clothing, and put a label on him. They refused him food and said he would get nourishment first from tubes stuck in his body, then from mysterious, monochromatic mush that they insisted was edible and just what he needed. They said to relax, that they were taking good care of him.

The metaphor is, alas, apt. Medical settings are quite alien for most of us, and medical professionals sometimes report feeling the same way when they become patients. When we are removed from familiar surroundings, we cannot rely on our "autopilot" to take care of the basics, leaving the majority of our attention for important tasks. Instead we are anxious and hypervigilant, and our cognitive skills, including memory, generally perform far from optimally. When we are unable to care for ourselves or our loved ones on our own, but have to defer to others for knowledge and skill, we can feel powerless, ineffective, and intimidated. We may feel that we are being unfavorably evaluated by others as well. We become acutely aware of the power differential between the professionals and the patient.

Generally, admission to the hospital is an emotion-arousing, anxiety-provoking event, often even for veteran families who have dealt repeatedly with the medical system. Despite having developed trusting relationships with certain individual professionals and generally knowing the routine, there is often the sensation that something could go wrong this time. There is also a knowledge that sometimes procedures hurt, staff focus on something other than the family's needs, privacy is a lost luxury, and small, even petty, irritations may mount before the patient is discharged.

Recent developments in the health insurance system in the United States have changed some aspects of the experience of chronic illness as well. First, most patients can no longer go to any doctor they choose, regardless of relationship, reputation, or expertise. Instead they are restricted to a list of providers. Second, the relationship of the physician with the third-party payer and, hence, the family, has changed. Instead of a physician choosing whether to accept a company's payment for the patient's treatment, the company chooses not only who they will reimburse, but also which procedures are acceptable. Surgeries require advance approval under most circumstances, and length of hospital stay is often out of the hands of the physician. Choice of prescriptions and treatments may be limited as well. The physician is no longer the ultimate power. Some patients have commented that when the control lay with the physician, they knew they had to choose someone they could trust, but now the power is held by someone faceless who does not even know who they are and has no obvious investment in them. The family may have no power to choose who makes decisions. On the other hand, many managed care companies have tried to address some of the concerns of the chronically ill by assigning case managers who come to know about the patient and are empowered to make decisions that might otherwise violate normal regulations. Case managers can become excellent allies for families and therapists.

A related issue for many persons with chronic medical conditions is that they use up their maximum coverage and are left with no insurance coverage for future illnesses. Chronic medical conditions are expensive, with costs that can reach into the hundreds of thousands of dollars per year or more. (Medical costs of people with chronic diseases account for more than 60% of the nation's medical care costs, according to the Robert Wood Johnson Foundation [1994]). Without coverage, individuals may be left to contemplate how to pay the enormous bills out of pocket or may turn to public programs such as Medicaid or Medicare. Because of income limitations to the programs, for some people, chronic illness may force a choice between maintaining employment, even on a part-time basis, and having medical coverage. Young adults with chronic illnesses have sometimes chosen to cohabit rather than marry, because the potential spouse cannot provide coverage for them and makes too much money for them to maintain their publicly funded coverage. One young couple had a church wedding ceremony complete with clergy, meaningful vows, and a reception but skipped the marriage license rather than lose coverage for the bride, who had cystic fibrosis. Only their parents and people within the health care system knew their secret. In other families, parents have not left low-paying or frustrating jobs because of difficulties gaining insurance for their chronically ill children with a "preexisting condition." People who work for small or self-insured companies may be pressured to leave jobs if the costs of care for a family member creates financial stress for the organization or dramatically increases the rates for other employees. The current health care funding arrangements can work against a family having power or control of aspects of their lives that seem separate from someone's illness.

Characteristics of the Medical Condition

Just as the characteristics of the family influence the frame in which they place the illness experience, some attributes of the medical condition itself influence the family's experiences and the meanings they attach to them. Rolland's (1994) writings have been especially informative in this regard. The attributes of the condition help to define the coping that is required of the family and individual. One of the first tasks of therapy should be to assess the family's understanding of these characteristics and the implications for them. Many times the understandings are incorrect or reflect other distortions, underlining the importance of clear, frequent, and ongoing communication between the therapist and the patients' primary care physician or specialist.

Nature of Onset

The first attributes of the medical condition that can play a role in shaping family response is the nature of the onset. There are three main categories in this regard: acute, insidious, and congenital. Examples of the acute category are traumatic brain injuries, myocardial infarctions, and sometimes diseases such as epilepsy or diabetes. In these instances, emotional and practical changes to the family system are compressed and the family is called upon to cope rapidly. Role flexibility and problem solving are useful family attributes, especially when paired with rapid identification of resources. Therapeutic intervention may be useful to deal with emotions blocking coping, keep families focused, and deal with conflict within the system. Therapists are often helpful in the role of educator and communicator. They have the distance to address the normative aspects of the experience and provide at least a sketch of an emotional road map for the family. Therapists, especially those who work frequently with specific physicians or persons with particular disorders, often can serve as translators, helping family members to understand the messages of the medical staff.

Insidious conditions with a more gradual onset (e.g., Alzheimer's, some forms of arthritis) allow the luxury of slower pace of coping but are often characterized by longer periods of uncertainty or misattributions, especially if the diagnosis is not clear for some time. Families that have difficulty with ambiguity or who have a history of coping in rather practical, if intellectualized, ways may have more difficulties with this situation. The therapist's role as mediator and clarifier may take precedence here. Having the luxury of time allows the therapist to work toward empowering the family to communicate with medical personnel themselves. Identifying what information is desired, determining what the family wants to tell medical professionals, and role playing talking to the physician can all be useful.

Congenital-onset conditions (e.g., birth defects of all natures, early diagnosis of genetic diseases such as cystic fibrosis and sickle-cell disease) tend to have different characteristics. The infant patient has no identifiable reaction to the condition per se, but the rest of the family, usually including extended family, responds strongly. The family may be shocked, depending on family history and prenatal diagnosis, but is almost always sad and disappointed. There is loss of the hoped-for, dreamed-of child; for some families, mourning is a necessary part of the process which enables them to attach to the infant that has arrived. Many families are reluctant to become attached to a child they fear may die. Helping the parents and grandparents especially to mobilize their strengths to approach the baby, identify their fears, support each other, and share their loss can allow attachment to occur. Because many babies with congenital anomalies are hospitalized longer than most newborns, often in the intimidating environment of the newborn intensive care unit, many families do not experience the baby as "theirs." Learning to participate in the care of the infant, providing breast milk if the child can use it, and holding the little one are all ways of claiming the baby as part of their family, not the hospital's. Nurses can be helpful and supportive allies in these endeavors. It is not unusual to see photos of family members in the isolettes or small plastic cribs of the babies. Parents often acknowledge that the pictures are meaningless to the baby, but see the photos as a way of showing family involvement to personnel who might come when they are absent. They are declaring to themselves, other parents, and the medical staff that the baby is part of their family.

Permanence

A second dimension of the medical condition which any family must face is the question of permanence of the condition. Often this is not clear at first and may be ambiguous for some time. The lack of clarity may lead to family members developing expectations that are at odds with each others'. Ambiguity about permanence makes the time line of expected coping far more blurry. Many people feel secure in their abilities to rise to a time-limited challenge with a positive outcome but doubt their capacity to permanently reorganize their families. This particular attribute also seems to influence in a profound fashion the meaning constructed for the condition. Therapist comfort with spiritual and existential issues is often helpful in addressing this issue. Hospital chaplains or other clergy can also be helpful in addressing these issues.

Another aspect of the dimension of permanence is the move from crisis to chronic mode for the family. Many of the solutions developed with an eye toward managing a short-term crisis need to be reevaluated as permanence becomes apparent. The kind of indulgence a child may receive during an acute, serious illness may contribute to very unpleasant behaviors and unbalanced parent/child power if maintained for long. Many women who have given up education, marriage, or careers to help out with a crisis have found themselves still locked into that pattern years later because the family did not recognize and reevaluate its coping strategies.

Cause

A third attribute of the medical condition that shapes family reaction is its cause. Again, there are three rough categories: (a) the cause is identifiable but it is external to the family; (b) the cause is identifiable and it is internal to the family; or (c) there is no identifiable cause in that it seems a random or chance event. In some ways, the identifiable and external cause is the easiest to deal with, although the force seen as causal may be the target of considerable anger. These are most often situations in which trauma or allegations of mishandling are involved. When the cause is identifiable and internal to the family, expressions of anger become more complicated. Other feelings such as guilt, sadness, and existential bewilderment may come into play more often. Meanings tend to be constructed differently when the cause is seen as genetic (there are now over 2,800 genetic diagnoses) than when the cause is a family member's behavior or neglect. Genetics are usually still seen as out of a person's control, but blaming may still occur, especially if there is tension between the two sides of a family. Information that the genetic condition is recessive, requiring contributions from both sides of the family, may not alter the belief that the condition came from the other side of the family. An interesting variation is the belief that the disorder may have come from both sides, but that the contribution of the other side of the family was greater.

Although therapists can be helpful in addressing family dynamics, often it is useful to address the question behind the desire to find a cause: Simply, why did this happen and to this person? Do bad things happen to good people? Is there a reason for the condition beyond the identifiable cause? If a person was injured in a car accident, why did the accident occur? If grandmother has a stroke, what does it mean in the grand scheme of things? Spiritual and existential issues abound, demanding respect for any of the related frameworks that people use to try to construct meanings for their worlds and events. Religion is one of the most common of these frameworks.

Apparently random happenings that result in chronic medical conditions are often the hardest events for which to find meanings. Although the issues are similar to those outlined previously, there is a tendency for family members to work very hard to find a cause, even if it is at the expense of blaming one or more family members, perhaps themselves. It seems to be a common human characteristic to prefer any cause to not knowing why something important happened.

Course

Rolland's (1994) writings on the fourth dimension of medical conditions, the course of the condition, shed light on the shaping influence of the very nature of the condition. He and others have categorized the course of medical conditions as progressive, constant, relapsing, or mixed. Coping with and adapting to each of these calls on different family strengths. Progressive conditions bring fairly steady declines in the health and/or capabilities of the person with the disease, although rates of deterioration vary widely. Examples of progressive conditions include cystic fibrosis, metastasized cancer, Alzheimer's disease, and muscular dystrophy. With each stage of decline, the family is called upon to reorganize itself to deal with a new level of disability. Almost inevitably, the signs of the new level of function bring new meanings and high levels of uncertainty. For many families with a member with cystic fibrosis, beginning home oxygen is a frightening and meaningful development. When oxygen during exertion is introduced and/or when the change is made to 24-hour oxygen, families often see the patient as moving closer to death, step by step. During the "long haul," families sometimes run out of energy or other resources. In very slow declines, there may be growing resentment - and exhaustion. Haley (1997) found that many people who take care of persons with advanced Alzheimer's at home spend more than 60 hours a week in caretaking activities or supervision. Further, they sustain this level of involvement for 6 to 7 years on average. Therapists can be helpful by being supportive, helping to separate the disease from the person, and accepting negative feelings toward the patient and the disease. Therapists also can have the objectivity to watch for the family reorganizing in ways that result in one member being "stuck" with caregiving when other alternatives could be available. Directly addressing gender-role influences is often important for this discussion, because most often women are the primary caretakers. Knowing practical options, such as how to access respite care organizations or home health care agencies, can be helpful as well.

In contrast, when a family member's condition is relatively stable and the symptoms constant, such as after partial recovery from a stroke, spinal cord injuries, or amputations, fewer reorganizations are required of the family. The degree of caring required for an individual also makes a difference for the exhaustion level over time. There is generally less ambiguity for the family under these circumstances.

On the other hand, relapsing conditions such as sickle-cell anemia, Crohn's disease, migraines, or vertebral disk problems are marked by periods of stability, perhaps even health, punctuated by periods of varying levels of symptoms and incapacity. The possibility of relapse is ever present, demanding great flexibility and even creativity of families. Members are "on-call" at all times, presenting a challenge that increases over time. The lack of predictability is a major issue and prevents long-term planning. Even short-term planning is often gradually abandoned in the face of repeated disappointments. The sense of loss of control over life may contribute to a loss of self-efficacy and self-esteem as individuals and as a family as a whole. Helping families to find a segment of existence where they can have control and helping them develop contingency arrangements so that planning can still be carried out can be particularly helpful in these circumstances.

The conditions with mixed courses have more pronounced ups and downs than the others but usually still have an overall downward direction. Examples of this kind of disorder are multiple sclerosis, lupus, some cardiovascular diseases, and some cancers. Families living with this kind of condition are faced with a combination of the need to be "on-call" and the long, sometimes exhausting adjustments and coping of the progressive conditions. The twin issues of predictability and sense of control are almost always a part of these sessions. In general, predictability tends to reduce stress and to make coping easier. Helping families to activate their resources to seize what control they can is a useful strategy.

Outcome

The fifth important aspect of the medical condition is its outcome, with the risk and rate of mortality from the condition being among the most important features. Families frequently reorganize themselves and set priorities in direct relation to their understanding of the prognosis, which may or may not match that held by medical personnel. Misunderstanding can lead to lack of necessary action, overprotection, or shock and/or resentment at the actual outcome. How quickly death or recovery is expected also helps to form an often unspoken time line for family coping. Often when death is believed to be imminent, there is considerable mobilization of the family; sometimes, such mobilization may be the first evidence of impending death that a patient receives. On the other hand, when death from the condition is expected at an indeterminate point in the future, coping through denial becomes much easier. More than a few adults who grew up having cystic fibrosis (CF) have expressed surprise and disbelief when they realized that they were nearing death from the disease. Despite years of clinic visits, medications, breathing treatments, hospitalizations, increasing symptoms, deaths of other CF patients, and knowledge of prognosis, they never really believed that they would die from the disease and thus were unprepared psychologically. Although dealing with death and dying is a topic far too broad to attempt to cover in this contribution, the fact that a condition is considered life-threatening or fatal does influence family system responses.

Another aspect of outcome is the degree of incapacitation that the individual with the condition experiences and the expectations the family holds for that individual's role. Family expectations have been shown to relate to response to rehabilitation. For example, when the family expects the patient to have a responsible and autonomous role, the individual is likely to gain more from rehabilitation than when the family expects little recovery. Similarly, accurate expectations and information can reduce resentment. For example, the husband of a woman who used oxygen because of chronic obstructive pulmonary disease (COPD) viewed her as "lazy and irresponsible" because she "wouldn't even run the vacuum cleaner." It took the intervention of medical professionals for the husband to understand that that particular household task is very difficult for a lot of people with breathing difficulties. The therapist was then able to help them negotiate what kind of household tasks were reasonable for her and what it took for both of them to feel that she was a contributing member of the team.

Another important feature is the nature of the person's incapacitation. Is the person physically, cognitively, emotionally, vocationally, and/or socially impaired? Although all of these are difficult and demand different adaptations of the family, changes in the patient that leave his or her personality or relational capacity substantially altered bring particularly challenging problems, highlighting the family as a unit of care. The basic issue becomes: When is a person psychologically in or out of the family system? Spouses of persons with Alzheimer's reported a greater need for support than spouses caring for patients with Parkinson's disease who did not have cognitive impairment (Monahan & Hooker, 1997). Boss et al. (1990) found that when Alzheimer's patients were physically present, needing care but not emotionally available or responsive, caregivers were more at risk for depression. It was the meanings caregivers assigned to changes in behavior of elderly family members that made a difference in the levels of distress the caregivers themselves experienced. People who felt their family members were emotionally demanding and dependent were more distressed than caregivers who thought of them as disturbed or disabled. Attributing the changes in personality to the medical condition made the characteristics less aversive than when caregivers viewed the changes as willful (Deimling & Bass, 1986; Gilleard, Boyde, & Watt, 1982). The role of the therapist is to examine attributions and meanings to help the family find those that are accurate but supportive of both coping and family relationships. Coming to grips with the loss of the person they had known while being faced with caring for a less pleasant, more demanding, and more unpredictable person can be a useful focus for therapy. As mentioned previously, respite care can be helpful, although alternative caregivers for persons with behavioral/emotional components to their conditions can be harder to find.

A different kind of outcome, which also brings complicated challenges to coping, involves a family member appearing physically, especially facially, anomalous. Although the most common conditions that bring these challenges are facial clefts, others include trauma, amputation, burns, and cancer-related treatment. In Western cultures, physically attractive people are likely to be seen as "good" people who are attractive to others as partners, friends, students, and employees (Berscheid, 1981). People are uncomfortable with and curious about those who stand out as looking different. There exists a large and reliable body of literature supporting the conclusion that physical attractiveness is one of the dimensions central to social judgments (e.g., Berscheid & Walster, 1974). Family members often experience the pain of observing reactions of strangers in public, even if the patient is unaware. Family members may collude to avoid photographs and public situations with the family member whose appearance has changed. Working with families to reframe the staring, questions, or comments as signs of ignorance on the part of the observer rather than reflections on the family member can open new methods of coping. Similarly, referring families to support organizations such as "About Face" or "Wide Smiles" can provide alternative coping models and strategies as well. Physical differences can change the quality of the individual's and family's life more than the change in function by itself would predict.

Lifestyle Change

The last dimension of medical conditions to be discussed here is the degree of change to the family lifestyle that is involved in caring for the condition. One aspect of this is the time commitment involved. Although some chronic conditions require no more than extra physician contact and/or a few pills, others demand hours per day. Some treatment regimens, like those for cystic fibrosis, HIV infection, and diabetes, can demand careful scheduling of treatments, medications, and meals. Other conditions require close supervision of the patient and much physical labor and body contact. Demands that bear so directly on at least two members of the family at any time require practical adaptations. More importantly, the medical conditions and treatments may also require changes in family identity. For example, families that were physically active and whose members enjoyed outdoor activities may have to limit or reshape what they do together, sometimes forcing a choice between either the once-perceived unit of family or that aspect of family identity.

There are other, often more difficult kinds of lifestyle changes that bring more ambiguity to the family situation. These are changes in health related behaviors that are known to be mediated by the family (Sallis & Nader, 1988). For example, following a heart attack, a man may be advised to give up smoking and change his diet. These behavior changes are not unique to the disorder in the same way as, say, insulin would be for the treatment of diabetes.

The target behaviors may have been bones of contention in the family prior to the heart attack and may bear the undercurrent of blame for it as well. Because failure to adhere to treatment recommendations is a common problem in medicine, the therapist should assume that there are breakdowns in the family's adherence and work to help the family overcome barriers. Possible barriers include the meaning of adherence for family members, role inflexibility, practical obstacles, misinformation, and deliberate quality-of-life decisions.

The meanings for adherence are often the most difficult to address, but change at that level may be the only one that makes a meaningful difference. As an example, for some men, the diet, smoking, drinking, or physical labor changes that are recommended challenge their definitions of themselves as men and as providers for their families. On the other hand, for some women, not taking care of their husbands by making the changes challenges their definitions of themselves as caretakers for the family. The opposing forces can worsen both family tension and health related behaviors.

Misunderstandings of treatment regimens are so widespread that it is useful to have a copy of a written plan to follow when working with families. When there is lack of clarity as to treatment recommendations, working with the family members to outline the questions and different interpretations of the same words, then having a joint session with the physician, can be quite effective if the therapist and physician have a positive working relationship. In those meetings, the role of the therapist is to empower the family to address the issues, rather than speaking for them or the physician. At the same time, processing comments and repeating the questions and answers can be very useful because they can illuminate how these unclear situations occur and can perhaps be circumvented in the future. Those are also excellent occasions for clarifying who will be responsible for each element of treatment and how treatment demands can be scheduled into the family's life together. Because the chronic condition will likely go on much longer than contact with a therapist, teaching a template or overall problem-solving strategy to deal with treatment demands can reduce the need for services in the future.

Deaton (1985) coined the term "adaptive noncompliance" to describe nonadherence that is based on decisions made in the interest of quality of life. Families weigh the benefits of adherence against the variety of costs that could ensue. Costs can be financial but are more often related to side effects, fatigue, lack of perceived benefit, or intrusion into everyday life. Examining the family's decisional balance and asking members for consensus on level of care actually carried out can sometimes remedy this kind of nonadherence.

SUMMARY AND RECOMMENDATIONS

Steinglass and his colleagues (Gonzalez et al., 1989) summarized well the basic goal of working with families with a chronic medical condition: to find a place for the illness and to keep the illness in its place. It is likely that there are several tasks that can help with reaching this goal. The family

- comes to accept the diagnosis and its implications. This must be balanced in such a way that hope is not lost, but perhaps the wish redefined.
- learns to manage and deal with symptoms, practically and psychologically.
- constructs a meaning for the condition and resulting situation, but one that preserves competence and mastery for all members.
- keeps the condition from dominating family life except during crisis times.
- reevaluates its coping and problem solving as the condition and the family develops.
- establishes a trusting, cooperative relationship with the primary physician and other health care providers, while maintaining a presence as an equal partner in decision making as experts on this particular family and individual.

- adapts to dealing with the medical system in general, including the hospital environment, developing or maintaining an assertive and proactive stance with professionals. Optimally this includes learning a problem-solving strategy.
- balances realistic needs imposed by the medical condition with the need for autonomy.
- identifies and takes appropriate advantage of opportunities for growth through the experience of coping and living with chronic illness.

General Recommendations for Therapists

1. Screen all persons seen in therapy for chronic illness experiences, as one would any other potentially stressful life history events.
2. Keep close contact with the patient's primary care physician or most involved specialist.
3. Obtain information about the patient's disorder, medications, and treatment regimen from books, journals, the Internet, and relevant foundations. Read the literature about the psychological and social effects of the condition.
4. Never fake knowing about a disease or procedure to a family. This is the perfect way to end one's credibility.
5. Address the meanings of the illness and the changes it brings for the family.
6. Talk about role changes and evaluate them for utility, cost, and alternatives. Lay groundwork for second-order change, a change in how the rules are viewed. Watch especially for complementary roles that may be forcing the members to opposite extremes.
7. Assess the coping skills of the family and individual members. In many families, members cope in ways that are problematic to other members or are at least "out of sync." Developing alternatives and teaching new skills can be helpful, but maintain the family's position as experts on itself.
8. Assess and, if necessary, work on communication, first within the family, then between family members and health care personnel. Help family members to mobilize social and practical support and limit or rechannel dependency-inducing assistance. Legitimize and address assertion with medical professionals and insurance/health maintenance organizations (HMOs). In the course of therapy and in the context of the therapeutic relationship, deal with "taboo" topics, which, among others, often include sex and death.
9. If behavioral medicine is an area of expertise, when appropriate, use symptom management techniques and strategies. If these skills are not in your repertoire, develop contacts with others to whom you could refer patients if indicated.
10. Identify and refer to appropriate support agencies, preferably after consultation with medical personnel who may have options in place. Foundations related to various conditions are good sources of information and, sometimes, formal support groups. Others now have on-line support chat rooms. Families who do not own computers can access these groups at most public libraries.
11. Monitor family coping and resources. Help them find alternative coping methods and supplemental social, emotional, economic, and practical support.
12. While choosing situations carefully, therapists can serve as advocates for families, especially with the medical system and insurance/HMOs. Proactive education of HMO staff, especially case managers, is recommended so that it is very clear that your work has direct bearing on medical outcome. Forming a working alliance with case managers can expedite psychosocial care being viewed as important and related to the medical condition.
13. Know your limits. What baggage do you bring to the situation? How much of this kind of work can you engage in before hitting your personal threshold for burnout?

CONTRIBUTORS

Janet R. Schultz, PhD, ABPP, is currently Director of Clinical Training for the PsyD program at Xavier University in Cincinnati. Prior to that position, she was Director of the Division of Psychology of Children's Hospital Medical Center and Associate Professor of Pediatrics at the University of Cincinnati. Her specialty has been working with children and adults with chronic medical conditions, especially craniofacial anomalies, cystic fibrosis, hemophilia, and dermatologic problems. Dr. Schultz may be contacted at Xavier University, 3800 Victory Parkway, Cincinnati, OH 45207-6511. E-mail: schultzj@xavier.xu.edu

Melissa Foti, MA, is a doctoral candidate in the PsyD program at Xavier University. Her area of concentration is children and adolescents, with a special interest in pediatric psychology. Her dissertation research is in the area of physician-family communication. Ms. Foti can be reached at Xavier University, 3800 Victory Parkway, Cincinnati, OH 45207-6511. E-mail: mfoti@xavier.xu.edu

RESOURCES

Cited Resources

Bernstein, N. (1990). Objective bodily damage: Disfigurement and dignity. In T. F. Cash & T. Pruzinsky, *Body Images: Development, Deviance and Change* (pp. 131-148). New York: Guilford.

Berscheid, E. (1981). An overview of the psychological effects of physical attractiveness. In G. W. Lucker, K. A. Ribbens, & J. A. McNamara (Eds.), *Psychological Aspects of Facial Form* (pp. 1-24). Ann Arbor, MI: Center for Human Growth and Development.

Berscheid, E., & Walster, E. (1974). Physical attractiveness. In L. Berkowitz (Ed.), *Advances in Experimental Social Psychology* (Vol. 7, pp. 158-216). New York: Academic Press.

Boss, P., Caron, W., & Horbal, J. (1988). Alzheimer's disease and ambiguous loss. In C. Chilman, E. Nunnally, & F. Cox (Eds.), *Chronic Illness and Disability: Families in Trouble Series* (Vol. II, pp. 123-140). Beverly Hills, CA: Sage.

Boss, P., Caron, W., Horbal, J., & Mortimer, J. (1990). Predictors of depression in caregivers of dementia patients: Boundary ambiguity and mastery. *Family Process, 29,* 245-254.

Cohen, D., & Eisdorfer, C. (1986). *The Loss of Self: A Family Resource for the Care of Alzheimer's Disease and Related Disorders.* New York: W. W. Norton & Company.

Deaton, A. V. (1985). Adaptive noncompliance in pediatric asthma: The parent as expert. *Journal of Pediatric Psychology, 10,* 1-14.

Deimling, G., & Bass, D. (1986). Symptoms of mental impairment among elderly adults and their effects on family caregivers. *Journal of Gerontology, 41,* 778-784.

Engel, G. L. (1977). The need for a new medical model: A challenge for biomedicine. *Science, 196,* 129-136.

Engel, G. L. (1980). The clinical application of the biopsychosocial model. *American Journal of Psychiatry, 37,* 535-544.

Gilleard, C., Boyde, W., & Watt, G. (1982). Problems of caring for the elderly infirm at home. *Archives of Gerontology and Geriatrics, 1,* 151-158.

Gonzalez, S., Steinglass, P., & Reiss, D. (1989). Putting the illness in its place: Discussion groups for families with chronic medical illnesses. *Family Process, 28,* 69-87.

Haley, W. E. (1997). The family caregiver's role in Alzheimer's. *Neurology, 48*(Suppl. 6), S25-S29.

Hoffman, C., & Rice, D. P. (1995). *Estimates Based on the 1987 National Medical Expenditure Survey* [On-line]. San Francisco: University of California - Institute for Health & Aging, on the Robert Wood Johnson site. Available: www.rwjf.org/library/chrcare

McCubbin, H. I., & Patterson, J. M. (1982). Family adaptation to crises. In H. I. McCubbin, A. Cauble, & J. Patterson (Eds.), *Family Stress, Coping, and Social Support* (pp. 26-47). Springfield, IL: Charles C. Thomas.

Monahan, D. J., & Hooker, K. (1997). Caregiving and social support in two illness groups. *Social Work, 42,* 278-287.

National Cancer Institute. (1996). *Report of Clinical Trials.* Bethesda, MD: National Institute of Health.

National Center for Chronic Disease Prevention and Health Promotion. (1999). *Centers for Disease Control* [On-line]. Available: www.cdc.gov/nccdphp

National Center for Health Statistics. (1993). *Current Estimates from the National Health Interview Survey, 1993* [Vital & Health Statistics, Series 10 (No. 190), December, 1994]. Atlanta, GA: Branch of Centers for Disease Control.

Rando, T. (1984). *Grief, Dying, and Death: Clinical Interventions for Caregivers.* Champaign, IL: Research Press.

Ransom, D. C. (1983). On why it is useful to say that "The family is a unit of care" in family medicine. *Family Systems Medicine, 1,* 17-22.

Robert Wood Johnson Foundation. (1994). *Annual Report 1994.* Princeton, NJ: Author.

Roberts, M., & Wallander, J. (1992). *Family Issues in Pediatric Psychology.* Hillsdale, NJ: Lawrence Erlbaum.

Rolland, J. S. (1993). Mastering family challenges in serious illness and disability. In F. Walsh (Ed.), *Normal Family Processes* (2nd ed., pp. 444-473). New York: Guilford.

Rolland, J. S. (1994). *Families, Illness, and Disability.* New York: Basic Books.

Sallis, J. F., & Nader, P. R. (1988). Family determinants of health behaviors. In D. S. Gochman (Ed.), *Health Behavior: Emerging Research Perspectives* (pp. 107-124). New York: Plenum.

Sawa, R. (1985). *Family Dynamics for Physicians: Guidelines to Assessment and Treatment.* New York: Mellen.

Wynne, L. C., Shields, C. G., & Sirkin, M. (1992). Illness, family theory, and family therapy: I, Conceptual issues. *Family Process, 31,* 3-18.

Internet Sites

The Internet has many sites having to do with medical conditions; not all of them contain accurate information. There are more sites than could probably fit in this book, so only general information is provided. Below are some suggestions of potentially useful sites regarding chronic conditions:

- While the government has many useful sites, the Centers for Disease Control (http://www.cdc.gov) tends to have up-to-date information on a number of conditions.
- This site contains information on many medical problems (http://go.drkoop.com). There is a list of choices of conditions with information available.
- Foundations are generally excellent sources of information about their diseases. Many have sites on the Web as well. An example: www.mdausa.org for Muscular Dystrophy Association. Some foundations also have on-line chat/support groups.

Solution Focused Family of Origin Therapy

Terry D. Hargrave and Linda Metcalf

"Life can only be understood looking back, but must be lived forward."
S. Kierkegaard

Imagine how difficult it must be for two therapists who believe in and practice from two different theoretical models to come together in a therapy session to work with a patient. Linda Metcalf is a well established author, teacher, and practitioner of Solution Focused Therapy. Terry Hargrave is equally well known for his writing, teaching, and practice from a Family of Origin perspective. Although it was difficult to let go of our own theoretical and practice biases, we had known one another for years and liked each other's work. Dr. Metcalf works from a perspective of the present, looking for solutions instead of focusing on problems. In her practice, however, she had many patients who wanted to articulate something about the past. It was as if they wanted to make sense of things before they could implement a change in behavior that would lead to solution. Dr. Hargrave works from a perspective of the past, seeking to help the patient identify insight and understanding that will lead to different behaviors. Many of the patients with whom he worked, however, would seem to get stuck in an endless cycle of remembering past experiences, questioning why those things happened and then being unable to apply the insight to avoid present-day problems.

Dr. Metcalf became interested in how to use the past productively to help the patient find new meanings to the past. Dr. Hargrave became interested in how to become more efficient in translating patient insight about the past into new actions. As a result, we became committed to work together for a period of a year to forge new understanding about each other's perspectives, find possible mergers between our models, and experience the process of therapy from the new perspective. The result was a mutual discovery of the strengths of both models and an evolution of a new model. This contribution will review the basic concepts of the Solution Focused and Family of Origin models, how we merged the two models, and how we apply the model to various situations. In the end, we discovered how to make the Family of Origin model more efficient and action oriented while making the Solution Focused approach more oriented toward using information about the past.

TWO MODELS FROM OPPOSING PERSPECTIVES

Integration of any two perspectives is difficult, but these two models seemed to be diametrically opposed on almost every point. It will be helpful here to articulate some of the foundational concepts to both the Solution Focused and Family of Origin models, in order to fully appreciate the integration of the theories. First, let us review the Solution Focused model (de Shazer, 1988; Metcalf, 1995; O'Hanlon & Weiner-Davis, 1989).

Foundational Concepts of Solution Focused Therapy

A Nonpathological Approach Makes Problems Solvable

Solution Focused Therapy centers itself on the idea that pathology constructs a meaning in people's minds that results in problems. When the idea of pathology exists, therefore, people tend to focus on the problem and limit thinking about possible solutions. For example, if parents and teachers think about a child being active and needing special situations to learn, more solutions and changes will be forthcoming than if the child were thought to have a pathology such as Attention-Deficit/Hyperactivity Disorder.

There Is No Need to Promote Insight

Insight into the past tends to bring attention to the problem, resulting in a cognitive construction that limits solution. The Solution Focused model tries to eliminate cognitive construction about the past so there can be little inhibition to construction of positive solutions.

Patient's Goals Define the Course of Treatment

From a Solution Focused perspective, people come to therapy because they want problems eliminated. They do not want to know *why* problems occur so much as they want solutions. This approach focuses on actions that lead to behaviors that eliminate problems.

Every Complaint Pattern Contains Some Sort of Exception

No matter how complicated and persistent problems are, there are times when the problems are nonexistent or at least less severe. For instance, a parent may complain that an adolescent child is uncontrollable and always a problem. The Solution Focused therapist would form the basis for the construction of a solution by asking at what times the adolescent is under more control or when he or she is not as much of a problem. After the times and circumstances are identified, the therapist would work with the parent and adolescent to expand the exception to the problem into a pattern.

Complex Problems Do Not Call for Complex Solutions

Many times both therapists and patients construct the belief that if the problem has caused intense pain or distress, then the solution must be equally difficult and complex. The Solution Focused model calls attention to the fact that small changes in perceptions of behaviors, such as reframing a problem as a positive or doing more of the behavior when the problem is not noticed, can alleviate complex issues.

Success in Therapy Is Built by Focusing on Successes, Exceptions, and Skill Building

The Solution Focused therapist functions like a resource coach, calling patients' attention to their existing strengths and encouraging them to expand those strengths and resources into new applications to solve problems. For instance, if a person sought therapy because he or she was dealing with grief over a lost relationship, the therapist might call attention to the person's problem-solving skills in his or her career. Playing off the person's competence in one area, the therapist would then ask the patient to use those same skills in seeking or figuring out solutions to his or her grief.

The Solution Focused Therapy approach focuses so much on the solutions to problems because it is based on a foundation of social constructionism. In the simplest terms, social constructionism maintains that belief systems and behaviors are constructed cognitively by individuals or societies. These cognitive constructions can be beneficial at times, but may be harmful when the cognitive construction creates problems that defy solutions or limits choices that may be helpful. The Solution Focused approach seeks to create a new context for the social construction that is focused on new and productive behavior and does not limit choice. Another very similar approach to Solution Focused Therapy is the Narrative Therapy approach discussed by White and Epston (1990). The Narrative approach would seek solutions to past problems by modifying and changing the narrative or "story" that the individual or family has created surrounding the problem.

Contrasted with the Solution Focused approach, which maintains that the past tends to focus on the problems and impede new thinking about solutions, Family of Origin approaches try to direct the attention of the patient on the past in order to resolve issues that are seen to reoccur or complicate present situations. Presented here are some of the key concepts of Family of Origin therapy (Boszormenyi-Nagy & Krasner, 1986; Bowen, 1978; Hargrave & Anderson, 1992).

Key Concepts of Family of Origin Therapy

Pathology in Relationships Is Often Related to Unresolved Issues in One's Family of Origin

Family of Origin Therapy believes that there is pathology that exists with patients and relationships. These pathologies or dysfunctions relate to states such as low differentiation or emotional fusion (Bowen, 1978) or destructive entitlement due to relational imbalance (Boszormenyi-Nagy & Krasner, 1986). These pathologies or dysfunctions are seen as very often being a reflection of problems that originated in the patient's past. As a result, Family of Origin Therapy focuses on the past.

Insight and Reworking Old Family of Origin Relationships Is Necessary

Family of Origin work is seen by the therapist as necessary because of the belief that the patient has basic beliefs, has formed action patterns, or is seeking compensation because of early influential family relationships. Unless the past relationship is reworked or insight is gained, the patient is likely to not be able to give up unproductive beliefs, patterns, or motivations.

Therapy May Involve Probing into Areas Where a Patient May Not Be Conscious of Problems

Because the Family of Origin therapist believes that past relationships may be of significant influence on the patient's current relationships or problems, the therapist will focus on the past. The patient, however, may focus on current problems only and see the past as unrelated. For instance, a patient may be overcontrolling and possessive in a marital relationship and see his or her spouse as being uncooperative in reporting or doing what the patient has requested. The therapist, however, will likely see the overcontrolling behavior as a coping mechanism that the patient developed in childhood in order to compensate for a distant or uninvolved parent.

Resolving Past Relational Issues and Gaining Insight Promotes the Opportunity to Live More Successfully in Current Relationships

When the issues of the past are brought up in therapy, the therapist and patient are able to examine the past relational problems or trauma with adult insight. At the minimum, this type of insight reduces the patient's need to rely on old and dysfunctional coping mechanisms. In order to achieve maximum benefit, however, there are many situations in which the patient can be coached or encouraged by the therapist to confront the Family of Origin issues with new behavior. This confrontation can lead to dismantling the old beliefs, patterns, and motivations of the patient and enable him or her to live differently in current situations and relationships.

These two approaches are very different not only in the foundational concepts, but also in the technique of therapy. For instance, in the Solution Focused approach, reframing is considered to be very helpful. In Family of Origin work, however, insight is considered helpful but reframing is not. In order to proceed in gaining the benefits of both models, we had to develop a basic framework of concepts and techniques that was heuristically sound and fit with our own therapeutic work.

MELDING THE TWO APPROACHES

Our first task was to clearly identify and conceptualize each approach. The theoretical work of Keeney and Ross (1985) was very helpful in conceptualizing the *political* and *seman-*

tic frames. The semantic frame has to do with the way that people make *meaning* into constructions about beliefs about themselves, actions, and others. The political frame deals with the idea of *actions* and behaviors that people perform. It was most helpful for us to assume that traditional Solution Focused Therapy dealt primarily with helping people take *action* in order to deal with complaints and problems. In the same way, traditional Family of Origin Therapy deals primarily with helping people understand the *meaning* of what their families taught them to believe about relationships and how they were to act in relationships. The action or behavior frame, which is the focus of Solution Focused Therapy, is fairly straightforward and easy to understand. Actions and behaviors are either adaptive and functional or maladaptive and dysfunctional, depending on the situation. The Solution Focused therapist makes an effort to help the patient come to the point where he or she is unhindered by past cognitive constructions and is able to choose actions that are adaptive and functional.

The meaning or belief frame, however, was a little more difficult to articulate. Traditional constructivism maintains that beliefs and realities are cognitively or socially constructed and are not real. Family of Origin Therapy, which holds to very real ideas of functional and dysfunctional behavior that cut across situations, is difficult to meld with constructivism. For instance, emotional fusion, or losing one's ability to control choice by intellect, is held as a sign of dysfunction and low differentiation by a Family of Origin therapist.

We came to believe that people do construct meaning and reality. However, we believe they construct that meaning and reality in a consistent way. We believe that human beings have two basic, consistent constructs which demand meaning. In other words, people do construct meaning, but they are consistent in the way they construct meaning. These two constructs, around which people construct meaning, are *belief about self* and *belief about how to act in relationships*. In the context of relationships and reality, people will come up with consistent beliefs about who they are and how they are to act in relationships. We think of this in the same way that Chomsky (1972) explains the nativist theory of language acquisition. Chomsky states that we have a Language Acquisition Device or LAD which allows humans to access and make language in consistent ways. As a child is exposed to language, he or she will access the language in a consistent way around constructs that will allow for objects and actions as well as syntax and grammar. Even though children will speak different languages depending on which one they are exposed to, all children go about learning language in the LAD in the same sequence, development, and characteristics.

In the same way, we believe that humans have a consistent construct or device that requires them to make meaning around who they are and how they are to act in relationships. It is like newly born humans come into the world with two spools which have no thread. As a person experiences love or lack of nurture from important relationships, thread is wound onto the spool that delineates the person's belief about himself or herself. This basic construct surrounds the idea of "Who Am I?". As a result of early relationships, the person gains a sense that could encompass such beliefs as lovable/unlovable, valuable/worthless, precious/shameful, or special/ordinary. The beliefs about self are primarily formed through how the person is *loved*.

The other empty spool is the construct of how the person should act in relationships. Depending on how the person is treated, the thread of experience will wind on the spool in a way that will tell him or her what course of actions to take in future relationships. Depending on whether the individual is treated in a trustworthy or untrustworthy fashion, he or she will develop beliefs that will result in actions that are controlling/chaotic, expectations that are optimistic/pessimistic, actions that are giving/defending, or connections that are nurturing/withholding. The beliefs about how the person should act in relationships are primarily formed through how the person is treated in a *trustworthy* manner.

We believe that understanding this step was significant for the melding of the two models. From the Family of Origin perspective, this step meant that we boiled down the essential information about the past to two issues concerning the person's history of loving and trustworthy relationships. Problems such as excessive guilt or shame could be seen as reflecting difficulty with the construct of love. Issues such as dysfunctional behaviors and motivations could be seen as reflecting difficulty with the construct of trust. From the Solution Focused perspective, this step meant that we had to acknowledge that there were some constructs that were formed from past relationships that could not simply be reframed or ignored in preference for solution behaviors.

The result of this step led Dr. Hargrave to move to a more efficient pattern of dealing with meanings in the past and therefore become freer to help the patient become action oriented. Dr. Metcalf was able to integrate effective use of past meaning when patients became stuck. We realized, once again, that the semantic and political frames inform each other (Keeney & Ross, 1985). In other words, *actions* and efforts to adapt help form meaning, and *meanings* about self and relationships lead to eventual action. It was helpful for us to conceptualize the fact that the melding of the two approaches was actually seeking balance. Humans will both take actions and make meanings. Both frames can be helpful to people when seeking to make changes in therapy. There are many times, however, when therapy is not effective because the patient is either imbalanced and too focused on meaning or action.

The merging of the two models into one was done with the hope that a patient would receive empathy, compassion, and the confidence to change toward something productive, not just informative. We integrated questions into therapy sessions that assisted clients to explore their past (*meaning*) and then fast forwarded exceptions that they discovered and combined them with goals to the future (*actions*). We found that patients left the session with practical, helpful, *exceptional,* historical, and useful information that could be used in the present. We began to notice that the perceptions the patient had held all of his or her life were challenged. This opened up new possibilities of dealing with the patient's family from a different perspective. Dr. Hargrave talked with patients about how their lives were wound with meanings imposed on them by their family's way of trusting/not trusting and loving/not loving them. The clients seemed to appreciate these explanations, understanding, finally, the reasons for their current feelings. Dr. Metcalf spoke with the same patients about their abilities to cope and deal with such meanings in their lives. The therapeutic effort then focused on who they were today, who their families were, and reaching a consensus to do something different because the current strategy was not working (Metcalf, 1998).

BASIC ASSUMPTIONS AND APPLICATIONS OF SOLUTION FOCUSED FAMILY OF ORIGIN THERAPY

As we worked with patients, it became helpful for us to keep the basic assumptions of the approach in front of us and develop questions or statements that assisted us in getting to the important information. These assumptions and applications follow (Metcalf, 1998).

Assumptions of Solution Focused Family of Origin Therapy

1. It is most helpful for us to assume that a traditional Solution Focused Therapy approach can assist people in taking *ACTION* to deal with complaints or problems. This is done by asking a question such as:

    - What will you be doing when things are slightly better for you?

2. It is helpful for us to assume that traditional Family of Origin Therapy can assist people in understanding the *MEANING* of what their families taught them to believe about themselves and how they were to act in relationships. This can be done by asking questions such as:

    - When you are believing what your family taught you about yourself, how do you react, behave, and so forth?
    - How would you like to think/believe about yourself during those times that would help you do things differently?

- When you think about the pain that is bothering you today, what do you think went on in your family that helped the pain to grow?
- How did you think about yourself when this was occurring?

3. *MEANING* is constructed by people. Human beings have two basic consistent constructs around which meaning is constructed:

A. *Belief About Oneself:* Who am I? I am either

lovable	unlovable
valuable	worthless
precious	shameful
special	ordinary

- This belief about oneself is primarily constructed from how a person is loved.

B. *Belief About Relationships:* How should I be in relationships? Should I be

controlling	chaotic
optimistic	pessimistic
giving	defending
nurturing	withholding

- This belief about oneself is primarily constructed through how a person was treated in a trustworthy/justified manner.

4. A *balance* between taking appropriate *ACTIONS* to deal with life and constructing helpful *MEANINGS* concerning self and relationships is essential for individual and family health. If a patient does too much of either, the balance is thrown off and satisfaction may lessen. In the past, Family of Origin Therapy attempted to clarify the meanings, assuming that insightful understanding would give the patient a reason to change his or her life. Solution Focused Therapy focused on helping the patient take actions, assuming that change in any behavior will cause change in another person, place, and event. Together, they construct questions such as:

- How could you begin to think about yourself so that you will act differently in the near future with your spouse? (meanings)
- What will you be doing in that situation, specifically? (actions)
- When you think of how you want things to be with your son, and how different that is from your relationship with your father, what beliefs would you have to take on so that this new relationship happens? (meanings)
- As you construct this new relationship with your son, what would your father see you doing differently, if he were watching on the sidelines? (actions)
- How do you suppose you will feel as you teach your son to carry on a new legacy in relationships between father and son? (meanings and actions)

ACTIONS Efforts to adapt functional behavior	**BALANCE**	**MEANINGS** Constructed beliefs about self and relationships

one's efforts to adapt .... one's constructed beliefs about self
one's attempt to be functional .... one's understanding of oneself
behavior in relationships .... the perception of relationships

5. *MEANINGS* concerning the self and relationships affect the *ACTIONS* a person takes in solving problems. The *ACTIONS* taken in solving problems and relating serve to construct additional *MEANINGS.* When a person is thinking differently about himself or herself, new behaviors will evolve into new meanings.
6. It is reasonable to expect families to treat their members in a loving and trustworthy manner which would promote healthy or functional individuals in terms of what they believe about themselves and how they are motivated to interact in relationships.
7. Individuals have strengths, resources, and abilities that give them certain abilities to adapt new and functional *ACTIONS* and control dysfunctional and problematic behavior. Understanding and recognizing one's strengths and resources is often made difficult by the timeless construction of personhood by one's family. Moving slowly, and recognizing fruitless efforts to change one's family as actions that *are not working* keeps the patient more solution focused instead of problem focused. Questions alluding to this idea for a patient, stuck on confronting a parent regarding abuse, might be:

    - Talking to and confronting your mother regarding the sexual abuse caused by her husband, your step-dad, seems to leave you unhappy and distanced from your mother, whom you say you love very much. Is this strategy working for you at this time or has it worked in the past?
    - I wonder what actions on your part would show your mom the depth of your concern to get back into life?

Goals of Solution Focused Family of Origin Therapy

The goals of this melded therapy are simple. First, our desire is to help the patients focus on exceptions to problems and on increasing their behavior options. The identification of such resources and exceptions will alter the meaning of patients' personhood and offer them an opportunity to practice the new behaviors in a safe environment. This will help them to take new actions more readily. Second, we want to assist patients in their construction of new meanings in situations. Insight, as well as small, productive, new actions taken with relationships, will promote the rewriting of such meanings. When patients have difficulty in putting strength, resources, and ability toward solutions, it may be the result of the problematic construction around the meanings and *beliefs* of the person and relationships. New meanings must always be balanced by the client taking constructive and adaptive new actions. *Balance between actions and meanings are essential or else the patient may become stuck in old beliefs and/or unproductive actions.*

TECHNIQUES OF SOLUTION FOCUSED FAMILY OF ORIGIN THERAPY

The Shifting Belief Frame: Rewind the Past

The primary focus of this technique is the intent to use meaning constructed in a family of origin to call attention to a similar meaning or action occurring in a present relationship. Many times, patients who have experienced some violation of love and trust in the past will have a tendency to react and feel in similar ways when confronted with circumstances that remind them of the past. For instance, a young father who was dissatisfied and angry about the relationship with his own father struggled off and on with depression. He had identified that his depression was often brought on when he remembered how little his father cared for him. When attempts were made to work with this man from strictly a Solution Focused approach, he showed no improvement at all.

As the therapists in the case, we switched from a traditional Solution Focused approach to incorporate the elements of Family of Origin discussed previously. We discovered that the man had a son to whom he considered himself very close. He also believed he was a very good father and contrasted himself often with his own father. It became clear that the father had very specific actions and meanings associated with both his family of origin and family of procreation. In the father's family of origin, the patient had a constructed meaning of feeling devalued by his father because of past violations of love and trust. He in turn took actions that were directed at staying away from the father and showing resentment. In his relationship with his own son, however, the patient had a constructed meaning of believing he was a worthy, trustworthy, and good father. This led him to take actions toward his own son to be nurturing and involved.

In the shifting belief frame technique, therapists use the strengths observed in one generation to improve conditions in another generation. In the same way, beliefs and meanings learned in one generation are used to direct the patient to insight in another generation. In this case, we praised the patient for being a good father, but asked if there might be any times that his own son might feel a lack of love or nurture from him. The patient reported that his son would likely feel that way when he was depressed or very busy with work. We then asked if he was still nurturing when he was depressed or busy. He answered that even though he felt love for his son, he probably did not show it when he was feeling bad. We then took this frame from the patient's family of origin and used it to focus on the insight that he might be sowing the seeds of the same type of feeling with his son that was given to him by his own father. The patient quickly confirmed this as a concern and said that even though he was trying to convince himself otherwise, he knew that at times he might commit the same errors for which he was angry with his father. This insight made explicit the meaning that was complicating the patient's depression. He was not only feeling bad about his own relationship with his father, which made him feel devalued, but he also felt bad and devalued as his behavior reminded him of his unloving and untrustworthy father.

We then shifted to the actions that the patient took with his own son. Although there were times when the father was absent, he gave many examples of how he tried to be nurturing in spending time with his son. He described his ability to be close to his son as one of being "buddies." We commented that this was indeed a strength, and we listed some of the techniques and skills the patient used to be a buddy to his son. After articulating the strengths in the current generational relationship with his son, we started discussing ways the patient could use some of those same skills to become a "buddy" to his father. Instead of using the old frame of expectation the patient had of what his father should be, we asked if a "buddy"-type relationship could also work between him and his father. In this way, we as the therapists were using current actions as strengths to apply to the past, which in turn affected the old meanings the son had constructed around his father. Although tentative at first, the patient began to think of different ways that he could relate to his father in this way. Consistent with both Solution Focused and Family of Origin Therapies, the therapists used these small insights and gains to successfully expand the patient's relationship with his father and reconstruct the meaning that the patient had always placed on his relationship with the father.

Using this technique, the therapist is actually searching for strengths and resources across generational lines. Once these are found, the therapist ties these strengths and resources to the past, present, and future. Likewise, when the therapist discovers a weakness or harmful meaning, he or she tries to draw the patient to insight on how these meanings can play out in the past, present, or future. In the preceding case, we took great care to balance the objectives of both moving the patient toward appropriate action and reconstructing meaning. This technique not only helps patients focus on new options, but also allows them to confront meanings that may not be helpful.

Searching for Exceptions: Fast Forward to the Future

In many cases, it is helpful for the therapist to utilize Solution Focused questioning, which is designed to identify exceptions and new possibilities and to focus the attention of the patient on past meanings. Using this technique with patients who struggle with being stuck on past meanings, the therapist will ask questions that help patients project themselves into the future facing a similar situation. Following are some questions that we have found helpful in bringing these past issues into a new light for patients:

- It is 20 years in the future. Your son/daughter confronts you on an issue that he/she does not understand. How would you hope you would respond? What would you hope happens with that situation? How might that same technique be helpful with your own parent at this time?
- When you believe in yourself the way this person did, even though he/she left you with the weaknesses you describe, what would he/she say he/she believed about you at the time in his/her own way? When you look at the resources you just described to me, how might your living these resources more *fully* contribute to new beliefs of that person toward you?
- Now that you recognize that some of your weaknesses have evolved in your family and you realize the strengths also found in your family, place yourself on the scale below in terms of strength or weakness.

  1 2 3 4 5 6 7 8 9 10
  weakness strength

  Where would you say you might have been when you were not living your life in the manner that you desire? What were you doing when the weaknesses took over? What do you do at times when the strengths reign? Where would you like to be before our next conversation? What could you do on a small scale to that point? What would you need to begin believing about yourself to move to that point?

We also have found it helpful to ask patients to "fast forward" a year, to a time where they have *re-taught* those persons to see them differently. The therapist can encourage this process by describing how he or she would be treating his or her children, spouse, relationships, careers, and so on, as if each day, he or she were the patient's audience, watching and learning every move.

SUMMARY

We have found that we discover more about this model the more we work with patients. The assumptions and strategies in the Solution Focused Family of Origin model allow the therapist to combine two very different models of therapy to utilize the strengths and resources of one generation (present or future) and redress issues of belief and relationship from another generation (past). In addition, the model gives the therapist a platform to point out that efforts to deal ineffectively with one generation (usually the past) will be ineffective in another generation (usually the future). In this way, the therapist encourages patients to open up the past beliefs about personhood and relationship to the new possibilities that work more efficiently in the present and future. Patients are more likely to be less defensive concerning the past. They are encouraged to explore contaminating past beliefs and to slowly experiment with healthier beliefs that can prove to be more productive in current and future generations. Finally, the need for balance between the actions and meanings of patients can direct the therapist to imbalances that tend to trap patients in past unresolved issues or unproductive patterns.

We have found in our work that this model has achieved the goal we had for wanting to work efficiently on issues of the past while moving forward to actions that solve problems. However, we also feel that there is much more work to be done in the area of developing the theoretical core of the model as well as techniques that apply to and help patients.

CONTRIBUTORS

Terry D. Hargrave, PhD, is currently Professor of Psychology at Amarillo College in Amarillo, Texas. He is author of several articles and several books on Family of Origin Therapy including, *Families and Forgiveness: Healing Wounds in the Intergenerational Family.* He is a frequent presenter at national and international conferences. He is also in private practice. Dr. Hargrave may be contacted at P.O. Box 447, Amarillo, TX 79178.

Linda Metcalf, PhD, is currently in private practice in Arlington, Texas. She has authored several books on Solution Focused Therapy including *Solution Focused Group Therapy.* She is well known for her applications of Solution Focused Therapy to school, student, and parent populations. She is a frequent presenter at national and international conferences. Dr. Metcalf can be reached at 5126 Bridgewater, Arlington, TX 76017.

RESOURCES

Boszormenyi-Nagy, I., & Krasner, B. (1986). *Between Give and Take: A Clinical Guide to Contextual Therapy.* New York: Brunner/Mazel.

Bowen, M. (1978). *Family Therapy in Clinical Practice.* New York: Jason Aronson.

Chomsky, N. (1972). *Language and Mind.* New York: Harcourt Brace Jovanovich.

de Shazer, S. (1988). *Clues: Investigating Solutions in Brief Therapy.* New York: Norton.

Hargrave, T. D., & Anderson, W. T. (1992). *Finishing Well: Aging and Reparation in the Intergenerational Family.* New York: Brunner/Mazel.

Keeney, B. P., & Ross, J. M. (1985). *Mind in Therapy: Constructing Systemic Family Therapies.* New York: Basic Books.

Metcalf, L. (1995). *Counseling Toward Solutions.* New York: The Center for Applied Research in Education.

Metcalf, L. (1998). *Solution Focused Group Therapy.* New York: The Free Press.

O'Hanlon, W. H., & Weiner-Davis, M. (1989). *In Search of Solutions.* New York: Norton.

White, M., & Epston, D. (1990). *Narrative Means to Therapeutic Ends.* New York: Norton.

The Assessment and Treatment Of Erection Dysfunction

Frederick L. Peterson, Jr.

This contribution introduces mental health professionals to the current therapies for erection dysfunction (ED), from behavioral and mechanical to pharmacological. ED is defined as the inability to achieve or maintain an erection of sufficient rigidity and duration to permit satisfactory sexual performance (National Institutes of Health [NIH] Consensus Development Panel on Impotence, 1993). The objective is to have mental health professionals develop a general understanding of how to respond with clients complaining of ED from the context of the multidisciplinary field of sex therapy. Assessment and treatment options are discussed, inclusive of considerations from several disciplines. Relevant cultural diversity issues are also presented. Because there are few published research studies on homosexual men with ED (primarily case reports), this contribution discusses the assessment and treatment of heterosexual men with ED, although many, if not most, of the interventions would likely be effective with men of any sexual orientation.

When treating ED, as well as any sexual dysfunction, one should always practice within the scope of one's competency. This contribution is intended to provide an intermediate level of understanding for the assessment and treatment of ED. Providing all information needed for proficiency in treating ED is well beyond the scope of this contribution. Mental health professionals who wish to pursue advanced skills in sex therapy are encouraged to join the membership of the American Association of Sex Educators, Counselors and Therapists (ASSECT), which is an accrediting body offering four levels of certification of practice. Additionally, readers are referred to the ASSECT Code of Ethics, which is useful in advancing the status of sex education, therapy, supervision, and research (ASSECT, 1993).

INTRODUCTION TO ERECTION DYSFUNCTION

At a 1993 Consensus Conference on Impotence at the National Institutes of Health, the term "impotence" was declared obsolete in favor of the more neutral as well as precise term "erection dysfunction." ED in the United States has been clinically defined by the *Diagnostic and Statistical Manual of Mental Disorders* (*DSM-IV*; American Psychiatric Association [APA], 1994) as the inability to get or maintain an erection suitable for intercourse. One of the best recent prevalence studies was conducted in 1992 by the National Health and Social Life Survey (NHSLS), involving a national probability sample of 1,410 men aged 18 to 59. The NHSLS estimated a point prevalence of approximately 5% and a lifetime prevalence of approximately 10% (Laumann, Paik, & Rosen, 1999).

The Massachusetts Male Aging Study (MMAS), a large longitudinal study following men aged 40 to 70, reported findings consistent with the NHSLS. The MMAS found 10% of that sample having "complete impotence" and approximately 35% reporting "moderate to complete erectile dysfunction" (Feldman et al., 1994). If considering any level of erectile functioning (even mild and temporary), then the prevalence increases to 52% (Feldman et al., 1994). These studies and others demonstrate a consistent association between aging and erectile dysfunction for men. In general, the incidence and severity of ED increases as men age and are also affected by men's health status (Laumann et al., 1999; Masters, Johnson, & Kolodny, 1995).

Traditional approaches to understanding ED emphasized a division between two types of ED based on causality: physical (often called "organic") or psychological. Physical causes include causal factors that are pharmacological (such as use of antihypertensives), endocrinologic (diabetes), neurologic (spinal cord injury), "lifestyle" choices (smoking), or related to penile disease or trauma. Psychological risk factors for ED include factors such as sexual trauma history, depression, anxiety, guilt, or having significant conflict with one's sexual partner.

An integrated systems perspective has evolved which views the division of causal factors into "physical or psychological" as artificial and not reflecting the true nature of the client's experience. Although identification of the contributing factors to ED is paramount, most cases of ED have a multicausal etiology ("mixed etiology"), and causal factors often have reciprocal influences upon one another. For example, a significant percentage of men who develop diabetes mellitus will experience some level of erectile dysfunction. A man who has a predisposition for developing diabetes and who also has clinical depression may exacerbate the development of diabetes. He does this by not exercising, failing to follow a healthy diet, abusing alcohol to self-medicate, and becoming obese. Once the diabetes becomes severe enough to cause ED, he may become more depressed, develop marital discord, and experience heightened anxiety when his partner leaves him. In a case like this, as well as most, patient satisfaction and outcome may be improved with counseling even when the sexual dysfunction is secondary to a medical condition or mixed etiology (American Association of Clinical Endocrinologists [AACE], 1998; NIH, 1993).

THE ASSESSMENT PROCESS FOR ERECTION FUNCTION

The comprehensive assessment of ED is a complex process, which requires multidisciplinary input and review. This section informs mental health professionals of their role in this process and what to consider from the perspective of other disciplines. Comprehensive assessment includes a review of presenting complaints and the couple's expectations (including desired outcomes), psychosexual history, substance uses, standardized measurement of the severity of ED, psychological assessment of personality factors if indicated (depression), and medical examination/measurement if there is indication of medical conditions/factors contributing to the presenting complaint. Determining if the patient is clinically depressed, has a sexual trauma history, experiences anxiety and/or guilt regarding sex, or reports partner conflict are also key factors in the assessment of ED.

Assessment of ED, unless it is solely of psychogenic etiology, usually requires multiple sessions. Single-session assessment of ED by mental health professionals usually is not effective unless it is an extended-time single session (2-4 hours) and/or a low-complexity case, such as performance anxiety as the sole causal factor. Moderate- to high-complexity cases usually require multiple sessions to allow detailed developmental histories to be taken from both individuals and conferring with other healthcare providers for medical evaluations.

It is recommended that the assessment process be comprised of two to three assessment sessions followed by a results-sharing conference. If multiple-session assessment is to occur, this structure is best communicated to a client prior to the first face-to-face meeting. Multiple-session assessment allows more time for an in-depth evaluation of the client's medical, social, and psychosexual history. Because there is an emphasis on the relationship as well as the dysfunction in sex therapy, both the identified client and his partner should be involved in the assessment, including individual assessment without the other present. A sexual development history should be completed with both the male client and his partner. With heterosexual couples, this individual time allows for his, her, and their view of the problem to be explored.

The psychosexual history and interview are important to include with every client (NIH, 1993). A family-of-origin review, how the client learned about sex, family rules about communicating about sex, masturbatory history, first sexual contacts (same and opposite sex as well as animal contacts), sexual functioning with principle sexual partners, extramarital affairs, frequency of naturally occurring erections, and previous experiences with ED and what has been tried to resolve it should be included in the psychosocial history. Although standardized self-report instruments (discussed later) also measure severity of the ED, comparing both partners' subjective estimates on specific behavioral elements of ED (i.e., percentage of time attempts at intercourse are unsuccessful, time before erection is lost) is recommended. The content and frequency of current sexual fantasies should be explored to determine the degree of confluence between fantasy life and behavioral sexual expression.

It is important to note that most complaints of not achieving or maintaining erections suitable for intercourse do lend themselves to the diagnosis of ED, and it is a matter of assessing the level of severity. Clients do anxiously present themselves with situational erectile difficulties that are transient in nature, such as not achieving an erection after heavy use of alcohol, a day of strenuous exercise resulting in fatigue, or being with a new sexual partner. At times, these clients do not meet the duration criteria for a diagnosis of ED, and spontaneous remission often occurs.

Standardized self-report measures have an important role in the assessing complaints of ED and moving from presenting complaints to a diagnosis. Highly recommended is the International Index of Erectile Functioning (IIEF), a 15-item, self-administered scale useful as one evaluation strategy in a comprehensive assessment of ED. The scale has been normed cross-culturally (10 languages), is psychometrically sound with high reliability and validity, and demonstrates sensitivity and specificity for detecting changes in erectile functioning (Rosen et al., 1997).

Assessment of Psychological Etiological Factors in Erection Dysfunction

The objective of this section is to describe the process of evaluating five psychological factors associated with ED. A patient may be in need of sex therapy when there is coexisting concern the patient is clinically depressed, has a sexual trauma history, experiences anxiety and/or guilt regarding sex, or reports conflict with his partner. Findings from further evaluation of these risk factors may lead to an array of psychosexual interventions designed to achieve symptom relief and allow the patient to enjoy his optimal level of sexual health (discussed later).

There are six questions useful to mental health professionals related to screening patients for psychological risk factors for ED. The first two questions indicate further in-depth evaluation if answered in the affirmative. These questions are:

Q1. Do you have naturally occurring erections in the morning, and can you get an erection by yourself (via masturbation)?

Q2. Have you ever been sexually molested or sexually assaulted, either as a child or as an adult?

The last four questions are answered on the following 4-point scale: 0 = no, not at all; 1 = yes, seldom; 2 = yes, quite a bit; 3 = yes, frequently. An answer of "2" or "3" on any of these four questions indicates further evaluation and possible treatment. These four questions are:

Q3. Do you feel depressed?

Q4. Do you feel nervous or anxious regarding sex?

Q5. Do you feel guilty regarding sex?

Q6. Do you have significant conflict with your partner regarding sex?

A client's report of regularly waking up in the mornings with an erection is usually, but not always, a sign that the patient has normal neurologic and vascular function. This information is often used to indicate that complaints of ED have a psychogenic basis. Beware that self-report is not always reliable; nocturnal penile tumescence and rigidity (NPTR) testing is still recommended by some authorities (Montague, 1998). Additionally, those who oppose

NPTR testing argue that sleep erections may be different in their causal mechanisms from erections occurring in response to sexual stimulation (Montague, 1998). NPTR is discussed in a later section under medical etiology factors in the assessment of ED. If the patient reports morning erections *and* reports that he is able to masturbate to satisfaction (able to get and maintain erection, experience orgasm and ejaculation), then it is highly likely there is a psychogenic basis to his complaints of ED when he is with his partner.

If the patient has a sexual abuse history, a careful evaluation of the trauma nature and severity is in order. Sexual dysfunction may be a long-term sequelae of sexual trauma. Laumann et al. (1999) reported that male victims of adult-child sexual contact are three times more likely to experience erectile dysfunction. This is most often the case if the patient had a female perpetrator and/or the patient is engaging in sexual activity similar in nature to the original sexual abuse.

If it is found that sexual trauma is related to the complaints of ED, then intensive psychotherapy focusing upon trauma resolution is indicated. The process of trauma resolution may be short- or long-term, depending upon the complexity of the case. Factors that increase case complexity include younger age of onset of the abuse, longer duration of the abuse, greater number of perpetrators, and degree of force and violence used. Cases in which there was mild to moderate levels of severity of these factors are likely to find ways for the male survivor to feel safe and overcome the ED provided he has an understanding partner willing to participate in the therapy process. Severe degrees of these factors indicate a poor prognosis for overcoming ED. However, it is to be understood that sexual trauma, by itself, may not be related to the presenting complaint of ED and may not require psychotherapy focused on resolution of trauma issues.

Because a patient's complaint of ED may be related to depression, a standardized screening for depression is recommended, such as the Beck Depression Inventory (BDI). BDI scores of 1 to 10 indicate a normal range of affect, but a score of 22+ indicates a severe level of depression, which likely needs treatment to resolve. Care should be taken not to exacerbate complaints of ED by prescribing antidepressants, which may further suppress erectile response (Beck, Steer, & Brown, 1996).

Commonly, anxiety or guilt may serve as psychogenic obstacles to erectile response. The patient's anxiety may be more specifically related to sex and frequently referred to as "performance anxiety" concerning whether or not he will get and maintain an erection when with his partner. Guilt related to sex is most often associated with strict religious training that typically has a specific view of sexuality as something a man does only for procreation and within the confines of marriage. Men who have been widowed sometimes have transient experience with ED when they start dating again. The same is true for some men who have extramarital affairs or during and after a divorce.

Anger and resentment between the couple may be expressed sexually by avoidance of sexual relations, sometimes perceived as punishment by one individual of the other. These perceptions often manifest in the history, especially when interviewing each person individually. If significant relationship conflict does exist, it needs to be resolved at least to a point where the couple mutually desires and is ready for physical intimacy.

Assessment of Substance Use Etiological Factors in Erection Dysfunction

Sometimes referred to as "lifestyle factors," substance use should always be a part of the assessment of ED. Patients should usually be referred for specialty treatment when they have an addiction to alcohol, tobacco, or illegal drugs, which have adverse effects on erectile functioning. Addictions to substances, whether legal addictions (alcohol and tobacco) or illegal addictions (amphetamines, cocaine, heroin, marijuana, morphine, or steroids) represent risk factors for ED. These six illicit drugs are listed because they have been found to have adverse effects on erectile response (Kolodny, 1985; Process of Care Panel of the University of Medicine and Dentistry, New Jersey, 1998; Wilson, 1988).

As tobacco use is a significant risk factor for ED (Shabsigh et al., 1991), all patients should be assessed for their use of tobacco products (not just cigarettes). All patients who are smoking should be referred to an intensive smoking cessation program if cessation efforts fail in the primary care or private practice setting (AACE, 1998; Agency for Health Care Policy and Research [AHCPR], 1996). Addressing clients' smoking status and assisting them to be tobacco free is within the professional role of psychologists (Wetter et al., 1998) and psychiatrists (APA, 1996). This is true for all clients (not just clients complaining of ED), as smoking is widely considered the number one preventable cause of premature disability and death in the United States (AHCPR, 1996).

Patients with addictions to alcohol and/or drugs should be referred for further assessment and treatment by a polysubstance abuse program (Masters et al., 1995; NIH, 1993). There are four questions useful to mental health professionals related to screening patients for addictions as risk factors associated with ED. These questions are referred to as the "CAGE" assessment and are most often used to differentiate between social drinking and alcoholism:

Q1. C - Have you thought that you should "CUT" down on your alcohol (or drug) use lately?

Q2. A - Have you been "ANNOYED" recently about being criticized for your alcohol (or drug) use?

Q3. G - Have you felt "GUILTY" about your alcohol (or drug) use?

Q4. E - Do you need an "EYE OPENER" in the morning by using alcohol (and/or drugs) to get going?

An affirmative response to two of the four questions indicates referral to Alcoholic's Anonymous (AA) and/or an addiction treatment program. It is important to note that patients commonly minimize their alcohol/drug use during assessment.

If the patient has addiction to alcohol only, then a referral to an alcohol abuse treatment program and active participation in AA would be indicated. Most frequently, patients have coexisting addictions to alcohol and drugs. Often, the only addiction treatment program available is a polysubstance abuse program; the referral reflects this practical reality regardless of the drug of choice. The referral to a polysubstance abuse treatment program and/or AA would be appropriate with reevaluation of ED in 6 months.

Assessment of Medical Etiological Factors in Erection Dysfunction

When assessing ED, it is important for mental health professionals to have at least some basic understanding of medical and laboratory procedures in the assessment process. This is particularly important when working in a multidisciplinary setting. For example, medical providers may ask the mental health provider what specific questions are of concern or even what specific laboratory results they are interested in receiving. A general medical history and examination, laboratory tests, review of medications, and specific endocrine, neurology, and urology examinations may be needed depending on the particular patient. The medical history and examination should be a routine part of the assessment of ED, even with men presenting with what looks to be a clear case of ED caused by a psychological factor (the patient reports waking up with morning erections daily but complains of performance anxiety). Laboratory evaluation is often employed. Both laboratory evaluations and other specialty examinations described below may or may not be indicated depending upon the results of the medical history and exam.

The medical history should include questions relative to all risk factors for ED and medical conditions associated with ED. An assessment of all current medications should be done (especially antidepressants, antihypertensives, and heart medications), as they may be a reversible cause of the ED. The medical provider should be looking for any risk factors for atherosclerosis, prior surgeries associated with ED, neurological and endocrinologic illnesses, and any history of pelvic and/or penile trauma (AACE, 1998; Department of Veterans Affairs [DVA], 1999; NIH, 1993).

A focused physical examination follows the history, may confirm findings from the history, and should emphasize the genitourinary, vascular, and neurologic systems. Important findings include abnormal penile or testicular anatomy, prostate pathology, neuropathy/radiculopathy, occlusive or aneurysmal vascular disease, or stigmata of endocrinologic disease, such as lack of secondary sexual characteristics, small testes, and enlarged breasts (AACE, 1998; DVA, 1999; NIH, 1993).

Clients often ask mental health providers about the relationship between testosterone and libido. It is important to note that a history of decreased libido does not predict low testosterone (Govier, McClure, & Kramer-Levien, 1996) and that low testosterone is found to be a contributing factor for ED in as few as 3% to 6% of cases (Buvat & Lemaire, 1997, Heaton, 1998). Unfortunately, there is not a standardized laboratory panel that is widely accepted to evaluate ED. NIH recommends a moderate work-up with measurement of testosterone in all patients, and serum prolactin, complete blood count, urinalysis, creatinine, fasting lipid profile, fasting blood sugar, and thyroid function testing in many patients (DVA, 1999; NIH, 1993).

Specialized medical testing is sometimes used in the diagnosis of ED. Mental health professionals should be aware that these diagnostic measures exist and are sometimes recommended by medical providers. These medical diagnostic measures include nocturnal penile tumescence testing or NPT, nocturnal penile tumescence and rigidity testing or NPTR, test injections of vasodilators, cavernosometry, cavernosography, and duplex ultrasonography (especially color duplex Doppler ultrasound or CDDU). Mental health professionals do not need to understand these procedures in detail but should be knowledgeable enough about them to engage in discussions of the results with patients and medical specialists (for detailed information, readers are referred to Broderick, 1998; Montague, 1998).

Ending the Assessment With a Results-Sharing Conference

Once all assessment information is collected, a results-sharing conference should conclude the assessment process. A results-sharing conference includes at least three elements. First, the therapist should share the results of standardized measures and summarize what he or she has heard from the client. This is an important opportunity for the therapist to check the accuracy of what he or she has heard and correct any misperceptions. In multidisciplinary settings, ideally several healthcare professionals are present to discuss the results and answer patient questions. More typically it is one healthcare provider, often the mental health professional, sharing results from all sources after receiving letters from the medical providers. This information may be results of the medical and psychosexual histories, physical exams, the IIEF, NPTR testing, depression and anxiety screens (BDI), and any specialty testing.

Secondly, the therapist should share the conclusions drawn from what was shared by the client. Here the client should be told the diagnosis, the type of ED (mixed, organic, psychogenic), and the causes and severity of the ED. Sometimes the complaints of difficulties with erections may be associated with other sexual disorders, such as inhibited sexual desire or rapid (premature) ejaculation. If other sexual disorders are present, they should be discussed at this point. Care should be given to use language the clients understand, take into consideration cultural factors that may affect the interaction (discussed in detail later), and check the accuracy of the client's understanding of what has been said.

Finally, recommendations should be shared which are likely to lead to resolution of ED. The results, conclusions, and recommendations may be shared with the couple in written form of a draft treatment plan. The draft treatment plan outlines key elements of the assessment (such as etiological factors of the ED), desired treatment outcomes, specific treatment goals, recommended treatment strategies to assist the couple in achieving their goals (inclusive of appropriate patient education on sexual health), evaluative criteria (by which clients will know progress is being made and a treatment end point is defined), and their client rights and responsibilities which include all obligatory information to be shared with clients via professional ethics.

TREATMENT STRATEGIES FOR ERECTION DYSFUNCTION

Treatment of ED should always be based upon a foundation of a comprehensive assessment and adequate patient education. Whether this patient education is integrated into the assessment process (sometimes as part of the results sharing) or as part of the treatment process (more commonly) varies according to healthcare setting and provider. Recommended components of patient education for couples seeking professional help for ED include the following: typical communication and relationship strains couples experience when dealing with ED, anatomy and physiology of male and female sexual response, causes and types of ED, and all treatment options for ED whether or not that particular healthcare setting provides all treatment options.

Generally in medical practices (whether primary care or urology offices), medical providers treat complaints of ED with the tools they know and do not provide patient education about all treatment options. As incentives to practice in multidisciplinary fashion continue (from accrediting agencies to consumer demand for better service), physicians will be increasingly relying on mental health and other professionals to assist in the education and treatment of their patients with ED. However, many patients' first inquiries for professional help are with mental health providers. Many of these professionals successfully treat patients with ED with psychogenic causes without ever consulting medical colleagues. If they are treating patients with mixed etiologies, they are doing so with the risk of not providing comprehensive care and increasing the likelihood of less-than-optimal treatment outcome.

There are several considerations that guide the selections of treatment of ED. The first question the provider should ask is if there is sufficient severity and duration of the problem to require treatment. Most times the answer will be in the affirmative. Occasionally, couples will seek out your assistance about their concerns, yet they are within a normal range of functioning or may have a mild level of severity. Appropriate interventions may include helping the clients normalize their situation or perhaps engage in some therapy designed at enhancing their present level of sexual satisfaction as opposed to treating them for a sexual disorder.

Secondly, before any treatment is initiated, are there any reversible causes of ED that can account for the presenting complaints? If so, working with appropriate professional colleagues to make changes in those factors would be in order. Third, noninvasive (lower risk) treatment options are considered before more invasive (higher risk) options. Considering risk, the treatment options for ED are prioritized into first-, second-, and third-line therapies. Reversibility, cost, and ease of administration are also considerations.

Selection of treatments should be made on a combination of client preference, appropriateness of treatment for etiologic base of ED, medical conditions that may rule out some options, and patient reimbursement factors such as out-of-pocket costs (Process of Care Panel, 1998).

Interventions With Reversible Causes

Specifically, consider four factors: prescription medication use, nonprescription drug use (including legal addictive drugs of alcohol and tobacco), hormonal replacement, and penile anatomical abnormalities. Very commonly, prescription medications have unintended adverse effects on erectile functioning (as well as sexual desire, ejaculation, and orgasm). In particular, antihypertensives, antidepressants, antiarrythmics, antiandrogens, and H2 blockers most often are suspect. The patient will need to work with the prescribing healthcare provider to explore if adjusting a dosage or substituting another medication may relieve the ED.

Before the physiological mechanisms for erections were well understood, testosterone used to be one of the most widely prescribed drugs for ED, sometimes used indiscriminately. Today, it is understood that testosterone does not have a direct effect on erectile response, although it does influence libido, which in turn may alter erection function. Although low testosterone level as a causal factor for ED has a low hit rate (3%-6%), it is reasonable to use supplemental testosterone if low sex libido is part of the presenting complaints (DVA, 1999; Heaton, 1998).

Abnormalities of the penis, anatomically, may adversely affect erectile ability and may be reversible, especially in younger men under age 45 who have suffered penile trauma. Microsurgical revascularization of the penis is usually what is most helpful, particularly if the ED stems primarily from an arterial occlusion without veno-occlusive dysfunction (Process of Care Panel, 1998). Peyronie's disease, which causes devastating penile deformity and affects up to 2% of men, is not to be confused as a reversible cause of ED. Men with Peyronie's disease, usually affected between the age 40 to 60, should always be referred to a urologist (Levine, 1998).

For any clients who are smoking, referrals should be made to specialized smoking cessation programs employing the AHCPR guidelines, which incorporate behavioral, educational, and nicotine replacement therapies and oral medications as treatment options. Clients using alcohol and/or drugs should be asked to abstain from use to evaluate whether the drug has an acute effect on their sexual performance. Those unable or unwilling to abstain should be referred for further assessment and treatment by a polysubstance abuse program (Masters et al., 1995; NIH, 1993). Addictions to substances represent risk factors for ED whether they are illegal addictions or legal addictions such as alcohol and tobacco.

Questions sometimes arise with providers and patients as to the "staging of treatment" or which addiction should be treated first (and if treatment of ED should proceed if addictive behaviors continue). Generally, treatment of addictions to illegal drugs is prioritized over treatment of legal addictions. As is often the case, if a patient is addicted to alcohol and illicit drugs, treatment for these addictions should be prioritized over smoking cessation. Patients often report that it is more difficult to give up smoking than overcoming their addictions to alcohol or illicit drugs. Concurrent treatment of drug, alcohol, and nicotine addictions is not recommended unless the patient participates in a highly structured inpatient or residential program.

First-Line Therapies - Sex Therapy, Vacuum Constriction Devices, and Oral Medications

Sex therapy, vacuum constriction devices (VCDs), and oral medications are all considered first-line therapies because of the relative low risk for adverse events (considering medical contraindications). Sex therapy is indicated, likely the treatment of choice, for most psychogenic-based cases of ED and is considered an important adjunct therapy with most organic and mixed etiology-based cases of ED (ACCE, 1998; Masters et al., 1995; NIH, 1993). Sex therapy and VCD use do not involve any invasive procedures, while oral medications (such as sildenafil citrate) introduce substances into the body that may have adverse side effects in a minority of men (Padma-Nathan, 1998).

Undeniably, sildenafil (Viagra) has become extremely popular, with over 6 million prescriptions (50 million tablets) being distributed in the first 6 months after initial FDA approval in March 1998. Over half of these prescriptions were written by primary care physicians (55%) and only 20% to 24% by urologists. Clearly this indicates a major shift in the treatment of ED - from the domain of urologists and mental health specialists to primary care clinicians (Padma-Nathan, 1998). The implication is tremendous, as family medicine and general internal medicine physicians are being asked to practice sexual healthcare, an area in which most physicians have not received comprehensive training. Hence, there are expanding opportunities for mental health professionals who have proficiency, if not a specialty, in sexual health and sex therapy (Althof, 1998).

Sex Therapy

Sex therapy is the treatment of choice for most psychogenic-based cases of ED and can be an important adjunct therapy with most other cases of ED. Sex therapy focuses upon the five most common psychological factors associated with ED: sexual trauma, depression, anxiety, guilt, and marital discord. If sexual trauma is related to the complaints of ED, then intensive psychotherapy focusing upon trauma resolution is needed to break the bond between past trauma and present sexual functioning. The process of trauma resolution may be short- or long-term, depending upon the history of the trauma and complexity of the case. Paramount is the process of the patient finding ways to feel psychologically safe. Unfortunately, many male survivors experiencing severe ED never form long-term relationships nor come into treatment. When they do, partner education and participation in the therapy process is critical to treatment outcome. However, it is important to again note that sexual trauma, by itself, may not be related to the presenting complaint of ED and may not require psychotherapy focused on resolution of trauma issues.

When sexual trauma is pertinent to complaints of ED, it may be an underlying cause of depressive symptoms. When abuse history is not present and the patient's complaint of ED is related to depression, brief psychotherapy should be first employed to bring relief. If psychotherapy does not abate the depressive symptoms in the short term, psychotherapy and psychotropic medication may be combined for more intensive treatment. Again, care should be taken not to exacerbate complaints of ED by prescribing antidepressants, which may further suppress erectile response (AACE, 1998). When anxiety or guilt serve as a psychogenic obstacle to erectile response, they can be effectively treated through relaxation training, cognitive therapy, and behavioral prescriptions, described below (Kaplan, 1986; Masters et al., 1995).

As noted in the introduction, sex therapy represents the combination of psychotherapy and prescribed behavioral exercises (sometimes referred to behavioral prescriptions) which focus upon relaxation and skill acquisition related to sensual touch. Between talk therapy sessions, sexually related behavioral assignments are completed within the couple's own value system and the privacy of their own home. The most common of these behavioral prescriptions are referred to as "sensate focus" exercises; their effectiveness has been extensively studied (Masters et al., 1995).

Sensate focus is defined as graduated touching exercises (not necessarily sexual) assigned to couples in therapy to reduce anxiety and teach nonverbal communication skills (Masters et al., 1995). Sensate focus exercises create a "nondemand" touching encounter, force a couple to attend to sensual aspects of their bodies other than erogenous zones, and allow the patient to relax and "let Mother Nature take over" so he can once again enjoy erections with his partner. The series of touching exercises becomes increasingly sophisticated, progressively including the entire body, and may involve vaginal containment of the male.

Outcome research on behavioral sex therapy is mixed. There are few studies employing randomized assignment of subjects, use of placebo procedures, and large subject pools (Hawton, Catalan, & Fagg, 1992; Leeming & Brown, 1992). However, there are many well-designed evaluation studies of behavioral interventions using control groups with clinical populations. The Masters and Johnson Institute conducted some of the best evaluation studies with patients seeking treatment. Across all diagnoses involving over 2,300 cases, they reported a treatment success rate of 82%. Related specifically to cases of ED (over 700 cases), the success rate is 67% if the man with ED had never successfully had intercourse (what used to be called primary impotence). However, efficacy climbed to 80% if the man had prior experience with successful intercourse (what used to be called secondary impotence) (Masters et al., 1995).

Vacuum Constriction Devices

Invented in 1962, vacuum constriction devices (VCDs) have been a popular treatment choice for men with ED since the mid-80s, when they received FDA approval (1982) and were legitimized as medical treatments by some prominent urologists. Historically, VCDs were one of the first "alternative" therapies developed other than implants offered by urologists and sex therapy offered by mental health specialists. VCDs consist of a plastic cylinder that is placed over the flaccid penis, a pump that is used to create an erection through negative pressure (vacuum) in the cylinder, and a tension ring used to constrict venous blood flow out of the penis. Additionally, a patient education videotape is usually included with the device for proper instruction. Even better, the client is instructed in use by in vivo demonstration before leaving the clinic. Clients may use the VCD to achieve erection and keep the tension band on for no longer than 30 minutes. There are no restrictions on how many times the client may use the VCD per day or week.

Treatment outcome is good but contingent on appropriate patient education and motivation. Being nonpharmacological, VCDs have no drug interactions, and side effects are minimal. Side effects include occasional penile numbing, pivoting at the penile base, mild bruising from the tension ring, pain with orgasm, and decreased penile tumescence and ejaculation. The most frequent complaint by men using VCDs is the unnatural interruption of the act of making love to achieve an erection via use of the device (Trapp, 1998).

VCDs are referred to by many names, including vacuum tumescence device, external vacuum therapy, or, informally, "the pump." Manufacturers report high levels of patient satisfaction, but this may reflect initial patient response, not long-term satisfaction. Once only available by prescription, VCDs are being sold over the counter in drug stores. There are no published studies comparing the effectiveness of the prescription models to the nonprescription models. VCDs are a very popular treatment option at the VA Medical Center where the author coordinates a Sexual Health Clinic. A monthly clinic was established to handle referrals because of increasing consumer demand.

Oral Medications

As mentioned previously, the FDA approval and marketing of the first orally administered agent for the management of ED (sildenafil citrate) has not only provided a new aid to sexual health, but also has greatly changed the clinical practice of sexual health, particularly sexual medicine. A good example of this is the Department of Veterans Affairs (DVA), one of the largest healthcare systems in the world and one that primarily serves older men. Although ED has been a condition plaguing veterans long before establishment of the VA some 130 years ago, ED could be argued to be the most underdiagnosed medical condition in the VA, if not everywhere medicine is practiced. Not until the release of sildenafil and the subsequent consumer demand was there a sustained national focus within the VA on the topic of ED. A national VA technical advisory group was established and spent over a year developing practice guidelines for primary care management of erection dysfunction (DVA, 1999). As the contributing psychologist to this group, the author learned that the estimated cost of providing this single medication to veterans with appropriate medical need would be about \$300 to \$600 million, potentially up to 20% of the entire VA 1999 pharmacy budget.

Sildenafil is a potent and selective inhibitor of the predominant isoform (PDE5) in penile spongy tissue (corpora smooth muscle). Nitric oxide, a neurotransmitter released during sexual stimulation, increases cyclic guanosine monophosphate (cGMP), which in turn produces relaxation of penile smooth muscle, allowing the spongy tissue to fill with blood and become entrapped by venous occlusion. As sildenafil inhibits PDE5, it allows longer activity of cGMP, which continues to relax smooth muscle in the spongy tissue, in effect, amplifying the effects of the sexual stimulation (Padma-Nathan, 1998). In short, sildenafil increases the flow of blood into the penis and enhances sexual responsiveness.

The patient takes a tablet (25, 50, or 100 mg dosage range) about an hour before he expects to be sexually active. After 30 to 60 minutes, he has a 3- to 4-hour period of treatment effect (heightened sexual responsiveness). Sildenafil takes effect in combination with sexual stimulation and does not result in "instant erections," as some patients have expected. Efficacy is significant, as 57% to 83% of men report increased erectile response, regardless of the etiology (organic, psychogenic, or mixed), age, or baseline severity of the ED (Padma-Nathan, 1998). Most frequent side effects include headaches (16%), flushing (10%), upset stomach (7%), nasal congestion (4%), and disturbance to vision (blue hue, brightness sensitivity, and blurred vision in 2% to 3% of men) (Process of Care Panel, 1998). Men receiving nitrate therapy are absolutely contraindicated for use of sildenafil, as this drug interaction may result in potentially life-threatening hypotension. In addition, high risk patients/clinical conditions for adverse effects of sildenafil use include men on complex multidrug antihypertensive regimens, several subtypes of cardiac disease, retinal disorders, renal and hepatic impairment, and spinal cord injury above T5-6 at risk for autonomic dysreflexia (DVA, 1999).

There are two other oral medications for ED that will soon be available. Phentolamine is another vasoactive agent, which has an effect of increasing arterial blood flow into the penis and enhancing erections, although it has a different mechanism than sildenafil. Phentolamine is a peripheral alpha-adrenergic antagonist with equal affinity alpha-1 and alpha-2 receptors in corpus cavernosum. The advantage of oral phentolamine is expected to be in absorption time, as little as 20 minutes in the 40 mg dose, and fewer side effects, limited to nasal stuffiness and flushing (Process of Care Panel, 1998). Sublingual apomorphine (apomorphine SL) is a centrally active, dopamine agonist drug which also has rapid absorption and onset of action (20-30 minutes). Efficacy is reported at from 44% at low dosage (2 mg) to 61% at higher dosage (6 mg). Side effects range from mild nausea (up to 16% at 6 mg dose), dizziness (7%), sweating (7%), somnolence (6%), and yawning (5%) (Padma-Nathan et al., 1997).

Second-Line Therapies - Intracavernosal Injections and Intraurethral Suppository

Intracavernosal Injections

In 1982, surgeon Ronald Virag was performing a routine procedure when he noticed that the injection of a vasodilating drug (papaverine) into a pelvic artery produced an erection in the anesthetized patient. One year later, Dr. Giles Brindley dropped his pants and injected himself in front of an audience at the American Urological Association to demonstrate the immediate effectiveness of erectogenic drugs, producing an erection without aid of psychological or tactile stimulation. Soon after, vasoactive injections revolutionized the urologic diagnosis and treatment of ED by providing the first direct test of penile health and the first specific drug therapy for ED (Broderick, 1998).

Patients often refer to self-injection therapy as "the shot." For those who chose to withstand the "wince factor," an effective therapy was created that proved successful for 70% to 80% of men. As dozens of men have told this writer, the exchange of 5 minutes of discomfort for a sustained erection of 60 to 90 minutes is a good trade, especially for those men who have not had an erection - let alone intercourse - in several years. The two medications used for injections are prostaglandin E1-alprostadil sterile powder and alprostadil alfadex (AACE, 1998). Appropriate dosing usually occurs in the physician's office to ensure proper patient instruction and erectile response. In 10 to 20 minutes, a sustained erection is produced which usually does not subside with orgasm or ejaculation. Full and natural tumescence is enjoyed independent of sexual desire (Montague et al., 1996).

Besides the "wince factor," the disadvantages include being limited to three injections per week, developing scar tissue at injection sites, needing to have good dexterity, ability to learn the multiple steps involved in self-injection, and risk of overdose producing priapism in less than 1% (Process of Care Panel, 1998). When the patient injects too high a dose or has an atypical reaction, priapism can result, with the patient having to report to the nearest emergency room if the erection lasts longer than 4 hours. Intracorporal injection therapy may be unsuitable in patients with inadequate hand dexterity (due to arthritis), visual impairment (due to diabetic neuropathy), or difficulty gaining sufficient access to the penis, such as with obesity (DVA, 1999).

Intraurethral Suppository

Intraurethral suppository therapy uses the same drug used in self-injection (alprostadil), but employs a different route of administration. A small plastic dispensing applicator is lubricated and inserted into the urethra meatus (the urinary opening at the tip of the penis). This method of administration is generally more acceptable than injection (AACE, 1998). These dispensing devices come individually and sterilely wrapped with a premeasured dosage ranging from 125 to 1,000 micrograms. Once fully inserted (approximately 2 inches), a small suppository of the medication in semisolid pellet form is deposited into the penis for absorption. The dispenser is extracted from the urethra and thrown away. As with the injected vasodilator, a sustained erection will develop which may last approximately an hour (AACE, 1998).

Absorption into the spongy tissue of the penis is 80% complete within 10 minutes. Soon after, an erection occurs (10-20 minutes). Approximately 65% of men using this therapy in the physician's office achieved erections suitable for intercourse, while efficacy dropped to

50% of men being able to complete intercourse when using the therapy at home (Process of Care Panel, 1998). Although transient penile discomfort may occur with most men, 5% to 10% of patients will have substantial pain that will preclude any further use of this form of medication administration. Priapism may also occur with urethral suppository use of vasodilators, although this is rare. Some clinicians give patients medications (adrenergic agents such as ephedrine) in case of the erection lasting more than 2 hours. If the erection is sustained after 4 hours, aggressive and immediate treatment is necessary (AACE, 1998).

Third-Line Therapy - Surgery

As mentioned previously, surgical rearterialization of the penis or venous litgation for venous leakage is sometimes performed on younger males. But after a review of the high rate of failure for these procedures, NIH issued a statement suggesting these procedure be done only as part of research protocols (NIH, 1993). Of course, special cases involving destruction or severe injury to the penile artery in men under 45 years of age after trauma or radiation therapy may indicate specific consideration of revascularization surgery as the treatment of choice (AACE, 1998).

Penile implants were introduced in 1972 with semirigid prostheses being inserted into the physical space where corpora tissue naturally lies. Implants are always the "last resort" intervention because they are the most invasive of all treatments and because the man will permanently lose any ability to have unassisted erections (as a result of having the corpus cavernosum removed). This is why many urologists will not consider patients for penile prostheses if they have had any naturally occurring erections in the last 6 months.

Over the last two decades, the semirigid rod has been the more common model implanted. Treatment failures attributable to infection, extrusion, or mechanical failure (especially in patients with diabetes) previously was as high as 36% (AACE, 1998). The technology over the last 25 years has greatly advanced. There are now several subtypes of the two general categories of implants: semirigid and hydraulic prostheses. Semirigid prostheses come in two subtypes: more popular malleable rods or the mechanical type with articulating segments made out of high molecular weight polyethylene. Hydraulic prostheses come in 1- to 3-piece models (Mulcahy, 1998).

As hydraulic implant designs improved, they have come to be seen as the "Cadillac model" with higher patient satisfaction ratings. A disadvantage of the multiple component hydraulic prostheses is there are more parts to malfunction. The overall satisfaction rate is high, with 80% of men and their partners reporting that they are happy with the results of the implants (Fallon & Ghanem, 1990). Complaints of implant recipients include some reports of diminished penile sensitivity and the implant resulting in an erection that is shorter than the natural erection (Mulcahy, 1998).

CULTURAL COMPETENCE IN SEX THERAPY

The review of assessment issues and treatment options for ED is the easy part. Let's talk about putting it all together in the real world. A client walks into your first meeting and identifies himself as a gay Hispanic male who has erectile dysfunction because he wants to become a heterosexual female through gender reassignment surgery. Clinical practice almost always differs from textbook examples of treatment application as this recent case example from the author's practice illustrates. To be effective providing sex therapy, mental health professionals must appreciate the complex role culture plays in psychosocial perspectives and approaches to patient care. Mental health professionals engaged in sex therapy need to endeavor to be culturally competent by continually attempting to increase awareness of cultural norms of the different ethnic groups, the gay and lesbian community, and the transvestite/transsexual (TVTS) subculture. This is commonly done through client interaction but may also be enhanced by participating in a group's community activity when possible (e.g., gay pride dinner).

Of course, cultural competence in sex therapy is not limited to differences in sexual orientation but also includes religious and ethnic diversity. In 1990, the U.S. Census counted minority groups as one-fourth the entire census; minority groups are expected to compose more than half of the U.S. population in about 40 years. Some states, such as California, are already making the shift to the status of ethnic pluralism where no one ethnic group has a majority (The New York Times, 1998).

Cultural competence is important in sex therapy because it helps to build the provider-patient relationship. When patients feel they are being treated with respect, they may increase their response to the therapist. Cultural competency can increase job satisfaction by making work more interesting via learning more about clients and preparing healthcare facilities to meet accrediting standards set by the Joint Commission for Accreditation of Healthcare Organizations.

Developing cultural competence in sex therapy DOES NOT mean knowing everything about every, or even a single, cultural group with whom you work. Cultural competence does mean being aware that cultural factors can influence the healthcare behavior of both the provider and patient as well as taking appropriate steps to learn about each patient's cultural influences. Dr. Pope-Davis, of the University of Maryland, has a simple two-step formula for cultural competence. First, ask patients for help in understanding the value system and norms from which they come. Secondly, ensure that patients feel that any cultural differences they may have with the clinician are respected and acknowledged within the therapy process. If we follow these two steps, we become more culturally competent and, hence, more effective addressing clients' sexual concerns when their backgrounds differ from our own. Readers are referred to the Center for Cross-Cultural Health (612-624-6930; http://www.umn.edu.ccch), the Office of Minority Health Resource Center (800-444-6472; http://www.omhrc.gov), and Ponterotto and Pedersen (1993) for additional information.

ERECTION DYSFUNCTION IN THE FUTURE

The future treatment of ED may pose intriguing possibilities. In the near future, molecular biology will be used to study ED in penile smooth muscle cells and make needle biopsy a routine procedure in the differential diagnosis of ED, determining whether etiology is organic, psychological, or mixed (Christ, 1998). Many more selective oral agents will be developed based upon the expanding knowledge of smooth muscle cells. With the potential of the human genome project identifying tens of thousands of genes which play a role in penile tumescence and rigidity (which could be transferred), the future of genetic therapy for ED may be promising (Christ, 1998). There is a serious dearth of research comparing the efficacy of different treatments in large-sample, randomized studies. In the new century, the clinical management of ED will hopefully benefit from empirical investigation of the most effective treatment regime, combining several clinical interventions from across disciplines. Finally, it is conceivable that erection dysfunction will become 100% correctable, if not eventually eradicated, in America.

CONTRIBUTOR

Frederick L. Peterson, Jr., PsyD, is health psychologist at the Veterans Healthcare System of Ohio, Dayton Campus, where he coordinates a Sexual Health Clinic and the Smoking Cessation Programs. He completed postdoctorate training as a Clinical Fellow at the Masters and Johnson Institute. Research interests include sex therapy, tobacco use treatment, and the effects of masculinity-related personality factors on health. He holds four academic appointments at Wright State University, including the School of Professional Psychology and the School of Medicine (Psychiatry). Dr. Peterson may be contacted at Mental Health Care Line, VA Medical Center, Dayton, OH 45428. E-mail: Peterson.Frederick@Dayton.va.gov

RESOURCES

Agency for Health Care Policy and Research (AHCPR). (1996). *Clinical Practice Guidelines on Smoking Cessation* (Centers for Disease Control and Prevention, Publication No. 18). Washington, DC: U.S. Government Printing Office.

Althof, S. (1998). New roles for mental health professionals in the treatment of erectile dysfunction. *Journal of Sex Education and Therapy, 23*(3), 229-231.

American Association of Clinical Endocrinologists (AACE). (1998). AACE Clinical Practice Guidelines for the Evaluation and Treatment of Male Sexual Dysfunction. *Endocrine Practice, 4*(4), 220-235.

American Association of Sex Educators, Counselors and Therapists (AASECT). (1993). *ASSECT Code of Ethics.* Mount Vernon, IA: Author.

American Psychiatric Association (APA). (1994). *Diagnostic and Statistical Manual of Mental Disorders* (4th ed.). Washington, DC: Author.

American Psychiatric Association (APA). (1996). *Clinical Practice Guidelines for Smoking Cessation* [Special supplement edition]. Washington, DC: Author.

Beck, A., Steer, R., & Brown, G. (1996). *Beck Depression Inventory Manual.* San Antonio, TX: The Psychological Corporation.

Broderick, G. (1998). Impotence and penile vascular testing: Who are these men and how do we evaluate the etiology and severity of their complaints? *Journal of Sex Education and Therapy, 23*(3), 197-206.

Buvat, J., & Lemaire, A. (1997). Endocrine screening in 10,022 men with erectile dysfunction: Clinical significance and cost effective strategy. *Journal of Urology, 158,* 1764-1767.

Christ, G. (1998). The control of corporal smooth muscle tone, the coordination of penile erection, and the etiology of erectile dysfunction: The devil is in the details. *Journal of Sex Education and Therapy, 23*(3), 187-193.

Department of Veterans Affairs (DVA). (1999). *The Primary Care Management of Erectile Dysfunction* (Published by the Pharmacy Benefits Management Strategic Healthcare Group and the Medical Advisory Panel, Publication No. 99-0014). Washington, DC: U.S. Government Printing Office.

Fallon, B., & Ghanem, H. (1990). Sexual performance and satisfaction with penile prostheses in impotence with various etiology. *International Journal of Impotence Research, 2,* 35-42.

Feldman, H. A., Goldstein, I., Hatzichristou, D. G., Krane, R. J., & McKinlay, J. B. (1994). Impotence and its medical and psychological correlates: Results of the Massachusetts Male Aging Study. *Journal of Urology, 151,* 54-61.

Govier, F. E., McClure, D. R., & Kramer-Levien, D. (1996). Endocrine screening for sexual dysfunction using free testosterone determination. *Journal of Urology, 156,* 405-409.

Hawton, K., Catalan, J., & Fagg, J. (1992). Sex therapy for erectile dysfunction: Characteristics of couples, treatment outcome and prognostic factors. *Archives of Sexual Behavior, 21,* 161-175.

Heaton, J. (1998). Androgens, andropause and erectile function. *Journal of Sex Education and Therapy, 23*(3), 232-235.

Kaplan, H. (1986). Psychosexual dysfunctions. In A. M. Cooper, A. J. Frances, & M. H. Sacks (Eds.), *Personality Disorders and Neurosis* (pp. 467-479). Philadelphia: Lippincott.

Kolodny, R. (1985). The clinical management of sexual problems in substance abusers. In T. Bratter & G. Forrest (Eds.), *Current Management of Alcoholism and Substance Abuse* (pp. 594-622). New York: Free Press.

Laumann, E., Paik, A., & Rosen, R. (1999). Sexual dysfunction in the United States: Prevalence and predictors. *Journal of American Medical Association, 281*(6), 537-544.

Leeming, A., & Brown, P. (1992). An eclectic or integrative approach to sex therapy? *Journal of Sexual and Marital Therapy, 7*(3), 283-293.

Levine, L. (1998). Peyronie's disease: A brief review of a difficult sexual dysfunction problem. *Journal of Sex Education and Therapy, 23*(3), 226-228.

Masters, W., Johnson, V., & Kolodny, R. (1995). *Human Sexuality.* New York: Harper-Collins.

Montague, D. (1998). Erectile dysfunction: The rational utilization of diagnostic testing. *Journal of Sex Education and Therapy, 23*(3), 194-196.

Montague, D., Barada, J., Belker, A., Levine, L., Nadig, P., Roehrborn, C., Sharlip, I., & Bennett, A. (1996). Clinical guidelines panel on erection dysfunction: Summary report on the treatment of organic erectile dysfunction. *Journal of Urology, 56,* 2007-2011.

Mulcahy, J. (1998). Review of penile implants. *Journal of Sex Education and Therapy, 23*(3), 220-225.

The New York Times. (1998). *The New York Times Almanac.* New York: Penguin Reference.

NIH Consensus Development Panel on Impotence (1993). NIH Consensus Conference on Impotence. *Journal of American Medical Association, 270*(1), 83-90.

Padma-Nathan, H. (1998). The pharmacologic management of erection dysfunction: Sildenafil citrate (Viagra). *Journal of Sex Education and Therapy, 23*(3), 209-218.

Padma-Nathan, H., Auerbach, S., Lewis, R., Lewand, M., & Perdok, R. (1997, April). *Efficacy and Safety of Apomorphine SL vs. Placebo for Male Erectile Dysfunction (MED).* Paper presented at the annual meeting of the American Urology Association, New York, NY.

Ponterotto, J., & Pedersen, P. (1993). *Preventing Prejudice: A Guide for Counselors and Educators.* Newbury Park, CA: Sage.

Process of Care Panel of the University of Medicine and Dentistry, New Jersey. (1998). *The Process of Care Model for the Evaluation and Treatment of Erectile Dysfunction.* Unpublished manuscript used for continuing education, UMDNJ-Center for Continuing Education, Princeton, NJ.

Rosen, R., Riley, A., Wagner, G., Osterloh, I., Kirkpatrick, J., & Mishra, A. (1997). The international index of erectile function (IIEF): A multidimensional scale for assessment and erectile dysfunction. *Urology, 49*(6), 822-830.

Shabsigh, R., Fishman, I., Schum, C., & Dunn, J. (1991). Cigarette smoking and other vascular risk factors in vasculoganic impotence. *Urology, 38*(3), 227-231.

Trapp, J. (1998). External vacuum therapy: A historical review. *Journal of Sex Education and Therapy, 23*(3), 217-220.

Wetter, D., Fiore, M., Gritz, E., Lando, H., Stitzer, M., Hasselblad, V., & Baker, T. (1998). The Agency for Health Care Policy and Research smoking cessation clinical practice guideline: Findings and implications for psychologists. *American Psychologist, 53*(6), 657-669.

Wilson, J. (1988). Androgen abuse by athletes. *Endocrine Reviews, 9,* 181-199.

Integration of Psychotherapy and Medication in the Treatment of Severe Personality Disorders

Paulette Marie Gillig

Medication is sometimes helpful in the treatment of severe personality disorders. This is because biological factors, such as temperament, likely play an important role in the emotional and cognitive coping styles that ultimately shape a personality (Digman, 1990; Rothbart & Ahadi, 1994; Widiger & Sanderson, 1994, 1997). Some of the underlying dimensions that influence the development of personality, such as aggression and emotional sensitivity to separation, are partly biologically inherited (Nigg & Goldsmith, 1994), have a basis in physiology, and therefore may be amenable to biological interventions such as medication (Coccaro et al., 1990; Siever & Davis, 1991).

Individuals who develop severe personality disorders experience extreme or stereotyped responses to common situations, partly because of certain biological vulnerabilities. These biological vulnerabilities may be shared with other individuals who develop more acute disorders having similar symptoms. It has been proposed that the symptoms of some severe personality disorders overlap substantially with Axis I disorders and even with some neurological conditions such as Tourette's syndrome. Some severe personality disorders could therefore be part of "spectrums" of disorders that reflect common biological vulnerabilities (Siever & Davis, 1991). According to this conceptualization, severe personality disorders may be manifestations of "subthreshold" anxiety disorders, depressive disorders, impulse control disorders, and the like. If this reasoning is correct, medication that is effective in managing the symptoms of acute disorders within the spectrum also may be effective in managing similar chronic symptoms experienced in that "spectrum."

The fact that biological interventions such as medication may be of help to persons with severe personality disorders does not disprove or even challenge the complementary view that developmental experiences, other learning, and the nature of the individual's cognitive processes are of critical importance in the development, manifestation, and treatment of severe personality disorders (Cloninger, Svrakic, & Przybeck, 1993). The cause of a severe personality disorder may not necessarily determine how best to treat it with medication. The choice of medication, at least at this point in time, really is very much symptom-based. Therefore, when we are considering treating an individual who has a severe personality disorder with medication, it is critical that we have a clear qualitative and quantitative idea about the target symptoms to be addressed.

It is important to keep in mind also that, unfortunately, some of the most severe personality disorders, such as Schizoid, Histrionic, Narcissistic, Dependent, and Obsessive-Compulsive Personality Disorder, do not respond particularly well to treatment with medication, even though their (possibly) related Axis I disorders do respond. It may be that we have overlooked some important factor in our classification of those particular severe personality disorders, because although superficially they seem similar to some Axis I disorders, they do not respond to medication that would be expected to treat those Axis I disorders (Kalus, Bernstein, & Siever, 1993).

GENERAL PRINCIPLES REGARDING ASSESSMENT FOR POSSIBLE MEDICATION REFERRAL

The Importance of Differential Diagnosis

Psychiatric History

The clinical interview, if done in a systematic manner, is the best way to uncover recurring personality patterns and therefore a severe personality disorder. Behavior that occurred earlier in life is very important, because a severe personality disorder will have been present since adolescence.

A careful clinical interview usually will allow you to make the differential diagnosis between most Axis I disorders (which will have been superimposed upon the personality structure) and severe personality disorders. Treatment of the Axis I disorder must be done first or in conjunction with treatment of the severe personality disorder. The clinical interview of a truthful person who is a good historian will clarify whether or not some intervening medical condition or treatment, or abuse of drugs or alcohol, may be affecting behavior. If the history is not reliable, of course third-party corroboration is essential.

Family history may reveal biological vulnerability to certain conditions. Medical history, including past or current illnesses or medications, is important, because these may be causing the current symptoms. In the case of impulsivity or aggression, a medical evaluation is needed to rule out seizures or other brain disorders such as degenerative disorders.

Clinical Challenges

As I reflect on my own clinical experiences, the most difficult differential diagnoses of severe personality disorders have occurred when I have been taking the clinical history of a person who had *both* a severe personality disorder and some other related psychiatric or medical condition. I have learned to avoid premature closure when I uncover the first condition afflicting a person. Medical students and physicians often are relieved when they can make a mental health diagnosis and "turf" a challenging patient to a mental health professional. However, there is nothing about having a mental illness or personality disorder that protects a person from getting heart disease, diabetes, multiple sclerosis, or breast cancer. In fact, people with mental illness have a higher incidence of many medical illnesses.

I sometimes have had difficulty differentiating Bipolar Affective Disorder (especially cyclothymia) from Borderline Personality Disorder because affective lability is present in both. Fortunately, the medication management is somewhat similar.

Recurrent substance abuse is also a challenge, because it may be present in a person with a severe personality disorder who is self-medicating. I always ask such a person, "What illicit drugs that you have taken have seemed to help you feel better?" Sometimes I can get an idea of the biological underpinning of such a person's personality disorder by finding out what has helped them "on the street." Also, when the individual realizes that I am not trying to find out about drug use in order to criticize, the person often is more forthcoming with this information.

Another challenge for me has been determining whether or not a severe personality disorder was present in a person who was receiving medication such as steroids. This could be a person with a kidney transplant, ulcerative colitis, multiple sclerosis, and so forth. Neurological conditions affecting the brain can change the apparent "personality." A frontal lobe glioma was overlooked (by others) in a man who presented with personality *changes*. The key word to this differential diagnosis: personality *changes*. Personality disorders do not suddenly appear and then disappear.

The mentally retarded person who is acting out in some way may or may not have a severe personality disorder. A helpful rule of thumb for me has been to ask myself: Is the mentally retarded person's behavior appropriate for the age of cognitive development with the superimposed challenges that puberty may have caused, or is it not?

I have been challenged when evaluating a person of a different culture, especially when ritual religious practices are part of the culture. In one situation, a person's very religious family had a very religious relative probated to the hospital out of concern for the person's safety while practicing religious rituals. Was the patient behaving appropriately within that cultural context? I was besieged by clerics who argued that this individual's religious practices were completely correct, which was true. It was helpful in this case to stop being distracted by culturally based practices, where I could make a serious mistake due to my own value judgments. Instead, I decided to move my focus to the nature of the individual's interpersonal relationships, which is the essence of making a personality disorder diagnosis. (Yes, there was a severe personality disorder present, I concluded, but it did not respond to medication.)

Finally, although Posttraumatic Stress Disorder may predispose some persons to develop Borderline Personality Disorder (Gunderson & Sabo, 1993), often I have been impressed by the remission of "personality" symptoms when the Axis I disorder has been treated.

General Principles of Medication Management

Medication management of someone with a severe personality disorder is difficult when the person is medically ill, especially with renal or hepatic failure, or if the metabolism has been altered by other medications. If I am going to prescribe a mood stabilizer for such an individual, I naturally will try to select one that is metabolized by an organ system that is relatively intact. I might choose lithium for a person who is in liver failure (because it is excreted mainly via the kidney) and sodium valproate in a person who is in kidney failure (because it is metabolized in the liver). It is essential that I know a detailed medical history and exactly what medications the person is taking and at what doses. I also will need to know about any abnormal laboratory studies.

In general, medication doses may need to increase at times of stress and decrease if toxic side effects outweigh the benefit. The difficulties inherent in establishing a therapeutic alliance with someone who has a severe personality disorder and so who therefore has serious problems with interpersonal relationships may make medication compliance problematic. With the more impulsive or acting-out individual, one naturally worries about overdoses.

Operational Definition of Symptoms

It is important to operationally define, qualitatively and quantitatively, each target symptom for each psychotropic to be taken. Examples of potential target symptoms include impulsiveness and compulsiveness; affective instability, including rage, anger, depression, low self-worth, anhedonia, or high responsiveness or low responsiveness; aggressiveness toward self or others; anxiety; slower habituation to new stimuli (which may be manifested in fear of separation or social phobia); abnormalities in perceptual or cognitive organization (such as transient psychotic episodes, ideas of reference, or paranoid projections); and the use of primitive defenses (such as periods of dissociation, splitting, denial, lack of a conscience, rigid conscience, idealization, or devaluation).

Professional Collaboration Between Psychotherapist and Pharmacotherapist for Severe Personality Disordered Clients Requiring Medication

When referring a severe personality disordered individual to another practitioner for medication evaluation, it is important to find out first the client's attitude about taking medication for symptoms. A number of these persons are concerned about altering their intrinsic "self," because they view their symptoms as a manifestation of their "self." This concern goes to the core of an individual's identity and therefore may be of greatest concern for the person with Borderline Personality Disorder or Narcissistic Personality Disorder. If possible, this issue needs to be worked through (or at least, addressed) before the person is referred. Also, Histrionic or Dependent patients may become resentful at a medication referral because they fear giving up the manifestations of their symptoms, perceiving no other way of getting their needs met.

Referral for medication management may be perceived by the person as abandonment by a psychotherapist who has "given up" on the patient. If this occurs, the stage is set for splitting between the therapist and the physician (Meyer & Simon, 1999). The little tablets or capsules of medication also can come to represent the prescribing physician (or the therapist) and act as transitional objects.

Medication also can become a "ticket" for continuing therapy. One of my patients absolutely refused to discontinue a medication I had prescribed despite severe side effects. This was because she thought that if she did not take any medicine, she could no longer see me. Clearly, discussion of the meaning of taking medication must become integrated into therapy.

On the other hand, a person who is suffering severe symptoms may come to wonder why the therapist who does not make a medication referral is not obtaining all the help that may potentially be available. The Paranoid patient will (naturally) distrust both being referred for medication and not being referred for medication. A frank, low-key discourse on risks and benefits of taking medication will be the most helpful approach here, without the therapist seeming to be overly invested in the client's decision about this matter.

When more than one professional is involved in the care of an individual, it is important for the treatment team to be clear about the specific clinical duty of each clinician. In a collaborative relationship there is a shared responsibility for the patient's care *in accordance with the qualifications of each therapist's discipline and abilities*. However, the person prescribing medication cannot evade responsibility by delegating the oversight of the medication to another member of the treatment team. Although it is critically important that the psychotherapist report any new medical problems to the prescriber, it is the responsibility of the prescriber to independently ensure that medications are being prescribed and used appropriately by the patient and that the medical history is complete (American Psychiatric Association, 1980; Bradley, 1990; Ellison & Smith, 1989).

In contrast to medication management, when there is more than one professional involved in treatment, it is very difficult to establish separable psychological arenas that are one clinician's sole, independent responsibility. Psychopharmacology inevitably involves psychotherapy in some way, and the clinical focus and responsibilities of therapist and psychopharmacologist will have multiple overlaps, as will the duties of clinical risk assessment and intervention with a patient's potential for suicide, violence, or impulsive behavior.

By virtue of their disorders, severely personality disordered individuals will have difficulties when relating to most members of the treatment team; these difficulties will need to be addressed by the team as a whole. The team must communicate regularly about each case. They must take care not to become part of the patient's "split" and fight political turf battles or compete with each other about who is the "good parent." When a person comes into one's office and describes all the "uncaring and incompetent" professionals with whom that person has had previous contact, one should visualize a long list of professionals stretching backward and forward throughout infinity, with one's own name soon to be displayed prominently in the center.

PSYCHOTHERAPY AND MEDICATION FOR THE TREATMENT OF SPECIFIC PERSONALITY DISORDERS

Personality disorders are grouped into three clusters based on descriptive similarities within the *DSM-IV* (American Psychiatric Association, 1994). Cluster A includes the Paranoid, Schizoid, and Schizotypal Personality Disorders, and individuals with these disorders are described as appearing "odd or eccentric." Cluster B includes the Antisocial, Borderline, Histrionic, and Narcissistic Personality Disorders, and these individuals are described as "dramatic, emotional, or erratic." Cluster C includes the Avoidant, Dependent, and Obsessive-Compulsive Personality Disorders. Individuals with these disorders often appear "anxious or fearful." This clustering system has serious limitations, and individuals with co-occurring personality disorders may cross clusters.

Cluster A: Paranoid, Schizoid, and Schizotypal Personality Disorders

Paranoid Personality Disorder

There is some scientific evidence that there is a genetic relationship between Paranoid Personality Disorder, Schizophrenia, and Schizotypal Personality Disorder (Nigg & Goldsmith, 1994; Siever & Davis, 1991). Individuals with Paranoid Personality Disorder often develop the Axis I disorders of Substance Abuse, Obsessive-Compulsive Disorder, and anxiety-based disorders such as Agoraphobia. They often experience depression.

Because their suspiciousness and distrust are ego-syntonic (due to their worldview), they more likely will come to a clinic or office for treatment of associated anxiety, mood or substance-related disorders, trouble controlling their anger, or various personal, legal, or situational problems attributable to poor interpersonal relationships. When discussing medication for treatment of related symptoms, it is better to be especially forthright and precise, so they do not feel something is being withheld.

There is some evidence that neuroleptics may be helpful if there is frank psychotic ideation. However, the more common presentation of nonpsychotic suspiciousness does not appear to be responsive to medication; in fact, suggestions about medication use may cause the individual to feel that you are trying to suppress or control legitimate concerns (Widiger & Sanderson, 1997).

In my clinical experience doing medication management with such patients, I have found that it was an error to allow the individual to reveal too much during the initial interview. I now use several sessions to obtain enough information to determine whether medication may be helpful. When I have rushed this process, the patient acted compliant within the interview but incorporated me into a threatening worldview. Becoming suspicious about my "real" motivation for learning so much, the patient has either "fired" me or dropped out of treatment.

Schizoid Personality Disorder

Persons with Schizoid Personality Disorder convey a sense of social detachment and restricted emotional expression (Kalus et al., 1993). This disorder does not tend to be genetically related to schizophrenia and may be better understood as a manifestation of extreme introversion, a temperament that does have a genetic basis. However, because the main symptom is that of a very low apparent ability to experience positive affect, some have suggested that Schizoid Personality Disorder represents the manifestation of subthreshold negative symptoms of Schizophrenia, and that Schizotypal Personality Disorder (below) represents subthreshold positive symptoms of Schizophrenia. Unfortunately, Schizoid Personality Disorder does not respond well even to the newer atypical neuroleptics which usually are more successful than earlier medications in targeting the negative symptoms of Schizophrenia.

The major distinction between Schizoid Personality Disorder and Avoidant Personality Disorder (which seems to be anxiety based) is the absence of an intense desire for intimate social relationships in the person with Schizoid Personality Disorder. These individuals can appear "depressed" at times, but most often this appearance really seems to reflect an anhedonic detachment without depression.

In my clinical experience, although patients with Schizoid Personality Disorder have looked more responsive to me and to other staff when they have received antidepressant medication (usually a serotonin reuptake inhibitor), curiously the patients themselves have not reported feeling any better. They have had no idea what I was talking about when I said they looked better, and they almost always discontinued their medication but did continue wanting to come back to see me. This latter fact has caused me to wonder whether the problem is not so much that these persons do not desire intimate social relationships but rather that they have difficulty conceptualizing how to go about having a relationship or what it might mean to their lives.

Schizotypal Personality Disorder

People who have Schizotypal Personality Disorder actually feel acute discomfort about close relationships. There is a genetic association between Schizotypal Personality Disorder and Schizophrenia. Persons with either of these disorders have deficits in the cognitive processes of attention and selection (Siever & Davis, 1991; Siever, Bernstein, & Silverman, 1991). This makes it very difficult for them to relate properly to their environment. Naturally, they feel a great deal of discomfort in social situations and therefore isolate themselves.

Schizotypal Personality Disorder must be differentiated from some of the symptoms of temporal lobe epilepsy, but this is not difficult because the symptoms of epilepsy occur episodically. Schizotypal Personality Disorder may be present in persons who also are diagnosed as having Borderline Personality Disorder. Unlike the person who exclusively has Borderline Personality Disorder, the person with Schizotypal Personality Disorder has enduring cognitive-perceptual aberrations that are not confined to periods of stress or intense anxiety.

As noted previously, Schizotypal Personality Disorder can be thought of as a subsyndromal manifestation of some of the positive symptoms of Schizophrenia, and as such may respond to neuroleptic medication in low doses (Goldberg, S. C. Schultz, & P. M. Schultz, 1986). This is true even if many of the symptoms (such as social isolation) seem anxiety based. Because of the risk of tardive dyskinesia and other side effects, it is probably better to taper neuroleptics during times when the patient is less distressed. The newer antipsychotics and antidepressant medications are also being studied for use in this condition (Siever & Davis, 1991; Trestman, deVegvar, & Siever, 1995).

Cluster B: Antisocial, Borderline, Histrionic, and Narcissistic Personality Disorders

Antisocial Personality Disorder

Persons with Antisocial Personality Disorder are impulsive and display aggression and a disregard for social norms. Impulsivity that leads to aggression is a dimension of behavior that likely is heritable. It also is seen in the Axis I disorders of Intermittent Explosive Disorder, Bipolar Affective Disorder, and Conduct Disorder (Myers, Stewart, & Brown, 1998). Evidence for a genetic factor associated with Antisocial Personality Disorder is stronger than for most psychiatric disorders, including Bipolar Disorder and Schizophrenia.

These individuals tend to have a low baseline arousal level, especially when confronted with potential painful stimuli (Fowles & Missel, 1994). It has been postulated that this is why they develop less fear-based guilt about the consequences of ignoring social norms and laws (Kochanska, 1991). Two-thirds of persons with Antisocial Personality Disorder have an associated Substance Abuse Disorder, which further decreases impulse control (Sher & Trull, 1994).

Antisocial Personality Disorder is the most difficult personality disorder to treat. Outpatient therapy is rarely successful. Therapy works best when it is backed up by the threat of real consequences for continued antisocial acts, especially for those individuals who have psychopathic traits (Agee, 1979; R. D. Hare, S. D. Hare, & Harpur, 1991). Utilitarian approaches that focus on the value of a behavior pattern that conforms to social norms usually are the best approach for a number of these persons, rather than those that attempt to arouse fear or guilt or build a "conscience."

Because the person with Antisocial Personality Disorder often does not readily accept responsibility for behavior, the individual often will readily accept the idea that medication should control symptoms. This fact has positive and negative aspects. Comorbid conditions, such as depression, irritability leading to aggression, anxiety, and substance abuse may in fact respond to medication, and this can indirectly reduce antisocial behavior and its associated propensity for violence (Coccaro & Kavoussi, 1997). On the other hand, one does not desire to excuse responsibility for behavior. In my clinical practice, I have been impressed by the number of persons with Antisocial Personality Disorder who have been depressed and who have responded well to antidepressant medication in terms of affect and their ability to better control emotional outbursts and impulsivity.

Also, I have found that a large number of these persons suffer from Attention Deficit Disorder and have responded to treatment for this disorder. In fact, Antisocial Personality Disorder is sometimes considered a neurodevelopmental abnormality, and it is often associated with minor physical anomalies, hyperactivity, and learning disabilities.

Serotonin reuptake inhibitors and mood stabilizers have been helpful in those persons who are suffering associated affective symptoms. Benzodiazepines should be avoided in this population because they may cause disinhibition and also because these persons have a tendency toward substance abuse. Stimulants or other medications useful with comorbid Attention Deficit Disorder also have proved to be helpful. Some persons with apparent Antisocial Personality Disorder may in fact be adults with residual Attention Deficit Disorder, with impulsivity, irritability, mood lability, difficulty focusing, and subtle learning disabilities attributable to Attention Deficit Disorder.

Borderline Personality Disorder

The person with Borderline Personality Disorder tends to display a pattern of impulsivity, mood instability, unstable and unsatisfying interpersonal relationships, and an unstable self-image. The mood instability of Borderline Personality Disorder probably is a genetically based trait. Because these persons are impulsive, they have trouble controlling their quick and intense anger and may do physically self-damaging acts. Their selective recall of emotionally charged events may be related to their intense rage, which may distort their registration and thus their memory of an event.

Borderline Personality pathology plays a very significant role in the suicide of people in their 20s. The stressors surrounding the suicides are often fairly mild, and it is postulated that this could reflect a lower threshold for suicide in Borderline patients (Gunderson & Phillips, 1991).

When treating depressive symptoms in these individuals, results are better with the serotonin reuptake inhibitors than with tricyclic antidepressants. There is some evidence that self-injury behavior may be reduced by treating Borderline patients with serotonin reuptake inhibitors (Markovitz, Calabrese, & S. C. Schultz, 1991).

Those patients experiencing decreased energy, hypersomnia, and hyperphagia sometimes respond best to the antidepressants known as monoamine oxidase inhibitors. Benzodiazepines are not a good choice because of the potential for behavioral dyscontrol (Markovitz et al., 1991; Stein, Simeon, & Frenkel, 1995).

Lithium reduces mood instability and is associated with a decrease in aggressive acting out. It is especially effective in those Borderline individuals who have a relative with Bipolar Affective Disorder. Anticonvulsants such as sodium valproate and carbamazepine also are helpful in stabilizing affective lability, increasing the capacity to delay impulsive action, and also, to some extent, improving brief psychotic episodes (Hollander, 1999).

Patients with behavioral dyscontrol, or physical and verbal aggression respond well to monoamine oxidase inhibitors and almost as well to a neuroleptic or a mood stabilizer such as carbamazepine. Their symptoms worsen with benzodiazepines in terms of increased severity in episodes of behavioral dyscontrol (Stein et al., 1995).

Some studies have revealed a substantial overlap between Borderline Personality Disorder and Schizotypal Personality Disorder. For patients with both disorders, the atypical and typical neuroleptics are equally effective for subtle psychotic symptoms (suspiciousness), and may also have mood-stabilizing qualities in these individuals, reducing depression and interpersonal sensitivity (S. C. Schultz, 1999).

In my clinical practice, I have found it useful to determine whether an individual Borderline patient has predominantly affective or psychotic symptoms. Having discerned this emphasis, I proceed to try to manage the most prominent symptoms (Groves, 1987). I do not treat transient symptoms or those that can be ameliorated with supportive psychotherapy.

Although I am not the primary psychotherapist in many cases, when I feel that the patient trusts that I care, I have not been shy about explicitly letting the person know that our relationship is valuable to me. I explain that it does distress me when the person does things that may be harmful to himself or herself. I advise the person that misuse of medication can be especially harmful, and I don't want to ever feel I have done anything that hurt the person. Although this may seem simplistic, I have found that my little auxiliary ego has sometimes either prevented the person from acting out or prompted the person to call immediately when having done so. I believe that when the individual feels in great pain, and also has temporarily lost sight of a coordinated and nonfragmented personal identity, the person has been able to substitute the esteem I have for their own lost sense of self-worth.

Having dealt with treatment resistance issues, including resistance to taking medications correctly, the psychotherapist usually proceeds toward teaching the patient coping skills for management of and reactions to stress, including how to cope with feelings of identity diffusion and how to improve interpersonal relationships. Dialectical behavioral therapy (Robins, 1999) has been found to be especially helpful in persons with suicide-related behaviors such as suicidal ideation, hopelessness, anger directed at self or others, dissociation, and risky behaviors. In one study, by the 4th month of treatment, only 25% of patients were still taking medication compared with 60% in the control group. The use of the emergency room and inpatient psychiatric hospitalization both also declined (Robins, 1999).

Histrionic Personality Disorder

The individual with Histrionic Personality Disorder displays excessive emotionality and attention-seeking behavior. These persons have great difficulty delaying gratification. Histrionic Personality Disorder may share a genetic disposition toward impulsivity or sensation seeking which also characterizes persons with Antisocial Personality Disorder. The Histrionic person's symptoms worsen when he or she perceives a threat to physical attractiveness or bodily integrity; thus, medical illness and hospitalization can be especially difficult for that person.

Although this disorder is difficult to treat with medication, some symptoms may respond to treatment with antidepressants, especially mood reactivity, hypersomnia, and rejection sensitivity.

Narcissistic Personality Disorder

Narcissistic Personality Disordered persons have a pervasive behavioral and thought pattern of grandiosity, a need for admiration, and a lack of empathy with others. They tend to idealize and then devalue others and are preoccupied with conflicts and insecurities about their self-worth. They do seek treatment for Substance Abuse, and intervention with medication may be helpful here. Although they often present with depressive symptoms, I have not found antidepressant medication to be especially helpful for this group of patients, although I continue to try it when depression is present and they agree to take medication. I have found that the depressed Narcissistic individual can be unpredictable and represent a high suicide risk. In a few instances in my own practice, psychological testing has revealed a subtle psychoticlike thought disorder in these individuals when they have been severely stressed. However, unlike patients with Borderline Personality Disorder, they have not responded well to low-dose neuroleptics. Unfortunately, when a medication treatment approach does not work, they tend to devalue the pharmacotherapist and sometimes generalize this to the psychotherapist.

There is no known pharmacological approach to the overall treatment of Narcissistic Personality Disorder at this time (Widiger & Sanderson, 1994).

Cluster C: Avoidant, Dependent, and Obsessive-Compulsive Personality Disorders

Avoidant Personality Disorder

Persons with Avoidant Personality Disorder have an increased level of tonic sympathetic nervous system activity, higher levels of cortical arousal, and slower habituation to new stimuli (Claridge, 1985; Cloninger et al., 1993; Gray, 1982; Pilkonis, 1984; Siever & Davis, 1991). Avoidant Personality Disorder and Dependent Personality Disorder may coexist with Major Depression and Obsessive-Compulsive Disorder, and symptoms of apparent Avoidant Personality Disorder may remit with treatment of associated Axis I disorders. The most effective medications for persons with Avoidant Personality Disorder are the monoamine oxidase inhibitors and serotonin reuptake inhibitors for depressive symptoms (Liebowitz, Hollander, & Schneider, 1986) and beta-adrenergic receptor antagonists for treatment of sympathetic nervous system hyperarousal (Gorman, Liebowitz, & Fyer, 1985). If the patient does not abuse the medication and become dependent on it, benzodiazepines also are helpful. Buspirone has also been effective for treating anxiety associated with this disorder.

Effective psychotherapy approaches involve social skills training and systematic desensitization of specific fears, as well as learning how to deal with insecurities and fears through cognitive techniques. Group therapies may help the person practice more assertive behaviors and develop increased self-confidence. Medication may be necessary to help the person deal with feelings of intense social anxiety, so that the person can benefit from psychotherapy.

Dependent Personality Disorder

The individual with Dependent Personality Disorder experiences a need to be taken care of that leads to submissive behavior and fear of separation (Hirschfeld, Shea, & Weise, 1989). This disorder may be the result of an interaction between an anxious-inhibited temperament (Livesley, Schroeder, & Jackson, 1990; Matheny, 1989) and an insecure attachment to a parental figure (van den Boom, 1989) that can occur for a variety of reasons. Dependent Personality Disorder is often seen in mentally retarded persons and also in others who have suffered since childhood from a serious general medical disorder. Taking a medical history is very important when evaluating and treating these persons.

Dependent Personality Disorder is often associated with mood or anxiety disorders, and treatment of these associated disorders may be helpful to the person, although there is no pharmacological approach known to treat the personality disorder itself. The relationship with the psychotherapist or pharmacotherapist may become an end in itself for the patient. This can be a problem if it results in the person becoming less than straightforward about symptom resolution or medication use. It is important to set some limits on these patients at the outset so that the person's expectations for contact do not exceed what the professional is able or willing to do over the long run. I have found that these persons actually respond well to limits once they feel assured that they will not be abandoned. I explain that ours is a continuing relationship and they should not "use me up" all at once.

Obsessive-Compulsive Personality Disorder

Obsessive-Compulsive Personality Disorder differs from the Axis I "Obsessive-Compulsive Disorder" in that Obsessive-Compulsive Personality Disorder is not characterized by the presence of obsessions or compulsions. Instead, it involves a pervasive pattern of preoccupation with orderliness, perfectionism, and control, and begins in early adulthood. There may be a genetically inherited trait of obsessionality related to the development of this disorder. Obsessive-Compulsive Personality Disorder involves rigid behavior patterns that are somewhat ego-syntonic to the person.

Persons with Obsessive-Compulsive Personality Disorder may be prone to anxiety, feelings of hostility, and physical disorders related to constant worry. Depression may develop in middle age or when career problems occur. These symptoms can be treated.

Pharmacologic treatment involves treatment of associated Axis I disorders involving anxiety or depression. Unlike the obsessions and compulsions of the Axis I disorder, which may respond to medication, the preoccupation with orderliness and perfectionism of the person with Obsessive-Compulsive Personality Disorder does not respond to any known treatment with medication (Nestadt, Romanoski, & Chahal, 1991; Oldham & Frosch, 1991; Pfol & Blum, 1991; Widiger & Sanderson, 1994).

THE MENTALLY RETARDED/DEVELOPMENTALLY DISABLED CLIENT WITH A SEVERE PERSONALITY DISORDER

Personality disorders can be present in mentally retarded patients. The most common are Dependent Personality Disorder, which may manifest itself both with passive and aggressive features, and Borderline Personality Disorder, which is the most difficult to diagnose and treat.

Mentally Retardation, Borderline Personality Disorder, Psychotherapy, and Pharmacotherapy

Mentally retarded patients are at a special risk for Borderline Personality Disorder because of their poverty of interpersonal relationships, impaired object relations, poorly internalized controls, and poor coping skills.

The diagnosis of Borderline Personality Disorder in mentally retarded persons is conceptually the same as with persons with normal intelligence, but the clinical presentation and history may be different (Hurley & Sovner, 1988; Silka & Hauser, 1997). In mentally retarded individuals, the volatile nature of relationships is the most obvious clinical feature associated with Borderline Personality Disorder, and it is sometimes dismissed as "cognitive immaturity" without appreciation of its diagnostic significance. The impulsive behavior of the mentally retarded person with Borderline Personality Disorder, although more concrete than in persons of normal intelligence, is goal directed, in contrast to the more global impulsive behavior stemming from central nervous system dysfunction alone. When stressed, the Borderline patient with mental retardation, if verbal, will tend to have directed verbal tirades rather than exclusively manifesting physical aggressiveness.

Bizarre identity disturbances may occur in mentally retarded persons with a Borderline Personality Disorder, but the thought content may be more concrete than that seen in patients with normal intelligence. For example, a mentally retarded person with Borderline Personality Disorder may demonstrate a confused sexual identity by sometimes stating that he is a man and other times stating that he is a woman. Fear of abandonment may present as constant unreasonable demands on staff for exclusive attention. Mood lability, which can be a sign of central nervous system dysfunction as well as Borderline Personality Disorder or other affective disorder, is a nonspecific but treatable finding.

Buspirone and the serotonin reuptake inhibitors have been used effectively to treat the anxiety (Stavrakaki & Mintsioulis, 1997) sometimes present in mentally retarded persons with Borderline Personality Disorder. Anxiety can present in these patients with increased aggressivity, agitation, obsessive-compulsive phenomena, and insomnia. Buspirone is especially helpful in those persons who also have Attention Deficit Disorder, as it may also increase their attention span (Khreim & Mikkelsen, 1997).

The affective symptoms of Borderline Personality Disorder are underrecognized in retarded persons, and antidepressants and lithium are probably underprescribed. Lithium reduces self-mutilating and hyperactive aggressive behavior, and if affective symptoms such as rage and fury are present, it is likely that there may be a good response to lithium.

Depakote also is useful for the treatment of the mood lability associated with Borderline Personality Disorder in mentally retarded persons as is carbamazepine. Carbamazepine can be used for persistent overactivity or associated bipolar disorder, which may be present along with Borderline Personality Disorder in these individuals. Carbamazepine also tends to be a superior anticonvulsant in mentally retarded persons who also have a Seizure Disorder.

CONTRIBUTOR

Paulette Marie Gillig, MD, PhD, is currently an Associate Professor of Psychiatry at Wright State University. She also is the Chief Clinical Officer of the Logan-Champaign Counties Mental Health, Drug and Alcohol Services Board, and holds the Ohio Department of Mental Health Professorship in Rural Psychiatry. Dr. Gillig earned a PhD in experimental social psychology prior to attending medical school. After graduating with her MD degree, Dr. Gillig completed an internship in internal medicine and residencies in neurology and psychiatry. She also is board-certified in geriatric psychiatry. This year, Dr. Gillig was awarded the only Golden Apple Teaching Award by the psychiatry residents in her department. Her current research publications are in the areas of human service delivery systems, psychiatric emergencies, and violence-related issues. She sits on the Committee on Poverty, Homelessness, and Mental Illness of the American Psychiatric Association, and chairs the Committee on Minority and Underrepresented Psychiatrists of the Ohio Psychiatric Association. Dr. Gillig may be contacted at Wright State University School of Medicine, Department of Psychiatry, P.O. Box 927, Dayton, OH 45401.

RESOURCES

Agee, V. L. (1979). *Treatment of the Violent Incorrigible Adolescent.* Lexington, MA: D. C. Heath and Company.

American Psychiatric Association. (1980). *Guidelines for Psychiatrists in Consultative, Supervisory or Collaborative Relationships With Nonmedical Therapists.* Washington, DC: Author.

American Psychiatric Association. (1994). *Diagnostic and Statistical Manual of Mental Disorders* (4th ed.). Washington, DC: Author.

Bradley, S. S. (1990). Nonphysician psychotherapist-physician pharmacotherapist: A new model for concurrent treatment. *Psychiatric Clinics of North America, 12,* 307-322.

Claridge, G. (1985). *Origins of Mental Illness.* New York: Blackwell.

Cloninger, C. R., Svrakic, D. M., & Przybeck, T. R. (1993). A psychobiological model of temperament and character. *Archives of General Psychiatry, 50,* 975-990.

Coccaro, E. F., Astill, J. L., Szeeley, P. J., & Malkowicx, D. E. (1990). Serotonin in personality disorder. *Psychiatric Annals, 20,* 587-592.

Coccaro, E. F., & Kavoussi, R. J. (1997). Fluoxetine and impulsive aggressive behavior in personality-disordered subjects. *Archives of General Psychiatry, 54,* 1081-1088.

Digman, J. M. (1990). Personality structure: Emergence of the five-factor model. *Annual Review of Psychology, 41,* 417-440.

Ellison, J., & Smith, J. (1989). Intertherapist conflict in combined treatment. In J. Ellison (Ed.), *The Psychotherapist's Guide to Pharmacotherapy* (pp. 96-115). Chicago: Year Book Medical Publishers.

Fowles, D. C., & Missel, K. A. (1994). Electrodermal hyporeactivity, motivation, and psychopathy: Theoretical issues. In D. C. Fowles, P. B. Sutker, & S. H. Goodman (Eds.), *Progress in Experimental Personality and Psychopathology Research* (pp. 263-283). New York: Springer.

Goldberg, S. C., Schultz, S. C., & Schultz, P. M. (1986). Borderline and schizotypal personality disorders treated with low-dose thiothixene versus placebo. *Archives of General Psychiatry, 43,* 680-686.

Gorman, J. M., Liebowitz, M. R., & Fyer, A. J. (1985). Treatment of social phobia with atenolol. *Journal of Clinical Psychopharmacology, 5,* 298-301.

Gray, J. A. (1982). *The Neuropsychology of Anxiety.* Oxford, England: Oxford University Press.

Groves, J. E. (1987). Borderline patients. In T. P. Hackett & N. H. Cassem (Eds.), *Handbook of General Hospital Psychiatry* (pp. 185-207). Littleton, MA: PSG Publishing Company.

Gunderson, J. G., & Phillips, K. A. (1991). Borderline personality disorder and depression: A current overview of the interface. *American Journal of Psychiatry, 148,* 967-975

Gunderson, J. G., & Sabo, A. N. (1993). The phenomenological and conceptual interface between borderline personality disorder and PTSD. *American Journal of Psychiatry, 150,* 19-27.

Hare, R. D., Hare, S. D., & Harpur, T. J. (1991). Psychopathy and the DSM-IV criteria for antisocial personality disorder. *Journal of Abnormal Psychology, 100,* 391-398.

Hirshfeld, R. M. A., Shea, M. T., & Weise, R. (1989). Dependent personality disorder: Perspectives for DSM-IV. *Journal of Personality Disorders, 5,* 135-149.

Hollander, E. (1999). Managing aggressive behavior in patients with obsessive-compulsive disorder and borderline personality disorder. *Journal of Clinical Psychiatry, 15*(Suppl. 2), 38-44.

Hurley, A. D., & Sovner, R. (1988). The clinical characteristics and management of borderline personality disorder in mentally retarded persons. *Psychiatric Aspects of Mental Retardation Reviews, 7,* 42-50.

Kalus, O., Bernstein, D. P., & Siever, L. J. (1993). Schizoid personality disorder: A review of current status and implications for DSM-IV. *Journal of Personality Disorders, 7,* 43-52.

Khreim, I., & Mikkelsen, E. (1997). Implications of a clinical study of anxiety disorders in persons with mental retardation. *Psychiatric Annals, 27,* 182-189.

Kochanska, G. (1991). Socialization and temperament in the development of guilt and conscience. *Child Development, 62,* 1379-1392.

Liebowitz, M. R., Hollander, E., & Schneider, F. (1986). Reversible and irreversible monoamine oxidase inhibitors in other psychiatric disorders. *Acta Psychiatrica Scandinavia, 20*(Suppl. 360), 29-34.

Livesley, W. J., Schroeder, M. L., & Jackson, D. N. (1990). Dependent personality disorder and attachment problems. *Journal of Personality Disorders, 4,* 232-240.

Markovitz, P. J., Calabrese, J. R., & Schultz, S. C. (1991). Fluoxetine in the treatment of borderline and schizotypal personality disorders. *American Journal of Psychiatry, 148,* 1064-1067.

Matheny, A. P. (1989). Children's behavioral inhibition over age and across situations: Genetic similarity for a trait during change. *Journal of Personality, 57,* 215-235.

Meyer, D. J., & Simon, R. I. (1999). Split treatment: Clarity between psychiatrists and psychotherapists. *Psychiatric Annals, 29,* 241-245.

Myers, M. G., Stewart, D. G., & Brown, S. A. (1998). Progression from conduct disorder to antisocial personality disorder following treatment for adolescent substance abuse. *American Journal of Psychiatry, 155,* 479-485.

Nestadt, G., Romanoski, A. J., & Chahal, R. (1990). An epidemiological study of histrionic personality disorder. *Psychological Medicine, 20,* 413-422.

Nigg, J. R., & Goldsmith, H. H. (1994). Genetics of personality disorders: Perspectives from personality and psychopathology research. *Psychological Bulletin, 115,* 346-380.

Oldham, J. M., & Frosch, W. A. (1991). Compulsive personality disorder. In R. Michels (Ed.), *Psychiatry, Volume 1* (pp. 1-8). Philadelphia: J. B. Lippincott.

Pfol, B., & Blum, N. (1991). Obsessive-compulsive personality disorder: A review of available data and recommendations for DSM-IV. *Journal of Personality Disorders, 5,* 363-375.

Pilkonis, P. A. (1984). Avoidant and schizoid personality disorders. In H. E. Adams & P. B. Sutker (Eds.), *Comprehensive Handbook of Psychopathology* (pp. 479-494). New York: Plenum Publishing.

Robins, C. (1999, January). Integrating dialectical behavioral therapy into the treatment of borderline personality disorder. *Clinical Psychiatry News*, p. 38.

Rothbart, M. K., & Ahadi, S. A. (1994). Temperament and the development of personality. *Journal of Abnormal Psychology, 103,* 55-66.

Schultz, S. C. (1999). The use of atypical antipsychotics in borderline personality disorder. *The Journal of Psychotic Disorders, II,* 8-9.

Sher, K. J., & Trull, T. J. (1994). Personality and disinhibitory psychopathology: Alcoholism and antisocial personality disorder. *Journal of Abnormal Psychology, 103,* 92-102.

Siever, L. J., Bernstein, D., & Silverman, J. M. (1991). Schizotypal personality disorder: A review of its current status. *Journal of Personality Disorders, 5,* 178-193.

Siever, L. J., & Davis, K. L. (1991). A psychobiological perspective on the personality disorders. *American Journal of Psychiatry, 148,* 1647-1658.

Silka, V. R., & Hauser, M. J. (1997). Psychiatric assessment of the person with mental retardation. *Psychiatric Annals, 27,* 162-169.

Stavrakaki, C., & Mintsioulis, M. D. (1997). The efficacy of antidepressant medication for individuals with mental retardation. *Psychiatric Annals, 27,* 198-206.

Stein, D. J., Simeon, D., & Frenkel, M. (1995). An open trial of valproate in borderline personality disorder. *Journal of Clinical Psychiatry, 56,* 506-510.

Trestman, R. L., deVegvar, M., & Siever, L. J. (1995). Treatment of personality disorders. In A. F. Schatzberg & C. B. Nemeroff (Eds.), *Textbook of Psychopharmacology* (pp. 753-768). Washington, DC: The American Psychiatric Press.

van den Boom, D. C. (1989). Neonatal irritability and the development of attachment. In G. A. Kohnstamm, J. E. Bates, & M. K. Rothbart (Eds.), *Temperament in Childhood* (pp. 299-318). Chichester, England: John Wiley & Sons.

Widiger, T. A., & Sanderson, C. J. (1994). Towards a dimensional model of personality disorders in DSM-IV and DSM-V. In W. J. Livesley (Ed.), *DSM-IV Personality Disorders* (pp. 433-458). New York: Guilford Press.

Widiger, T. A., & Sanderson, C. J. (1997). Personality disorders. In A. Tasman, J. Kay, & J. A. Lieberman (Eds.), *Psychiatry* (pp. 1291-1317). Philadelphia: W. B. Saunders Co.

A Cognitive-Experiential Model of Dream Interpretation for Couples*

Misty R. Kolchakian and Clara E. Hill

Imagine that a couple come to therapy with a dream in which one partner cheats on the other partner. Or imagine that a couple bring in a dream that they both were in a car accident but only one partner gets hurt. Or, as a more pleasant example, imagine that a couple come to therapy with a dream about feeding cake to one another on their wedding day. Most likely, in each of these three scenarios, the wheels may begin to turn in the therapist's head and he or she might wonder what to do with this information. Should the therapist ignore the dream and stick to waking-life concerns, or could the dream help the couple learn more about their relationship?

We support the notion that dream interpretation is one useful way for couples to learn about themselves, their partners, and their relationships. Bynum (1993) suggested that couples should be encouraged to share their dreams as a method of becoming closer to and more differentiated from one another. Furthermore, sharing dreams with one's partner can demonstrate the capacity and desire for closeness through the willingness to take risks and expose oneself to one's partner, thus deepening the overall level of communication. Fielding (1967) also noted that therapists should attend to the reporting of the interpersonal dream as a mode of communication between members of a couple. Often, the relationship between the couple is represented in the dream, and the dream can communicate affect in a manner that can be deciphered by the partner (Perlmutter & Babineau, 1983). It may be easier and less threatening for the dreamer to tell his or her partner about a potential difficulty in the relationship through the images in the dream, as it can be asserted that he or she did not have control over what occurred in the dream.

Often, the couple's dreams may not pertain to their relationship as clearly as the examples indicated previously. However, Delaney (1993) noted that intrapersonal dreams (i.e., dreams about oneself) may be just as important to interpret in couples therapy as interpersonal dreams (i.e., dreams about one's relationship or partner) because the partners can learn important information about one another as individuals. Delaney further suggested that working with dreams in couples therapy allows both partners to begin to learn the process of sharing dreams so that they can take this method outside of therapy to help prevent difficulties and sustain their relationship.

Although the use of dreams in therapy is not a new phenomenon, few models have been described in enough depth to ensure that therapists are employing the methods as recommended. Assuming that the therapist or the couple consider the dream to be potentially important and worthy of attention, it seems important for the therapist to know how to work with the dream so that the couple can gain something from the process. Hence, we modified the Hill (1996) cognitive-experiential model of working with dreams with individuals to working with couples.

*We would like to extend our gratitude to Julie Quimby, Aaron Rochlen, Teresa Wonnell, and Jason Zack for reading drafts of this contribution. Additionally, we would like to acknowledge Aaron Rochlen for his contribution as the therapist in the included case scenario.

THE HILL METHOD FOR COUPLES DREAM INTERPRETATION

The Hill (1996) cognitive-experiential model of dream interpretation integrates humanistic/experiential, psychoanalytic, cognitive/behavioral, and gestalt theories. This model provides carefully delineated procedures for using dream interpretation and is the only one that has empirical evidence to substantiate its use.

There are two major components of the model: a cognitive component and an experiential component. The cognitive component of the model suggests examining the dream units to understand a client's thoughts. The therapist facilitates the client in decoding the meaning of the dream and finding an understanding of the dream that best fits for the client. This model assumes that only the client can decipher the "true" meaning of the dream, given that dreams are personal and thus cannot be understood through standard means such as dream dictionaries or universal symbols. Thus, the therapist does not act as an "expert" who relays the accurate interpretation of the dream to the client, but rather the therapist works collaboratively with the client to construct a meaning that best fits for the client. Dreamers make the ultimate decision about what the dream means.

The experiential component emphasizes the importance of affect throughout the interpretation process as the client attempts to understand his or her dream. The client needs to be emotionally involved in the process of dream interpretation to gain an understanding of the dream. Gendlin (1962) noted the importance of "experiencing" in therapy to help clients change. Furthermore, a cognitive understanding of the issues presented in therapy is necessary but often not sufficient to achieve therapeutic goals. The client's emotions must also be involved to facilitate change.

The Hill model involves the three stages of exploration, insight, and action. In the exploration stage, the therapist works with the client to describe and associate to each of the images as well as to express feelings about the images of the client's dream. Describing and associating to the images helps the client get back into the experience of the dream by giving greater detail about the images and what other thoughts or feelings the images might introduce. Once the images have been discussed in some depth, the therapist and client attempt to achieve some understanding of the dream and its meaning during the insight stage. Once insight into the client's thoughts or feelings is obtained, the therapist can work with the client in the action stage to explore how the client would like to change or whether the client would find change desirable. The action involves considering how to change the dream and then how to translate those changes into actual changes the dreamer can make in his or her life. Throughout the interpretation process, the nondreaming partner is asked to project onto the dreaming partner's dream "as if it were his or her own" in each of the three stages. Thus, by the end of the dream interpretation process, the partner will have also progressed through exploration, insight, and action stages and considered what the dream means for him or her as an individual. This process helps to ensure that the nondreaming partner is not interpreting the meaning of the partner's dream for the partner, but rather is listening empathically and thinking of a meaning for himself or herself.

Approximately two-thirds of the dream session focuses on the dreamer and one-third focuses on the dreamer's partner. We suggest that each couple have at least two sessions, so that each member of the couple has the opportunity to present a dream. In this way, equal attention can be given to each partner, thereby reducing the likelihood of therapist bias toward one member of the couple. Table 1 (p. 87) presents a comparison of the Hill model for use with individuals (see also Hill, 1996; Hill & Rochlen, 1999) and the adapted model for use with couples. Although specific procedures are suggested, therapists can deviate somewhat from the guidelines by using their clinical judgment for the particular couples with whom they are working.

In this contribution we describe each stage of the Hill model for couples and give a case example to illustrate the techniques. For this example, the member of the couple who brought

TABLE 1: Procedures for the Hill Models of Dream Interpretation

Hill Model for Individuals	Hill Model for Couples
Exploration Stage 1. Ask client to retell dream in present tense 2. Ask how client felt about the dream after waking 3. If dream length is appropriate, go through each image sequentially: a. discuss feelings about the image b. describe in more detail c. associate to image 4. Ask about triggers from waking life (can be done as you go along) 5. (Optional) Evoke emotional arousal by reflecting or intensifying feelings 6. (Optional) Work with conflicts	***Exploration Stage*** 1. Discuss what will happen in session 2. Ask dreamer to retell dream in present tense 3. Ask how dreamer felt about the dream after waking 4. Ask how partner would feel after waking (if it were his or her own dream) 5. Go through each image sequentially: a. discuss feelings about the image b. describe in more detail c. associate to image d. partner associates to image "as if it were own dream" 6. Ask about triggers from waking life (can be done as you go along) 7. (Optional) Evoke emotional arousal by reflecting or intensifying feelings 8. (Optional) Work with conflicts
Insight Stage 1. Restate dream using the associations given by client 2. Ask client about meaning of the dream 3. Collaborate with client to understand dream using one of four possible levels: a. Dream as experience in and of itself b. Relation to current waking events c. Relation to past memories d. Parts of self 4. Have client summarize meaning of the dream	***Insight Stage*** 1. (Optional) Restate dream using the associations given by client 2. Ask dreamer about meaning of the dream 3. Collaborate with dreamer to understand dream using one of four possible levels: a. Dream as experience in and of itself b. Relation to current waking events c. Relation to past memories d. Parts of self 4. Ask partner about meaning of the dream "as if it were own dream" 5. Collaborate with partner on one of four levels (shorter) 6. Collaborate with couple to understand dream as parts of relationship 7. Ask each member of couple to summarize what he or she learned about self, partner, and relationship
Action Stage 1. Choose one or more types of action: a. Changing the dream in fantasy or while dreaming b. Continued work on dream c. Behavioral or life changes 2. Have client summarize what he or she learned from dream	***Action Stage*** 1. Ask dreamer how he or she would change the dream (in fantasy) 2. Ask how the change relates to waking life (what waking-life changes can be made) 3. Do steps 1 and 2 for the partner 4. Ask about possible change in the relationship 5. Have each member of the couple summarize what he or she learned from dream and process the experience

in the dream will be referred to as the dreamer and the other member will be referred to as the partner. To protect the confidentiality of the couple, pseudonyms will be used (John is the dreamer and Jane is the partner). Furthermore, note that the text that follows has been shortened and modified slightly for readability and for further protection of the couple's confidentiality. John and Jane agreed to participate in a single dream interpretation session in partial fulfillment of research credits for an undergraduate psychology course. They granted permission to recount information from their session for the purposes of this contribution.

John and Jane were both 18-year-old first-year undergraduate students. They had known one another for approximately 4 years but had been involved in an exclusive relationship for approximately 2 years. The current relationship is John's first, whereas it is Jane's third, and neither John nor Jane has previously been married. They reported that their intent to marry one another was very serious, and thus they seemed very interested in learning more about their relationship.

The Exploration Stage

The purpose of the exploration stage is to reimmerse the dreamer in the images and feelings in the dream by having him or her describe and associate to each of the images of the dream. The therapist should not allow the partners to interpret the dream for one another because this could make the dreamer feel that his or her partner is in a superior, more knowledgeable position. Instead, the partner should be asked to project onto the dream "as if it were his or her own dream." In this way, the partner learns about both the dreamer and himself or herself.

The exploration stage begins by asking the dreamer to retell the dream in the present tense, and then the dreamer is asked how he or she felt upon waking from that dream. The present tense is used to help clients reimmerse themselves in the dream as if it were happening at that moment, thus facilitating recall of both the events and the feelings in the dream.

John described the following dream in the first of two sessions:

> My dream is very similar to the movie *Father of the Bride*. I'm in that house; it's a huge house. I start off in the foyer wearing a tuxedo, and everyone around me is nicely dressed like it's a special occasion. I look up this nice staircase and I see many people there. Then I turn and I go into this big dining room. It's been converted into a room with brown tables and seats all around. It's kind of like the little reception after a wedding. I'm looking around and I can't seem to find my table so I just go from table to table to table looking for where my seat is supposed to be. They're not labeled or anything, and eventually I turn and I see the table I'm supposed to be at. It's the biggest round table and it's in the middle of this big room. My parents and Jane's parents are sitting down next to one another. With everyone looking at me, I start walking over there to sit down and then I have a feeling that someone is missing. I start looking around for Jane. The whole time I knew I was looking for her, but I couldn't find her. Then I get a feeling that she is behind me. I get the feeling she is coming out from a kitchen door because I kind of get this image of someone wearing a wedding dress with a kitchen behind her. I never actually see Jane's face, I just see the image of a bride. I start to turn around to look at her and I wake up.

Therapist: When you woke up, how did you feel?

Dreamer: It was just like a normal dream for me. I've had other dreams where I was actually in the wedding ceremony itself and I was at the top waiting for her to come down the aisle. I knew I was getting married to her, but I never actually see her face. Whenever I've had a dream that has something to do with a wedding, I never see her face. But I know, mentally, that I'm supposed to be marrying her. It's happened before and I just have felt like maybe it's not set in stone yet that I'm supposed to marry her.

Next, the therapist asks the partner how he or she would have felt after waking if this were his or her own dream. The purpose of asking this question early in the session is to help orient the partner to thinking of the dream "as if it were his or her own" so that the partner can begin to put himself or herself in the dreamer's shoes.

Therapist: So Jane, if this were your dream, what kind of feelings come up for you?
Partner: I think that I would have been disappointed that I hadn't seen the person's face. I would feel incomplete because that's the climax and it never occurred so I would feel inadequate at the end.

The next step in the exploration stage is to ask the dreamer to describe each image in greater detail and then to associate to that image. Images can be concrete such as people, places, or things, or they can be abstract such as actions or feelings. An association, as defined by Johnson (1986) is "any word, idea, mental picture, feeling, or memory that pops into your mind when you look at the image in the dream" (p. 52). The therapist can elicit associations from clients by asking if the images remind them of anything or by asking what comes to mind when they think about the images. It is helpful to proceed through the images sequentially by asking the dreamer to describe and associate to each image separately before moving on to the next image. Going through the images sequentially assists the dreamer in becoming involved in the dream and allows him or her to reach deeper depths of understanding for each of the separate images.

Therapist: Let's start with that scene when you walk into the room. Tell me more about that.
Dreamer: Well, first there aren't many people sitting around. There are just a few people here and there sitting at tables. As I walk into the room, there are a couple of tables in front of me and a couple of tables to the right. I walk to the right, and I visit every table as I'm going. Time moves pretty quickly because more people are sitting as I go along, and then suddenly I turn around and my parents are sitting there. The tables look similar to ones at a football banquet in high school, very large round tables that seat about 10 or so.
Therapist: And how about your parents, were they sitting looking at you?
Dreamer: Uh huh, they were sitting right next to each other and looking at me. Both my parents and her parents.

Once the dreamer has fully described and associated to the first image, the partner is asked for his or her associations (but not descriptions, given that it is not his or her dream). Generally, the therapist does not ask the partner for as much detail as he or she tries to elicit from the dreamer. It is important for the partner to avoid attempting to interpret the dream for the dreamer (e.g., "Well, I think his dream shows him that. . . ."). Instead, it is essential to say to the partner, "If this were your dream, what associations would *you* have to the image?").

Therapist: How about for you, Jane, if this were your dream, what associations would you have to both of your parents sitting at a table?
Partner: When he said that our parents were sitting next to each other, I thought of a time when we were at an athletic banquet together and our parents were sitting next to each other.
Therapist: What was that experience like for you?
Partner: It was unnerving because our parents are not alike at all and don't have any of the same interests, nothing. You're always on pins and needles because you don't know if someone is going to say something to offend the other person. And we get really, really scared. We just want the situation to end. So if I saw that, I would be uncomfortable.

The therapist then proceeds through some of the other major images in a similar manner, beginning with the dreamer and then switching to the partner. Also, if appropriate, the therapist can ask the dreamer and partner for any waking-life triggers that come to mind when considering the particular images. Waking-life triggers can be discussed with respect to each of the images either as the client describes and associates to the individual image or after the client has described and associated to all the images of the dream.

Therapist: Okay, I wanted to ask you about that door, can you describe that door, or the walking through the door a little bit more?

Dreamer: The door was already open. It's kind of a cream kind of color with wood panels. As for her walking through the door, it's just like a normal doorway, and in the background you can see the kitchen with the pots hanging and stuff. But she's walking through gracefully and elegantly and she's standing up tall. You know, holding herself up high like she's really happy and proud.

Therapist: So pretend I'm from Mars, and I don't know what an open door is. What is that?

Dreamer: Kind of like acceptance or allowing a person to come into my life. It's like something new is coming into my life too because if I think of coming through a door into a room, I think of that room as being my life and another room as being outside of my life. When she comes in through my door, you could figuratively say that would be the marrying part.

Therapist: So what is your open door right now? Where are you entering?

Dreamer: My goal right now is basically to educate myself here at college and to prepare myself to get a good job once I get out of college. Another goal of mine is to make our relationship better and to make it progress and go further.

Therapist: How about your open door, Jane?

Partner: To me an open door is something everyone can pass through. It's an entranceway. Just something to walk through to discovery, to enlightenment.

Therapist: So it's something new and surprising, too.

Partner: Right, it's a pathway into something different.

Therapist: Where is your pathway into something different right now?

Partner: My pathway is that I want to be a journalist. I want hopefully to get into sports journalism, doing personal profiles, background stories, and historical stories.

Therapist: John, what is this new door that you mentioned of wanting to strengthen your relationship? What do you consider to be the new door in your relationship?

Dreamer: I feel like we have talked about marriage, and we both feel like we will get married. Now is just a time for preparing ourselves to get up to that stage where we can get married. And that's what we're doing now. That's what our new doorway is. It's the time when we are getting to know each other and getting to understand what we have been through, who we are, and where we're going. Now it's like, our relationship has evolved into a more mature relationship that is ready for marriage. Like maybe a more spiritual one.

Therapist: How do you feel about that, Jane?

Partner: I think in our relationship, we're not through the door; we're right in the entrance way and we're not quite ready to step down into the room that the door precedes. I think that we're waiting. It's like waiting for a cue to come in. Sort of a transition, but it seems like we're going to be waiting there for a long time. That's similar to a feeling of desperation. If I had a dream that I was standing at a door, it kind of feels like I couldn't go through it yet.

Therapist: Okay. So let's move away from the specific objects for a moment because there seem to be two things that you're searching for. First, you are searching for your table and looking around and your name isn't on any of them. What does that kind of feeling or experience bring up for you?

Dreamer: It's kind of like I'm out of place, like maybe I wasn't supposed to be in that setting. It was awkward because sometimes when I get into a formal situation where everyone is dressed up, I kind of feel a little different from everyone else because I'm not dressed up as much, I kind of feel like when you get into a formal situation a lot of times people are faking their emotions and stuff like that. You know?

Therapist: And being all cordial.

Dreamer: Yeah, and being all cordial. Acting nice to people that they normally wouldn't because they don't really like them. I don't act like that. If I don't like a person, I let them know. So, I kind of feel like I don't fit in as well as other people do in formal situations. So maybe that's why I couldn't find my seat.

Therapist: What about for you, Jane, if you're searching around and trying to find a table?

Partner: Oh gosh, I think it's really desperation. It's comparable to looking for this room. I couldn't find it and I was getting really frustrated and I just feel like giving up, but then you know that you can't give up because you have to go through with it. And you have to find where it is you have to go. So basically it's desperation.

Therapist: Okay, John, the second thing you seem to be looking for in the dream is Jane. And that's really the grand theme here, looking for a face that you're familiar with that doesn't appear. So what are your feelings about that? Feelings and recollections of looking for Jane?

Dreamer: It's like an annoyance because I never actually do see her face and it's like she's supposed to be there and I don't know where she is. I am constantly looking for her, but I can never find her and it's frustrating. This theme is something that has come up in my dreams in the past couple months.

Therapist: Now let's take a step back for a second. Pretend I'm from Mars and I have no idea what a face is. Try to describe it in words.

This technique of asking the client to describe an image as if the therapist has never heard of it before helps to move the client away from the literal meaning of the word so that he or she can get in touch with what the image might represent for him or her personally. This method can be particularly useful with images that are very common in waking life (e.g., face, door, table, etc.) and with clients who are not very psychologically minded because it forces them to think about what the image represents or symbolizes.

Dreamer: A face is basically the structure of the head in the front. It's the nose, eyes, lips, ears, jaw, cheeks, the way the head is constructed. That's how you identify a person. If I saw your face, I could tell who you were and who you weren't.

Therapist: So the face is critical, the essence of a human being, that makes them unique.

Dreamer: Yes.

Therapist: So what is the essence that makes Jane unique?

Dreamer: The best thing is her attitude toward everything. She's always so loving.

At this point, the therapist can move to the relationship level where members of the couple speak to one another about how their relationship might fit in with the images of the dream. We suggest having members of a couple speak directly to one another rather than *about* one another (e.g., Instead of saying, "She is so loving," say "You are so loving"). Referring to the partner directly can help bring affect into the session for both partners and helps the speaker see his or her partner as a person with thoughts and feelings. Although moving to the relationship level is not essential in this particular stage of the model, the therapist chose this direction with this couple because the dream seemed highly relevant to the relationship.

Therapist: You can speak to her directly. . . .

Dreamer: You're so caring and loving and understanding. You've just got the greatest smile in the world. It's just everything about you that I'm attracted to. It's not just one feature like you're smart. I value an intelligent person, but that's not the only reason. It's a combination of everything that you are. And that's why I love you.

Partner: (blushing and laughing nervously) Okay, and that's why I'm getting red.

Therapist: Okay Jane, let's work a little bit with you in terms of looking for a face and not finding it.

Partner: I think it would be a feeling of desperation. Because when you have expectations and they're not fulfilled, it would make me feel lost because you don't have something that you identify with, it's not there. So you feel empty because that's the person's identity. You don't know who they are without their face and their expressions.

Therapist: And if you see John with no face, with his essence missing, how does that make you feel?

Partner: Empty, because the whole essence in our relationship interaction is with eye contact and speaking and if he didn't have a face and an identity, I wouldn't have something to identify with, something to recognize.

Therapist: So you want to know the person who he is?

Partner: Right.

Therapist: Hearing you two describe it is kind of interesting because I get a sense of urgency in wanting to identify and to find that face.

Dreamer: Well I didn't get to see her at all really. It's kind of like I'm looking at my parents but then I turn and I don't see her. It's kind of like I'm stepping outside of my body and taking a look, but I don't actually see her with my own eyes.

Therapist: But you have the sense that someone is coming through the door.

Dreamer: Yes, I have the sense that someone is coming through the door! And then it's kind of like I stepped out of my body, took a look, and it's her but it's not her face.

Therapist: Maybe as you described earlier, you were feeling kind of incomplete. Not only by not being with Jane, but with that sense of not belonging.

Thus far, the clients discussed waking-life triggers only minimally during the exploration of each image, so the therapist asked about waking-life triggers for the important images after going through all of the images.

Therapist: Now that you have associated to searching for something, are there any instances in waking life that you can recollect where you have been looking around for your place to fit in, or maybe not feeling exactly like you belong with the rest of these people?

Dreamer: At first when I would go to family events at her house with all of her different family members, it felt like I didn't know them. I didn't know how they act. I would just stand back and watch to see how they would act toward each other and toward me. Because I don't know if they really accept me or not, but you have to interact with them so they can accept you. The first time I met her parents I felt very cautious. My hands were sweaty, and I felt very nervous. Then I noticed that there were about 20 people at her house, and I didn't know what to do, didn't know where to go, didn't know where to sit, and didn't know who to talk to.

Therapist: It sounds similar to your feelings in the dream. How about for you, Jane?

Partner: When I first came here, I was in a cluster which means that I have the same people in three or four of my classes. And once we got into smaller groups of about 20 of us, I found that there were no girls that I got along with. I only got along with the guys, and I was wondering how come all of these other girls were getting along, but I didn't get along with any of them. I really felt out of place. I was wondering what my role was and why I didn't fit in with any of the girls, and why I only fit in with the guys.

The Insight Stage

The insight stage builds upon information gained in the exploration stage. During the insight stage, the members of the couple get the chance to reflect upon the significance of the dream for them as individuals and as members of a relationship. They are encouraged to arrive at new understandings of the meaning of the dream. To assess what the dream might mean for them as individuals, Hill (1996) suggests four possible levels of interpretation. First, considering the dream as an experience in and of itself may help clients learn more about who they are and the intensity of their wishes without assuming that the dream represents something else. Second, considering the dream in relation to current waking events may help clients understand how they feel about events in waking life. Third, considering the dream in relation to past memories can help clients understand their reaction to the waking event in relation to past memories. Fourth, considering the parts of the dream as parts of self may help the dreamer or partner gain insight into different parts of their personality. Usually, only the level that seems most appropriate for the person is discussed in any given session. There is not one "right" level of interpretation, and thus therapists can use their clinical intuition about which level would be most appropriate. The therapist can select a different level for each member of the couple (i.e., the therapist can go to the level of the dream as an experience in and of itself for one partner and go to the level of the dream as parts of oneself for the other partner).

In addition, a fifth level of interpretation (parts of relationship) has been added to the insight stage so that couples can learn more about their relationship. In other words, both members of the couple can be asked what the dream means with regard to their relationship. This is probably the most important step in the model for couples because this is where the couple can learn the most about each other's feelings through direct communication with each other about the relationship. The couple is asked to turn and face each other for this part of the dream interpretation process to facilitate open and direct communication. This level of dream interpretation is most salient when couples can directly see the relevance of the dream to their relationship. However, even if the dream does not seem to be directly related, members of the couple can still learn more about themselves and their partners, thus learning more about their relationship. In the case of John and Jane, the dream seems directly relevant to their relationship.

Therapist: Okay, I think that we are ready to move on to the next stage. John, what do you think this dream means for you?

Dreamer: Basically it's something in our future that is going to happen in that I want it to happen, but it's not quite set in stone yet. Maybe we won't actually get married or maybe it's just so far away that we're not ready for it yet. But it's something that I want and something that I'm not going to get quite yet, like I have to turn more for me to see her face.

John is easily able to come up with an initial interpretation due to thorough exploration in the previous stage. If, however, John struggled to create a meaning, the therapist can begin to offer suggestions to help the dreamer on the basis of information gained in the exploration stage. One technique to help the client come up with his or her own meaning is to restate the dream using the associations given by the client (e.g., "You started in this room that reminded you of a football banquet room and then you get the feeling that Jane is coming through the door, which makes you think of giving someone permission to enter your life," etc.). Because John was able to move quickly to insight, the therapist moved on to working toward greater understanding of the dream.

Therapist: You've got to turn more?

Dreamer: Well, I turn a little bit and then I wake up. Maybe as we get older I'll turn more and we'll be able to get closer and closer to that point that we're going to get married and I'll be able to, hopefully, be able to dream and see her face. But it's not quite happening yet.

Therapist: Is that what comes to mind when you think of searching for Jane and for the tables?

Dreamer: Yes, it's kind of like I'm searching to be complete. I'm searching for me being able to go home, sit down, and know where I'm going. I want to see her face and not question whether it's really her or not. I know it's her, but I don't really have proof, and it's like I'm searching for it to be resolved.

Therapist: A quest for the unknown!

Dreamer: Yeah.

Therapist: Jane, if this were *your* dream, what would it mean for *you*?

Here, the therapist has a decision to make. Because the dream is interpersonal and involves images of both partners, the therapist uses his or her best judgment to decide whether to ask the partner to reverse roles or to consider the dream "as is." In other words, Jane could be asked to think of herself as John who does not see her face or to be herself walking through the door and not being seen. In either case, the partner will reflect upon the dream's significance and learn more about himself or herself. It may also be helpful to directly ask the partner which direction he or she wishes to go. In the case of Jane, she chose to reverse roles.

Partner: Okay, if I was John, and I was turning around seeing myself come through the door, I wouldn't feel like I was ready to see my face yet. I would know it's me, but it's like I'm almost not complete until I get married. Marriage is how your relationship becomes complete. So maybe it's not time to see the face yet.

Therapist: So, you recognize this dream as kind of a sign, not as a sense of urgency, but as a sign of where you are at right now?

Partner: Right.

Therapist: And what I'm hearing from John is "Just get me there, I'm tired of being lost, I just want to see the face already, this is irritating."

Note that the therapist reflects upon what each member of the couple has stated, recognizing that there are some important differences between the ways they view the dream. When the therapist points out this differentiation, it allows the partners to recognize that they may have different perspectives but they can still empathize with how the other person is feeling.

Partner: I think if it were me, I'd be a little bit more understanding of not seeing the face immediately and knowing that I'm just going to have to wait just a little bit. But I would still feel frustrated and wonder why it is happening. I guess it's almost scary because you get that far and then it's left up in the air. So you're scared because you don't know if it's going to turn out the way you want it to, whether it's going to be him, or if it's going to be someone else who you just completely don't know yet. And that's sort of terrifying because it's like everything that I'm working for may not turn out.

Therapist: Yeah, and do you see some of that for you, some of that uncertainty?

Partner: Yeah, not so much for me, but from outside of the relationship, like where is my career going to take me and what is going to happen to my family? Life may take me in different directions. What's going to happen with his career and with his family.

Therapist: Yeah, that's good. Since your own existence is unknown in the dream, you feel that there is some uncertainty in your relationship. Sometimes people can gain personal understanding in hearing someone else's interpretations. So, based on what Jane shared with you, does that bring any new understanding to where you're at, John?

Dreamer: It gives me understanding as a couple, since I know that she feels like it's the time in between where you're waiting. It makes me feel like we're right where we should be in our relationship.

Therapist: Okay, you guys are doing great. Let's see here. We've talked a lot about this dream as an experience in and of itself and how it relates to your relationship. Sometimes we work with the assumption that images in the dream are a representation of yourself, like a part of yourself. John, the theme of incompleteness really stood out in the dream as far as how you were searching for the table and searching for your partner. What do you see as being incomplete in yourself that you're seeking to fulfill?

Note that the therapist covers more than one of the four individual levels in the insight stage, because the therapist viewed two levels (the dream as an experience and the parts of the dream as parts of self) as being equally important for this couple. One word of caution is to note the couple's energy level during this phase of the model, because many steps remain to be covered. This couple seem particularly engaged in the dream interpretation process, however, so moving to another level made sense.

Dreamer: The only thing that really feels incomplete is having someone, having her (turns to Jane). Having you. It's the one thing that I want. I want to be married to you, and I want to know that your focus is there. Just like I'll always have you and have your love. That's the one thing I'm searching for. I'm just searching for a guarantee that I'll have you and have your love. I guess that's what marriage is . . . like I love you and there is nothing that is going to change that. So I guess that's what I'm kind of searching for, that guarantee.

Partner: Yeah, it's almost exactly the same for me. I'm kind of uncertain about the future. It's like I don't want to be alone. I want to have a family, I want to have a house, and I want to have a husband. I want to be able to culminate all of that together and have a wonderful life. But, I also do feel like without having a complete commitment with you, you can go away. Like tomorrow you could meet someone and leave me. If I were married to you, there would be less chance of that, even though you could still do that technically. But still, I would feel better in my heart. I think I would be more stable.

Therapist: How did it feel to hear that, John?

Dreamer: Well, I've known that, and it's like I'm constantly telling you, "I don't want to be with anyone else, I want to be with you." I can understand your feeling, but I wish it weren't there because I'm not worried about you going off with some other guy. I'm sure that you want to be with me. I just wish that you didn't doubt yourself or doubt me.

Partner: You are really a cocky and bullheaded person. I always feel like you're so confident, and I don't feel that way. So obviously, I'm inadequate in some way. I think that your head is just so big sometimes, and mine is not as big. So I feel like why don't I have this complex where I'm completely confident that no one is going to leave me and that you don't want anyone else, just like you are with me.

Here is an example of Jane recognizing that she and John have differences and wondering if it is acceptable or healthy to be less confident than John. She initially seems to view this difference as somewhat threatening for their relationship, and she wants to feel the same way he does (i.e., be more confident and cocky) for fear that he may leave her. She also seems angry at John for being so "cocky" and "confident."

Dreamer: Just because you don't have as much confidence as I do doesn't mean that you can't be sure that I want to be with you and that I'm not going to want to go off with some other girl.

Partner: Right, but that's my interpretation of it.

Therapist: That's all right. It's an important thing because you both may be feeling similar things but may be interpreting it differently as far as how the other person is seeing it. It's good to talk about it.

The therapist makes sure to point out that it is acceptable for each of them to have different perspectives or interpretations of the same feelings. At this point, as a way of summarizing the insight stage, the therapist asks each partner what he or she has learned about the other partner.

Therapist: So what did you learn about Jane from working with this dream today?

Dreamer: She knows a lot about me. When I started explaining my dream, I noticed that she feels almost exactly the same way I do. We often know what the other person is thinking. She knows me but I don't know her as well. I feel like she's perfect because this is what being real is. What? (to Jane)

Partner: I'm just not used to people saying these things about me. I learned that you are a lot more complex emotionally than you seem to be on the surface. You have a lot of complex feelings that you don't show or talk about. And I think that I would like it a lot better if you would show it. I would feel like you would know me better if we talked about things more. Because, I could show you more of me if you showed me more of you. That would make me feel better. Basically, I've just learned that you're trying. You're at least trying.

Therapist: Is that why you looked surprised and laughed sometimes when he was sharing some of his emotional feelings with you?

Partner: I've heard it in little bits and pieces but not when it all comes together, so it's kind of overwhelming when it all comes together.

Dreamer: Because I've never actually said all that stuff.

Partner: Yeah, not at one time. It kind of gets lost in other things sometimes.

Therapist: How so?

Partner: Well, like the thing you said when I pointed out that the other girl is nicer looking than me. You said to me, "I don't want her, I just want you." But then you go on to reprimand me and I lose the "I just want you" because you go so far into it.

Dreamer: I complicate things often. I tell you why you shouldn't think that way.

Partner: Yeah, why I'm wrong!

Dreamer: Yeah, I do that to try to boost your self-confidence!

Partner: This just confuses me.

Dreamer: Since we've been together, I've always been the cocky one, the one who is confident. I'm sure of what I'm doing, and it seems like she questions herself more and she's not sure of herself as much and she has nowhere near the amount of self-confidence as I do. I want her to be more confident because I know that she can do it. (to Jane) I *know* you can do whatever you want.

Therapist: You have a lot more confidence in her than she sees.

Dreamer: I have a lot more confidence in you than you have in yourself. You question yourself too much. I feel that sometimes if you just acted on your instincts, you wouldn't be questioning yourself.

Partner: But then I feel like the reason you don't question yourself is because when I've seen you interact with other people and other people interact with you, they're more likely to compliment you than they are to compliment me. And that is troubling for me sometimes because I wonder why aren't they complimenting me for something that is comparable? It always seems like people are more likely to agree with you. I think you have a warmer personality than I do. As far as getting along with other people, I get along with certain kinds of people. Everybody can get along with you.

It is interesting to note that the roles that these clients presented in the beginning of the session seem to have changed. More specifically, John seemed to feel somewhat vulnerable and insecure early in the session, whereas Jane now appears more vulnerable and needy. Both John and Jane seem to have learned something new about themselves and each other in the process and are thus ready to move into the next stage.

The Action Stage

After gaining a sense of what the dream means for each partner individually and for their relationship, the therapist moves into the action stage. In this stage, couples can begin to work on change at the individual level by discussing how they might change the dream or how they would envision a sequel to the dream if they do not want to change the dream. Changing the dream is a relatively unthreatening way to introduce the action stage because participants are just fantasizing. If clients can begin to see that they have some control over their dreams (and their lives), then making changes in waking life often seems more possible. Once they have decided how to change the dream, the therapist helps the couple turn these changes into specific behavioral changes that they can make in their waking lives. Therapists do not need to force change or be invested in whether clients change, but rather they should simply help clients assess whether change would be desirable and what changes would be consistent with the insights gained in the previous stage. Clients may decide that change is unnecessary or undesirable; however, it is helpful for clients to explore the possibilities of change. A complete unwillingness to examine change could suggest passivity, depression, or denial on the part of the clients. Again, therapists should rely on their clinical intuition to assess whether or how much they suggest change.

In addition, the action stage encourages couples to consider how they can improve or maintain the relationship given the insights they discovered in the previous stage. Again, the improvement of the relationship may not be a major focus in the action stage for some couples when there are few images in the dream which clearly pertain to the relationship. In short, therapists should attempt to help the clients explore the possibility of change in their individual lives and in their relationship with their partner.

Therapist: All right, we're going to move into the action stage. John, if you were to have this dream again, tell me how you would change the dream.

Dreamer: I would turn around and see her.

Therapist: Tell us exactly how it would happen.

Dreamer: (to Jane) I would turn around, I would see you, you would be smiling, you would be glowing, like you always are, and we would walk hand in hand to the table and sit down and have a good time.

Therapist: How about the scene with your parents and her parents? What would you like to change?

Dreamer: Actually, I would like it if they could be sitting next to each other, and we would not have to be worried about it.

Therapist: You would like that peace of mind.

Dreamer: Yeah, I would like it if I could just look over to them and not be worried about what they're going to say to each other. I wouldn't have to worry about whether my parents would accept her parents or whether they would have conflicts. It's like no matter how much Jane and I get along together, our parents don't get along at all. And they most likely won't, but I would like it to be at the point where we don't have to worry about it.

Therapist: Jane, how would you change the dream if you could?

Partner: I would want us to see each other's faces. I would want to have a celebration, but I would like it to be more family-oriented in terms of the parents. I would like to have them together and us not have to worry about them. I would like to get to the point where they can interact and not have to worry about anything bad coming out of it, a cordial interaction that's not forced. I don't like situations where people are fake. If I were going to have the ceremony and the reception, I would want everything to be natural. I would want the best to come out of everyone.

Therapist: So, you would like to see each other's faces and you would like for your parents to get along in the dream. How do those changes that you noted represent changes that you can make in your waking life and potentially with your relationship?

Partner: I guess we should make more of an effort to talk things through more so that there are not misconceptions. Maybe we shouldn't force our families together so much, sort of get to a point where we're understanding that our families have differences and that they might not ever get along. We just might have to deal with it, rather than always have that hope that somehow they'll get along. And I think we need to talk more. Or you need to talk more to me so that I can talk more to you. I'm more likely to tell you how I'm feeling than you are, and I'm much more likely to elaborate. Even if you do tell me how you're feeling, I'll say "why" and you'll say "because" and that's it. If you'd elaborate on that "because," maybe we'd have a better understanding of each other.

Therapist: Do you see that as potentially pushing you toward moving through that door?

Here the therapist ties the discussion back to the images in the dream so that the couple can gain more understanding of what the dream means for their relationship. It is important for the therapist to help the couple consider changes that are specific and concrete so that they are more likely to remember the changes after they leave the session.

Partner: Right.
Therapist: (to John) What do you think about what she just said?
Dreamer: I agree with the need for communication because at times I do have trouble communicating with you. But at times, you also have trouble communicating with me.
Partner: Right back at me, right?
Dreamer: Yes. It's not just me. But I do have to admit that I have more of a problem than you do. We both think communication is a problem. So resolving it is, communicating more is symbolic of the changes that would help us get toward that goal of getting married. And also if we talked more and got a better understanding of each other and a better understanding of our families, then maybe we would not force them to interact with each other, but when they do interact, make it easier on them if they know more about each other.
Therapist: So one change is opening the channels of communication and taking time to talk more about feelings that you're having about each other. The second change is not to push the relationship with your parents.
Dreamer: Yeah.
Partner: Yeah, just sit back and let it happen.
Dreamer: Yeah, hopefully they'll just be able to sit back and act naturally around each other. I don't know if they do. I've never asked them. All of it seems like something that will come with time.
Therapist: Well said. That was the next thing I was going to ask you about. It almost seems like a change in the way you're summarizing the situation as being comfortable with making slow changes and understanding and accepting where you are now. Obviously, it would be nice to be at the end stage and have your goals being met. But maybe some of those other things will improve by not having that sense of urgency. Is that fair to say?
Dreamer: Yeah, I mean, I've always felt like you shouldn't rush into marriage. You should let things fall into place. You should understand the person and know as much as you can about the person before you get into marriage. So that when you get into marriage and you're living together, there's fewer conflicts. So I want to be absolutely sure . . . (to Jane) and I'm pretty sure.
Therapist: Jane?
Partner: (Laughing nervously) I forgot the question.
Therapist: He summarized being comfortable staying where you're at now without feeling a sense of urgency to move to the next level.
Partner: You're a person who likes to leave things alone, and I'm the kind of person who is impatient. I like to get the ball rolling. That's what makes us different. It's not like I want to get married tomorrow, but I wish I knew what was going to happen because then I'd feel better.
Therapist: You'd have that sense of security.
Partner: Yeah, security. That's how we're different because I'm the impatient one. I need to know so that I can go on. I like being on a schedule, not too much of a schedule, but enough so that I'm sorted out. And you just fly by the seat of your pants and sometimes it puts me on pins and needles. It makes everything so uncertain and that just makes me uncomfortable.
Therapist: So do you want to change and let some of that go a little bit?
Partner: I want to change but I want him to change a little bit, too.
Therapist: So maybe move toward that common ground. And how can you do that?
Partner: Well, I guess I can relax a little more and be a little more confident about our relationship and bring that into more confidence for myself. And you, since you like

to wait everything out, if you're still going to do that, just don't be as ambiguous with your feelings. If you have goals, if you're thinking about marriage, it's okay to talk about it. It's not going to curse you. He has this thing where he can't say the word "marriage."

Dreamer: I had the toughest time. She's like "What, can't you say the word, the 'm' word?"

Partner: He would just shiver (laughing).

Dreamer: That kind of made me feel uneasy.

Therapist: So you can say the word now.

Dreamer: Yeah, I can say the word now, and I don't have a problem saying it.

Partner: It took a long time.

Dreamer: Yeah, it was a long time.

Therapist: So would you agree with those steps?

Dreamer: Mmm hmm.

Both Jane and John have collaborated in coming up with changes they can begin to make in their relationship on the basis of what they each have learned about their own and their partner's needs. John has agreed to communicate more with Jane about his feelings. Jane has agreed to attempt to relax and feel more confident in the relationship and with herself when he does open up to her with his feelings. At this point, they seem ready to discuss what they have learned from the dream interpretation process.

Therapist: I think it is really critical in this last part of this stage to really think about what you've learned about yourself and how can you use that to make some concrete changes. I think a lot of it, and some of what you've done already, is just sharing and being open and secure with each other, that you're not going to take off. Is that true?

Partner: Yeah.

Dreamer: You bet.

Therapist: That kind of understanding can go a long way. You can use this dream to remind each other of these things with your relationship and as individuals. Remember what this dream told you is you need to take some time out to try to see each other's faces a little bit more. Maybe we could end with both of you summarizing what you have learned from this process.

Dreamer: I learned that I need to stop trying to push our families together and that we should let our families' relationship and our own relationship progress naturally. I've learned that Jane would like me to be more expressive of my feelings so that she does not have to guess how I feel about her and the direction of our relationship. This session also reinforced our commitment to each other.

Therapist: Great. Jane?

Partner: I think I need to be more patient and relaxed in my relationship with John and trust in how he feels about me. I learned how much he really is trying and how much he really cares for me. I also learned that we both want to move through the door, so to speak, someday, but that the time is not right now and I should not try to force it. Also, similar to what John said, I should stop worrying about how our families relate and not expect drastic improvements in their communication any time soon.

CONCLUSIONS

Dream interpretation with couples can be a useful experience in and of itself or it can be included as a part of the therapy process. We are not advocating that dream interpretation replace traditional therapy, but rather we are suggesting that dream interpretation is one useful method to use within therapy for helping couples communicate more openly and clearly, to learn more about themselves, their partners, and their relationship.

We recommend that therapists remain open to couples who mention having an important dream because this may represent an indication or "marker" that they are willing to work with the dream. Better yet, early in the course of therapy, therapists can inform clients that they are open to working with dreams with the couple. Often, clients are not aware that discussing and/or interpreting dreams is an option in couples therapy, and they need to be informed of the potential advantages of such a method. We also suggest that therapists begin the process of interpretation at the beginning of sessions, as it typically takes at least an hour to do, especially when working with couples as opposed to individuals.

The amount of information that a therapist can gain quickly from a couple using this method is impressive (consider how much you just learned about this couple!). Important issues that a couple are facing surface rapidly during the interpretation process. It is especially important for the therapist to not allow the partners to become each other's therapists but instead to help them differentiate themselves from each other or understand their differences.

The benefits of working with dreams in individual therapy (Cogar & Hill, 1992; Diemer et al., 1996; Heaton et al., 1998; Hill, Diemer, & Heaton, 1997; Hill et al., 1993; Hill, Nakayama, & Wonnell, 1998) and group therapy (Falk & Hill, 1995) have been shown empirically. Dream interpretation seems to result in increased insight and self-understanding. We are currently studying dream interpretation with couples (Kolchakian & Hill, 1999), and we encourage other researchers to conduct empirical research to determine the effects of dream interpretation with couples.

In this contribution, we hope that we have conveyed some of the benefits of working with dreams in couples therapy and some of the excitement involved in this approach. The Hill method can be used with both unmarried and married couples to help them communicate more openly and clearly; learn more about themselves, their partners, and their relationships; and recognize that having a sense of "differentness" from one's partner can contribute to a healthy relationship.

We end the contribution with a quote from Jane during a follow-up phone interview 1 month after the dream session. She reported, "I do not think that the progress we have made in the past month would have occurred if we had not had these dream interpretation sessions. It was like a light bulb went on with every new thing that I heard." We hope that other couples benefit from dream interpretation in a similar way.

CONTRIBUTORS

Misty R. Kolchakian, MS, is a graduate student in the counseling psychology program at the University of Maryland. Her master's thesis is an evaluation of the efficacy of dream interpretation for couples. Ms. Kolchakian may be contacted at the Department of Psychology, University of Maryland, College Park, MD 20742.

Clara E. Hill, PhD, is a professor in the Department of Psychology at the University of Maryland. She received her doctorate in counseling psychology from Southern Illinois University in 1974. She is a past editor of the *Journal of Counseling Psychology* and is a past president of the Society for Psychotherapy Research. She has published extensively on the process and outcome of psychotherapy, dream interpretation, and therapist training. She has written three books (*Therapist Techniques and Client Outcomes: Eight Cases of Brief Psychotherapy,* 1989, Sage; *Working With Dreams in Psychotherapy*, 1996, Guilford; and *Helping Skills: Facilitating Exploration, Insight, and Action*, 1999, American Psychological Association). Dr. Hill can be contacted at the Department of Psychology, University of Maryland, College Park, MD 20742.

RESOURCES

Bynum, E. B. (1993). *Families and the Interpretation of Dreams: Awakening the Intimate Web*. New York: Harrington Park Press.

Cogar, M. C., & Hill, C. E. (1992). Examining the effects of brief individual dream interpretation. *Dreaming, 2*(4), 239-248.

Delaney, G. (1993). *New Directions in Dream Interpretation*. Albany, NY: State University of New York Press.

Diemer, R. A., Lobell, L. K., Vivino, B. L., & Hill, C. E. (1996). Comparison of dream interpretation, event interpretation, and unstructured sessions in brief therapy. *Journal of Counseling Psychology, 43*(1), 99-112.

Falk, D. R., & Hill, C. E. (1995). The effectiveness of dream interpretation groups for women undergoing a divorce transition. *Dreaming, 5*(1), 29-42.

Fielding, B. (1967). Dreams in group psychotherapy. *Psychotherapy: Theory, Research, and Practice, 4,* 74-77.

Gendlin, E. (1962). *Let Your Body Interpret Your Dream.* Wilmette, IL: Chiron.

Heaton, K. J., Hill, C. E., Petersen, D. A., Rochlen, A. B., & Zack, J. S. (1998). A comparison of therapist-facilitated and self-guided dream interpretation sessions. *Journal of Counseling Psychology, 45*(1), 115-122.

Hill, C. E. (1996). *Working With Dreams in Psychotherapy.* New York: Guilford.

Hill, C. E., Diemer, R. A., & Heaton, K. J. (1997). Dream interpretation sessions: Who volunteers, who benefits, and what volunteer clients view as most and least helpful. *Journal of Counseling Psychology, 44*(1), 53-62.

Hill, C. E., Diemer, R. A., Hess, S., Hillyer, A., & Seeman, R. (1993). Are the effects of dream interpretation on session quality, insight, and emotions due to the dream itself, to projection, or to the interpretation process? *Dreaming, 3*(4), 269-280.

Hill, C. E., Nakayama, E. Y., & Wonnell, T. L. (1998). The effects of description, association, or combined description/association in exploring dream images. *Dreaming, 8*(1), 1-13.

Hill, C. E., & Rochlen, A. B. (1999). A cognitive-experiential model for working with dreams in psychotherapy. In L. VandeCreek & T. L. Jackson (Eds.), *Innovations in Clinical Practice: A Source Book* (Vol. 17, pp. 467-480). Sarasota, FL: Professional Resource Press.

Johnson, R. (1986). *Inner Work.* San Francisco: Harper & Row.

Kolchakian, M. R., & Hill, C. E. (1999). *The Effectiveness of the Hill Dream Interpretation Method for Working With Couples.* Unpublished master's thesis, University of Maryland at College Park.

Perlmutter, R. A., & Babineau, R. (1983). The use of dreams in couples therapy. *Psychiatry, 46,* 66-72.

Parent-Child Interaction Therapy

Amy D. Herschell, Vicki A. Lumley, and Cheryl B. McNeil

Bradley,* who was described by his teachers and parents as aggressive, noncompliant, and hyperactive, was waiting with his mother in the waiting room. As the therapist opened her office door, she could hear Bradley screaming and whining as his mother patiently tried to calm him. After taking a deep breath and pausing for a moment, the therapist bravely walked down the hall to meet her new client. Immediately apparent by the condition of the waiting room was that in the 10 minutes Bradley and his mother had waited, he had played with each available toy, drawn in crayon on the table, taken office supplies from the receptionist's desk, and not put one toy back where he found it. As the therapist introduced herself, Bradley's mother began to apologize for his behavior as she had done with others countless times before.

Many therapists are encountering situations similar to the one described here. Children are most often referred to psychological clinics for disruptive behavior which can be challenging to treat (e.g., Kazdin, Seigel, & Bass, 1990; Schuhmann et al., 1996; Wells & Forehand, 1985). Typically, these children do not present with one or even two difficult behaviors. Instead, on average, a child referred for disruptive behavior comes to the clinic with 23 separate problem behaviors (McNeil et al., 1991). To add to this challenge, therapists are finding themselves in an era of managed care and increased accountability. Not only do therapists need to treat disruptive children, but that treatment needs to be time-efficient, cost-efficient, and empirically supported.

THEORETICAL AND EMPIRICAL FOUNDATIONS FOR PARENT-CHILD INTERACTION THERAPY

Parent-Child Interaction Therapy (PCIT; Eyberg & Matarazzo, 1980; Eyberg & Robinson, 1982; Hembree-Kigin & McNeil, 1995) is a short-term, empirically supported intervention designed for families with children between the ages of 2 and 7 years who are experiencing a broad range of behavior problems. This structured program is divided into two phases. The first phase emphasizes the parent-child relationship, and the second phase concentrates on establishing a structured, consistent discipline program. Each phase contains multiple components and is designed to impact both the parents' and the child's behavior (Eyberg & Boggs, 1998).

Originally developed by Dr. Sheila Eyberg (Eyberg & Boggs, 1989; Eyberg, Boggs, & Algina, 1995; Eyberg & Robinson, 1982; Hembree-Kigin & McNeil, 1995) and modeled after Hanf's (1969) two-stage approach, PCIT is a blend of operant theory, traditional psychotherapy, and early child developmental psychology (Eyberg, 1988). Two fundamental assumptions underlie PCIT. The first assumption is that problem behaviors are established and maintained by the child's interaction with the parent (Eyberg & Boggs, 1998). Second is the assumption

*Names and identifying characteristics of persons in all case examples have been disguised thoroughly to protect privacy.

that noncompliance is a key issue and may be the initial behavior that leads to antisocial behavior in adolescence and adulthood (Forehand & McMahon, 1981). Drawing from these assumptions, the goal of treatment in the first phase of PCIT is to teach parents skills that will change their negative interaction style with their child. Specific, constructive skills are taught in order to replace negative interaction patterns with more positive, warm, and loving interactions. The second phase of PCIT focuses on establishing child compliance and assisting the parents to gain control over their child's disruptive behavior (Foote, Eyberg, & Schuhmann, 1998).

For most families, the full course of treatment can be conducted in 12 to 14 weekly, 1-hour sessions. One session is devoted to a pretreatment assessment of child and family functioning and feedback. Approximately five sessions are spent on the first phase of the program which includes one session for teaching behavioral play therapy skills to the parents and four sessions coaching the parents in behavioral play therapy skills. The second phase of treatment typically occurs over the remaining eight sessions and includes teaching discipline skills to the parents, coaching discipline skills, and assessing the child and family functioning at post-treatment. Booster sessions are scheduled as needed. Typically, these sessions are held at 1, 3, 6, and 12 months to enhance maintenance of parenting skills and to address new problems. This treatment model is consistent with managed care's short-term treatment philosophy and emphasizes systematic assessment on a regular basis so that services can be based on that assessment (Kazdin, 1997). In this contribution, we provide an overview of the clinical skills and procedures used in PCIT. For a more detailed description, see Hembree-Kigin and McNeil (1995).

Outcome research on PCIT has demonstrated statistically and clinically significant improvements in child conduct-problem behavior (e.g., Eisenstadt et al., 1993; Eyberg et al., 1995; Eyberg & Robinson, 1982; Zangwill, 1984). This research has demonstrated that PCIT improves parenting skills and reduces child disruptive behaviors from outside normal limits to within normal limits in clinic (Eisenstadt et al., 1993; Schuhmann et al., 1998), home (Boggs, 1990; Zangwill, 1984), and school (McNeil et al., 1991) settings. Parents report that PCIT has helped to improve the behavior of untreated siblings (Brestan et al., 1997; Eyberg & Robinson, 1982). In addition to finding that PCIT is effective in helping them to manage behavior, parents also report high levels of satisfaction with the content and process of PCIT (Schuhmann et al., 1998) and report less distress as their child's behavior improves (Eyberg & Robinson, 1982). Follow-up studies have reported that treatment gains maintain up to 2 years after therapy is terminated (Newcomb et al., 1990; Schuhmann et al., 1998).

PCIT was originally developed to treat children with disruptive behaviors common to oppositional defiant disorder, conduct disorder, or attention-deficit/hyperactivity disorder, and has been demonstrated to be effective with these populations. However, PCIT has also been successfully applied to children with developmental delays (Eyberg & Matarrazzo, 1975) and histories of abuse (Urquiza & McNeil, 1996). Research and clinical experience also has suggested there are certain populations with whom PCIT is less successful. These include families whose parents are actively abusing substances or those who are experiencing severe psychopathology (e.g., depression). PCIT also appears to be less effective with children who are over age 7. Families with severe marital discord or that are extremely chaotic may also be less responsive to PCIT (Hembree-Kigin & McNeil, 1995; McNeil & Herschell, 1998).

THE STRUCTURE OF PCIT

Session 1

The first step in PCIT is to evaluate the needs of the child and the family so that treatment can be tailored accordingly. In addition, a formal evaluation provides baseline data that can be used to measure progress as treatment advances. Data are collected throughout the course of treatment, which is essential for objectively determining readiness to proceed through the treatment components.

To begin the evaluation, a semistructured interview is conducted with the parents while the child plays in the room. The interview provides information on the specific behaviors of concern, currently used discipline strategies, family stressors, and the child's developmental, medical, and psychosocial history. Permitting the child to play in the room provides an informal opportunity for direct observation of the child's behavior and the parent-child interaction. The evaluation also consists of a number of parent-report and teacher-report measures, as well as a structured observation of the parent-child interaction using the Dyadic Parent-Child Interaction Coding System (DPICS-II) developed by Eyberg and Robinson (1983) and revised by Eyberg et al. (1994). For children who are attending school, a classroom observation is recommended.

Preliminary feedback regarding the results is provided to the parents at the conclusion of the first session, and a more in-depth feedback session is scheduled. An overview of PCIT is provided along with a rationale for the behavioral play therapy and discipline components.

Child-Directed Interaction (CDI) Didactic

The second session consists of a didactic in which the parents attend the session without the child and receive information regarding the behavioral play therapy skills. During this session the therapist continues to build rapport and provides a more detailed conceptualization and additional educational information. Because regular attendance is crucial for successful treatment, an attendance contract can be introduced during this session. As determined by the evaluation, the specific goals of the therapy are described. In general, in addition to improving the parent-child relationship, the outcome for the child is often increased self-esteem, improved attention span, decreased anger, and improved frustration tolerance.

To achieve these outcomes, parents are instructed to engage in 5 minutes of "special playtime" with their child at home every day. The term "playtime" can be misleading to parents and should be explained. Parents are taught a number of relationship-enhancing skills that are essential for interacting with children with disruptive behaviors. The idea is that these special children require "specialized parenting" and that the specialized skills are implemented within the context of play. In other words, this special playtime is a therapeutic exercise and should be presented as such.

In two-parent families, it is important that each parent participates individually in a 5-minute playtime with the child. During the special playtime the child is encouraged to lead the activity, which is conducive to the child demonstrating desirable behaviors. In addition to teaching children more prosocial skills, a primary purpose of this special playtime is for parents to practice the therapeutic skills. Because the time is brief, the parents are better able to maintain high quality when executing the skills. Importantly, by practicing the skills daily, it is likely that the skills will become overlearned and the parents will begin to use the skills throughout the day.

Completing this daily "homework" is very important. If the parents are not completely involved and dedicated to all aspects of the therapy process, treatment will not be successful. Because homework is so important, each subsequent session will begin with a review of homework from the previous week, for which parents are expected to have completed a daily recording sheet. Beginning with this homework review, each session is structured similarly so as to establish a clear and predictable routine. This structure seems to maximize parental participation.

After the description of the special playtime, parents are taught the behavioral play therapy skills. The skills fall into two categories: actions to avoid and actions to perform. The actions to avoid describe what parents should refrain from doing. They include: "Avoid Giving Commands," "Avoid Asking Questions," and "Avoid Criticisms." It is important for parents to avoid giving commands and asking questions so that the child stays in the lead. Criticisms should be avoided for a number of reasons. Criticisms may produce an increase in the child's undesirable behaviors (because the child receives negative attention), and they cause an unpleasant interaction that possibly can damage the child's self-esteem. Descriptions and examples of each of these "Don't" skills are provided for the parents.

Parents are next taught the actions to perform, which are presented using the acronym P-R-I-D-E and are presented in Table 1 (p. 106). The first skill is *Praise*. There are two types of praise: general (unlabeled) praise, which conveys approval without indicating a specific action for which the child is being praised, and specific (labeled) praise, in which a specific de-

TABLE 1: PRIDE Skills for Parents

Praise desirable behaviors
Reflect appropriate speech
Imitate play
Describe appropriate activity
Enthusiasm!

sirable behavior is identified. "Good job!" is an example of an unlabeled praise, and "Good job putting away your toys" is an example of a labeled praise. Labeled praises are preferred to unlabeled praises, because they tell the child which behaviors the parents would like to see in the future.

The second skill parents are taught to use is *Reflection.* This skill entails repeating the basic content of the child's statement. By verbally imitating the child in this manner, parents demonstrate that they are paying careful attention and are interested in what the child is saying. Reflections allow the child to remain in the lead and typically have the effect of encouraging the child to talk about thoughts and feelings.

Next parents are taught to *Imitate* the child's play, the third "Do" skill. As with reflection, imitation conveys the parents' interest in what the child is doing. In addition, imitating the child facilitates the child imitating the parent, which is important for teaching prosocial skills like turn-taking.

The fourth skill parents are taught is *Description.* Essentially, this skill entails providing a running commentary on the child's actions. Doing so can improve the child's attention and organization of thoughts, and also keeps the child in the lead. Furthermore, by describing the child's appropriate play, the parent is providing positive attention and conveying interest in the activity, which can enhance the child's self-esteem.

Finally, parents are encouraged to display *Enthusiasm* when using the aforementioned skills. It is believed that enthusiasm magnifies the attention and interest shown by the parents, thereby making the interaction more rewarding for the child.

Once these skills have been learned, the goal is to use the skills to increase the child's desirable behaviors and prevent behavior problems. This goal is accomplished through the use of "strategic attention." First, behaviors that the parents would like to occur more often are identified. Then, the parents watch for these behaviors and apply the "Do" skills. The point is to "catch the child being good" and reward the desirable behaviors with positive attention. To maximize the utility of this strategy, "selective ignoring" is also employed. With this strategy, behaviors that the parents would like to see decrease are identified, and those behaviors are actively ignored. By providing positive attention for appropriate behaviors, while at the same time ignoring the inappropriate behaviors, it becomes more likely that the child will demonstrate the appropriate behaviors.

To teach these skills the therapist first models them, then the parents participate in role-play practice. Parents are then asked to agree to engage in the daily special playtime with their child and are given recording sheets to keep track daily of whether they engaged in the playtime and what problems, if any, arose. A handout that summarizes the skills presented in this session is provided to parents as a learning aid. Importantly, parents are active participants in this and all subsequent sessions; the therapist functions in a facilitative rather than a prescriptive role.

CDI Coaching

After the parents have received instruction regarding the behavioral play therapy skills, the next step is to coach them in using the skills. The coaching session begins with a 5- to 10-

minute check-in that includes a discussion of the special playtime homework and a review of the skills presented in the previous session. After observing and coding the parents for 5 minutes, the therapist then coaches the parents in the use of the skills, following certain guidelines that maximize the effectiveness of coaching. These guidelines are contained in Table 2 (below). Through coaching, the therapist is able to increase parents' use of the skills, including strategic attention and selective ignoring. The therapist also is able to guide the parents through any instances of aggressive or destructive behavior demonstrated by the child, which is addressed more thoroughly in the discipline portion of the therapy program. The coaching session concludes with a 10-minute wrap-up in which the therapist provides feedback on the parents' skill level and discusses homework for the forthcoming week.

TABLE 2: Coaching Statements Guidelines and Clarifying Examples

Guideline	Example
1. Coaching statements should be clear and concise.	"Just ignore that. Go ahead and turn away. Great ignoring."
2. The therapist should use lay language.	"Earlier you praised sharing. Now she's sharing more. See, praise works!"
3. The therapist should provide feedback to the parents after each parent verbalization. This helps to develop a rhythm between the therapist and parents so that the parents learn when to pause and listen for feedback. Essentially, the parents say something, the therapist provides feedback, the parents say something else, the therapist responds, and so on.	*Parent:* "That's a spotted leopard." *Therapist:* "Good teaching while still letting her lead." *Parent:* "You're good at drawing animals." *Therapist:* "Nice specific praise. That's great for her self-esteem."
4. Try to connect content of session to situations outside of the clinic.	"Good job of waiting and letting her figure that out for herself. This will help her work more independently at school."
5. Save "minilectures" for when there is a brief pause to explain important processes occurring during the session.	"Let's pause for a minute and talk about what just happened. He was bossy and demanded that you hand him the block. You did a great job of not rewarding the bossiness. Instead, you waited until he asked more politely. Then, you gave him what he wanted. Now he's learning that being polite gets him what he wants and being bossy does not pay off. Super job of teaching him better behavior!"

Parents participate in coaching sessions in this manner until their skills reach a predetermined criterion level (i.e., mastery criteria). The mastery criteria are set very high (e.g., providing 15 praises in 5 minutes) because the goal is for parents to overpractice and overlearn the skills so that they will generalize throughout the day. To determine whether parents have met mastery criteria, objective data are collected at the beginning of each session while parents engage in behavioral play therapy without coaching. When parents have achieved criterion performance, they progress to the discipline phase of the program.

Parent-Directed Interaction (PDI) Didactic

The discipline phase of the program begins with a session during which parents attend the session without the child and learn to deliver effective commands and praise child compliance. First, parents are taught about the importance of structure for children with disruptive behavior, which requires consistency, predictability, and follow-through on the part of the parents. Because giving good instructions is an important skill, parents are given rules to follow when issuing instructions (Hembree-Kigin & McNeil, 1995); these rules are presented in Table 3 (below).

TABLE 3: Guidelines for Giving Good Instructions

- Use direct commands, and be specific.
- Use positively stated commands (tell your child what *to do* instead of what *not to do*).
- Give commands one at a time.
- Use a neutral tone of voice.
- Demonstrate politeness and respect.
- Save commands for things you are *sure* your child can do.
- Avoid overusing commands.
- Use gestures.
- *Always* issue a consequence for compliance and noncompliance.
- Use only age-appropriate commands.
- Provide choices with older children.

A consideration when teaching parents to deliver good instructions is how to determine when the child is being compliant. Although it may seem an easy determination, there are instances in which compliance is questionable. For example, the child might partially comply with the instruction, comply with a bad attitude, or respond by doing something slightly different from what the parents requested. Guidelines have been developed for responding to these and other questionable child responses, and parents are trained on how to handle these situations.

Also during this session, parents learn a strategy known as the "broken record" technique. Specifically, when the child fails to comply or argues with the parent following a command, the parent repeats the command up to three times (like a broken record). The parent repeats the command using the same words and same tone of voice while maintaining a neutral facial expression. As homework, parents are instructed to practice delivering commands and praising compliance and to practice use of the broken record technique during their "special playtime."

During the following session, parents are coached in issuing commands, using praise and other rewards, and employing the broken record technique. As homework, parents are instructed to continue practicing these skills.

At this point in the course of therapy, parents are introduced to time-out as a strategy for addressing noncompliance. It is common for parents to be somewhat skeptical, as most have tried some form of time-out by this point with little success. However, time-out has been demonstrated to be effective in managing even extreme disruptive behaviors. Furthermore, there are many advantages to using time-out as a discipline strategy: (a) Children will behave appropriately to avoid time-out because it is boring and keeps them from fun activities (this is particularly true for very active children, because time-out means that they have to sit still with no stimulation); (b) time-out can be applied immediately following undesirable behavior; (c) unlike physical punishment, time-out can be used many times during the day without harm; (d) time-out does not model aggressive behavior; and (e) time-out is used in many schools, and consistency between home and school is important.

Although many parents will insist that time-out will not work for their child, the time-out taught in PCIT is different from what most parents have learned. In PCIT, children rehearse time-out before actually receiving a time-out. Also, parents learn to institute a "two-choices statement." To avoid repeated commands or arguments, the parents simply tell the child, "You have two choices. You can either (the command) or go to time-out." At the same time, the parents hold up two fingers as a visual cue. Because predictability, consistency, and follow-through are important, the parents are instructed to never issue a two-choices statement unless fully prepared to implement a time-out. As a result, the child will eventually comply at the sight of the two fingers and the issuance of the two-choices statement.

Parents receive guidance on logistical issues pertaining to time-out (e.g., what type of chair to use, the length of time-out) and are taught to respond effectively to problems that may arise during the course of a time-out. It is likely that parents who are disenchanted with time-out have become so because of child behaviors such as refusal to go to time-out, failure to stay in time-out, or disruptive behavior while in time-out. Parents are taught how to respond to these and other difficult situations. For instances of serious time-out infractions committed by the child (i.e., escape from time-out; rocking, scooting, or standing on the time-out chair; or self-injurious behavior), backups to time-out are taught according to the specific needs of the child and parents. Potential backups include a two-chair hold procedure (McNeil, 1996; McNeil et al., 1994a, 1994b, 1994c), use of a time-out room, or restriction of privileges.

Importantly, time-out does not end until the child complies with the original instruction. Following through in this manner is vital to the child learning that noncompliance will not result in escape from the command. Parents learn how to respond to all possible outcomes that could occur when the original command is reissued. Finally, parents are taught to then provide an additional instruction as a means of overteaching compliance.

Compliance is emphasized with young children who demonstrate disruptive behavior, because noncompliance often precedes more severe behaviors. Accordingly, parents are taught to apply time-out only following noncompliance. Although a child might demonstrate numerous challenging behaviors in addition to noncompliance, it is important to remember that many misbehaviors can be addressed using a command. By using time-out only following noncompliance, the child is able to more quickly learn the contingency.

The therapist and parent then role-play a time-out scenario. Parents are given a diagram that displays the discipline steps to become familiar with before the next session. Parents are instructed *not* to attempt a time-out prior to the next session, as an unsuccessful time-out could set a poor precedent. Instead, parents will attempt their first time-out during a session under the direction of the therapist. As homework, parents are instructed to continue with the daily special playtime, as well as practicing the use of good commands, the broken record technique, and praising compliance.

PDI Coaching

Before beginning discipline coaching, the therapist reviews the discipline strategies with the parents and asks whether they are prepared to implement the time-out procedure. This point is important, because the first time-out can be very intense and, consequently, emotional for the parents. This may be particularly likely with a child with a long history of noncompliance, because there will *finally* be consistent consequences for noncompliant behavior.

When ready, the parents explain to the child what is about to happen. Specifically, the therapist coaches the parents to tell the child about the new rules and consequences, model the procedures, then walk through the procedure with the child, who is fully aware that this is just practice.

The parents and child then engage in behavioral play therapy, coached by the therapist. Play therapy and discipline skills are used in conjunction during this session, with the parents using the play therapy skills and interspersing commands as directed by the therapist. After 5 to 10 minutes of play therapy, the therapist gradually introduces instructions that the parents are to give the child. Notably, it is important that during discipline coaching the therapist is very directive, telling the parents exactly what to say. The demands placed on the child are gradually increased, making it more likely that noncompliance and, therefore, a time-out, will occur. A time-out is desirable in this situation, so that the parents can receive coaching for administering the time-out. If a time-out does not occur, the parents can still be given applicable homework.

If the child does fail to comply with an instruction and the two-choices warning, the time-out procedure is instituted. Again, the therapist is very directive when instructing the parents. To ensure that the time-out progresses smoothly, the therapist issues only one instruction at a time, using positively stated instructions and praising the parents for following through. In addition to telling the parents what to say, the therapist also tells the parents what to do (e.g., "Use a neutral tone of voice" or "Get up quickly and take her by the hand"). It is also important for the therapist to provide support, guidance about how to relax and manage anger, and reassurance, as this can be a very emotional experience for parents. Following these guidelines, the therapist coaches the parents through the time-out exactly as described during the instructional session. The session will not end until compliance is achieved and both the child and parent are able to calm down through the use of play therapy. It is important for the therapist to provide debriefing as needed. Having completed a successful time-out, parents are then given a discipline homework assignment to complete before the next session.

Progressing Through the Discipline Program

After the initial discipline coaching session, families must master a series of six steps for successful completion of the program. Coaching and homework continue to be employed throughout the steps, each of which takes a week, on average, to master. As the steps progress, coaching becomes less and less directive in order to promote parental autonomy.

Step 1 involves minding exercises. The goals are for the child to comply with commands in the context of play and to display a good attitude when minding, for the parents to give good instructions and follow-through with time-out following child noncompliance, and for the child to remain in time-out. The goal of overpracticing the command-compliance-praise sequence in both the clinic and home is to allow the child to experience countless positive experiences with minding so that compliance becomes an overlearned habit.

During Step 2 the focus is on "real-life" directions. The goal is for child compliance to generalize from the play context to real-life circumstances.

Step 3 focuses on the application of skills throughout the day, and siblings are included in the session. Including siblings helps the parents to have a consistent discipline program that can be used with each child, helps the siblings to learn the discipline procedures, improves generalization to the home by having the parents attending to both children, and also provides more material for the sessions.

During Step 4 the parents learn to establish house rules, which entails establishing one or two standing rules in order to eliminate repeating commands and to deal with behaviors that parents want the child to "stop" doing (e.g., hurting others, using profanity). Once a rule has been established and the child informed, breaking the rule results in an immediate time-out with no warning. This strategy is used only as a last resort after less restrictive approaches have been attempted (e.g., praising an opposite behavior like playing gently, using a positively stated, incompatible command).

The focus of Step 5 is discipline in public settings. Parents are taught how to use time-out to address problems such as misbehavior in the car and running away in public areas. Often the therapist will coach the parents and child in public settings (e.g., waiting room, cafeteria).

Finally, in Step 6 any remaining developmental or behavioral issues are addressed. At this point, individual and marital problems that have become evident can be addressed.

The Last Session

Therapy is considered complete when the presenting problems have disappeared or diminished substantially, as determined by both the therapist and the parents. At that point a posttreatment evaluation is conducted to document progress as well as identify any remaining problem areas. The assessment consists of the same measures that were conducted prior to treatment. During the feedback pre- to posttreatment improvements are highlighted, with video data used when available to clearly illustrate successes. During this session the focus is on celebrating treatment accomplishments. To achieve this objective the therapist can provide tangible rewards to the child and certificates of achievement to the parents. Finally, to facilitate maintenance of treatment gains, "booster" sessions are scheduled with the family. During these sessions parents receive coaching in play therapy and discipline skills and engage in problem solving with the therapist regarding current areas of concern.

CASE ILLUSTRATION

In this next section, we will describe PCIT in more detail through a case description. In a session-by-session format, we will briefly discuss session goals, content, and homework assignments.

Background Information

Bradley is a 4-year-old boy who was referred for treatment by his Head Start teacher. In the classroom he had been exhibiting behaviors such as hurting peers (e.g., hitting, name calling, spitting), climbing on furniture, talking disrespectfully to adults, and getting out of his seat during structured activities. At home Bradley frequently argued with his mother, initiated verbal and physical fights with his sister, and refused to comply with parental requests. His mother indicated that his behavior had always been a problem, but she thought he would grow out of it. She sought treatment because she had recently found Bradley attempting to set a fire in their home. Also, his behavior was so disruptive at Head Start that his teacher was concerned about the other children in the classroom. The teacher had mentioned to Bradley's mother that Head Start may not be able to provide services if Bradley continued to disrupt the classroom and hurt other children.

Session 1 - Conducting the Intake Evaluation (1-1/2 Hours)

Session Goals

The first session provides a valuable opportunity for the therapist to give as well as receive information. Parents often come to therapy looking for solutions to unanswered questions and sometimes have misconceptions about why their child is behaving disruptively. For example, parents may think their child acts out because the child is innately bad or because they are incompetent as parents. One of our goals for the first session is to help parents reverse any misconceptions and feel as if they have learned something new about their child or situation.

Specific goals for the first session include (a) building rapport; (b) conducting a brief clinical interview during which an understanding of the current problem, developmental pathway, and appropriateness for treatment is gained; (c) providing the parents with information about PCIT and a rationale for why it is an appropriate treatment for them (if it is appropriate for them); (d) completing necessary office paperwork (e.g., description of clinic policies and procedures, billing contract); (e) reviewing limits of confidentiality; (f) asking parents for consent and child for assent to treatment; (g) completing at least two standardized assessment measures: The Eyberg Child Behavior Inventory (ECBI; Eyberg, in press-a), Dyadic Parent-Child Interaction Coding System-II (DPICS-II; Eyberg et al., 1994); and (h) asking the parents to have the teacher complete the Sutter-Eyberg Student Behavior Inventory (SESBI: Eyberg, in press-b). The DPICS-II assessment should be videotaped so that clients can view the tape at the end of treatment.

Content of Session

During this first session, Ms. Douglas reported that Bradley was and had always been a difficult child. In fact, Ms. Douglas reported that Bradley was very active, did not comply with her requests, talked to her in a disrespectful manner, and was frequently physically aggressive with his older sister. Additionally, Ms. Douglas reported that Bradley had broken objects (e.g., his mother's glasses, toilet cover, and windows), attempted to set a fire, and hurt animals. Ms. Douglas reported using a number of different behavior management strategies with Bradley but did not experience success in changing his behavior. She mentioned that she felt like a failure because she had quit working in order to be a full-time mom, but still could not manage Bradley's behavior.

The therapist responded to this by saying, "Ms. Douglas, it sounds like Bradley's behavior has been difficult in a number of situations and that you are not the only person who has had difficulty in managing him. In fact, it sounds to me like you are doing the best you can in a very difficult situation. One reason I think that is because you came here today. Bradley is very lucky to have a mom who is so dedicated to him and trying to make things better. I think I can help you make the situation better because there are some special skills that I can teach you to manage his behavior. These skills have been developed with children just like Bradley. They are specialized skills for children, like Bradley, with special behavioral needs. I would like to tell you a little bit about these skills and services that we can provide and then hear what you think. How does that sound?" The therapist went on to explain what PCIT is and why it would be appropriate for Ms. Douglas and Bradley.

Session 2 - Teaching Behavioral Play Therapy Skills (1 Hour)

Session Goals

The second session is attended by the parents only and is usually an active didactic session in which the therapist teaches parents behavioral play therapy skills. This instruction typically contains multiple examples, role-plays, discussions, and handouts. Specific goals for this session include (a) describing the goals of play therapy, (b) introducing and discussing the importance of daily homework, (c) teaching the skills to avoid and skills to perform, (d) discussing the use of strategic attention and selective ignoring, and (e) problem solving the logistics of play therapy at home. An attendance contract may also be introduced during this session (see McNeil & Herschell, 1998, for an example).

Content of Session

Through role-plays, active discussions, and frequent questions, the therapist taught Ms. Douglas skills to use, skills to avoid, and strategic attention/selective ignoring. When the therapist mentioned praise as a skill to use, Ms. Douglas quickly responded by saying, "I've tried that with Bradley and it made him worse." Nodding, the therapist responded by saying, "You're right, and I'm impressed that you are so in tune to Bradley's behavior. Praise does seem to make some children's behavior more disruptive, but let's look at it from Bradley's perspective. Let's say he is coloring a picture and his teacher says, "Bradley, you are doing a great job staying in the lines. What is Bradley immediately going to do?" Ms. Douglas replied, "He will scribble all over the page to irritate her." Therapist: "Exactly, because he likes to get a reaction from people. We talked last time about some children needing more attention or stimulation than others. Bradley seems to be a child who needs to be very active and get a lot of stimulation. When he scribbles instead of continuing to color in the lines, what do you think the teacher's reaction is?" Mom: "Well, he gets irritated like anyone would." Therapist: "It is tough not to react to the scribbling, but that reaction is what Bradley works for. Right now, Bradley may be getting more attention for negative behavior than for positive behavior. By using the skills that we are talking about today, you can reverse that pattern so that Bradley gets more attention for positive behaviors than for negative behaviors."

Homework

Ms. Douglas was asked to conduct a daily 5-minute play therapy session at home, which would provide Bradley with the attention he needed and Ms. Douglas with an opportunity to practice her newly learned skills. She also was given a homework form to record whether she had held the play therapy session each day and whether there were any problems during the play therapy time.

Sessions 3 Through 6 - Coaching Behavioral Play Therapy (1 Hour Per Session)

Session Goals

Sessions 3 through 6 are attended by the parents and their child. As previously discussed, during each of these sessions, parents are directly coached by the therapist in the use of the behavioral play therapy skills. Each session is structured similarly such that parents first meet with the therapist for approximately 10 minutes to discuss completion of homework and any relevant issues that came up during the previous week. Next, the therapist records and then coaches the parents in the play therapy skills. If one parent attends, he or she is coached for approximately 40 minutes. If two parents attend, each is coached for approximately 20 minutes. In the remaining 10 minutes, the therapist meets with the parents and provides specific feedback on skills they are using well and skills that could be improved. Specific goals for these sessions include (a) helping parents improve their play therapy skills and achieve mastery criteria, (b) recording and closely monitoring parents' skill acquisition, and (c) providing frequent, positive, high quality feedback on parents' performance through coaching.

Content of Sessions

Each session began with the therapist asking for Ms. Douglas to return her homework sheet and to describe the previous week's progress. For 3 out of 4 weeks Ms. Douglas reported completing homework for 6 out of 7 days. For the remaining session, Ms. Douglas reported completing homework 5 out of 7 days. Ms. Douglas was praised for her diligence and commitment to treatment. After this brief check-in, Ms. Douglas was coached in the use of play therapy skills for approximately 40 minutes. A 10-minute check-out was also part of each session so that the therapist could provide Ms. Douglas with feedback and make suggestions for skills Ms. Douglas should focus on during the daily 5-minute play time. In part because of Ms. Douglas' commitment to completing homework and receptiveness to feedback, her skills reached mastery criteria after four sessions.

As therapy progressed and Ms. Douglas' skills improved, Bradley appeared to enjoy the special playtime more. During the first coaching session, he had difficulty remaining in his seat. The therapist coached Ms. Douglas to ignore Bradley when he ran around the room, to redirect him back to the table by describing her own play enthusiastically, and then to give him a labeled praise when he finally did sit in his seat. By the last coaching session, Bradley was able to remain seated 95% of the time. Additionally, he was less critical of his mother, more willing to share his toys, and used manners more frequently.

Homework

Ms. Douglas was asked to continue conducting 5-minute play therapy sessions each day and record these times on homework forms.

Session 7 - Teaching Commands, Compliance, and Consequences (1 Hour)

Session Goals

This session is attended by the parents only and begins the second phase of treatment which is oriented toward establishing a clear, predictable, consistent discipline program. Specific goals for this session include (a) teaching the parents how to give effective commands, (b) helping the parents to distinguish between compliance and noncompliance, (c) discussing the value of praising compliance, and (d) instructing the parents on how to provide a specific consequence for noncompliance (i.e., the broken record technique).

Content of Session

After teaching Ms. Douglas how to give effective commands, determine compliance, and praise compliance, the therapist introduced the broken record technique. The therapist began by saying, "Do you think that Bradley is going to comply with every instruction you give him?" Ms. Douglas smiled and said, "No." The therapist responded by saying, "I thought you might say that. We need to have an idea of what to do when he doesn't do what you ask him. Later we will talk about a more confrontive way to get him to listen, but today I would like to talk about a strategy we call the 'broken record.' We call it that because when Bradley doesn't comply, that is how I want you to act - like a broken record. I think it might be better to explain the technique by using an example. Can you think of a time when Bradley didn't listen?" Ms. Douglas said, "Sure. I can think of a lot of times. One was when we were getting ready to come here today. I asked Bradley to get his coat and he said 'No' and then refused to get it." Therapist: "Okay, if you were to use the broken record technique with this situation, you would first use a good command. What would be a good command for this situation?" Ms. Douglas: "Bradley, please put your coat on." Therapist: "Great. That is a very clear and direct command. Using the broken record technique, you would give the command, point, and wait 5, long, quiet seconds with a neutral face, and then see if Bradley was making a reasonable attempt to do what you asked. If he was not, you would repeat the command again, pointing and using the same words in a neutral, calm tone. Again, you would wait to see if Bradley was going to listen. If not, you would repeat the command again with the same words and tone of voice. Using this technique, you should repeat the command up to three times. Typically children respond by the third time because they want you to stop being so boring and robotic and to give them some rewarding attention. If Bradley does not listen after the third time, either ignore it or physically help him to comply, and we will talk about another strategy in a couple of weeks that will help him to listen even better to your instructions."

Homework

Ms. Douglas was asked to continue the 5-minute play therapy sessions and practice using good instructions, determining compliance, and providing an appropriate consequence (i.e., enthusiastic, specific praise for compliance, and the broken record technique for noncompliance).

Session 8 - Coaching Commands, Compliance, and Consequences (1 Hour)

Session Goals

During this session parents are coached in using good instructions and providing consistent consequences with their child. The play format provides a developmentally appropriate environment for parents to issue commands and then use their good play therapy skills to manage their child's response. Goals include (a) helping the parents give effective commands, (b) assisting the parents to determine compliance, (c) distinguishing a clear and neutral tone of voice, and (d) continuing to refine play therapy skills.

Content of Session

The session began with a brief check-in during which Ms. Douglas reported no problems with the previous week's homework assignment or significant issues since the last session. After approximately 5 minutes of coaching play therapy skills, the therapist said, "Ms. Douglas, I'd like you to say, Bradley, we're going to practice listening now. Please hand me the red block." Ms. Douglas repeated the command using the same words as the therapist, opened her hand, and pointed to the block so that the command was clear. Therapist: "Perfect. That was a clear, direct command and a great physical reminder. Now let's wait 5 seconds to determine compliance. You are being very patient. Okay, it looks like Bradley is not going to listen. Please repeat the command again in the same neutral, calm tone." Ms. Douglas repeated the command and pointing gesture. Therapist: "That was very calm and clear and you used the same words. Great job. Again, we want to wait 5 seconds. Looks like he is still not listening. Please repeat the command again using the calm and clear tone." Ms. Douglas repeated the command for the third time in the same manner. Bradley handed her the block and Ms. Douglas said "Thank you." Therapist: "Thank you for what?" Ms. Douglas: "Thank you for handing me the red block. I like it when you listen to me, Bradley." Therapist: "Great labeled praise. Those labeled praises tell Bradley exactly what he did that you liked."

Homework

Like the week before, Ms. Douglas was asked to complete 5 minutes of play therapy a day and to practice giving effective commands, determining compliance, and providing appropriate consequences within the play therapy situation.

Session 9 - Teaching Time-Out (1 Hour)

Session Goals

Session nine is attended by the parents only and consists of instruction on the use of a time-out procedure. Goals for this session include (a) teaching the parents a two-choices statement and visual signal, (b) discussing structural and logistical issues associated with time-out (e.g., placement of the time-out chair, choosing the time-out chair, length of time-out), (c) reviewing what may happen on the way to time-out, (d) discussing how to handle misbehavior in time-out, and (e) determining an appropriate back-up consequence if the child will not stay in time-out.

Content of Session

After discussing the procedure of how to get Bradley to time-out, the therapist said, "Let's talk about how to handle Bradley when he misbehaves in time-out. I want you to ignore everything he *says* during time-out. I know some things he says are hard to ignore, like swearing and name calling, but for now I want you to try your best to ignore his verbalizations. On the other hand, there are some things that Bradley might do in time-out that should not be ignored. You should not ignore Bradley if he gets out of time-out, if he stands on the time-out chair, if he rocks the time-out chair, if he scoots the time-out chair, or if he intentionally tries to hurt himself to the point of making bruises or drawing blood. If he does any of these five things, we need to implement a consequence. I would recommend a back-up time-out room as a consequence for Bradley. How do you feel about that?" Ms. Douglas responded by saying, "I'm not sure what you mean. Do you mean that he would go to his room?" The therapist clarified by saying, "In the clinic we have a room specially designed as a time-out room. It's right next to the play room, is completely empty, and has a window so that Bradley can see you and know that he is safe. At home you would want to use a room that is safe and relatively free of toys or things that Bradley could get into. Do you have a room that you might be able to use as a time-out room?" Ms. Douglas appeared to think about the question for a few moments and then commented by saying, "Maybe I could use our laundry room. There isn't much in that room." The therapist cautioned by saying, "That may be a good room. You just want to make sure that there is nothing there that Bradley could hurt himself with or damage. Tell me more about the room."

Homework

Ms. Douglas promised *not* to use the time-out procedure discussed during the session for the following week. We asked her to make this promise because we wanted to ensure that her first time-out went well. Ms. Douglas was asked to continue conducting 5 minutes of play therapy a day, practicing effective commands, praising compliance, and using the broken record technique.

Session 10 - Coaching Time-Out (1 Hour)

Session Goals

Because Session 10 is typically the session during which the first time-out occurs, the goals of the session include (a) guiding the parents step-by-step through the time-out procedure so that they begin to establish a "routine" of discipline, (b) providing the parents with supportive comments so that the parents feel more confident and secure in imposing limitations, and (c) ending the session with the child complying with all parental requests.

Content of Session

To begin the session, the therapist coached Ms. Douglas to use stickers to encourage Bradley to practice sitting appropriately in time-out. All of the rules of time-out were reviewed with Bradley. Then, after approximately 5 minutes of coaching play therapy skills, Ms. Douglas was instructed by the therapist to say, "Bradley, we're going to practice listening now. Please pick up that piece of Play-Doh that fell off the table." Ms. Douglas repeated the command, pointed to the Play-Doh, and then waited for Bradley to comply. When he did not, the therapist instructed Ms. Douglas to use a neutral tone of voice and say, "Bradley, you have two choices. You can either pick up the piece of Play-Doh that fell off the table or go to time-out." As Ms. Douglas said this, she held up two fingers and then pointed to the Play-Doh. In response, Bradley screamed "No!" With a confident and reassuring tone of voice, the therapist said, "Ms. Douglas, please stand up, lead Bradley to the time-out chair, and say, 'Since you didn't choose to listen, you have to sit on the time-out chair'." After Ms. Douglas had done this and Bradley was on the time-out chair, the therapist said, "Ms. Douglas, please say to Bradley, 'Stay on the chair until I tell you to get up,' and quickly walk away." Immediately after Ms. Douglas did as she was instructed, Bradley got off the chair. The therapist quickly said, "Ms. Douglas, he is off the chair. Please go over to him and say, 'Bradley, if you get off the chair again, you'll have to go to the time-out room,' and then walk away." Ms. Douglas did as the therapist asked and again Bradley immediately defied her by getting out of the chair. The therapist responded by saying, "Bradley is off the chair again. Please go over to him and say, 'You got off the chair again so you have to go to the time-out room' and lead him to the room."

Therapist: "Carefully put Bradley in the time-out room and close the door." After Ms. Douglas had placed Bradley in the time-out room, he began to tantrum. As he was crying, the therapist reassured Ms. Douglas that Bradley was okay, praised her for remaining calm during a challenging situation, and reminded Ms. Douglas of the importance of following through with the discipline procedure so that Bradley could learn clear consequences for his behavior. The therapist emphasized the long-term benefits of him learning to listen. After Bradley had been in the time-out room for 3 minutes, the therapist instructed Ms. Douglas to go to the time-out room and say, 'Bradley are you ready to sit on the time-out chair?' Bradley nodded his head and went to the chair. After he was seated, Ms. Douglas said, "Stay on the chair until I tell you to get up," then quickly stepped away from the chair.

After Bradley was sitting in the chair for only 10 seconds, the therapist instructed Ms. Douglas to go back and say, "Bradley, since you are sitting on the chair, are you ready to pick up the Play-Doh?" Bradley nodded and Ms. Douglas pointed to the Play-Doh. After Bradley picked it up, Ms. Douglas responded by simply saying "Thank you" and giving him a similar command, "Bradley, please pick up the Lego that fell off the table." After Bradley complied with the second instruction, Ms. Douglas enthusiastically praised him by saying, "Bradley, thank you for doing what I asked you to do so quickly. When you listen like that, you don't have to go to time-out. Instead we can play together! In fact, now we can play with anything you want." The therapist explained to Ms. Douglas the importance of praising Bradley when he does what she asks after her first request so that he would learn that positive attention would follow compliance. The play therapy was used to reduce Bradley's anger, calm Ms. Douglas, and help Bradley and his mother enjoy being together before the end of the session.

Homework

Ms. Douglas was asked to practice "minding exercises" each day. Ms. Douglas was asked to conduct their special playtime for 10 minutes and throughout that time to give Bradley approximately five commands. Before beginning minding exercises, Ms. Douglas was told to review and practice the time-out procedures with Bradley. She was to begin each command by saying, "Bradley, we are going to practice listening." Ms. Douglas was instructed to determine compliance and then provide the appropriate consequence.

Session 11 - Coaching Time-Out (1 Hour)

Session Goals

This session is similar to the previous week's session in that the focus is guiding parents through the time-out procedure. However, as the session progresses, the therapist becomes less directive and assists the parents in becoming confident in their ability to implement the time-out procedure on their own. Specific goals include (a) fostering independence, (b) providing support to the parents when needed, and (c) problem-solving difficulties in implementing time-out at home.

Content of Session

During the beginning of the session, Ms. Douglas mentioned that Bradley was having a difficult time staying in time-out at home. Most of his time-outs resulted in him being placed in the back-up room. The therapist suggested using a star chart to help Bradley learn to sit on the time-out chair. Together Ms. Douglas and the therapist developed the following plan: Bradley would have the opportunity to earn a star every day for the next week. If he earned a star, it would be placed on a colorful chart hung on the refrigerator. Stars could be earned two ways: (a) by having no time-outs for an entire day or (b) if there was a time-out, by sitting in the time-out chair and not having to go to the back-up room. Before his bedtime each day, if Bradley had earned a star, he and his mother would place the star on the chart and his mother would tell him how proud she was. He would also get to pick a small prize out of a grab bag. In addition, if he got 6 out of the 7 available stars, Bradley would be able to pick one of three special prizes which his mother determined (e.g., having lunch at his favorite restaurant, inviting a friend over to play, making homemade Play-Doh). Ms. Douglas was instructed to remind Bradley throughout the day of the star chart and the associated rewards.

Homework

In addition to the 5 minutes of play therapy each day, Ms. Douglas was asked to give Bradley three preselected commands throughout the day. She was asked to begin these commands with, "We are going to practice listening now," determine compliance, and provide the appropriate consequence (i.e., praise for compliance, time-out for noncompliance).

Session 12 - Coaching Time-Out (1 Hour)

Session Goals

Parents are invited to bring their other children to participate in this session. Goals for Session 12 include (a) coaching the parent in using skills with two or three children present, (b) setting up a "no hurting" house rule in the clinic, (c) role-playing time-out with siblings, and (d) conducting minding exercises with siblings.

Content of Session

Ms. Douglas, Bradley, and his older sister, Kerry, attended this session. Ms. Douglas was coached in using behavioral play therapy and discipline skills. With both children present, the therapist was able to help Ms. Douglas use the play therapy format as a developmentally appropriate medium to teach social skills such as sharing, turn-taking, and using good manners. Also during this session, the therapist helped Ms. Douglas establish a "no hurting" house rule. If either child hurt someone, he or she was given an automatic time-out. At this point, the therapist also began to prepare Ms. Douglas and Bradley for the end of treatment by highlighting the amount of progress that had been made and mentioning that only a few more sessions would be needed.

Homework

Ms. Douglas was asked to use time-out for all noncompliance with a two-choices statement and to begin instructions with, "We're going to practice listening now."

Session 13 - Teaching and Coaching Time-Out in Public (1 Hour)

Session Goals

Session 13 has two main goals: (a) practicing time-out in public using a time-out towel and (b) teaching the parent to set up a house rule of "no hurting" at home.

Content of Session

After a brief check-in, the therapist explained that during this session they would talk about time-out in public and then practice the skill. The therapist reviewed a procedure for applying discipline techniques to public situations, which included reviewing rules of behavior with Bradley before entering a public place and using time-out as a consequence for misbehavior in public. To help Bradley learn that time-out could be instituted in public, Ms. Bradley was asked to carry a small towel (i.e., time-out towel) with her and use it instead of a chair. Next, the therapist accompanied Ms. Douglas and Bradley to a nearby store and coached Ms. Douglas through the procedure. To conclude the session, the group came back to the clinic where the therapist listened to Ms. Douglas' reactions, provided feedback, and provided information about applying the "no hurting" rule at home. The therapist emphasized that the "no hurting" rule would be most effective if used in combination with frequent labeled praise for times when Ms. Douglas caught her children playing gently. Additionally, the therapist mentioned again that sessions would soon be ending. If the week went well, the next session would be the last.

Homework

Ms. Douglas was asked to continue the 5 minutes of play therapy with Bradley each day. Additionally, she was asked to practice time-out in public three times before the next session. These practice times involved going somewhere with the primary purpose of using time-out in public. Ms. Douglas mentioned during Session 13 that Bradley misbehaves in the grocery store. As a practice session, Ms. Douglas was asked to take Bradley to the grocery store. On the way to the store, Ms. Douglas was to review with Bradley the rules for the store (e.g., listening to his mother, not hurting other people) and the consequences for following or breaking the rules. Once they got to the store, Ms. Douglas was instructed to follow-through with the consequences she had mentioned to Bradley.

Session 14 - Handling Future Behavior Problems

Session Goals

Session 14 is typically the last session. It is helpful to have the parents complete an ECBI before the session begins so that the therapist has an objective measure to help determine treatment termination. Goals for this session include (a) reviewing the pretreatment videotape and discussing treatment gains, (b) setting up a booster session, (c) discussing common pitfalls (e.g., stopping play therapy, not following through with a two-choices statement), and (d) identifying signs of regression.

Content of Session

After the therapist scored Ms. Douglas' ECBI and determined that Bradley's behaviors were reported to be similar to his same-aged peers, the therapist asked Ms. Douglas to talk about any differences she noticed in Bradley's behavior. Ms. Douglas mentioned that Bradley was now listening to her, getting along with his sister, and using good manners, whereas he had not done these things before. The therapist asked Ms. Douglas to explain why his behavior changed to make sure that she understood the connection between her own behavior and Bradley's. Next, Ms. Douglas, Bradley, and the therapist reviewed videotapes of the mother-son interaction at pre- and posttreatment. During this review, the therapist highlighted improvements and sensitively pointed out how both the parent's and child's behavior changed. Also during this session, Ms. Douglas was given information on how to detect treatment regression and to handle future behavior problems. An exercise was conducted in which Ms. Douglas was asked to use strategies other than time-out to handle such misbehaviors as leaving the yard, screaming while playing video games, and tattling. To end the session, a 1-month booster session was scheduled, Ms. Douglas was invited to call if she had any further questions or concerns, and Ms. Douglas and Bradley were given certificates to acknowledge their excellent attendance, participation, and completion of PCIT.

SUMMARY AND CONCLUSION

Considering the climate of managed care and the era of accountability in which clinicians are finding themselves, it has become increasingly important to implement time- and cost-effective treatment strategies that produce noticeable benefits for clients. Parent-Child Interaction Therapy (PCIT) offers a viable option for early intervention for behavior disorders. PCIT is an empirically supported intervention program for families with young children who are experiencing a wide range of behavior problems. This approach relies on systematic assessment of parents' skill acquisition and progression through treatment only after skills have reached a predetermined level. PCIT is a short-term approach that can be completed in 12 to 14 weeks and often results in clinically significant improvements in both child behavior and parenting skill.

CONTRIBUTORS

Amy D. Herschell, MA, received her masters in clinical psychology from West Virginia University, and is currently pursuing a doctoral degree in child clinical psychology at the same university. Ms. Herschell's clinical and research interests are focused on teaching parents and teachers effective strategies for managing disruptive behavior exhibited by young children. Ms. Herschell can be contacted at Department of Psychology, West Virginia University, P.O. Box 6040, Morgantown, WV 26506-6040. E-mail: ahersche@wvu.edu

Vicki A. Lumley, MS, received her masters in clinical psychology from North Dakota State University, and is currently a doctoral candidate in the child clinical psychology program at West Virginia University. Her current research and clinical interests are in the areas of developmental disabilities, applied behavior analysis, and treatment of disruptive behavior disorders. Ms. Lumley may be contacted at the Department of Psychology, West Virginia University, P.O. Box 6040, Morgantown, WV 26506-6040. E-mail: vlumley@wvu.edu

Cheryl B. McNeil, PhD, is an Assistant Professor of Psychology in the Child Clinical Program at West Virginia University. Her clinical and research interests are focused on program development and evaluation, specifically with regard to managing the disruptive behaviors of young children in both the home and school settings. Dr. McNeil has co-authored two books (*Parent-Child Interaction Therapy* and *Short-Term Play Therapy for Disruptive Children*), a continuing education audio and video package (*Working With Oppositional Defiant Disorder in Children*), and a classroom management program (*The ADHD Classroom Kit*). Dr. McNeil can be contacted at the Department of Psychology, West Virginia University, P.O. Box 6040, Morgantown, WV 26506-6040. E-mail: cmcneil@wvu.edu

RESOURCES

Boggs, S. R. (1990). *Generalization of Treatment to the Home Setting: Direct Observation Analysis.* Unpublished manuscript, University of Florida, Gainesville, FL.

Brestan, E., Eyberg, S. M., Boggs, S., & Algina, J. (1997). Parent-child interaction therapy: Parent perceptions of untreated siblings. *Child and Family Behavior Therapy, 19,* 13-28.

Eisenstadt, T. H., Eyberg, S. M., McNeil, C. B., Newcomb, K., & Funderburk, B. (1993). Parent-child interaction therapy with behavior problem children: Relative effectiveness of two stages and overall treatment outcome. *Journal of Child Clinical Psychology, 22,* 42-51.

Eyberg, S. M. (1988). Parent-child interaction therapy: Integration of traditional and behavioral concerns. *Child and Family Behavior Therapy, 10,* 33-46.

Eyberg, S. M. (in press-a). *Eyberg Child Behavior Inventory: Professional Manual.* Odessa, FL: Psychological Assessment Resources.

Eyberg, S. M. (in press-b). *Sutter-Eyberg Student Behavior Inventory: Professional Manual.* Odessa, FL: Psychological Assessment Resources.

Eyberg, S. M., Bessmer, J., Newcomb, K., Edwards, D., & Robinson, E. (1994). *Dyadic Parent-Child Interaction Coding System - II: A Manual.* Unpublished manuscript, University of Florida, Gainesville, FL.

Eyberg, S. M., & Boggs, S. R. (1989). Parent training for oppositional preschoolers. In C. E. Schafer & J. M. Briesmeister (Eds.), *Handbook of Parent Training: Parents as Co-Therapists for Children's Behavior Problems* (pp. 105-132). New York: Wiley.

Eyberg, S. M., & Boggs, S. R. (1998). Parent-Child Interaction Therapy: A psychosocial intervention for the treatment of young conduct-disordered children. In C. E. Schaefer & J. M. Briesmeister (Eds.), *Handbook of Parent Training: Parents as Co-Therapists for Children's Behavior Problems* (2nd ed., pp. 61-97). New York: Wiley.

Eyberg, S. M., Boggs, S. R., & Algina, J. (1995). Parent-child interaction therapy: A psychosocial model for the treatment of young children with conduct problem behavior and their families. *Psychopharmacology Bulletin, 31,* 83-91.

Eyberg, S. M., & Matarazzo, R. G. (1975, April). *Efficiency in Teaching Child Management Skills: Individual Parent-Child Interaction Training Versus Group Didactic Training.* Paper presented at the annual meeting of the Western Psychological Association, Sacramento, CA.

Eyberg, S. M., & Matarazzo, R. G. (1980). Training parents as therapists: A comparison between individual parent-child interaction training and parent group didactic training. *Journal of Clinical Psychology, 36,* 492-499.

Eyberg, S. M., & Robinson, E. A. (1982). Parent-child interaction training: Effects on family functioning. *Journal of Clinical Child Psychology, 11,* 130-137.

Eyberg, S. M., & Robinson, E. A. (1983). *Dyadic Parent-Child Interaction Coding System: A Manual. Psychological Documents, 13,* Ms. No. 2582. (Available from Social and Behavior Sciences Documents, Select Press, P.O. Box 9838, San Rafael, CA 94912.)

Foote, R., Eyberg, S. M., & Schuhmann, E. (1998). Parent-child interaction approaches to the treatment of child behavior problems. In T. Ollendick & R. Prinz (Eds.), *Advances in Clinical Child Psychology* (Vol. 20, pp. 125-151). New York: Plenum.

Forehand, R. L., & McMahon, R. J. (1981). *Helping the Noncompliant Child: A Clinician's Guide to Parent Training.* New York: Guilford.

Hanf, C. (1969). *A Two-Stage Program for Modifying Maternal Controlling During Mother-Child Interaction.* Paper presented at the meeting of the Western Psychological Association, Vancouver, British Columbia, Canada.

Hembree-Kigin, T. L., & McNeil, C. B. (1995). *Parent-Child Interaction Therapy.* New York: Plenum.

Kazdin, A. E. (1997). A model for developing effective treatments: Progression and interplay of theory, research, and practice. *Journal of Clinical Child Psychology, 26,* 114-129.

Kazdin, A. E., Seigel, T. C., & Bass, D. (1990). Drawing upon clinical practice to inform research on child and adolescent psychotherapy: A survey of practitioners. *Professional Psychology: Research and Practice, 21,* 189-198.

McNeil, C. B. (1996). Aversive-nonaversive issue: Tip of the iceberg. *Child and Family Behavior Therapy, 18*(2), 17-23.

McNeil, C. B., Clemens-Mowrer, L., Gurwitch, R. H., & Funderburk, B. W. (1994a). Authors' response to Lutzker's evaluation. *Child and Family Behavior Therapy, 16*(4), 37-46.

McNeil, C. B., Clemens-Mowrer, L., Gurwitch, R. H., & Funderburk, B. W. (1994b). Assessment of a new procedure to prevent timeout escape in preschoolers: Authors' response to Lutzker's rejoinder. *Child and Family Behavior Therapy, 16*(4), 51-56.

McNeil, C. B., Clemens-Mowrer, L., Gurwitch, R. H., & Funderburk, B. W. (1994c). Assessment of a new procedure to prevent timeout escape in preschoolers. *Child and Family Behavior Therapy, 16*(3), 27-35.

McNeil, C. B., Eyberg, S. M., Eisenstadt, T. H., Newcomb, K., & Funderburk, B. W. (1991). Parent-child interaction therapy with behavior problem children: Generalization of treatment effects to the school setting. *Journal of Clinical Child Psychology, 20,* 140-151.

McNeil, C. B., & Herschell, A. H. (1998). Treating multi-problem, high-stress families: Suggested strategies for practitioners. *Family Relations: Interdisciplinary Journal of Applied Family Studies, 47,* 259-262.

Newcomb, K., Eyberg, S. M., Funderburk, B. W., Eisenstadt (Hembree-Kigin), T. H., & McNeil, C. B. (1990, August). *Parent-Child Interaction Therapy: Maintenance of Treatment Gains at 8 Months and 1 and 1/2 Years.* Paper presented at the annual meeting of the American Psychological Association, San Francisco.

Schuhmann, E. M., Durning, P. E., Eyberg, S. M., & Boggs, S. R. (1996). Screening for conduct problem behavior in pediatric settings using the Eyberg Child Behavior Inventory. *Ambulatory Child Health, 2,* 35-41.

Schuhmann, E., Foote, R., Eyberg, S. M., Boggs, S., & Algina, J. (1998). Parent-child interaction therapy: Interim report of a randomized trial with short-term maintenance. *Journal of Clinical Child Psychology, 27,* 34-45.

Urquiza, A. J., & McNeil, C. B. (1996). Parent-child interaction therapy: Potential applications for physically abusive families. *Child Maltreatment, 1,* 134-144.

Wells, K. C., & Forehand, R. (1985). Conduct and oppositional disorders. In P. H. Bornstein & A. E. Kazdin (Eds.), *Handbook of Clinical Behavior Therapy With Children* (pp. 128-265). Homewood, IL: Dorsey Press.

Zangwill, W. M. (1984). An evaluation of a parent training program. *Child and Family Behavior Therapy, 5,* 1-16.

Assessment and Treatment of Chronic Headaches in Adolescents

Vanessa K. Jensen and Dunya T. Yaldoo

INTRODUCTION

The occasional headache is common among individuals of all ages and is typically managed independently and successfully. Severe recurrent headaches, however, can interfere with daily activities and severely limit an adolescent's ability to function in his or her life. Until recently, research regarding etiology, related factors, and treatment of persistent headaches was largely conducted with adults, with pediatric practices extrapolated from adult findings. In the last decade, however, there has been a surge in the study of chronic pain in adolescents, including chronic headache (P. J. Norton et al., 1999). This research has continued to demonstrate the often serious and impairing nature of chronic headache as well as the effectiveness of biobehavioral interventions.

Incidence and Impact

Headaches are common in children, adolescents, and adults, although exact incidence is difficult to verify due to limitations in diagnostic categorization. Recent studies have supported the incidence of frequent nonmigrainous headache in the child and adolescent population as approximately 2.5% (Newacheck & Taylor, 1992), with an increased incidence with age (Egger, Angold, & Costello, 1998). By age 13, 82% of teens have reported some form of headache in their previous 12 months, and 14% to 17% of adolescents report some degree of recurrent headache (Sillanpaa, 1983). The incidence of childhood migraine also increases with age, with a preadolescent rate of 3% (Abu-Arefeh & Russell, 1995; Sillanpaa, 1983) and adolescent rates ranging from 7% to 11% (Prensky & Sommer, 1979; Sillanpaa, 1983). New cases of migraine in boys peak in preadolescence and, in girls, in mid to late adolescence (Stang et al., 1992).

Approximately 1% of all school days missed appears to be related to headache pain (Collin, Hockaday, & Waters, 1985), and several hundred thousand school days are estimated to be missed each month due to pediatric migraine (Stang & Osterhaus, 1993). Including all headache types, more boys than girls experience headache in the preschool to early elementary school years. By early adolescence, the incidence has shifted, with a greater number of girls than boys reporting headache (Abu-Arefeh & Russell, 1995; Bille, 1962; Mortimer, Kay, & Jaron, 1992; Sillanpaa, 1983).

Classification and Diagnosis

Lack of diagnostic reliability and validity has created problems with outcome measurement and limits the generalizability of results of treatment research. Historically, headaches have been classified as either migraine or tension-type based upon the presence or absence of autonomic nervous system symptoms and the quality of the pain, regardless of the age of the patient (Ad Hoc Committee on the Classification of Headache, 1962). Modifications to these criteria that considered the different presentation of pediatric headache improved diagnostic sensitivity and specificity but have not been uniformly accepted (Gladstein et al., 1993). Unfortunately, the recent criteria introduced by the Headache Classification Committee of the International Headache Society (1988) were created without consideration of the pediatric population. Recommendations to improve the utility of this system with the youth population have been suggested, including altering criteria for headache duration and number of autonomic nervous system symptoms required for migraine diagnosis (Gladstein et al., 1993; Maytal et al., 1997).

Headaches can be classified along dichotomous variables of incidence (acute or recurrent) and course (progressive or nonprogressive) (see Table 1 below). Headaches that become progressively more severe over time (whether acute or recurrent) should be considered suspicious for some type of organicity, either infectious or neoplastic, and require complete medical evaluation. Nonprogressive headaches may be acute in course, as with migraine or tension headache, or recurrent, as with chronic daily headache (also called chronic nonprogressive or recurrent daily headache). A "mixed headache" condition includes a combination of intermittent migraine and chronic headache. Although the Headache Classification Committee of the International Headache Society (1988) also utilizes the category of cluster headaches, these are relatively rare in childhood and adolescence and will not be discussed further here.

TABLE 1: Classification of Headaches by Incidence and Course

	Progressive	**Nonprogressive**
Acute	Suspect organicity Refer for medical evaluation	Tension or migraine
Recurrent	Suspect organicity Refer for medical evaluation	Chronic recurrent (chronic daily)

Migraine headaches are distinct from other headaches in their physiologic mechanism, frequency, and presentation. They are associated with a variety of autonomic system prodromal symptoms (an aura), including nausea, vomiting, phonophobia, photophobia, and/or other visual disturbances. A number of triggers are associated with migraines, including changes in temperature, weather, bright lights, and hormones, and there is a strong hereditary component. Stress and distress have also been associated with precipitation, exacerbation, or maintenance of migraine (Carlsson, Larsson, & Mark, 1996).

Chronic daily headache is a less well-understood disorder. Such headaches may occur several times per week or be present continuously, possibly lasting days to months. The symptom pattern may continue for many years. Chronic headaches can easily be distinguished from migraines by intensity, duration, and presence or absence of related symptoms, even when both occur in the same patient, as in those with mixed headache. In practice, patients presenting with chronic headache, particularly of greater than 6 months duration, seem to share many social and behavioral features. Many appear to maintain high academic standards and have a history of academic and vocational successes, have strict expectations regarding behavior of self and others, and establish a greater than typical degree of distance from others socially. Such observations do not indicate etiology but, rather, suggest relationships among various factors and pain presentations that must be explored in planning treatment.

Observations of patterns of behavior and symptoms among patients has led to the conceptualization of chronic headaches as a somatoform disorder (*Diagnostic and Statistical Manual of Mental Disorders [DSM-IV],* American Psychiatric Association [APA], 1994). This provides a framework for understanding the complex set of symptoms that are associated with pediatric headache and leads logically to effective treatment planning. Attention is drawn away from etiology and toward the reaching of functional goals, including decreasing distress and increasing day-to-day activities. For all diagnoses within the somatoform category, it is important for the clinician to understand (and communicate to the patient and family) that the pain symptoms are not intentional but, rather, psychological factors may play a complex role in the development, maintenance, and/or resolution of the pain.

Etiology, Related Factors, and Comorbidity

Although the etiology of recurrent headache in either children or adults is not entirely understood, research with adults has suggested a genetic component, stronger for women than men, for both tension and migraine headaches (Honkasalo et al., 1995; Larsson, Bille, & Pederson, 1995). There may be an inherited headache predisposition, which may be triggered by a variety of biological (e.g., puberty) or psychosocial (e.g., stress) factors, with individual headache course moderated by multiple individual difference variables (e.g., personality and coping style).

Multiple familial factors appear to predict an increased likelihood of pediatric headache. Gulhati and Minty (1998) found that parents of children with headache, particularly mothers, were more likely than controls to report extensive childhood and adulthood illness histories. Mothers of children with headache were also more likely to report the loss of their own mothers due to death, express feelings of loneliness, and express concerns about serious disease in themselves with reluctance to accept medical reassurance.

Among children, Aromaa et al. (1998) found that a number of factors appear to predict an increased likelihood of chronic headaches at age 6, including global health or feeding problems in infancy or sleep difficulties or depressive symptomatology at age 3. Children with behavioral problems, increased fatigue, and concentration difficulties at age 5 are also more likely to experience persistent headaches at age 6, as are those who were considered highly social. Adolescents with headache often report school stresses and social difficulties and have a greater number of school absences than controls (Metsahonkala, Sillanpaa, & Tuominen, 1998). In clinical practice, there appears to be a relationship among parental expectations, social adjustment, peer pressure, and recurrent headache. Some adolescents with recurrent headache, including both males and females, seem to hold high standards for self and others, may be somewhat socially naïve, and have difficulty tolerating other opinions and views. Parents tend to report these teens as exceptionally "good" children, often excelling in academics, engaging in no behavioral difficulties, and generally well mannered and well behaved (Jensen et al., 1998).

Well-designed epidemiological studies of adults with headaches have demonstrated a common coexistence of depression or anxiety. An association between migraine and depression has been shown in women (Morrison & Price, 1989) and between panic disorder and migraine (Stewart, Breslau, & Keck, 1994). Among children and adolescents, there have been a number of clinical studies and a few epidemiological studies of headache and psychopathology, although most have been methodologically flawed, using nonvalidated measures of psychiatric symptoms. Pine, Cohen, and Brook (1996), using validated diagnostic criteria, found that headaches were twice as common in depressed adolescents as in their nondepressed peers. Comorbidity has been reported between migraine headaches and depression or anxiety in children and adolescents (Guidetti et al., 1998). Egger et al. (1998) found an association between headaches and internalizing disorders specific to girls: Girls who met *Diagnostic and Statistical Manual of Mental Disorders (3rd ed. rev.)* (*DSM-III-R*; APA, 1987) criteria for a depressive disorder had a four times higher prevalence of headaches than did girls who were not depressed. Additionally, girls with an anxiety disorder had a three times higher prevalence of headaches than their nonanxious female peers. Egger et al. further found that boys who met criteria for conduct disorder experienced twice as many headaches as boys without conduct disorder.

ASSESSMENT

The assessment of patients with recurrent headaches takes on a particular tone because of the patient's frequently intense belief that the symptoms are not psychological. Patients (and their families) referred for evaluation and treatment of headaches are often quite clear in their impression that their headaches represent a physiological problem that cannot be addressed via psychological treatment. For this reason the orientation of the examiner to headaches (and pain disorders in general) must be well communicated to the patient and family at the start, as a means of gaining trust and establishing a common goal. From this perspective, the purpose of the evaluation is to assess current functioning and concerns and to shift the perspective of the patient and family from a strictly medical to a psychological/habit focus. At that time, a workable treatment plan can be developed. The core components of the assessment process are interviews with the patient and parent(s) and review of history and records, although standardized psychological testing may also be utilized, based upon the clinical situation.

Interviews

Clinical interviews are invaluable in understanding headache pain as perceived by the patient and family. Variables such as the age of the patient, chronicity of symptoms, and type of headache must be considered. The patient who has seen many different professionals for his or her pain and found each lacking presents a different clinical picture (and different treatment issues) when compared to the patient who is just entering his or her first attempt at symptom relief. As well, treatment issues will be slightly different for the patient with moderate level recurrent pain versus the patient with a severe incapacitating migraine every 2 weeks coupled with mild daily headache. Regardless of type, it is generally more effective to begin the evaluation by focusing on more concrete, pain-related, and medical information, gradually moving toward exploration of the impact of the pain and behaviors surrounding the pain (precipitating factors and reactions), and finally exploring more personal issues of social, emotional, and family functioning.

Throughout the initial interviews, the clinician will also be able to acquire information regarding the patient and family that are not necessarily directly questioned, such as the family's attitude toward health and illness, their views of health care professionals, and the role of thoughts, feelings, and behaviors in pain symptoms. Parent response to patient symptoms and complaints (even during the office visit) add to the data set. Issues of secondary gain and inadvertent reinforcement of symptoms may be played out in the office evaluation. Overall, particular attention should be given to the patient and family orientation toward illness versus health, individual and family attitude toward achievement and success, the adolescent's general development and the family's response to this, signs of family stress or conflict, and family interaction.

Initially, the patient and parents are seen jointly, at least briefly, with the goal of clarifying the purpose and process of the assessment and finding a common ground to enlist the involvement of the patient and parents as a part of the "treatment team." This arrangement also permits observation of interactions between parents and the adolescent. The family may need to be frequently reassured, directly and indirectly, that the pain is indeed real and that no one doubts the patient's distress. Still, the availability of psychological and behavioral strategies that can assist in managing and/or decreasing the patient's pain must be continually communicated.

Next, the parents are generally met with privately. The parent interview can follow a structured or semistructured format, depending upon the preference of the examiner. The more structured the format, the more comfortable the parents generally tend to be and the less defensive they may be regarding their child's complaints. There are a number of structured interviews available that are frequently utilized in assessing pain and pain disorders among both children and adolescents, including the Pediatric Pain Questionnaire (PPQ; Tesler et al., 1983) and the Varni-Thompson Pediatric Pain Questionnaire (VTPPQ; Varni, Thompson, & Hanson, 1987), both of which assess sensory, affective, and evaluative dimensions of chronic pain. Regardless of whether a structured or semistructured format is utilized, however, the principal areas necessary to assess are situational, familial, and emotional factors relevant to the pain, as well as sensory dimensions of the pain. In practices where chronic pain represents a large portion of referrals, such a system allows for systematic collection of data and comparisons across patients. The majority of office-based clinicians will likely follow a less-structured process, similar to that used with other patients. In this situation, the clinician must take care to keep the pain and pain issues central in order to keep rapport with the patient and family. Components of the interview should include a specific history of the pain and surrounding variables, an assessment of the impact of the pain on the patient and family, information on any previous attempts at treatment (medical and behavioral), history of similar complaints in the patient or family members, and a thorough developmental history (including academic, psychosocial, and family functioning). The interview should also provide some indication of the parents' response to the symptoms, including a "moment to moment" recollection of "what happens" when the patient reports significant pain. An underlying, although often not spoken, purpose in this historical review with the parents is to identify any comorbid psychological difficulties in the patient or family.

The patient portion of the interview allows for further rapport building and identification of issues that may not have been raised by the patient in the presence of parents, or by the parents alone. Typically, discussion of "factual" information is a helpful entrée, unless the patient has already expressed concerns about or interest in psychological issues. History should minimally include information regarding school (including academic, extracurricular, and social activities), other activities (sports, community, religious, and/or social), family relationships, and general emotional state. Assessing the adolescent's understanding of the medical aspects of his or her pain may be useful, querying specifics regarding the symptoms and obtaining a thorough pain history and timeline. A "moment to moment" recall of events surrounding an episode of pain is again useful, using a "What happens then?" model, which can show the impact of the pain on routine daily functioning. Open-ended questions may be difficult for some patients who are less than pleased with being at the appointment, and a "checklist" approach can be useful. Such lists can be used in assessing what patients have tried for relief of pain (e.g., closing your eyes, going to a dark room, eating/drinking certain things, thinking certain things, talking to someone, taking specific medications, doing things to distract yourself, etc.). With this nonchallenging approach, the clinician gains credibility, which may move the patient toward a more problem-solving view that is more open to attempting behavioral or psychological interventions.

Psychological Testing

In most clinical settings, the individual and parental interviews, along with supporting data from records, will provide the core assessment of patients with chronic headaches. Screening for other behavioral and/or psychological difficulties is recommended through a broad-band rating scale. At times, self-report measures of specific symptoms, such as anxiety and depression, can quantify information obtained by history. In practice, formal psychological testing and assessment is not typically necessary or feasible for "routine" cases. However, if the interview or history raises questions of significant comorbid psychological disorders or if treatment is not progressing as expected, formal assessment of personality, psychopathology, or specific symptomatology may be helpful.

Broad-band behavior rating scales that are completed by the patient, parents, and/or teachers, such as the Behavior Assessment System for Children (BASC; Reynolds & Kamphaus, 1992) or the Child Behavior Checklist (CBCL; Achenbach, 1991), are useful for screening. These measures allow for rapid review of a range of behavioral and psychological symptoms and provide information on the perceptions of multiple informants. Symptom-specific measures, such as the Children's Depression Inventory (CDI; Kovacs, 1992) or the Revised Children's Manifest Anxiety Scale (RCMAS; Reynolds & Richmond, 1985), can add information regarding the patient's perception of severity of psychological symptoms, although results should be viewed with caution. Such self-report rating scales maintain a high degree of face validity (starting with their names), and patients may view the questionnaire as evidence that the clinician thinks the pain is "not real" but, rather, is the result of anxiety or depression. Additionally, many patients appear unable or unwilling to openly endorse symptoms of psychological distress.

For patients who have not been successful in previous attempts at treatment or in those with clear comorbid symptoms, detailed diagnostic evaluation may be beneficial. General measures of psychological functioning, such as the MMPI-Adolescent (MMPI-A; Butcher & Williams, 1989) and the Personality Inventory for Children-Revised (PIC-R; Lachar, 1981), have been used with this population. Recent research on the MMPI-A has been generally consistent with earlier data with adults, finding that adolescent headache patients, as a group, show elevations on the Hypochondriasis, Depression, and/or Hysteria clinical scales (Jensen et al., 1998). Jensen et al. also found a response style on the PIC-R (a parent-completed, empirically derived measure of global social, emotional, cognitive, and behavioral functioning) suggestive of defensiveness on the part of the parent. Psychological testing can add a dimension not always available from interview or self-report checklists, both of which may be biased by social desirability (Jensen & Rothner, 1995).

INTERVENTION

Although most adolescents have dealt with an occasional tension headache without significant life impact, treatment of chronic headaches is much more challenging. Patients with recurrent pain have typically tried (although not necessarily systematically or thoroughly) a number of pharmacological and nonpharmacological treatments and are often entrenched in maladaptive behavioral and emotional patterns. Regardless of the underlying etiology of the pain, to be successful in pain relief, intervention must move the patient (and family) away from the role of passive recipient of treatment and toward a role as an active and solution-oriented participant in their care. Cognitive-behavioral interventions can be presented as effective and efficient options for reducing headache symptoms. A variety of research supported techniques can be utilized, depending upon the individual patient's needs and the expertise of the clinician.

Research-Supported Intervention

Although few well-controlled studies unequivocally support any one treatment for chronic headache in children and adolescents, the collective data clearly support that cognitive-behavioral techniques are effective in reducing pain and for increasing daily functioning (Holden, Deichmann, & Levy, 1999; Lipchik & Holroyd, 1999). Most programs utilize biofeedback, relaxation, or other self-regulation techniques; behavioral contingency management; and/or other cognitive-behavioral interventions.

Most research has studied psychophysiological treatments, specifically biofeedback and relaxation training/self-hypnosis. These treatments have been found to be more effective than attention-placebo or no treatment groups in reducing symptoms (Larsson & Melin, 1988; Richter et al., 1986; Williamson, Baker, & Cubic, 1993). EMG biofeedback has been effective in decreasing pain (Bussone et al., 1998; Williamson et al., 1993) as has thermal biofeedback (Burke & Andrasik, 1989; Labbé & Williamson, 1983, 1984). Relaxation training decreases pain (Larsson & Melin, 1986; McGrath et al., 1992) and may increase general stress management skills (Engel, Rapoff, & Pressman, 1992). A recent review of the scientific literature found significant support for psychological treatment of recurrent headache in children and adolescents, particularly utilizing relaxation/self-hypnosis (Holden et al., 1999). A behavioral contingency management component, which teaches parents to systematically reinforce appropriate, nonpain behaviors while extinguishing pain behaviors, has also been effective in treating adolescents with headache (Beames, Sanders, & Bor, 1992). Although data are less clear regarding the efficacy of other cognitive-behavioral interventions, such as self-monitoring and problem-solving, such strategies are often embedded within the psychophysiological interventions, and clinical protocols often rely on multiple techniques. Limited data are available on the comparative efficacy of interventions.

Pharmacological Treatment

Pharmacological management of headache pain can be can be divided into (a) prophylactic treatment, (b) abortive measures, and (c) symptom control (Rothner, 1989). Although research has not demonstrated the efficacy of many of these medications in children, they are frequently used in clinical practice based upon empirical evidence and research with adults (Holden et al., 1998). Prophylactic medications, including beta blockers, calcium-channel blockers, antihistamines, and antidepressants, are typically initiated when the headaches are significantly interfering with the patient's daily functioning and the patient has not responded to symptomatic or abortive treatment. Increasingly, amitriptyline (a tricyclic antidepressant) has been used prophylactically in patients with either migraine or chronic headache, both with and without comorbid depression. The effect on headache appears independent of any antidepressant effect (Rothner, 1989), and the dosages used are typically lower than that which would be used to achieve therapeutic antidepressant levels.

Serotonin agonists, such as subcutaneous or oral somatriptan (Imitrex), are used for severe migraine, as is dihydroergotamine (DHE; Holden et al., 1998). Abortive medications used to decrease existing pain or to relieve related symptoms include analgesics (aspirin, acetaminophen, or ibuprofen), antiemetics (for associated nausea and vomiting), or sedatives. In general, narcotics and tranquilizing medications are avoided in children and adolescents (Rothner, 1989). There is limited research that addresses the relative efficacy of medications compared to psychological interventions, and medical and psychological treatments are often utilized together in clinical practice, particularly when pain is interfering with daily functioning.

A Three-Part Cognitive-Behavioral Headache Treatment Program

In clinical practice, a combination of empirically supported treatment techniques is recommended, including (a) self-regulation (biofeedback, self-hypnosis, or relaxation training), (b) cognitive-behavioral self-management, and (c) behavioral contingency management. This self-management approach is similar to that used in the management of other chronic disorders, such as diabetes or asthma, teaching the patient to take preventive actions, identify potential triggers, and create a menu of actions to reduce symptoms and improve functioning. Coordination with the patient's medical care practitioner is advised in order to provide the most effective patient care possible, as well as to continually educate the medical practitioner of the role of psychological treatment in treating the patient's pain.

Many adolescents with the primary complaint of chronic headache appear skeptical of psychological interventions. An initial focus on the more concrete components of treatment is generally better accepted, thus resulting in greater patient and family compliance. Thus, self-regulation training is typically taught first, with self-management and contingency management taught more gradually.

Self-Regulation Training

Although biofeedback and self-hypnosis are empirically proven interventions for headache pain, relatively few clinicians have the training and equipment necessary to use these as a primary treatment. Instead, teaching general relaxation training is recommended, including diaphragmatic breathing, progressive muscle relaxation (PMR), and/or autogenic relaxation. Starting with diaphragmatic breathing first is encouraged, as most other programs (e.g., PMR) utilize breathing as one component. An initial focus on breathing can provide the patient with an experience of mastery and success and increase patient trust in the clinician and intervention. The sample script on page 131 is geared at early to mid adolescence, although the wording can easily be adjusted for older or younger patients. Depending upon the needs of the patient and his or her response, other techniques can be introduced to further develop relaxation skills, such as PMR or imagery. EMG or thermal biofeedback or self-hypnosis can also be ıtilized if the clinician is appropriately trained.

After the initial instruction and practice of the breathing techniques, the patient should be given positive feedback in an age-appropriate manner, and a plan for home practice should be established. Generally, daily practice is encouraged, preferably several times per day, with the techniques first mastered in nonstressful situations. Building relaxation exercises into the patient's daily routine increases compliance, and the patient can be instructed to practice at set times or specific situations, such as upon awakening, after school, or at bedtime. The patient should initially practice for about 5 minutes per session. As the basic techniques are mastered, suggestions can be added during office rehearsal, such as reminding the patient that as he or she breathes out, the heart rate slows and muscles relax, decreasing any feelings of discomfort. Once a relaxed state is achieved in only a few breaths, practice can be shortened. Including diaphragmatic breathing in an adolescent's routine in a less intrusive way should be encouraged, making this type of relaxation more automatic. Such practice can be done in a few minutes or less before or after each meal, each time the patient gets into a car, at the start of each new class, and so on. This type of daily stress management, involving practice, consistency, and active participation, is often contrary to what patients expect, imagining that something will be done *to them.*

Cognitive-Behavioral Self-Management

Self-management strategies are frequently used in teaching self-care to patients with chronic illnesses and/or disabilities. A similar approach can be extremely useful in teaching adolescent patients to manage their headaches more effectively and independently. Such intervention capitalizes on most adolescents' desire for greater independence and seems to decrease the likelihood of inadvertent reinforcement from the environment.

An essential aspect of self-management is regular data monitoring regarding a patient's pain symptoms and daily functioning. In order to track progress and identify possible contributing or maintaining factors, a headache diary is recommended, which can be prepared and given to the patient, or the patient can be given instructions on tracking headaches in a journal or notebook (sample diaries can be found in several of the on-line sites listed in the Resources section). In addition to tracking time, situation, and intensity, an "action taken/outcome" component to the diary allows for monitoring of patient use of specific techniques and their effectiveness. Activity avoidance, inadvertent environmental reinforcement, and patient coping can also become evident through diary review. The diary itself is often a vehicle for reinforcing patient compliance and active headache management.

Self-management begins with a detailed review of possible "triggers," such as physical or environmental factors or social or emotional stresses. In addition to the more concrete triggers of noise, bright light, specific foods, and so on, patients frequently appear to have difficulties with specific social or developmental situations and beliefs. Social intolerance (particularly of others who have different values and resulting behaviors), ambivalence regarding adolescent independence, management of school and extracurricular activities, and a tendency toward a rigid, perfectionist self-view are often present. The clinician must be cautious in suggesting a relationship between such variables and the onset or maintenance of pain, particularly early in treatment. Once possible triggers are identified, options for managing triggers *prior to the onset of headaches* can be taught. Specific cognitive-behavioral techniques, such as thought stopping, distraction, active problem solving, and positive self-talk, are used, in addition to initiation of the previously taught self-regulation techniques. The specific set of strategies recommended for each patient will depend upon his or her needs, beliefs, and past history and should be outlined individually for each patient. Later in treatment, many adolescents are more ready and willing to explore the relationship between their own thoughts and feelings and subsequent headaches. Themes of perfectionism, irrational expectations of self and others, and frustration at others for not doing things "the right way" are common. An awareness of these links can help young people to alter their behaviors, in order to decrease perceived distress and ultimately decrease pain. Typically, the older and more intellectually capable the patient, the more likely he or she is to engage in this type of discussion with a positive outcome.

Behavioral Contingency Management

In the initial interviews with the patient and parents, the goal of moving the attention away from pain behaviors toward alternative wellness behaviors should have been made clear. In order to avoid inadvertently reinforcing pain behaviors, pain complaints should be actively ignored or handled in a prearranged manner (such as reminding the patient to follow his or her management plan). Increased attention should instead be given for health-focused, nonpain behaviors, such as increased daily activities, regular school attendance, and appropriate social activities. Parents often engage in ineffective behaviors, such as frequently asking the patient about pain or anticipating pain in certain situations (e.g., in hot weather, in bright lights, etc.). They may interpret specific observations as indicators of pain (e.g., each time the teen is lying down he must have a headache, or if she "looks tired" it must be related to her pain). Parents may further inadvertently reinforce the pain-avoidance cycle by suggesting that the patient should "take it easy" when they see possible triggers or indicators of pain.

Initially, it may be difficult for parents to alter their responses, particularly given their distress regarding the child's pain and concern that the child's symptoms may be misunderstood or not taken seriously. Parents are often afraid that health professionals have "missed" a serious physical illness; thorough medical evaluation is helpful in reassuring the patient and parents that all avenues for evaluation and treatment are being addressed and that all care providers are working in concert. Parents may need to be reminded that no one is disputing the patient's pain, but, rather, perceptions of pain can be altered when attention is paid to the symptoms (e.g., consider the child who obtains a cut and cries only *after* seeing it bleed or *after* someone comments on it). Parents themselves can usually understand that distraction is often an effective tool for managing discomfort and that increasing attention toward pain will likely increase distress.

For most adolescent patients, a clear behavioral plan for pain management can be established, including identifying goal behaviors and consequences for meeting or not meeting expectations. The younger the patient, the greater the parental role in the patient's care, and the more parents can influence behavior through behavioral contingencies. The first portion of the plan clarifies expected behaviors that will allow the patient to engage in social or other activities or rewards (i.e., sports, television, or computer access). The patient must attend school daily and participate in routine family and community activities in order to earn the rewards. The second component lists the expectations and allowable behaviors when the patient does not attend school due to pain. Typically, this translates into remaining at home with no television, phone calls, or visitors. Parents may initially consider this to be "punishment" and may express concerns about limiting activities, believing that the patient is already disengaged with peers and that any social activity is "good for him or her." A behavioral contingency program for pain management can instead be viewed as a positive reinforcement program, restructuring social activities (or sports or other extracurricular activities) as privileges to be earned by meeting behavioral expectations of school attendance and household chores. Much of the energy in this part of treatment is spent helping parents fully understand the importance of consistent responding and teaching patients to manage their headaches and how to function *in spite of them.* If parents are doubtful or less than fully committed, inadvertent reinforcement of pain behaviors is likely.

The pace at which interventions are introduced will vary. Our experience has been that treatment moves along more rapidly for patients who are older, more educated, and more psychologically open and whose parents are more educated, more physically and emotionally healthy, and less defensive regarding psychological treatment. For those having greater difficulty, a longer time will need to be spent teaching and reinforcing each concept or technique. Individualization of treatment is essential, despite a general framework from which to start. Table 2 (p. 130) offers a guide regarding treatment strategies through a 4- to 8-week intervention program.

SUMMARY

Headaches, whether acute or chronic, are a frequent occurrence among adolescents and represent growing areas of clinical and research interests. Although etiology is not entirely understood, multiple environmental and psychosocial stress factors appear to contribute to the maintenance of chronic headaches in adolescents. Moreover, comorbid psychiatric disorders (e.g., depression or anxiety) may exist. Comprehensive assessment of these youth is therefore required, with sensitivity to the possibility that the patient and family may be hesitant to accept a psychological conceptualization of the pain. Treatment, in order to be effective, must move the patient (and family) away from the role of passive recipient and toward a role as an active and solution-oriented participant in the intervention. Sufficient evidence exists from treatment outcome studies to support the efficacy of behaviorally based treatment strategies.

Although recent years have demonstrated a surge in the study of chronic pain in both children and adolescents (Norton et al., 1999), including chronic headache, continued research is clearly warranted. A particular and critical area of interest remains around headache classification and diagnosis, specific to the pediatric population. Which treatments are effective specific to headache type remains to be understood among youth. Additionally, it may be useful to compare behavioral interventions to pharmacological interventions among the pediatric population, whether used simultaneously or successively, and with respect to both short- and long-term treatment gains. This requires that research move beyond general efficacy trials to explore the efficiency and cost-effectiveness of behavioral interventions. These pursuits will be vital to the survival of nonpharmacological approaches to recurrent headache treatment in the future health care marketplace.

TABLE 2: Three-Part Cognitive-Behavioral Treatment Program

Evaluation and Beginning Treatment (1-2 Sessions*)
- Evaluation/diagnostic interview
- Self-regulation
  - Teach diaphragmatic breathing
- Cognitive management
  - Identify triggers, stresses, and target behaviors
  - Set up headache diary and monitoring
- Contingency management
  - Outline expectations for behavior during headache

Stage Two (1-2 Sessions*)
- Self-regulation
  - Review diaphragmatic breathing
  - Add imagery or PMR
- Cognitive management
  - Review diary, triggers, and outcome of breathing
  - Plan alternate behaviors (incompatible with headache)
  - Reinforce appropriate coping behaviors
- Contingency management
  - Review behavior during headaches
  - Contract for limitations on behavior if headaches occur

Stage Three (1-3 Sessions*)
- Self-regulation
  - Outline preferred self-regulation technique and practice
- Cognitive management
  - Review diary, triggers, and outcome
  - Teach self-talk and begin analysis of irrational beliefs
  - Teach alternate responses to distressing thoughts/feelings
- Contingency management
  - Review parent/patient compliance with contract
  - Modify plan to increase expectations as headaches decrease

Stage Four (1 or More Sessions*)
- Self-regulation
  - Review self-regulation technique and modify as needed
- Cognitive management
  - Review diary, triggers, and alternate responses used
  - Further exploration of relationships between thoughts and feelings and onset and/or maintenance of headaches
  - Relapse prevention
- Contingency management
  - Review progress and plan for relapse

***Note:** Number of sessions required at each stage will vary by patient and clinician.

Basic Diaphragmatic Breathing: Sample Script

One of the first things we are going to work on is breathing. We both know that you know how to breathe. But the way you breathe, actually the way we all breathe day to day, is not the best type of breathing to help get rid of your headaches.

Let's start by talking about what exactly your body does when you take a deep breath in. What part of your body moves? [Response is usually chest or lungs.] Right, your lungs fill up, expanding your chest - but what about the rest of your body? What else moves when you really inhale? [Response is usually shoulders or stomach.] Exactly! That's just what most people do - they lift their shoulders and suck in their stomachs, thinking that will help get a better breath. But what they are really doing is working their muscles in areas that actually make it HARDER to get a good breath. If your energy, blood, and oxygen are going to the large muscles in your shoulders and abdomen, then they are not working on filling your lungs.

Have you ever seen how a young baby or animal breathes? If you watch them closely, you'll see that they don't seem to breathe with their chest or shoulders but, rather, with their stomach area. They don't "suck in" their abdomen, but actually expand their bellies as they breathe in, using the muscle at the bottom of their lungs, the diaphragm. Their shoulders and other large muscles stay relaxed.

That's what you are going to do. It sounds easy but for most people it takes practice. It tends to feel like you are doing something wrong at first, because it's so different from what you are used to.

Let me show you. I start by relaxing my shoulders and chest area. I breathe in through my nose, trying to fill up the bottom of my lungs first, almost as if I was pouring water into a big balloon, filling up the bottom first. As my lungs fill from the bottom up, my stomach area expands, and my lungs gradually fill up to the top of my chest. Then I let the air out through my mouth with a soft "whooooo" sound. Let's try it.

Start by sitting comfortably, legs not crossed and arms on the arms of the chair. Relax your shoulders and neck. Take a deep breath in through your nose, filling up from the bottom of your lungs. Good . . . fill them all the way up keeping your shoulders relaxed. Good! Now slowly let the air out, like collapsing a balloon. Good! Let's try another. [Repeat.]

How do you feel? Some people feel a bit dizzy at first, with such a rush of oxygen to their system. That will go away in a few seconds. Can you feel the relaxed feeling in your shoulders and chest? Good. [Practice a few times with much positive reinforcement for approximations of success, shaping with each attempt.]

NOTE: The younger the patient, the more adaptation needed, with simplified language and more practice to shape the response to approximately accurate diaphragmatic breathing.

CONTRIBUTORS

Vanessa K. Jensen, PsyD, is the head of Pediatric Psychology at The Cleveland Clinic Foundation. Dr. Jensen specializes in the evaluation and treatment of children and adolescents with a range of difficulties, including chronic pain, chronic illness, autism, and eating disorders. She is active in state and national professional organizations and is involved in the education of medical and psychology residents and fellows. Dr. Jensen may be contacted at The Cleveland Clinic Foundation, Division of Pediatrics/Desk A120, 9500 Euclid Avenue, Cleveland, OH 44195.

Dunya T. Yaldoo, PhD, is a member of the staff at The Cleveland Clinic Foundation. Dr. Yaldoo completed her doctoral training in clinical psychology in 1998 at the University of Detroit Mercy. She specializes in the evaluation and treatment of children and adolescents with chronic pain and a wide range of chronic illnesses. She is a member of various professional organizations and continues to participate in empirical research. Dr. Yaldoo can be contacted at The Cleveland Clinic Foundation, Division of Pediatrics/Desk A120, 9500 Euclid Avenue, Cleveland, OH 44195.

RESOURCES

Cited Resources

Abu-Arefeh, I., & Russell, G. (1995). Prevalence of headache and migraine in school children. *BMJ, 309,* 765-769.

Achenbach, T. M. (1991). *Manual for the Child Behavior Checklist 4-18 and 1991 Profile.* Burlington, VT: University of Vermont, Department of Psychiatry.

Ad Hoc Committee on the Classification of Headache, National Institute of Neurological Diseases and Deafness. (1962). Classification of headache. *Neurology, 12,* 378-380.

American Psychiatric Association. (1987). *Diagnostic and Statistical Manual of Mental Disorders* (3rd ed. rev.). Washington, DC: Author.

American Psychiatric Association. (1994). *Diagnostic and Statistical Manual of Mental Disorders* (4th ed.). Washington, DC: Author.

Aromaa, M., Rautava, P., Helenius, H., & Sillanpaa, M. L. (1998). Factors of early life as predictors of headache in children at school entry. *Headache, 38*(1), 23-30.

Beames, L., Sanders, M. R., & Bor, W. (1992). The role of parent training in the cognitive behavioral treatment of children's headaches. *Behavioral Psychotherapy, 20,* 167-180.

Bille, B. S. (1962). Migraine in school children. *Acta Paediatrica Scandinavica, 51,* 1-51.

Burke, E. J., & Andrasik, F. (1989). Home- vs. clinic-based biofeedback treatment for pediatric migraine: Results of treatment through one year follow-up. *Headache, 29,* 343-440.

Bussone, G., Grazzi, L., D'Amico, D., Leone, M., & Andrasik, F. (1998). Biofeedback-assisted relaxation training for young adolescents with tension-type headache: A controlled study. *Cephalalgia, 18,* 463-467.

Butcher, J. N., & Williams, C. L. (1989). *Minnesota Multiphasic Personality Inventory-Adolescent.* Minneapolis, MN: University of Minnesota Press.

Carlsson, G., Larsson, B., & Mark, A. (1996). Psychosocial functioning in school children with recurrent headaches. *Headache, 36,* 77-82.

Collin, C., Hockaday, J. M., & Waters, W. E. (1985). Headache and school absence. *Archives of Disease in Childhood, 60,* 245-247.

Egger, H. L., Angold, A., & Costello, E. J. (1998). Headaches and psychopathology in children and adolescents. *Journal of the American Academy of Child and Adolescent Psychiatry, 37,* 951-958.

Engel, J. M., Rapoff, M. A., & Pressman, A. R. (1992). Long-term follow-up of relaxation training for pediatric headache disorders. *Headache, 32,* 152-156.

Gladstein, J., Holden, E. W., Peralta, L., & Raven, N. (1993). Diagnoses and symptom patterns in children presenting to a pediatric headache clinic. *Headache, 33,* 497-500.

Guidetti, V., Galli, F., Fabrizi, P., Giannantoni, A. S., Napoli, L., Bruni, O., & Trillo, S. (1998). Headache and psychiatric comorbidity: Clinical aspects and outcome in an 8-year follow-up study. *Cephalalgia, 18,* 455-462.

Gulhati, A., & Minty, B. (1998). Parental health attitudes, illnesses, and supports and the referral of school children to medical specialists. *Child: Care, Health, and Development, 24*(4), 295-313.

Headache Classification Committee of the International Headache Society. (1988). Classification and diagnostic criteria for headache disorders, cranial neuralgias and facial pain. *Cephalalgia, 8,* 9-28.

Holden, E. W., Deichmann, M. M., & Levy, J. D. (1999). Empirically supported treatments in pediatric psychology: Recurrent pediatric headaches. *Journal of Pediatric Psychology, 24*(2), 91-109.

Holden, E. W., Levy, J. D., Deichmann, M. M., & Gladstein, J. (1998). Recurrent pediatric headaches: Assessment and intervention. *Developmental and Behavioral Pediatrics, 19,* 109-116.

Honkasalo, M. L., Kaprio, J., Winter, T., Phlic, K. H., Sillanpaa, M., & Koskenvuo, M. (1995). Migraine and concomitant symptoms among 8,167 adult twin pairs. *Headache, 35,* 70-78.

Jensen, V. K., Reiter, S. L., Martin, B. A., & Lee, A. L. (1998). *Chronic Headache in Adolescents: Empirical Support for a Somatoform Profile.* Unpublished manuscript, The Cleveland Clinic Foundation, Cleveland, OH.

Jensen, V. K., & Rothner, A. D. (1995). Chronic nonprogressive headaches in children and adolescents. *Seminars in Pediatric Neurology, 2,* 151-158.

Kovacs, M. (1992). *Children's Depression Inventory.* Toronto, Canada: Multi-Health Systems, Inc.

Labbé, E. E., & Williamson, D. A. (1983). Temperature biofeedback in the treatment of children with migraine headaches. *Journal of Pediatric Psychology, 8,* 317-326.

Labbé, E. E., & Williamson, D. A. (1984). Treatment of childhood migraine using autogenic feedback training. *Journal of Consulting and Clinical Psychology, 52,* 968-976.

Lachar, D. (1981). *Personality Inventory for Children-Revised.* Los Angeles, CA: Western Psychological Services.

Larsson, B., Bille, B., & Pederson, N. L. (1995). Genetic influence in headaches: A Swedish twin study. *Headache, 35,* 513-519.

Larsson, B., & Melin, L. (1986). Chronic headaches in adolescents: Treatment in a school setting with relaxation training as compared with information-contact and self-registration. *Pain, 25,* 325-336.

Larsson, B., & Melin, L. (1988). The psychological treatment of recurrent headache in adolescents - short-term outcome and its prediction. *Headache, 28*(3), 187-195.

Lipchik, G. L., & Holroyd, K. A. (1999). Behavior therapy for headaches. *The Clinical Psychologist, 52,* 3-6.

Maytal, J., Young, M., Schechter, A., & Lipton, R. B. (1997). Pediatric migraine and the International Headache Society (IHS) criteria. *Neurology, 48,* 602-607.

McGrath, P. J., Humphreys, P., Keene, D., Goodman, J. T., Lascelles, M. A., Cunningham, S. J., & Firestone, P. (1992). The efficacy and efficiency of a self-administered treatment for adolescent migraine. *Pain, 49,* 321-324.

Metsahonkala, L., Sillanpaa, M., & Tuominen, J. (1998). Social environment and headache in 8- to 9-year-old children: A follow-up study. *Headache, 38*(3), 222-228.

Morrison, D. P., & Price, W. H. (1989). The prevalence of psychiatric disorder among female new referrals to a migraine clinic. *Psychological Medicine, 19,* 919-925.

Mortimer, M. J., Kay, J., & Jaron, A. (1992). Epidemiology of headache and childhood migraine in an urban general practice using Ad Hoc, Vahlquist, and IHS criteria. *Developmental Medicine and Child Neurology, 34,* 1095-1101.

Newacheck, P. W., & Taylor, W. R. (1992). Childhood chronic illness: Prevalence, severity and impact. *American Journal of Public Health, 82*(3), 364-371.

Norton, P. J., Asmundon, G. J. G., Norton, G. R., & Craig, K. D. (1999). Growing pain: 10-year research trends in the study of chronic pain and headache. *Pain, 79,* 59-65.

Pine, D. S., Cohen, P., & Brook, J. (1996). The association between major depression and headache: Results of a longitudinal epidemiologic study in youth. *Journal of Child and Adolescent Psychopharmacology, 6,* 153-164.

Prensky, A. L., & Sommer, D. (1979). Diagnosis and treatment of migraine in children. *Neurology, 29,* 506-510.

Reynolds, C. R., & Kamphaus, R. W. (1992). *Behavior Assessment System for Children (BASC).* Circle Pines, MN: American Guidance Service.

Reynolds, C. R., & Richmond, B. O. (1985). *Revised Children's Manifest Anxiety Scale Manual.* Los Angeles: Western Psychological Services.

Richter, I. L., McGrath, P. J., Humphreys, P. J., Goodman, J. T., Firestone, P., & Keene, D. (1986). Cognitive and relaxation treatment of pediatric migraine. *Pain, 25,* 195-203.

Rothner, A. D. (1989). Headaches in children and adolescents. *The Clinical Journal of Pain, 5,* 67-75.

Sillanpaa, M. (1983). Prevalence of headache in prepuberty. *Headache, 23,* 10-14.

Stang, P. E., & Osterhaus, J. T. (1993). Impact of migraine in the United States: Data from the National Health Interview Survey. *Headache, 33,* 29-35.

Stang, P. E., Yanagihara, T., Swanson, J. W., Beard, C. M., O'Fallon, W. M., Guess, H. A., & Melton, L. J. (1992). Incidence of migraine headache: A population-based study in Olmsted County, Minnesota. *Neurology, 42,* 1657-1662.

Stewart, W., Breslau, N., & Keck, P. E. (1994). Comorbidity of migraine and panic disorder. *Neurology, 44*(Suppl. 7), S23-S27.

Tesler, M., Ward, J., Savedra, M., Wegner, C., & Gibbons, P. (1983). Developing an instrument for eliciting children's description of pain. *Perceptual and Motor Skills, 56,* 315-321.

Varni, J. W., Thompson, K. L., & Hanson, V. (1987). The Varni-Thompson Pediatric Pain Questionnaire: I. Chronic musculoskeletal pain in juvenile rheumatoid arthritis. *Pain, 28,* 27-38.

Williamson, D. A., Baker, J. D., & Cubic, B. A. (1993). Advances in pediatric headache research. *Advances in Clinical Child Psychology, 15,* 275-304.

Resources for Patients and Families

American Council for Headache Education (ACHE). Nonprofit physician-patient program focusing on headache prevention and treatment with resources for both patient and health professional. (Telephone: 609-423-0258; http://www.achenet.org/)

Bensen, H., & Klipper, M. K. (1990). *The Relaxation Response.* New York: Avon Publishers.

Davis, M., Eshelman, E. R., & McKay, M. (1998). *Relaxation & Stress Reduction Workbook.* Oakland, CA: New Harbinger.

Excedrin Headache Resource Center. A website run by the pharmaceutical manufacturer that includes patient learning modules, a sample headache diary, and information on diagnosis and treatment. (http://www.excedrin.com/)

Journal of the American Medical Association (JAMA) Migraine/Information Center. Resource produced by the JAMA that includes resources for both patients and professionals. (http://www.ama-assn.org/special/migraine/migraine/htm)

National Headache Foundation (NHF). Resource for patients and professionals regarding types of headaches, diagnosis, and management of all types of headaches. (Telephone: 800-NHF-5552; http://www.headaches.org/)

Pain.Com. An on-line resource for patients and professionals that includes an on-line journal and general pain information. (http://www.pain.com/)

Assessment and Treatment of PTSD in Motor Vehicle Accident Survivors

Jillian C. Shipherd, J. Gayle Beck, Jessica L. Hamblen, and Jennifer B. Freeman

Within the last 10 years, an increasing number of clients have presented to treatment centers seeking assistance for posttraumatic stress reactions. Although an abundant amount has been written on Posttraumatic Stress Disorder (PTSD; American Psychiatric Association [APA], 1994) and posttrauma adjustment, the wide variety of available treatment approaches (Carlson, 1997; Wilson & Keane, 1997) can lead to confusion about how to conceptualize and implement successful therapy for individuals with PTSD. This is especially true given the diverse range of traumas that have been discussed within this literature (e.g., sexual assault, natural disasters, childhood sexual abuse, combat, violent crime). In this contribution, we will outline a cognitive-behavioral treatment approach which is targeted at individuals who are experiencing PTSD following a serious motor vehicle accident (MVA). This treatment approach is modeled after an intervention developed by Blanchard and colleagues (Blanchard & Hickling, 1997) and can be used in either an individual or small group format. Although there are currently no large-scale studies that examine which treatments are most effective for MVA-related PTSD, preliminary reports indicate that this cognitive-behavioral approach is effective, even for individuals who experienced severe accidents and withstood painful, extensive injuries (Hickling & Blanchard, 1997; Shipherd et al., 1999). Prior to describing this treatment, background about the presentation of PTSD following a motor vehicle accident (MVA), assessment of the disorder, and conceptualization of treatment will be reviewed.

DESCRIPTION OF PTSD FOLLOWING A MOTOR VEHICLE ACCIDENT

Although millions of MVAs occur each year (National Safety Council, 1993), it has not been until fairly recently that there was recognition of the psychological sequelae of accidents. Early writings documented that people often experienced considerable depression, fear of driving, generalized anxiety, and related phobias following a serious MVA (e.g., Parker, 1977; S. Taylor & Koch, 1995). Recently, there has been a growing interest in studying these aspects of posttrauma recovery and their relationship to PTSD.

The essential features of PTSD, as outlined by the *Diagnostic and Statistical Manual of Mental Disorders* (*DSM-IV*; American Psychiatric Association, 1994) require exposure to a life event that involves actual or threatened death (or threat to physical or psychological integrity), where the individual's emotional response included intense fear, helplessness, or horror. In addition, a collection of symptoms must be present for at least 1 month following the trauma. These symptoms are organized into three clusters: (a) reexperiencing symptoms, (b) avoidance and numbing symptoms, and (c) symptoms indicative of increased physiological arousal (see Table 1 below). PTSD shares many features with other anxiety disorders, such as heightened physiological arousal, but is distinguished by unique symptoms, such as reexperiencing phenomena (e.g., flashbacks) and emotional numbing. To be given the diagnosis, the constellation of symptoms must be disruptive and/or disturbing to the client.

TABLE 1: Diagnostic Criteria for Posttraumatic Stress Disorder*

Criteria A
The individual has been exposed to a trauma in which the following two characteristics were present:

1. The person directly experienced or watched an event that involved actual or threatened harm, injury, or death, and
2. The person's response to this event included intense fear, helplessness, or horror.

Criteria B
The trauma is reexperienced repetitively, as evidenced by one of the following symptoms:

1. recurrent and distressing recollections of the trauma
2. recurrent and distressing dreams of the event
3. acting or feeling as if the trauma was reoccurring (e.g., flashbacks)
4. emotional distress at exposure to cues that resemble an aspect of the trauma
5. physical reactions (e.g., palpitations) at exposure to cues that resemble an aspect of the trauma

Criteria C
Stimuli associated with the trauma are avoided and a general numbing of responsiveness is present, as evidenced by three of the following symptoms:

1. efforts to avoid thoughts, feelings, or conversations associated with the trauma
2. efforts to avoid activities, places, or people that prompt recollections of the trauma
3. difficulty recalling an important aspect of the trauma
4. drastically reduced interest in significant activities
5. feeling detached or estranged from others
6. restricted emotional feelings
7. a sense of foreshortened future

Criteria D
Persistent increased physiological arousal, as evidenced by two of the following symptoms:

1. trouble falling or staying asleep
2. angry outbursts or irritability
3. trouble concentrating
4. hypervigilance
5. exaggerated startle response

*Consistent with criteria in the *Diagnostic and Statistical Manual for Mental Disorders* (4th ed.; American Psychiatric Association, 1994).

Current estimates suggest that 6% to 40% of people involved in serious MVAs will report posttrauma problems of sufficient magnitude to receive a diagnosis of PTSD (e.g., Blanchard & Hickling, 1997; Kessler et al., 1994). These figures suggest that MVA-related PTSD may actually be more prevalent than previously believed. Despite these prevalence estimates, the survivor with PTSD may feel isolated by their symptoms, particularly if outside observers believe the accident was not especially life-threatening or horrifying. This sense of isolation may contribute to secondary problems, such as depression or substance use disorders (e.g., Blanchard et al., 1995), which further complicates the treatment of these individuals. Although specific discussion of the effect of these comorbid problems on treatment of PTSD is beyond the scope of this contribution, it is important to note that many MVA survivors report additional problems in multiple domains of their lives. In addition to psychological concerns, survivors may face the loss of occupational skills owing to permanent injuries, significant changes in their marital/romantic relationships, legal challenges, and chronic pain stemming from injuries sustained during the MVA. Fortunately, the use of careful pretreatment evaluation, combined with a problem-focused cognitive-behavioral treatment, can be helpful for relieving the distress and impairment caused by PTSD in these individuals despite their complicated presentation.

THE ASSESSMENT OF MOTOR VEHICLE ACCIDENT SURVIVORS

The initial step in management of the MVA survivor is a comprehensive evaluation. In many instances, this can be best accomplished in conjunction with the client's managing physician, particularly in those cases where substantial bodily injury occurred and/or the client reports chronic pain. Relevant domains of psychosocial assessment of MVA survivors as described below include (a) evaluation of posttrauma symptomatology; (b) evaluation of overall psychological functioning, including the presence of comorbid psychiatric disorders; and (c) evaluation of psychosocial influences to medical problems.

Evaluation of Posttrauma Symptomatology

Assessment of posttrauma symptomatology generally begins by asking clients to provide a detailed description of their accident. It is important to learn how the accident occurred, the number of vehicles and people involved, and the extent of sustained injuries. In many cases, clients may provide a flat, "objective" account of their MVA, possibly as the result of having re-told the story many times to police, attorneys, medical personnel, and friends. Sometimes, MVA survivors will have difficulty recounting specific aspects of the MVA or will become distressed while describing their MVA. These occurrences should alert the clinician to the presence of PTSD symptomatology.

Additionally, it is crucial to assess the client's initial emotional response to the MVA. Although this may be underplayed by the client, it is extremely important to evaluate the client's emotional response during or immediately following the MVA, given the importance of this feature in the diagnostic criteria for PTSD. We have encountered MVA survivors who were not emotionally overwhelmed by the accident per se, but felt helpless or terrified by events which they were exposed to in the emergency room or during related experiences following the accident. Although these individuals technically do not meet diagnostic criteria for MVA-related PTSD (because they do not satisfy Criteria A as noted in Table 1), it is possible that they may report the full constellation of PTSD symptoms and may benefit from an adapted version of the treatment program outlined in this contribution.

Evaluation of specific PTSD symptoms can be extremely challenging with MVA survivors. In particular, clients may not be able to discriminate between symptoms that are attributable to PTSD and those which are attributable to other physical or psychological conditions. For example, difficulty sleeping could be attributable to PTSD or to other comorbid conditions such as chronic pain or depression. One venue for assessing PTSD symptoms that can be extremely useful in this regard is a semistructured interview. A number of PTSD-specific interviews exist, such as the PTSD Interview (Watson et al., 1991), the Structured Interview for PTSD (Davidson, Smith, & Kudler, 1989), and the Clinician Administered PTSD Scale (CAPS; Blake et al., 1990). Among these choices, our clear preference is the CAPS, because the majority of published work with MVA survivors has utilized this interview. Other advantages of the CAPS are the inclusion of questions regarding the effect of PTSD symptoms on social and occupational functioning and its established psychometric support (Weathers et al., 1992). Additionally, the CAPS is distinguished by inclusion of standardized prompts to evaluate the frequency as well as the severity of each PTSD symptom. The CAPS in its entirety may be too involved for use outside of a research setting, but the prompt questions can be useful in any context.

During evaluation of PTSD symptoms, one must consider all three clusters of symptoms (reexperiencing, avoidance and numbing, and increased physiological arousal). Although *DSM-IV* is clear about the specific number of symptoms within each cluster that are required for a diagnosis, research suggests that individuals who fall slightly short of these criteria may still manifest significant distress and interference (Blanchard et al., 1996). It is also important to recognize that subsyndromal clients may subsequently develop PTSD, Delayed Onset (Buckley, Blanchard, & Hickling, 1996). Thus, careful attention to the evaluation of posttrauma symptomatology is an essential first step in working with an MVA survivor.

In addition to evaluation through diagnostic interviews, PTSD symptoms can also be documented with self-report measures. Several available self-report measures are useful in the assessment of posttrauma symptoms. Included in this category are the Los Angeles Symptom Checklist (L. A. King et al., 1995), the Mississippi Scale, which has both combat and civilian versions (Keane, Caddell, & K. L. Taylor, 1988), the Impact of Events Scale (IES; Horowitz, Wilner, & Alvarez, 1979), the Posttraumatic Symptom Scale - Self Report (PSS-SR; Foa et al., 1993), and the PTSD sub-scale of the Symptom-Checklist-90-Revised (SCL-90-Revised; Saunders, Arata, & Kilpatrick, 1990). Two of these instruments, the PSS-SR and the IES, are particularly useful for the evaluation of MVA-related PTSD in a clinical setting. The PSS-SR has the advantage of providing a brief, diagnosis-based assessment of the frequency (within the previous 2 weeks) of the 17 symptoms of PTSD as defined by the *DSM-IV*. This measure has good reliability and validity and has been used with a variety of trauma populations. The IES is one of the most widely used PTSD instruments and assesses the frequency of subjective distress as measured by intrusive and avoidance symptoms related to PTSD. Although there are numerous other self-report measures which have been developed for use with individuals with PTSD (e.g., Borkovec, Castonguay, & Newman, 1997; Wilson & Keane, 1997), there is little literature examining whether these scales are particularly valuable for individuals with MVA-related PTSD. As such, it is difficult to make recommendations about their utility with this population.

Evaluation of Overall Psychological Functioning

It is not surprising that many MVA survivors report numerous mental health problems. For example, the rate of additional psychiatric disorders in individuals with PTSD is significantly higher than in the general population (Kessler et al., 1995) and does not necessarily reflect psychopathology that existed before the trauma. As summarized by Blanchard and Hickling (1997), mood and anxiety disorders are quite common among samples of MVA survivors who are seeking psychological assistance. In our own work, we have noted relatively high rates of comorbid Major Depressive Disorder, Generalized Anxiety Disorder, and Specific Phobias of enclosed places (claustrophobia). In some respects, the presence of these comorbid diagnoses makes intuitive sense. For example, many MVA survivors report feeling as if they are a burden to family members and feel guilty because "a stronger person would be over this by now." As a result, depressed affect and social isolation often are seen in these clients. In addition, lifestyle changes, such as loss of employment, seem to contribute to heightened levels of generalized anxiety by fostering worries about finances, family functioning, and other related issues. Finally, some MVA survivors report claustrophobic-type fears, which are attributable to circumstances such as being strapped to a backboard immediately following the MVA or repeated experiences in a Magnetic Resonance Imaging (MRI) device. Clearly, it is important to evaluate comorbid disorders in these clients, particularly as these related issues may impact treatment.

In addition to comorbid Axis I diagnoses, a set of unique differential diagnosis issues arise in this population. Many MVA survivors (with and without PTSD) avoid driving in some fashion. This avoidance can be subtle, such as refusing to drive by the scene of the accident, or generalized, such as refusing to drive on any busy street. When MVA survivors drive, they often report feeling anxious and are hyper-alert. Although these are PTSD symptoms, they are also symptoms of a Specific Phobia of driving. Therefore, the clinician must make a determination as to which disorder better accounts for the avoidance symptoms. The presence of a traumatic event that precipitates the avoidance is not a determining factor in diagnosing PTSD rather than Specific Phobia. In fact, if the presenting symptoms primarily involve avoidance and do not include reexperiencing or numbing symptoms, it is likely that a diagnosis of Specific Phobia is more appropriate. Similar issues arise when considering other related anxiety problems, such as Panic Disorder, Social Phobia, and Generalized Anxiety Disorder. The use of careful questioning can facilitate a better understanding of the underlying fears and thus lead to an accurate diagnosis.

In addition to diagnostic interviewing, several standard self-report measures are useful when assessing comorbid symptoms in MVA survivors. For example, the Beck Depression Inventory (BDI; A. T. Beck et al., 1961) is designed to measure the behavioral manifestations of depression, and the State Trait Anxiety Inventory (STAI; Spielberger, Gorsuch, & Lushene, 1970) measures both transient and general levels of anxiety. These measures provide a quick screen for negative and/or anxious mood and can be administered periodically throughout treatment as a means to index the radiating effects of therapy.

Evaluation of Psychosocial Influences to Medical Problems

We recommend that clients with chronic pain and related medical problems be referred to appropriate specialists for medical management. However, it is important to recognize that there are instances where psychosocial factors can influence an individual's medical condition. Because many MVA survivors experience injuries with chronic effects, it is important to examine whether psychosocial factors are impacting a client's physical recovery. Blanchard and Hickling (1997) have noted that clients who report PTSD throughout a 12-month interval show less remission and recovery from their injuries. They posit that "long-lasting, nagging injuries . . . seem to impede psychological recovery" (p. 169). However, we argue that in addition to chronic pain complaints slowing psychological recovery, it is equally plausible that the reverse relationship is true. Thus, chronic PTSD symptomatology may impede physical recovery, particularly if psychiatric symptoms reduce a client's motivation to be compliant with physical therapy or rehabilitation efforts.

To date, no studies have sought to explore how PTSD and chronic injuries interrelate in MVA survivors. Although many therapists are aware of the profound effect of mood on the immune response (e.g., Irwin, 1988), the time required for wounds to heal (Kiecolt-Glaser et al., 1998), and related facets of physical functioning, it is important to be aware that MVA survivors may show changes in their physical functioning that parallel psychological changes. Depending on the client, one may want to utilize a standardized pain inventory, such as the Oswestry Low Back Pain Disability Questionnaire (Fairebank et al., 1980) or the Sickness Impact Profile (Roland & Martin, 1983). These measures provide a rapid means to evaluate a client's ongoing pain and disability, factors that may be important in determining the timing of specific components of treatment.

Thus, the initial evaluation of a MVA survivor may require a particularly thorough assessment. Specifically, careful psychiatric evaluation of Axis I disorders such as PTSD, related anxiety disorders, and depression is necessary, as well as a broad psychosocial evaluation. Finally, consideration of the role of medical problems may also be necessary, particularly for the client with considerable injuries and long-term disability. Ideally, this thorough assessment can help to refine the cognitive-behavioral treatment outlined below.

TREATMENT OF PTSD IN MOTOR VEHICLE ACCIDENT SURVIVORS

Treatment of PTSD in MVA survivors can seem like a daunting task within the context of the comorbid complaints described previously. However, our experiences have shown that a focused approach to treatment can assist clients in regaining emotional stability. Several important issues are reviewed in the following sections, including the underlying conceptualization of the disorder upon which the treatment program is based, a description of the approach to treatment, advice about overcoming common obstacles in the treatment of MVA-related PTSD, and an overview of the skills included in the treatment protocol.

Conceptualization of PTSD

According to the *DSM-IV* (APA, 1994), a diagnosis of PTSD is based on the development of symptoms from three clusters following the experience of a traumatic event (see Table 1, p. 136). However, our treatment program is based on a conceptualization of PTSD that includes four clusters of symptoms and follows the formulation originally presented by Blanchard and Hickling in 1997. These clusters include (a) cognitive symptoms such as intrusive thoughts, (b) behavioral symptoms such as avoidance of trauma cues, (c) physical symptoms such as hyperarousal, and (d) emotional symptoms, which can include emotional numbing and/or an increase in negative emotions such as irritability. We have found that clients readily adapt to this approach because they are experiencing significant interference from their emotional symptoms and classify them as worthy of direct intervention. In fact, for many clients, it is the emotional detachment and anger that prompts them to seek psychological counseling. This conceptualization of PTSD drives the treatment approach of addressing each of the four symptom clusters with specific techniques.

Approach to Treatment

This approach to the treatment of PTSD is based on teaching cognitive-behavioral strategies to assist clients in the management of their symptoms. Within the context of providing clients with the tools to master their own recovery, homework is essential. Through practice via homework, clients become experts at managing their own symptomatology. However, this approach is not designed to downplay the importance of the therapist or the therapeutic relationship. If the change that occurs through cognitive-behavioral treatment could be explained by simply making lifestyle changes, then PTSD sufferers would have made those changes long before coming to the therapist's office.

A skill-building approach can be empowering for MVA survivors who may have struggled for months or years to regain pre-accident functioning. Many MVA survivors feel as though their lives have been destroyed by events outside of their control (S. Taylor & Koch, 1995). The therapist can guide survivors down the path of recovery by providing techniques to improve their day-to-day living situation. Some expertise is needed in guiding clients through skill acquisition, as is the case with most cognitive-behavioral programs. In particular, the therapist should be attentive to subtle avoidance behaviors or other modifications of these therapeutic skills which diminish their effectiveness. The work in session includes teaching the rationale behind each of the skills, practicing the skills to ensure comprehension, and problem solving obstacles to their application. Each of these components is vital to the mastery of the individual skills.

It is important to recognize that all skills will not be equally effective for all clients. Some clients will find that certain skills are most useful while other techniques do not drastically improve their symptoms. Therapists should begin treatment with the expectation that all clients will attempt to learn each new skill and then determine which techniques are most helpful in their situation. In this way, clients can feel assured that if there are skills that they "just don't get" or that are less effective for them, the treatment package as a whole can still be beneficial.

Overcoming Obstacles Stemming from PTSD Impairment

Clients with PTSD may have difficulty learning the skills taught in session, in part due to interference from the PTSD symptomatology itself. For example, the presence of intrusive thoughts, sleeplessness, and hyperarousal may decrease a client's ability to focus and concentrate when learning new skills. Thus, the use of numerous handouts can be extremely helpful. With each new objective discussed in session, clients should be provided with a handout that describes in detail the overall concept. Written directions that describe each of the skills in a "how to" approach and include detailed descriptions of homework tasks are helpful for many clients. Similarly, audiotapes of relaxation procedures, imaginal exposure scenes, and any other in-session practices can be helpful in reminding the clients how to go about conducting their practice between sessions.

Overview of the Skills

Each of the skills described below is a part of this four-pronged treatment approach. As clients are educated about their symptomatology, skills are provided to address each of the areas where they are experiencing difficulty. Thus, the underlying basis for working with these clients is psychoeducation about the symptoms of PTSD. It is important for them to hear from a mental health provider that these symptoms are a normal response to trauma (such as MVAs). Many MVA survivors believe that they should be "over it" by now. It can be meaningful for clients to discover that the first 3 to 4 months following a MVA are often marked by PTSD symptoms which decline as a part of the natural recovery process (Kilpatrick, Veronen, & Resick, 1979; Rothbaum & Foa, 1993; Rothbaum et al., 1992; Steketee & Foa, 1987). This phase of recovery is considered acute PTSD in the *DSM-IV* nomenclature (APA, 1994). However, the large number of car accident survivors who continue to experience difficulty with these symptoms for several months or even years afterward are the most likely candidates for intervention. Continued distress and interference from PTSD symptomatology beyond 3 months posttrauma qualifies for a diagnosis of chronic PTSD (APA, 1994). Explanation of the symptoms of PTSD in the normalizing context of psychoeducation can also assist in building rapport with clients who already may have seen several different health care professionals and not had their concerns about emotional recovery addressed. This type of education can reassure clients that they are not "going crazy" and that there is an effective treatment available to address each of the symptom clusters as described below. An overview of the session organization is provided in Table 2 (p. 142).

Exposure

Exposure is designed to address the behavioral symptom of avoidance. Avoidance can be overt and readily apparent such as refusing to drive, or can be more subtle such as attempts to avoid thinking about the MVA.

The Accident Description. As one of the first steps, clients are asked to write out a detailed accident description. Although clients have been asked to describe their accident numerous times prior to beginning treatment, this may be the first occasion when they are purposely attempting to recall details of the incident for their own benefit. In this account, emotions, sensory experiences, consequences, and other details are just as important as the basic facts of the accident. The goal of this exposure is to have clients generate a complete version of their traumatic event. In general, more dramatic treatment effects can be realized with more detailed accounts, as the vivid imagery facilitates habituation of anxiety. In some cases, pertinent details may be remembered which become salient in overcoming unrealistic fears. One example of this is illustrated in the case of Sarah.*

> Sarah was involved in a motor vehicle accident when she was 8 months pregnant. Her truck was struck on the driver's side door by a car attempting to cross through an intersection. Sarah was trapped behind the steering wheel in her damaged truck for some time before the police extracted her from the vehicle. Although she had suffered a lower back injury, her primary concern at the time of her MVA was for the health of her unborn child. One year later when she came into treatment at our clinic, she reported significant PTSD symptomatology and chronic back pain. In addition, she reported a continued fear that the MVA may have harmed her baby in ways that could not be detected, but that would manifest as her child grew up. These fears were most pronounced when changing her baby's diapers and would sometimes precipitate crying spells. Although it was clear that her fear was somehow connected to her MVA, it was not until she had completed her accident description that her fears were explainable. When asked to complete her MVA description, Sarah remembered for the first time that during her accident a container of baby powder had exploded

---

*Names and identifying characteristics in all case examples have been changed to protect confidentiality.

TABLE 2: Overview of Sessions

Each session is about 90 minutes and begins with a review of the previous week, including homework, and ends with assignments for the coming week.

Session 1
A. Introduction to the therapy setting
B. Review of information discussed in the initial intake
C. Education about the symptoms of anxiety and PTSD
D. Overview of treatment including strategies to be covered
E. Homework assignment - Write out a detailed accident description.

Session 2
A. Reading the accident description
B. 16-muscle PMR
C. Homework assignments - Read MVA description two times daily, use 16-muscle PMR two times daily.

Session 3
A. Reading the accident description
B. Discussion of memories and avoidance
C. 7-muscle PMR
D. Homework assignments - Read MVA description two times daily, use 7-muscle PMR two times daily. Develop hierarchy.

Session 4
A. Learn imaginal and in vivo exposure
B. Learn cued relaxation
C. Homework assignments - Low level in vivo exposure two times daily, medium level imaginal exposure two times daily, use cue-controlled relaxation two times daily.

Session 5
A. Introduction to changing thought: Coping self-statements
B. Adding coping self-statements to imaginal exposure
C. Learn relaxation by recall
D. Homework assignments - Medium level in vivo exposure one time daily, medium-high level imaginal exposure two times daily using coping self-statements, use relaxation by recall as needed.

Session 6
A. Developing alternative explanations: The A-B-C-D method
B. Homework assignments - Medium level in vivo exposure one time daily, medium-high imaginal exposure two times daily, apply A-B-C-D method daily.

Session 7
A. Cognitive method: Logical errors
B. Using thought skills during imaginal exposure - moving up the hierarchy
C. Homework assignments - Medium level in vivo exposure one time daily, highest level imaginal exposure two times daily, using A-B-C-D records, address logical errors daily.

Session 8
A. Cognitive method: Decatastrophizing
B. Applying decatastrophizing to imaginal and in vivo exposure
C. Homework assignments - Medium-high in vivo exposure one time daily, highest level imaginal exposure two times daily, address catastrophic thoughts daily.

Session 9
A. Summary and review of cognitive techniques
B. Taking care of yourself: Scheduling and social support
C. Homework assignments - High level in vivo exposure one time daily, highest level imaginal exposure two times daily, schedule at least one additional social activity each day, reward self for completion.

Session 10
A. Depressed feelings
B. The importance of pleasant events
C. Homework assignments - High level in vivo exposure one time daily, schedule several activities each day for the purpose of mood elevation, including social activities, reward self for completion.

Session 11
A. Understanding irritability and anger
B. Applying A-B-C-D technique and assertiveness
C. Homework assignments - Highest level in vivo exposure one time daily, apply assertiveness and A-B-C-D method to daily interactions.

Session 12
A. Review of treatment
B. Discussion of termination issues

> and had saturated the inside of her truck with the distinctive powdery smell. It was not until she wrote out her accident description that it made sense to her why changing her baby's diaper was such a difficult task. Bolstered by the knowledge that she was not "going crazy," a series of exposure exercises remedied her fear.

It is normal for clients to want to avoid thinking about their accident (or certain aspects of it). However, it is one of the most dramatic steps that clients can take in facing their traumatic event and is a vital part of their emotional recovery. Research has shown that writing about traumas provides a method of emotional processing which helps the client come to terms with the traumatic event within the context of their own individual experiences (e.g., Pennebaker, 1989). Although this is a difficult task for the majority of clients, we often see dramatic changes in anxiety levels following repeated exposure to the detailed accident description. In the case described previously and for many others, this detailed account not only assists the client in regaining a sense of control over the event but also provides the clinician with beneficial details from the MVA that may have otherwise gone unreported.

It is important to understand that clients will be reluctant to engage in this process, yet the benefits from this type of exposure are clear. We ask clients to read their accident description out loud repeatedly until their anxiety is reduced to at least half of their initial rating on a 0 to 100 scale. We often pair the relaxation exercises with reading the accident description both in session and for daily homework. In this way, the relaxation exercises can aid the client in reducing the arousal brought on by reading their accident description.

Building a Hierarchy. Hierarchies are a useful tool when planning a strategy for how clients can learn to face feared situations. They consist of a rank-ordered list of avoided activities ranging in the amount of anxiety that the situations produce for each client based on a 0 to 100 scale. At the top of the list (100) are the most feared and avoided situations, such as driving by the accident scene. At the low end of the list are situations that are endured with some distress. At the midrange are combinations of activities that are frequently avoided but occasionally endured with distress or entered into only while accompanied by others.

Although constructing a list of avoided activities can seem like a straightforward task, several revisions usually are required. Most clients are readily able to generate examples of avoided activities for the top of the hierarchy. But clients often find it more difficult to generate examples for each of the gradiated levels. Typically, hierarchies consist of numerous divisions, by 10-point increments. The most common pitfall when developing a hierarchy is the inclusion of a situation that actually is comprised of several steps at different stages of the hierarchy. It is important to have numerous examples in order to insure that the exposure gradient is gradual. An incomplete hierarchy, especially one that only has examples of the most difficult situations, can lead to feelings of being overwhelmed and may result in failure once exposure begins. Instead, it is best to break more difficult situations down into several exposure steps as in the next example.

> Mark's MVA occurred at a fairly busy intersection of the city during the early evening rush hour. Since the accident, he has not needed to confront this intersection since it is not a route that he typically drives. At the top of the hierarchy, he initially put "driving past the accident scene." However, with the assistance of his therapist, he was able to expand his hierarchy by making his tasks more specific, including the following:
>
> 100 - Drive alone past the scene of the accident during evening rush hour
> 95 - Drive with his wife past the scene of the accident during evening rush hour
> 90 - Drive alone past the scene of the accident at a nonpeak time
> 80 - Drive with his wife past the scene of the accident at a nonpeak time

Hierarchies often need to be revised several times during the course of treatment. Some situations may initially be placed too low on the hierarchy and after several attempts at exposure, it is discovered that the activity should have a higher ranking. In these cases, the exposure assigned for homework should be switched to an item that is actually closer to the targeted level of difficulty and the situation attempted in the unsuccessful exposure should be given a new ranking. Similarly, if items are rated as more difficult than they actually are, then they will be easily mastered within days of the assignment. Clients should then be encouraged to move up to an item at the desired level for the remainder of the weekly homework practices.

Imaginal Exposure. Unfortunately, when people experience traumatic situations, the overwhelming fear associated with the accident also can become associated with reminders of the accident (Foa & Kozak, 1986). Because these emotions have become associated with specific behaviors such as driving, it is likely that your clients will have a long list of things they avoid or are able to do only while experiencing distress. Avoidance is part of the behavioral cluster of symptoms and is common in people with PTSD. This cognitive-behavioral program includes both imaginal and in vivo (real life) exposure in a two-stage process. The first stage is to confront situations in imagination. Once the first stage is mastered, the second stage is to test the situations in real life. Confronting difficult situations repeatedly in imagination helps clients feel comfortable when the time comes to attempt the process in real life. In this way, clients can rely on their own mastery experiences when confronting avoided situations in real life. Many clients have developed elaborate schemes to avoid difficult situations, as the case of Beth illustrates:

> Several years ago, Beth was struck from behind while waiting to make a left-hand turn. The person in the car behind her reportedly never applied his brakes. The impact was strong enough to knock Beth's car into two lanes of oncoming traffic where she was struck again by an oncoming car. Since the accident, Beth initially reported that she had no difficulty driving, although it took her longer to get places. When questioned about this, Beth revealed that she had developed elaborate routes of getting to various destinations. These pathways included numerous right-hand turns that eventually circled back to where she was going, but prevented her from making left-hand turns. Sometimes these routes took as long as an additional hour for her to arrive at a local destination.

Perhaps one of the best ways to learn that you really are safe in any given situation is to test out the situation. However, it would be unrealistic to expect that Beth would be able to begin making left-hand turns in real life without first mastering this situation in imagination. Imaginal exposure is a useful tool because it allows the therapist to guide the client through a mastery experience. This is particularly important in situations that are either impossible to create in real life (e.g., the original accident) or which are too scary initially for the client to confront in real life. It may have taken clients some time to perfect their avoidance of situations that remind them of their accident, so it will also take some time to un-learn this fear and avoidance. The best way to change a client's reaction to any given situation is by confronting the feared environment in a controlled manner.

In Vivo Exposure. Exposures that occur in real life (in vivo) are more frightening to most clients than imaginal exposures. Imaginal exposure is a useful tool for learning to confront feared situations. However, real-life exposure can be an even more powerful learning experience. Often, clients are reluctant to believe that their anxiety will reduce if they stay in a feared situation. However, once they are able to stay in a feared situation long enough for the process of habituation to take place, clients are often excited by their progress and become tempted to face more difficult challenges. In these situations, it is important to stress the reasoning behind gradual exposure, as clients will sometimes "bite off more than they can chew" and attempt their most difficult exposure following success with a lower-level exposure.

Typically, in vivo exposure begins at a very low hierarchy item. The therapist should identify an item from the hierarchy that the client reports already entering with some regularity but that creates distress (e.g., 10-30 on the hierarchy). By assigning a low-level exposure first, clients can gain a feeling of mastery over the skill and an appreciation for how quickly their fear can subside. Simple exercises such as a daily assignment of driving around the block can bolster the client for gradually moving up their list of feared situations.

Relaxation

The relaxation procedures described next are taught to address the physical symptoms of PTSD. Relaxation lowers the overall physiological arousal of clients through regular daily practice and provides a tool to utilize in stressful situations.

Progressive Muscle Relaxation (PMR). The skill taught to combat physical symptoms of PTSD (e.g., muscle tension) is Progressive Muscle Relaxation (PMR; Bernstein & Borkovec, 1973). This well-established technique is a useful tool for teaching clients about their own cycles of tension and relaxation. It is an active form of relaxation wherein clients are taught the difference between tension and relaxation. Initially, clients are asked first by the therapist and later by audiotaped instructions, to tense and then relax each of 16 major muscle groups. For each muscle group, tension onset begins at the therapist's request with the word "now" and is held for 5 to 7 seconds before instructions are given to relax the muscle group. The therapist uses a calm, soothing tone as he or she slowly guides clients through the tension-relaxation cycle. In subsequent sessions, PMR is made more portable for the client by combining muscle groups. Next, relaxation becomes associated with a cue, such as the word "Relax," which signals a remembrance of the feeling of tension draining away. Then, the tension phase of the procedure is eliminated while the cue for relaxation remains. In this way, the sensation of relaxation becomes quite accessible for the client at any given moment. For therapists who are unfamiliar with this procedure, a review of the original description (Bernstein & Borkovec, 1973) would be useful.

Despite the fact that treatment cases may include individuals who are suffering from chronic pain, our experiences indicate that these individuals are often able to complete the PMR exercises without modification. However, for clients who experience pain during this procedure, instructions should be given to stop tensing these specific muscles and to participate only in the relaxation component.

Cognitive Techniques

The cognitive techniques described below are a set of tools that clients can use to address maladaptive thoughts that may be contributing to the cycle of fear surrounding trauma-related cues. The identification of maladaptive thoughts is often the most difficult part of working with MVA survivors. In treatment, clients frequently remark that these thoughts are difficult to identify due both to their automatic nature and to the entrenched belief that negative outcomes are likely to occur in any given situation. Thus, these approaches require consistent practiced application to ensure a shift in the underlying maladaptive thoughts associated with MVA-related PTSD.

Coping Self-Statements. As an initial step toward explaining how cognitive skills can be valuable in combating anxiety, coping self-statements are useful. These statements are described as "the things you say to yourself to get through difficult situations." Often, these are positive reminders or affirmations of individual strengths. Clients are encouraged to generate examples of statements that they can utilize at three different time points. The first time point is when clients need to prepare for potentially stressful situations. For example, "This situation is not impossible - I can handle this." The second time point is when they are actually in the stressful situation and need to apply coping strategies. For example, "I'm in control" or "One step at a time." The third time point for applying coping self-statements is after the stressful situation is over. These statements generally serve as rewards such as "I knew I could handle it" or "I made a good effort." Individualized coping self-statements can also center around religious themes, the support of family and friends, or on individual assets. In each case, these statements are personalized and clients are encouraged to make them as user-friendly as possible. For an individual who has difficulty recalling these statements during times of stress, the use of index cards or Post-it notes as prompts may increase the accessibility of coping self-statements. In this way, clients have a readily available tool that can work well for a "quick fix" before, during, and after stressful situations.

Developing Alternative Explanations (A-B-C-D Method). This technique requires clients to challenge their previously held beliefs in order to expand the number of possible ways of looking at any one particular situation. It has been adapted from other cognitive interventions such as those used in the treatment of irrational beliefs (e.g., Ellis & Harper, 1975). The focus of this intervention is on unraveling the interrelationship between thoughts about a situation and the accompanying emotional responses. The initial step in changing an individual's feelings about a situation is to recognize the role that his or her thoughts play in the experience of anxiety. This relationship often can be difficult to unravel because emotional reactions happen so quickly. Thus, clients are told that in order to determine what is happening in these situations, they will need to try to slow things down in their own minds, so they can identify the elements of their reaction.

The first part of this process is the identification of Activating events (A's). These are situations where clients notice that they are feeling an increase in anxiety or discomfort. Using homework forms, clients are encouraged to identify situations where they become upset. Step 2 is to identify the Beliefs (B's) that clients have about the situation. This step can be one of the most difficult because it is unlikely that your clients will be used to considering what beliefs they are having about these stressful situations. Examples include thoughts such as "I've escaped being killed once but I won't be so lucky next time." Step 3 is often the easiest part, which is to list out the Consequences (C's). These consist of the emotions that your clients are experiencing about the activating event. Typical feelings may include emotions such as sad, anxious, scared, or angry. For clients who had difficulty identifying their underlying beliefs (B's), the types of feelings they list at this point can serve as clues for their underlying thoughts. The last step is to Develop alternative thoughts (D's) for each of the beliefs listed in the B's. Clients are encouraged to challenge the thoughts that they listed in Step 2 by considering them as hypotheses rather than facts, and to generate alternative thoughts that are just as likely to be true. Alternative thoughts could include, "Most accidents don't involve someone getting killed; if something bad happens it would probably be minor" or "I have been able to handle lots of things so far. I am a strong person." By developing alternative explanations, the client can begin to regain a sense of control over their emotions and to develop alternative views to the previously held anxious beliefs.

Logical Errors. Once clients begin to become accustomed to identifying their own maladaptive thoughts, some patterns may begin to emerge. PTSD often leads clients to make specific predictions about the future that are based on faulty logic. These predictions are called Logical Errors (e.g., A. T. Beck et al., 1979). Essentially, when clients are anxious, they are likely to rely on distorted ways of perceiving situations. A useful analogy is that clients view these situations through colored lenses. These lenses lead them to perceive things differently than they actually are. Thus, clients' experience of situations become "colored" by their anxious thoughts. Due to the experience of feeling frightened and out of control in their MVA, it is likely that driving situations will be most affected by the "colored lenses." Once identified, patterns of faulty logic such as filtering, all-or-none thinking, overgeneralizing, and personalization can be easily remedied (see Table 3, p. 147). Once clients are shown their predisposition toward making specific logical errors and shown how to combat these thoughts, they can more readily identify errors and correct them. Intervention is based on the specific type of logical error, as exemplified in the case of Brian.

> Brian would often come into sessions flustered by the drive into the treatment center. On several occasions, he reported that he was considering dropping out of treatment because the drive was too stressful. "People drive like maniacs in this town," he would say. "The drive here is awful, the cars must be going about 80 miles per hour and it's terrible the way they race past other cars without a care for who might get hurt."

TABLE 3: Logical Errors and Their Solutions

Type of Error	Solution
FILTERING - Characterized by tunnel vision, looking at only one element of a situation to the exclusion of everything else. Picking out a single detail instead of seeing the larger picture. *Key words: terrible, awful, disgusting, horrible.*	WIDEN YOUR PERSPECTIVE - For example: If you believe that you are going to be in a car accident because the cars around you are driving too fast, widen your perspective and realize that it is only the cars in the outside lane that are going fast.
POLARIZED THINKING - Insistence on dichotomous choices; perception of everything in terms of black or white, extremes, with very little room for middle ground. *Key words: either, or; if not x, then y.*	REMIND YOURSELF OF THE GRAY AREA - For example: If you believe that driving is not a safe means of travel, remind yourself of the gray area and remember that accidents are relatively infrequent.
OVERGENERALIZATION - Making broad, generalized conclusions based on a single incident or piece of evidence. Often couched in terms of absolute statements: "I'll never be able to drive safely again." Conclusions are based on one or two pieces of evidence and everything else is ignored. *Key words: all, every, none, never, always, everybody.*	REMEMBER EXCEPTIONS - Try to remember the specific instances that don't fit the generalization. For example: Try to remember all the times you have driven and not had an accident.
PERSONALIZATION - The tendency to relate everything to yourself. Major aspect is the habit of continually comparing yourself to others. "I'll never be able to be as comfortable on the road as he or she is." Basic thinking error is that you interpret every experience as a clue to your worth, skill, and value. *Key words: I'm not as. . . . I'm worse than. . . .*	NOTICE ALTERNATIVES - Try to determine what other people or factors might be responsible. For example: If you believe that your accident was all your fault, try to remember to determine what other people or factors might be responsible for the accident.
SHOULDS - Operate from a list of inflexible rules about how you should act and feel. As a result, you're often in a position of judging and finding fault. People irritate you. *Key words: should, ought.*	BE FLEXIBLE - Remind yourself to be flexible with the rules. For example: If you frequently say to yourself that you should feel better about the accident by now, remind yourself to be flexible with the rules and remember that you are making progress in treatment.

With some encouragement, Brian was able to realize that this type of thinking was an example of a logical error. Specifically, he decided that he was filtering his perceptions of driving to session. With practice, Brian learned to widen his perspective when driving and decided the following:

> "I guess what was happening is that I was just focusing on the one or two drivers that were scaring me. In reality, most of the other people on the road were going about the speed limit. In fact, the drive here is actually a pretty one since I drive past the river on the way in. I guess I was letting my fears get in the way of seeing how things really are."

Thus, Brian was able to see that his perception of the drive to the session was being colored by his negative interpretation of the situation. In effect, he was focused on the parts of the drive that were frightening without recognizing the positive aspects (e.g., most drivers were traveling at safe speeds, there was a beautiful view, etc.).

Decatastrophizing. One specific type of logical error that is particularly salient in MVA survivors is catastrophic thinking. Thus, we advise addressing this type of error seperately. Because these clients have experienced a traumatic event, they often believe that traumatic events occur more frequently than what prevalence data supports. For example, these clients are likely to believe that they will be injured or die in a future accident. In reality, the most frequent type of accident is the classic "fender bender," where injuries tend to be mild and there is only minor damage to the vehicles. Generating a realistic example of a typical MVA can be a useful experience for clients because it is a technique that stops them from predicting the worst and helps them to realize that most car accidents may be upsetting and annoying, but are not catastrophic events. Be aware that clients' initial attempts at generating an example of a "typical" car accident are likely to include reports of severe injury or car damage. The therapist's role is to challenge the likelihood of these occurrences to insure that clients come up with a truly realistic example. This example then can be used as an imaginal exposure scene. Correcting the client's perceptions of the type of accident that is likely to occur, along with bolstering their perceptions of their ability to deal with an accident, is the most effective approach with these clients.

Emotions

The techniques listed next are designed to address the emotional symptoms of PTSD. Each technique assists clients in managing negative emotions and increasing their experience of positive emotions.

Anger and Irritability. As mentioned earlier, anger is a symptom of PTSD. This symptom also can become compounded when issues such as chronic pain are present. Typically, people find anger to be a difficult emotion, perhaps because it is socially unacceptable to act on angry feelings. As a result, clients sometimes report feeling guilty about feeling angry. The approach described below teaches skills designed to manage anger in two different types of scenarios. In the first case, the client may believe that their anger is disproportionate to the given situation. In the second case, clients believe that their level of anger is appropriate, but they are unsure of how to express their feelings in a productive way.

The first skill applied to anger is the cognitive skill of the A-B-C-D method. This skill (as outlined previously) assists clients in combating anger in situations where the response is not appropriate. This approach encourages clients to combat irrational angry thoughts by developing alternative explanations. In this way, the client is reminded that their response (anger) to the situation (activating event or A) is guided by their beliefs (B's). By treating their beliefs as hypotheses rather than facts, it is possible to come up with other explanations or ways of looking at the situation. These new thoughts then influence the response to the situation and lessen angry feelings.

The second skill is applicable when anger is an appropriate reaction. This skill encourages clients to express their anger in socially acceptable ways that will maintain open communication with friends and family members. Feelings of anger can serve as a signal that a problematic situation has been encountered and can be an energizing force toward seeking a resolution. Within this context, clients are reminded that an assertive, rather than aggressive, response can help them regain a sense of control over the situation (e.g., Alberti & Emmons, 1982). In this way, others will be able to understand the client's needs and the lines of communication will remain open.

Depression. Depressed feelings are frequently reported by MVA survivors, as they adjust to changes in lifestyle that often accompany recovery. Unfortunately, this anticipated expression of depressed mood could become problematic if mood changes persist and/or if intense feelings of anhedonia, hopelessness, or despair arise. Interference often is noted in several areas including work performance, leisure activities, and interpersonal relationships.

One way of conceptualizing depression is a very simple but a powerful concept originally developed by Lewinsohn and colleagues (Lewinsohn & Clarke, 1984). In this model, depression is explained by an imbalance between negative and positive outcomes from interactions with the environment. At its core, this concept proposes that when an individual has more positive social interactions than negative, then he or she will feel good. Conversely, more negative interactions with the environment leads to feeling bad. One benefit of utilizing this straightforward approach to the conceptualization of depressed affect in MVA survivors is that it provides an uncomplicated approach to alleviation of the symptoms.

Because the underlying explanation for depressed mood is an imbalance between negative and positive interactions with the environment, the goal of treatment includes two components. The first is to magnify the quantity of positive interactions with the environment. This is most easily accomplished by scheduling additional pleasant activities on a daily basis. For individuals who have experienced a dramatic reduction in the type of activities which they are able to perform (due to physical injuries), a list of activities which they still enjoy should be generated which includes suggestions of new activities to try. The second goal is to improve the quality of positive interactions with the environment. This can be achieved either through encouraging clients to focus on positive feelings and intensify them through scheduling larger occasional rewards (e.g., going to the movies), or by rewarding themselves on a daily basis when they have positive interactions (e.g., praise self).

Although this approach to fighting depression may sound easy, it is sometimes difficult to implement. Implementation can be especially difficult if the client perceives the skill as "being selfish." Surprisingly, not all clients will be comfortable making happiness a priority in their day-to-day lives. This may be especially true for individuals whose life circumstances make this task difficult (e.g., single parents). Fortunately, the tasks assigned when learning this skill often include activities with other people, which may make this skill more palatable to clients who are initially uncomfortable with the concept. Similarly, clients are sometimes reluctant to implement rewards upon completion of intrinsically rewarding activities for the purpose of mood elevation. However, for individuals who seldom take time during their day for enjoyable activities, rewards can be an important method to increase the likelihood of engaging in pleasant activities in the future. Providing this rationale may assist clients in using rewards as a useful short-term tool to assist in the maintenance of treatment gains.

Emotional Numbing. Typically, people recognize that difficult times are easier to get through when they can rely on people around them. However, it is often difficult for MVA survivors to reach out to other people. This can be especially true for people with PTSD because one of the diagnostic features is feeling detached from other people and experiencing a restricted range of emotional responses. Unfortunately, isolation can only compound the problem by encouraging feelings of being detached and "out of sync" with friends and family. In the long run, the symptom of feeling distant from others becomes a self-fulfilling prophecy. We encourage clients to overcome their feelings of numbness and detachment by increasing the frequency of direct social activities such as team sports, or talking on the phone. Similarly, we encourage a decrease in the amount of time clients spend engaged in solitary or noninteractive activities (e.g., TV). Essentially, clients should plan to be near other people in situations where they might strike up a conversation (e.g., a bookstore). Again, clients can utilize a reward system when they increase contact with other people.

SUMMARY

In this contribution, we have attempted to identify and discuss the relevant issues for working with MVA survivors. Proper assessment, as discussed previously, is a valuable tool for understanding clients' mental health needs. A multimethod approach utilizing a combination of structured interview, physician reports, and self-report measures is highly recommended. In this way, a thorough evaluation of the survivor's posttrauma symptomatology, comorbid psychiatric issues, and psychosocial influences to medical problems is achieved.

For those cases where PTSD is the primary issue, we have described one approach to conceptualization and treatment. The available literature indicates that this approach is valid and addresses the relevant symptoms (Blanchard & Hickling, 1997; Hickling & Blanchard, 1997). Similarly, we have found this approach to be useful in our research on recovery following a MVA (Shipherd et al., 1999). Specifically, we have noticed that despite a complicated presentation, a narrow focus of treatment on PTSD symptoms is beneficial.

We encourage further exploration of these issues within the literature as the demand for services by this population continues to grow. Examination of the mechanism of action within protocols such as the one outlined earlier would be useful. In particular, it would be of interest to understand the circumstances that are favorable for the generalization of treatment effects to comorbid diagnoses.

CONTRIBUTORS

Jillian C. Shipherd, MA, is currently completing her dissertation at the State University of New York at Buffalo under the mentorship of J. Gayle Beck, PhD. Her grant-funded dissertation is an examination of intrusive thoughts in MVA survivors. She is also actively involved in the implementation of the PTSD treatment protocol described in this contribution. Her interests include the study of trauma recovery, anxiety disorders, and the treatment of PTSD. Ms. Shipherd may be contacted at the Department of Psychology, Park Hall, State University of New York at Buffalo, Buffalo, NY 14260.

J. Gayle Beck, PhD, completed her undergraduate training at Brown University and her graduate training at the State University of New York at Albany, where she worked with David Barlow, PhD. In 1994, Dr. Beck relocated from the University of Houston to the State University of New York at Buffalo, where she is an active faculty member of the clinical training program. Her research focuses on the etiology and treatment of adult anxiety disorders, particularly Panic Disorder and, more recently, PTSD. Dr. Beck has published extensively, with numerous empirical articles and chapters examining issues such as the interaction of physiological and psychological factors in anxiety and treatment efficacy. In addition to her research clinic, Dr. Beck maintains a private practice. Dr. Beck can be reached at the Department of Psychology, Park Hall, State University of New York at Buffalo, Buffalo, NY 14260.

Jessica L. Hamblen, MA, is currently at Dartmouth College completing her predoctoral internship in clinical psychology and will receive her PhD from the State University of New York at Buffalo. Her interests are in the areas of trauma, PTSD, and developmental psychopathology. Ms. Hamblen may be contacted at The Department of Veterans Affairs, National Center for PTSD (116D), Medical and Regional Office Center, White River Junction, VT 05009.

Jennifer B. Freeman, PhD, is currently a Postdoctoral Fellow at the Brown University School of Medicine in Providence, Rhode Island. She received her PhD in Clinical Psychology from the State University of New York at Buffalo and completed a Predoctoral Internship at the Brown University School of Medicine. She has special interests in the areas of child and adolescent anxiety disorders, Posttraumatic Stress Disorder, and information processing. Dr. Freeman can be contacted at Brown University School of Medicine, Rhode Island Hospital, Department of Child and Family Psychiatry - Potter Building, 593 Eddy Street, Providence, RI 02903.

RESOURCES

Alberti, R. E., & Emmons, M. L. (1982). *Your Perfect Right.* San Luis Obispo, CA: Impact Publishers.

American Psychiatric Association. (1994). *Diagnostic and Statistical Manual of Mental Disorders* (4th ed.). Washington, DC: Author.

Beck, A. T., Rush, A. J., Shaw, B. F., & Emery, G. (1979). *Cognitive Therapy of Depression.* New York: Guilford.

Beck, A. T., Ward, C. H., Mendelson, M., Mock, J., & Erbaugh, J. (1961). An inventory for measuring depression. *Archives of General Psychiatry, 4,* 561-571.

Bernstein, D. A., & Borkovec, T. A. (1973). *Progressive Relaxation Training: A Manual for the Helping Professions.* Champaign, IL: Research Press.

Blake, D., Weathers, F., Nagy, L., Kaloupek, D., Klauminzer, G., Charney, D., & Keane, T. (1990). *Clinician Administered PTSD Scale (CAPS).* Boston, MA: National Center for Post-Traumatic Stress Disorder, Behavioral Science Division.

Blanchard, E. B., & Hickling, E. J. (1997). *After the Crash: Assessment and Treatment of Motor Vehicle Accident Survivors.* Washington, DC: American Psychological Association.

Blanchard, E. B., Hickling, E. J., Taylor, A. E., Forneris, C. A., Loos, W. R., & Jaccard, J. (1996). Effects of varying scoring rules of the Clinician Administered PTSD Scale (CAPS) for the diagnosis of post-traumatic stress disorder in motor vehicle accident victims. *Behaviour Research and Therapy, 33,* 471-475.

Blanchard, E. B., Hickling, E. J., Taylor, A. E., & Loos, W. R. (1995). Psychiatric morbidity associated with motor vehicle accidents. *Journal of Nervous and Mental Disorders, 183,* 495-504.

Borkovec, T. D., Castonguay, L. G., & Newman, M. G. (1997). Measuring treatment outcome for Posttraumatic Stress Disorder and Social Phobia: A review of current instruments and recommendations for future research. In H. Strupp, L. Horowitz, & M. Lambert (Eds), *Measuring Patient Changes* (pp. 117-154). Washington, DC: American Psychological Association.

Buckley, T. C., Blanchard, E. B., & Hickling, E. J. (1996). A prospective examination of delayed onset PTSD secondary to motor vehicle accidents. *Journal of Abnormal Psychology, 105,* 617-625.

Carlson, E. (1997). *Trauma Assessments: A Clinician's Guide.* New York: Guilford.

Davidson, J., Smith, R., & Kudler, H. (1989). Validity and reliability of the DSM-III criteria for posttraumatic stress disorder: Experience with a structured interview. *Journal of Nervous and Mental Disorders, 177,* 336-341.

Ellis, A., & Harper, R. A. (1975). *A New Guide to Rational Living.* Hollywood, CA: Wilshire Book Company.

Fairebank, J., Couper, J., Davies, J., & O'Brien, J. (1980). The Oswestry Low Back Pain Disability Questionnaire. *Physiotherapy, 66,* 271-273.

Foa, E. B., & Kozak, M. J. (1986). Emotional processing of fear: Exposure to corrective information. *Psychological Bulletin, 99,* 20-35.

Foa, E. B., Riggs, D. S., Dancu, C. V., & Rothbaum, B. O. (1993). Reliability and validity of a brief instrument for assessing post-traumatic stress. *Journal of Traumatic Stress, 6,* 459-473.

Hickling, E. J., & Blanchard, E. B. (1997). The private practice psychologist and manual-based treatment: A case study in the treatment of post-traumatic stress disorder secondary to motor vehicle accidents. *Behaviour Research and Therapy, 35,* 191-203.

Horowitz, M., Wilner, N., & Alvarez, W. (1979). Impact of Events Scale: A measure of subjective distress. *Psychosomatic Medicine, 41,* 209-218.

Irwin, M. (1988). Depression and immune function. *Stress Medicine, 4,* 95-103.

Keane, T., Caddell, J. M., & Taylor, K. L. (1988). Mississippi Scale for Combat-Related Post-Traumatic Stress Disorder: Three studies in reliability and validity. *Journal of Consulting and Clinical Psychology, 56,* 85-90.

Kessler, R. C., McGonagle, K. A., Zhao, S., Nelson, C. B., Hughes, M., Eshleman, S., Wittchen, H-U., & Kendler, K. S. (1994). Lifetime and 12-month prevalence of DSM-III-R psychiatric disorders in the United States. *Archives of General Psychiatry, 51,* 8-19.

Kessler, R. C., Sonnega, A., Bromet, E., Hughes, M., & Nelson, C. B. (1995). Post-traumatic stress disorder in the National Comorbidity Survey. *Archives of General Psychiatry, 52,* 1048-1060.

Kiecolt-Glaser, J. K., Page, G., Marucha, P., MacCallum, R., & Glaser, R. (1998). Psychological influences on surgical recovery. *American Psychologist, 53,* 1209-1218.

Kilpatrick, D. G., Veronen, L. J., & Resick, P. A. (1979). The aftermath of rape: Recent empirical findings. *American Journal of Orthopsychiatry, 49,* 658-669.

King, L. A., King, D. W., Leskin, G., & Foy, D. W. (1995). The Los Angeles Symptom Checklist: A self-report measure of posttraumatic stress disorder. *Psychological Assessment, 2,* 1-17.

Lewinsohn, P. M., & Clarke, G. N. (1984). Group treatment of depressed individuals: The "Coping With Depression" course. *Advances in Behavior Research and Therapy, 6,* 99-114.

National Safety Council. (1993). The national accident fatality toll. *Traffic Safety, 93,* 15.

Parker, N. (1977). Accident litigants with neurotic symptoms. *Medical Journal of Australia, 2,* 318-322.

Pennebaker, J. W. (1989). Confession, inhibition, and disease. In L. Berkowitz (Ed.), *Advances in Experimental and Social Psychology* (Vol. 22, pp. 211-244). San Diego, CA: Academic Press.

Roland, M., & Martin, R. (1983). A study of the natural history of back pain. Part I: Development of a reliable and sensitive measure of disability in low-back pain. *Pain, 8,* 141-144.

Rothbaum, B. O., & Foa, E. B. (1993). Subtypes of Posttraumatic Stress Disorder and duration of symptoms. In J. R. T. Davidson & E. B. Foa (Eds.), *Posttraumatic Stress Disorder: DSM-IV and Beyond* (pp. 23-36). Washington, DC: American Psychiatric Press.

Rothbaum, B. O., Foa, E. B., Riggs, D., Murdock, T., & Walsh, W. (1992). A prospective examination of post-traumatic stress disorder in rape victims. *Journal of Traumatic Stress, 5,* 455-475.

Saunders, B. E., Arata, C. M., & Kilpatrick, D. G. (1990). Development of a crime-related post-traumatic stress scale for women within the Symptom Checklist-90-Revised. *Journal of Traumatic Stress, 3,* 439-448.

Shipherd, J. C., Beck, J. G., Hamblen, J. L., Freeman, J., & Lackner, J. (1999, November). *Cognitive Behavioral Treatment of PTSD: Do the Treatment Effects Generalize to Comorbid Chronic Pain?* Poster presented at the annual meeting of the Association for Advancement of Behavior Therapy, Toronto, CA.

Solomon, S. D., Gerrity, E. T., & Muff, A. M. (1992). Efficacy of treatments for Posttraumatic Stress Disorder: An empirical review. *Journal of the American Medical Association, 268,* 633-638.

Spielberger, C. D., Gorsuch, R. L., & Lushene, R. E. (1970). *Manual for the State Trait Anxiety Inventory (Self-Evaluation Questionnaire).* Palo Alto, CA: Consulting Psychologists Press.

Steketee, G., & Foa, E. B. (1987). Rape victims: Post-traumatic stress responses and their treatment: A review of the literature. *Journal of Anxiety Disorders, 1,* 69-86.

Taylor, S., & Koch, W. J. (1995). Anxiety disorders due to motor vehicle accidents: Nature and treatment. *Clinical Psychology Review, 15,* 721-738.

Watson, C. G., Juba, M., Manifold, V., Kucala, T., & Anderson, P. E. D. (1991). The PTSD Interview: Description, reliability, and concurrent validity of a DSM-III based technique. *Journal of Clinical Psychology, 47,* 179-188.

Weathers, F., Blake, D., Krinsley, K. E., Haddad, W., Huska, J., & Keane, T. M. (1992, November). *The Clinician Administered PTSD Scale: Reliability and Construct Validity.* Paper presented at the 26th annual meeting of the Association for the Advancement of Behavior Therapy, Boston, MA.

Wilson, J. P., & Keane, T. M. (1997). *Assessing Psychological Trauma and PTSD.* New York: Guilford.

Directed Family Therapy: Treatment for Divorcing Families in Conflict

Kevin D. Arnold and Jeff D. Sherrill

The domestic or family courts have adopted, by and large, an approach that encourages mediation of parenting disputes during divorce, and that appears to favor the use of shared parenting (or joint custody) over single-parent decision making. The use of shared parenting by courts has several purposes, including an attempted remedy to the possibility of instability experienced by divorced children, responsiveness to gender issues raised in the society regarding the fitness of both parents regardless of sex, and expediency on the part of courts to avoid making difficult decisions in which one parent or the other might otherwise be declared a "winner" (Benedek et al., 1998). Courts use reasoning that appears to rely on social science, as illustrated by the opinion in *Perotti v. Perotti* (Benedek et al., 1998): "The concept of 'joint custody' can serve to give the measure of psychological support and uplift to each parent that would communicate itself to the children in measures of mutual love, mutual attention, and mutual training" (p. 39).

The courts typically distinguish between the rights of parenting and physical access to the children. Usually, shared parenting refers to the joint decision-making process as a part of sharing the rights of parenting. Courts have also begun to consider dividing the time children spend with one parent or the other in models much like shared parenting (e.g., 50% with one parent, 50% with the other). The courts in many states appear to begin with the presumption that both parents have an equal right to parenting duties and residence of their children. For example, a review of the list of the status of joint custody across states (Emery, 1994) indicated that 22 states have some form of mandatory or strongly encouraging language in their statutes regarding parenting and divorce. It must be kept in mind that the point of shared parenting is not necessarily an equal distribution of time between the two parents. Instead, it is also the distribution of parental rights to both parents, presumably leading to a collaborative approach and joint decision making in many areas of their children's lives. For example, the Ohio Revised Code (ORC; Anderson Publishing Co., 1998) states: "As used in the Revised Code, 'shared parenting' means that the parents share, in the manner set forth in the plan for shared parenting that is approved by the court under division (D)(1) and described in division (K)(6) of this section, all or some of the aspects of physical and legal care of their children" (ORC 3109.04[J]). This definition presumes that the parents will collaborate and communicate.

Unfortunately, a fairly high number of parents who leave court with a shared parenting agreement do not have the emotional or behavioral skills to manage the interactions for successful shared parenting. According to Johnston and Roseby (1997), about 10% of divorcing couples cannot collaboratively reach resolution and must seek the court's help in remedying their disputes. Further, Johnston and Roseby (1997) indicated that these families consume a disproportionately high amount of court and therapeutic resources, and the conflicted couples have a markedly higher likelihood of producing children who are maladjusted. In some states, courts are to take into account the inability of the parents to cooperate when making decisions about shared parenting (Benedek et al., 1998), but in practice, it is probably far less likely to be considered than would be suggested by the summary of case law supplied by Benedek et al. As they stated: "it is a fact of life that a great many divorced spouses are so angry with each other that no useful cooperation can be expected of them; and it is not at all clear that the law should foster joint responsibility for a child if the price for that outcome is continuing and overt hostility undermining the child's happiness and at least complicating the child's development" (p. 46).

In order to assist the courts in providing justice with a therapeutic outcome, models have been developed to assist families who highly conflict in their efforts to parent their children postdivorce. Johnston and Roseby (1997) described four levels of intervention that imply four levels of conflict in these families (see Johnston & Roseby, 1997, pp. 225-248): (a) no or little disruptive conflict that benefit from parenting education, (b) parenting or custody disputes that benefit from mediation services or those of collaborative law (a form of nonadversarial legal services), (c) conflicts at an impasse in which ongoing disputes did not benefit from mediation, requiring more intensive interventions, and (d) high levels of conflict that persist after the settlement of the case. They recommend interventions that are based upon the level of conflict between the parents. They suggest that for those who are at the third level, interventions such as therapeutic mediation or custody evaluations be provided. At the fourth level, they recommend several intrusive interventions such as parenting coordination or arbitration.

Therapeutic mediation is defined as an explicit combination of mediation strategies and family therapy techniques. The therapy is designed to be child focused, with mediation of disputes delivered in the context of the therapy. Johnston and Roseby (1997) argue that the process should be largely confidential from the courts, with only status reports provided to the legal system. Parenting coordination is a more intrusive strategy in which the family is overseen by a coordinator whose role is to determine the best interest of the children and mediate disputes among conflicted couples in shared parenting arrangements. Further, the coordinator manages a number of interventions, including the children's therapy and interventions for the parents. Garrity and Baris (1994) described in detail the role and function of the parenting coordinator and recommended its use in cases where one parent has so disrupted the relationship of the other parent with the children that alienation from that parent is likely imminent or present.

Although these recommendations are fairly comprehensive, there is a model of intervention that would not be confidential from the courts, but instead would involve the attorneys and the courts through information sharing. This model, Directed Family Therapy, is described in this contribution. It was developed by Kevin Arnold and Jeff Sherrill, together with Attorney Stephen Daulton, in response to the ongoing litigation in which many families found themselves after divorce and under a shared parenting agreement. It is designed for couples at the third or fourth level of conflict in Garrity and Baris's model of conflict assessment, wherein the couples have ongoing conflict with threats to litigate (Level 3) or there are threats of violence with displays of intimidating behaviors and continual litigation (Level 4). At present the model incorporates a number of already accepted practices, with some methods not yet empirically tested. The overall model itself has not yet been assessed on the whole, but clinical case studies suggest its utility. The following information is provided first to inform the reader about the research on the effects of high conflict on children, and then to present an overview of the intervention model.

A RATIONALE FOR DIRECTED FAMILY THERAPY: EFFECTS OF HIGH INTERPARENTAL CONFLICT ON CHILDREN

The risk of negative outcomes to children when divorce occurs is greater than for those children whose parents do not divorce. According to Hetherington, Bridges, and Insabella (1998), risks to children of divorce include academic problems, externalizing and internalizing behaviors, poor social skills, low self-esteem, higher rates of dropping out, lower socioeconomic attainment, and marital instability later in life. Children of divorce are not only at greater risk for several of these negative outcomes, but the risk appears to cut across ethnic subgroups. Their review also suggests that any adjustment to remarriage after divorce may take as long as 5 to 7 years. However, of those who remarry, about one-fourth are likely to divorce again within 5 years, suggesting that for those children whose parent(s) remarry, 25% will not be able to adjust because their family changes before they have adjusted to the first divorce.

Johnston and Roseby (1997) recounted a plethora of negative outcomes for children when exposed to interparental conflict that includes verbal abuse, positioning the child to be alienated from one parent, and/or mild forms of physical confrontations such as shoving. For example, they describe outcomes such as hypervigilance, avoidance of complexity and emotions, overconcern with caretaking by the parent(s), and taking on responsibility for the conflicts. They argue that the long-term effect is the development of cognitive scripts, or schemas, that then become these children's automatic way of processing information and behaving in relationships with others, presumably into adulthood.

In clinical and legal practices, reports abound of frequent conflicts between parents (and among other interested parties such as grandparents or surrogate parents) who have histories of predivorce conflicts. This fact appears to be due to the requirement that co-parents maintain their relationship as parents with one another while all other aspects of their previous relationship are likely to be severed. Although we as professionals can distinguish the differences among such roles, divorced or estranged parents who have a history of conflicts and disputes within the context of other family functions and roles cannot. As Maccoby and Mnookin (1992) pointed out, shared parenting requires communication between two people who have decided to sever their relationships. In our experience, the conflicts regarding parenting and other roles previously shared between the parents continue despite the artificial court order that directs them to collaborate. Thus shared parenting provides an excellent opportunity for many conflicted couples to continue to fight when attempting to parent their children, thus exposing those children to high levels of conflict as well. Maccoby and Mnookin (1992) reported that conflicted parents early in their separation continue to report conflict several years later; many of these conflicts result in continued legal conflicts. They further point out that only about one-fourth of divorced parents develop collaborative relationships despite the shared parenting model, and about the same number remain quite confrontational and conflicted.

The literature also suggests that the frequency and intensity of conflicts between parents affect negatively the adjustment of their children. The review by Davies and Cummings (1994) indicated that exposure to parental conflicts leads to problems with emotional dysregulation and arousal, guilt, anxiety, and behavioral problems. In their book, Cummings and Davies (1994) pointed out the relationship between frequency of conflicts, mode of conflict expression, intensity, content, and conflict resolution and negative child adjustment. Within the divorce context, Buchanan, Maccoby, and Dornbusch (1996) reported negative effects for ongoing parental conflict on adolescent school adjustment and several aspects of overall adjustment in teenagers. However, there can be a mediating effect of resolution to conflicts that improves the impact on children (Cummings & Davies, 1994). Therefore, it seems that the imposition of increased opportunities for conflict (i.e., shared parenting) for already conflicted postseparation or postdecree couples would predictively have a deleterious effect on their children. These findings suggest that reduction of frequency and intensity of conflict and the development of postdivorce parenting skills to mediate and resolve those conflicts will improve children's adjustment.

In fact, two recent studies of the effects of conflict on divorced children indicate that such interventions might be useful. First, Davies and Cummings (1994) indicated that one of the core elements in predicting negative outcomes from conflict is the degree to which the conflict leads the child to experience a sense of threat to the attachment to parents. The model argues that if the conflicts occur, but the parents resolve the conflicts and do so by either modeling conflict resolution skills for the children, or discussing later with the children the fact that they have reached a solution to the conflict (see Cummings & Wilson, 1999), then the negative effects of the conflict can be somewhat ameliorated. Thus a therapeutic model that develops for parents the capacity to resolve conflicts would promote a decrease in the degree of threat experienced to the attachments.

Second, Hetherington (1999) indicated that maladjustment is also predicted by the degree of parentification that is caused by the parents. She defined parentification as the process of placing children into parental roles such as performing child care duties that are typical only of a mother or father. She described two types of parentification: instrumental and emotional. The former is assignment of age-inappropriate tasks to a child that are traditionally the domain of the parent (e.g., care of siblings), while the latter is the use of the child as an emotional support or confident by the parent. Her results indicate that the effect of parentification is negative to children of divorce. Because the dynamic in parentification includes a failure to see children as the needy parties in the dyad, instead then subjugating their emotional needs in the service of the parents, an intervention model that reconnects the parent to their role and to their children's emotional needs would be expected to decrease the probability of parentification.

THE MODEL OF DIRECTED FAMILY THERAPY

As indicated in Lyster (1996), many states encourage or require mediation as a dispute resolution strategy for divorcing parents. However, the most highly conflicted couples are unlikely to stay in mediation. Often, to perpetuate their conflicts, these parents will force litigation regarding the custody of their children, regardless of the effect of such conflicts on the emotional well-being of the children. However, custody evaluations are often counterproductive to therapeutic efforts, providing couples with more information with which to carry on their chronic power and intimacy struggles. Custody battles and custody evaluations encourage contentious couples to continue the power struggle in hopes of winning control of the parenting process and proving the other parent "bad," thus perpetuating the alienation process (see Garrity & Baris, 1994). These processes inadvertently allow them to avoid the reality that children need the attachment to both parents to increase the likelihood that they will develop in a healthy fashion, and that high levels of chronic conflict damage children. It is unlikely that typical divorce-oriented family therapy will be effective in these cases. In fact, Garrity and Baris (1994) argued that often naïve family or child therapists enter into these family systems unaware of the high degree of triangulation that is likely to occur. They often become unwitting pawns as they allow one or both parents to enmesh them into the conflicts. Further, when the shroud of confidentiality is placed around therapy with such couples, and no court order exists, even seasoned therapists are caught off guard when the parties feel no barrier to continuing the verbal attacks on each other. Confidentiality protects such parents from any accountability for their lack of concern for their children or their open hatred of each other, and therapy becomes either an unwitting accomplice to their conflicts or a short-lived event that is ended by one or both parents. Because of the need to focus on the children, to provide long-term therapy, and to create consequences or barriers to malevolent behaviors, the model now known as Directed Family Therapy is offered.

Directed Family Therapy, which is a combination of schema-focused therapy (Young, 1994), integrative couple therapy (Jacobson & Christensen, 1996), and traditional cognitive-behavioral therapy, validates a parent's feelings as well as, at the same time, confronting them with the need to minimize conflict and resolve the issues involved in postdecree parenting. Directed Family Therapy provides a structure for conflicted parents to experiment with different parenting plans under the supervision of a psychologist. The psychologist can also serve the role of consultant, helping the parents evaluate the impact of various plans on their children, while encouraging them to talk and to minimize and manage their conflict. Directed Family Therapy, which has structured procedures and a therapeutic component, directs parents to focus on the best interests of the children. Based on that focus, it directs their energy toward reducing the dysfunctional relationship dynamics that heretofore have been almost unalterable.

Directed Family Therapy has several goals. The primary goal is the establishment of a cordial, businesslike relationship between the parents that promotes shared parenting of the decisions regarding their children. In conjunction with that goal, Directed Family Therapy promotes decision making that is in the best interest of the children, not the parents. Also, the model is intended to structure needed changes to the parenting plan as time and circumstances change over time, with the provision of feedback to the parents and the court about the children's adjustment as the changes are implemented.

Structured Procedures

Collaboration of the Therapist and the Legal System

The judge or magistrate, guardian ad litem (GAL), and the attorneys for the parties all must agree that the particular family could benefit from Directed Family Therapy. It is preferred that the attorneys agree to court-ordered therapy, because it is unlikely that parents with this type of conflict history will willingly engage in a therapeutic process at all or for very long. The court order provides an increased likelihood that the parents will attend therapy, and the courts are included in the process at the onset. This latter factor is designed to enhance the chances that the court and the therapist can collaborate toward a common goal.

Limits to Confidentiality

Confidentiality is limited in Directed Family Therapy. Therapists, in their role as an advocate for the children's best interest, take an active role in delivering information to the courts. Typically, letters or verbal reports include factors such as the involvement of each parent in the therapy, their willingness to engage in suggested compromises regarding conflicts, their capacity to be focused on their children's well-being, and their ability to foster a relationship between their children and each other.

The limit to confidentiality serves several purposes. First, it allows the court to have access to information that would presumably be valuable should it need to make custody decisions. Second, it places on the parents a sense of responsibility for their actions. That is, if they continue to engage in alienating behaviors or vitriolic diatribes about the former spouse, or should either parent refuse to accept responsibility for his or her individual actions that harm their children, then the parent will no longer be able to appear as if he or she is the "good" parent in court while actively undermining the children's well-being in private. Third, it creates an active role for the psychologist in collaborating with the court, which presumably has far more authority to use adverse consequences in reaction to malevolent parental behaviors. The psychologist can therefore join with the court in planning a coordinated intervention, while at the same time relying on the court's authority to create a motivation to change, not unlike the use of the threat of arrest and prosecution as a motivator in the reduction of violent behaviors of male batterers (see Dutton, 1995).

Role Clarification

If litigation persists, and the Directed Family Therapist testifies in hearings or depositions, the role is clearly established by the psychologist. Although expertise in clinical assessment forms the basis of the testimony, it is not framed as expert testimony in the sense of an independent expert. The role is more of a fact witness testifying as to the facts of the clinical process and actions of the parties (see Greenberg & Shuman, 1997). Further, because the goal is to promote the outcome of functional shared parenting, the psychologist does not opine on ultimate issues such as custody, visitation schedules, or changes in residential status. Instead, the role is to provide insightful clinical data from the attempted therapy and allow the court to use those data to make such decisions.

Informed Consent

Directed Family Therapy employs written informed consent that reviews a number of issues (see pages 164-166). The written form addresses (a) the children's well-being as the target of the therapy; (b) limits on confidentiality; (c) definition of the roles of each parent and of the therapist; (d) definition of therapeutic expectations, techniques, and length; and (e) experimental nature of the treatment model. The parents are not permitted to participate in the therapy without signing an informed consent form prior to the first session. Before the initial session begins, the psychologist reviews the material in the informed consent form, providing an opportunity for questions. After the oral review is completed, and any questions are answered, the psychologist then countersigns the form to create a record of having thoroughly obtained informed consent for participation.

Therapeutic Methods

The following represents a combination of behaviorally oriented, directed psychotherapy and divorce mediation strategies. There is an emphasis on the use of acceptance/tolerance (Jacobson & Christensen, 1996), empathy, schema-focused (Young, 1994) or constructivist strategies, conflict resolution and problem solving, and communication skills development. In addition, when a power imbalance exists, assertiveness skills (Walen, DiGiuseppe, & Dryden, 1992) are also taught.

We believe that most conflicted families will need a minimum of 2 years in intensive Directed Family Therapy. Given a large and growing body of evidence on the difficulties children face in dissolving families, it seems reasonable to communicate to these families the need for substantial intervention. After the primary results of Directed Family Therapy are obtained, the psychologist will establish an ongoing consultative role to treat new or resurfacing problems.

In addition to the Directed Family Therapist, the model includes the option of a child therapist. As pointed out by Garrity and Baris (1994), children in high-conflict families often need a safe and validating therapist to aid them in the development of the self or identity. The children's therapist will need to remain neutral and work in direct conjunction with the Directed Family Therapist in order to decrease the probability that one of the two parents might triangulate the therapist against the other parent.

There are several therapeutic targets of the Directed Family Therapy model. First, both parents are a target of the direct interventions, with attendance at individual and joint sessions. When either parent is remarried or seriously involved with a significant other, then that person is often included, particularly if he or she aggravates the conflicts. Sometimes extended family members will contribute to the conflicts or place the children in the middle between one parent and the other. When that occurs, the extended family members are included in the therapy. Finally, the well-being of the children is the primary target, although the children are not typically seen by the Directed Family Therapist except during an evaluation session.

Assessment

The assessment of the divorced parents' relational dysfunction, and its effect on the children, requires a number of frameworks and strategies. First, the assessment should determine the core conflict issues that are typically not articulated during the assessment sessions. Instead, these core issues usually can be framed in terms of both the predivorce personal issues and facets of the divorce itself. For example, consider the example of parents in which the father presents with the core need of being idealized and valued, while the wife is dependent and conflict-avoidant. They are ordered into Directed Family Therapy because of conflicts over the mother's decision to change day care, made unilaterally after the father's refusal to consider the change in previous conversations. In this example, the wife left the husband, obtained the divorce, and then remarried. The father's predivorce issues might lead to a sense of extreme shame due to the perceived slight not only from the divorce, but also from his ex-spouse's remarriage. The mother's issues can create passive-aggressive avoidance in response to the demands of her ex-spouse that could lead to failed communication regarding their children's lives.

Second, the assessment should consider the factors regarding the structure of the marriage and divorce. Data should consider the power balance of the relationship prior to the divorce, as well as the levels of intimacy needs and the extent to which the needs were met. The psychologist should also investigate the dynamics of the divorce, such as the extent to which both agreed to the divorce, or the imbalance between one spouse's decision to leave that was a surprise to the other. In the latter cases, according to Emery (1994), one would anticipate that each parent would be at a different point in adjustment to the divorce, and might use either custody or financial issues to perpetuate the marriage through divorce and postdivorce conflicts.

Third, the degree of conflict between the parties should be assessed. Garrity and Baris (1994) have developed a five-level conflict assessment model using the following taxonomy: Minimal, Mild, Moderate, Moderately Severe, and Severe. For the purposes of Directed Family Therapy, differentiating between the four more severe levels will be most important. At the Mild level, the authors describe behaviors such as occasional fighting in front of the children, occasionally talking negatively about the other parent in front of the children, and sometimes questioning the children about the other parent. At the Moderate level, there is no history of threats of or actual physical violence, but there is one of verbal abuse. The negative portrayal of the other parent is extremely negative to the children, and threats are made from one parent to the other to limit the amount of time with the children or of repeated litigation. At this level, there are efforts by one or both parents to create an alienating union with the child. At the Moderately Severe level, the parents are a danger to each other, and there are threats of physical violence. Conflicts escalate to property damage and intimidation, as well as threats of removing the children altogether. Litigation at this level is ongoing and repetitive. One or both of the parents make continual efforts to alienate the children from the other parent, and the children exhibit signs of emotional or identity disturbances. At the Severe level, there exists physical or sexual abuse and disruptive levels of substance abuse, and one or both of the parents reveal serious psychopathology. Directed Family Therapy is designed for Mild, Moderate, and Moderately Severe levels of conflict, although its utility might be less at the Moderately Severe level depending on the degree of alienation between the children and one or both parents.

Fourth, the assessment should assess the degree to which the conflicts are perpetuated by outside influences. Typically, there are three types of such influences. First, one or both parents' attorney might be motivated to perpetuate the conflicts, with an overzealous desire to serve the client rather than the well-being of the children. Second, extended family members, usually grandparents, feel a need to reassert their control over one of the parents, and they use the conflicts as an opportunity to ingratiate themselves to their adult offspring. They will often berate the other parent or magnify the issues of a conflict in order to form the enmeshed bond with the parent, thus perpetuating the conflict to their own ends. Third, a significant other or stepparent may find a cooperative relationship with the other parent threatening to the new relationship, or may feel a need to bolster a partner's conflict stance in order to serve his or her own intimacy needs. In such cases, the stepparent may not only encourage ongoing conflicts, but may also try to take the place of the other parent, to the point of requiring the children to call him or her father or mother, or go by the stepparent's last name.

Fifth, the degree of maladjustment exhibited by the children should be assessed. The process is done in a relatively unstructured way, although the psychologist indicates to the children in an age-appropriate fashion that the purpose of the assessment is to let their mother and father know how the fighting makes them feel. The children are probed as to their reactions to various conflict-laden or alienating behaviors of each parent, and behavioral as well as affect descriptors are noted. Other signs of maladjustment are noted as well, such as peer conflicts, social withdrawal, somatic complaints, behavioral acting out, and academic underachievement or failure.

Finally, the assessment should identify the current presenting issues of conflict. Often, these will present as issues regarding one parent's claim that the other violated one of the parenting agreement stipulations, or that one or both have returned to the court to modify custody or visitation arrangements. Often secondary issues such as compensation for perceived wrongs or control of the other parent's behaviors become the argued subpoints to these oftentimes petty presenting issues. However, if one does not assess them, the risk is that an issue of substance might be overlooked, and the parent may conclude that the psychologist has already taken sides with the other parent.

The steps listed below are used to conduct the assessments.

Clinical Assessment of Individual Parents. Individual sessions are conducted with each parent to allow each to tell the "real story" without inhibition, to assess distorted beliefs about the other parent and level of understanding each has of his or her own maladaptive behaviors, and to identify individually based psychopathology contributing to the ongoing conflicts. Complete histories are taken both of the family of origin and of the marriage/divorce. In Directed Family Therapy, there is typically a minimal, if any, use of psychometric scales unless there is suspicion of serious psychopathology that is not readily diagnosable with the clinical assessment. Additionally, individual sessions are held with the children to allow them to express (a) their emotional reactions to parental conflict and (b) their wishes regarding resolution of residential/time conflicts and disagreements over child-rearing decisions.

Conjoint Assessment. A session with both parents is conducted to allow each to tell "their story," to observe the dynamics of their conflicts, and to identify the presenting conflict issues. Often the conflicts between the parents prohibit this session early in the work, and sometimes it is necessary to facilitate interparent communication through alternative means such as phone calls or written correspondence. At times, the communication occurs through the therapist. All of these data sources assist the psychologist in assessing the conjoint dynamics.

Assessment of Family Dynamics (Including Dynamics Among Extended Family Members and Parents/Children). Family sessions are conducted that permit the assessment of the role of extended family members or other partners in maintaining the conflict, the degree to which the parents place their children in the middle of conflicts, and the capacity of each parent to empathize with their children's distress resulting from the conflicts.

Empathy Induction

The role of empathy, or perspective-taking skills, is integral to many forms of therapy for abusive adults. For example, empathy induction is described in Dutton (1995) in his section on treatment of male batterers. The task for Directed Family Therapy is to induce empathy for the pain and suffering caused by each parent in the children's lives. This is accomplished by educating them on the effects of high-conflict divorce on children in general and through direct confrontation with the experiences of their children. Individual sessions with each parent are conducted that educates them on the effects of ongoing conflict on their children and assignment of reading materials that make these points. For example, the books by Garrity and Baris (1994) or Maccoby and Mnookin (1992) can be assigned, depending on the sophistication level of the parents. Both books provide a detailed description of the effects of high-conflict divorce on children, although that by Maccoby and Mnookin (1992) is far more technical.

Facilitation of parental perspective taking is introduced in individual sessions in order to promote empathy with their own children's reactions to the parental conflicts. During these individual sessions, the psychologist uses the parents' own early painful experiences to activate emotional reactions to parental conflict, then develops role-taking skills that promote empathy with their children's painful reactions (as identified from earlier assessment sessions with the children) to the present conflicts. The purpose of this stage of therapy is to promote awareness of painful reactions within the parents that will serve to inhibit their ongoing conflicts. Through empathy, parents are encouraged to decrease their role in inflicting pain on their children.

Identification and Management of Individual Issues as Represented in Marital or Divorce Conflict

In individual sessions, both parents are provided a schema-based construction of their own personal issues and a framework to understand how those issues affected the dynamics of their relationship with each other during the marriage and divorce (see Young & Gluhoski, 1996). In addition, the parents are taught to consider the core issues of the other parent. The purpose of understanding their own issues is to create a cognitive framework with which to conceptualize their actual, albeit maladaptive, motives. Once these are identified, then cognitive and schema-focused strategies are employed to modify the automatic thinking or pattern-driven affect and actions. An understanding of the other parent's issues is used to promote perspective taking, reduce demonization, and increase the possibility of softening statements during the communication and conflict management phase of treatment. Often, a constructivist framework (Mahoney, 1991) is explained to the parents, using metaphors such as computer operating systems or corrective lenses to explain the role of schemas in interpreting information, distorting reality based on earlier experiences, giving the information meaning, and guiding automatic reactions.

Explanations of automatic thinking and attribution errors provide a foundation for cognitive corrections. Parents are taught to recognize their anger and arousal as driven by cognitive distortions about the other parent, as well as about their own status as a wronged individual. These conceptualizations are then used to implement reality testing and corrections to the cognitive distortions.

A revised perspective of roles is also fostered during this stage of the treatment. Emery (1994) pointed out that a major role of adjustment to divorce is the parents' transition from the role of spouses to that of partners in the joint venture of child rearing. Often, the transition is impeded not only by premarriage issues as described earlier, but also by a failure to recognize that they are using marital role definitions to shape their understanding of their rights, boundaries, and functions postdivorce. An explicit description of this model is provided, with detailed descriptions of their behaviors or beliefs that are driven by these old roles. Once these roles have been acknowledged, the parents are assisted in determining reasons why new roles must be constructed. After the parents have developed motivation to reconceptualize their roles, the psychologist provides suggestions for new roles that are based on metaphors such as business-partner relationships, and the new roles are defined regarding structures, limits, and functions.

Individual Skill Development

During individual sessions, both parents are taught a specific set of skills regarding conflict management, assertiveness, and communication. The skills are taught as a set of basic social skills to promote their children's well-being and to support the new roles that they have defined for themselves.

Conflict management skills are taught using a didactic approach, using the behavioral strategies of Stuart (1980), the acceptance methods of Jacobson and Christensen (1996), and the validation strategies of Linehan (1993). The behavioral strategies first create for the parents a shift in perspective from conflicts based on past conflicts to one based on present problems to be solved. Questions are reshaped from "why" to "how" as the psychologist shifts the parents from requiring justification and blame assignment to asking what the problem really might be and how it might be solved in the best interest of their children. The framework of win-lose is reconstructed as win-win, with an emphasis on the children being the winners. Visual aids such as Venn diagrams are also used to promote the understanding of overlap between both parents' positions. Finally, the therapist structures conflicts into problems, while teaching the skills of identifying present problems, possible solutions, negotiation skills, mutual agreement on solutions, implementation of solutions in a stepwise fashion, and evaluation of the success of the solutions.

Acceptance and change skills in the Jacobson and Christensen (1996) model are not taught directly. In Directed Family Therapy, they are taught specifically as strategies to decrease conflict. The acceptance and change skills of making softening statements and role taking are both employed. The former utilizes statements that send to the other parent statements that describe the parent's possible mood state and likely causes for that mood state. The conflict is framed as a result of issues other than the one at hand, but the feelings are acknowledged in a nonjudgmental fashion. Often, during the individual sessions, this skill must be taught through modeling and role-play strategies, as it is initially too threatening for the parents. At the same time, when acceptance of the other parent's reactions is not feasible, the skill of tolerance is taught. Tolerance does not require the parent to understand the underlying motivations or feelings of the other parent, but it does create a nonthreatening framework that views the other's behaviors as nonthreatening even if irritating. The other parent's actions are seen as not requiring a response and simply as something to put up with from time to time in the interest of the children.

Finally, the disarming strategy of radical acceptance is taught (see Linehan, 1993). Radical acceptance promotes validation of the feelings of the other parent in an effort to reduce their intensity. The underlying theory is that intense emotional reactions are perpetuated by the invalidating reactions of others. When one of the parents uses comments such as "Of course you're upset." or "Given our past, how else would you feel?" the other parent's expectation of a conflicted reaction is not met, disrupting the conflict cycle and modifying their view of each other. By reducing the anger in the exchange in this manner, the conflicts can be decreased.

Assertiveness (see Walen et al., 1992) is taught directly to both parents using a modification that relies on the children's best interest. The parents are taught to conceptualize not only their own needs but also those of their children to create the basis of the "I" statements. They are then taught how to form "I" messages, ask for a specific action or compromise, and negotiate for a reasonable degree of the request to be met. They are also taught to recognize aggressive, passive, or indirect attempts to communicate so that they can replace these behaviors with assertiveness.

The Gottman et al. (1976) model for communication is used to teach communication skills. The parents are taught to understand a message's intent and impact, and how to determine if the intent and impact are consistent or if they instead are incongruent. They are given a framework that conceptualizes messages as distorted by the sender's schemas as well as those of the receiver, and are taught to recognize the probable distortions that might have occurred when a discrepancy between intent and impact occurs. Further, they are given skills in correcting such discrepancies through such strategies as identifying poor communication (e.g., throwing in the kitchen sink), calling time-out, setting agendas, and problem-solving strategies. They are asked to use these skills while in individual sessions during role-plays and reverse role-plays, as well as in vivo during actual conflicts out of the sessions. When in vivo opportunities are taken, the skills are reviewed in individual sessions to improve skill acquisition.

Joint Sessions

After the individual sessions have accomplished their purposes, joint sessions are held. A current conflict is selected by mutual decision, and it is negotiated by using the various techniques. The role of the psychologist is that of a mediator and consultant, providing feedback to each party while also identifying possible solutions to employ as behavioral experiments. At first, the use of experiments is crucial as a framework to decrease any threat the parents might feel by asking to compromise or collaborate with the other parent. The experiments then allow the therapist to identify problems with empathy, role taking, or the social skills, targeting these problems in an ongoing manner during the joint sessions. 'At times, the parents will negotiate a compromise on an issue, only to then balk after the session. During these times, the psychologist must decide if the issue should wait until the next session, or if it might be useful to use telephone consults in which the psychologist uses mediation skills to bring the parents back to a focus on their children and thus reach a compromise. When phone consults are used, the psychologist typically serves as a conduit through which the parents communicate with one another, as well as a reminder of the need to address the benefits that their positions offer to their children.

At times, the psychologist will be required to more directly facilitate an agreement on major issues through use of adapted mediation methods. When conflicts inhibit successful use of communication strategies, the psychologist may be required to introduce a framework of the possible issues that are driving the conflict and of possible solutions to those problems.

Through the use of nondirected mediation strategies, the psychologist generates communication about the suggestions, fosters the use of skills that promote compromise in the best interest of their children, and uses in vivo experiments that implement solutions produced by compromise or direction from the therapist.

Follow-Up and Relapse Prevention

Once the psychologist observes improvement in the parenting behaviors in conjoint sessions, and the children report a reduction of painful reactions to parental conflicts, the psychologist schedules regular check-up sessions to promote the maintenance of the external structure provided by therapy. The parents also agree to schedule as-needed sessions to prevent relapse when either one, or their children, identify a return of earlier unhealthy conflict patterns that do not ameliorate.

Failure of the Model

Not all couples will respond to Directed Family Therapy. Some couples lack the motivation or the basic personality structures to promote such fundamental shifts in their frameworks and behaviors. In other couples, one or both of the parents exhibit severe personality disturbances, psychopathology, or psychopathy. Regardless of the reasons, Directed Family Therapists must help parents manage their own schemas and not allow their need to succeed to overshadow the needs of the children. When success is unlikely, the therapy should be stopped and the court should intervene. In these cases, when the model fails, the psychologist should identify the most likely causes and report these to the attorneys, the parents, and the court. Again, the reporting should be designed to provide the clinical impressions and facts of the therapy, not expert opinions on parenting. The psychologist must not cross the line into the role reserved for the court itself.

Through the use of this model, the psychologist assists parents in creating a new set of interactional behaviors that promote conflict resolution and minimization of new conflicts that might harm the child. The authors' experience has been that, through the introduction of external structure and the skills training contained within this model, parents are able to modify their behaviors toward each other and thus reduce the negative effects of conflicts on their children. The role of the therapist is far more directed and dynamically oriented than that of a mediator. However, the need for external authority, as represented by the therapist's imposition of skills and possible conflict solutions, is seen as necessary in conflicted couples who, if left to their own strategies, would most likely engage in frequent and intense conflicts. Such a state would most certainly increase the probability that their children would develop maladaptive behaviors and psychopathology as adults.

Informed Consent to Participate In Directed Family Therapy

1. **Definitions**

Directed Family Therapy: Directed Family Therapy is a form of family therapy that is intended to reduce the conflicts between divorcing or postdivorce couples when collaborating to rear their children under a shared parenting agreement. Directed Family Counseling/Psychotherapy is directed at the two parents, and other family members if the therapist believes it necessary, although the children may become involved if that is determined by the therapist to be important. The treatment relies on individual work with each parent to have already been completed to a point at which basic skills in taking each other's perspectives and the children's perspectives, identifying one's own personal issues that affect the parenting conflicts, identifying "old baggage" that existed during the marriage/relationship which now interferes with shared parenting, skills in identifying a conflict when it occurs, deescalating anger while employing problem solving, and using healthy communication and conflict management skills while parenting. Directed Family Therapy then teaches both parties to employ these skills and abilities effectively in real-life situations during the couple's sessions.

Best Interest of the Child: For the purpose of Directed Family Therapy, the best interest of the child is served by both parents working in nonconflicted ways to rear him/her. The treatment relies on the research that indicates that ongoing conflict between parents increases the chances of children developing behavioral and emotional problems. Therefore, the therapy assumes that it is in the best interest of the child to reduce conflicts and replace these with healthy skills in conflict management and resolution.

Length of Treatment: The treatment is intended to be intensive during the initial phase in which the skills mentioned earlier are used more frequently and proficiently. The maintenance and follow-up phases continue throughout the children's later years until they become adults and the shared parenting agreement is no longer relevant. During the initial phase, weekly or bi-weekly sessions may be in order, but during the maintenance and follow-up phases, sessions may occur less often or on an as-needed basis.

Goal of Treatment: Although the parents are the targets of the treatment, improvement of the well-being of the children is the actual goal. Therefore, all counseling/therapy done during the treatment is not necessarily for the benefit of each parent, although such benefit may be derived, but instead is for the benefit of the children. In this regard, the counselor/therapist is treating the family through work with individuals or couples.

2. **Role of the Counselor/Therapist**

The counselor/therapist has as his/her role the reduction of stress and conflict as they impact on the children of each set of parents. The counselor/therapist may choose whatever strategies seem most appropriate to that end, even when those strategies might cause one or both of the parents discomfort. The therapist may be directive, meaning that specific strategies may be proposed, homework assignments may be given, and various solutions may be offered to problems. These shall be considered options or proposals, and should not be taken as guaranteed solutions. The counselor's/therapist's role is to shape the skills and abilities noted earlier to the specific needs of each couple and family so as to decrease the chances of their children developing behavioral and emotional problems.

_____ initial

3. Role of the Clients

The clients have, as their role, the duty to improve their skills at collaborating among themselves in ways that reduce and manage conflicts. They may attempt suggestions made by the counselor/therapist and report back on the utility of each one. They will work to understand the effect of high conflict and dispute levels on children and make efforts at understanding what their children go through when such conflicts occur. They will strive to parent their children and work together in a businesslike relationship that is directed at rearing their children in a shared way.

4. Limits of Confidentiality

In Directed Family Therapy, the role of the counselor/therapist is to serve the children's best interest, which at times may mean reporting to the court, the parties' attorneys, and/or the Guardian Ad Litem the progress of the therapy, the behavior of each parent in the therapy, clinical opinions about each parent's interest in parenting collaboratively, and other information that they waive their privilege and release this confidential information insofar as the counselor/therapist may reveal information about the therapy and about any and all clients related to this case to the court of jurisdiction, officers of the court with a direct interest in the case, and/or the Guardian Ad Litem, should the therapist deem it necessary to serve the best interest of the child, or should either party cause the case to be heard by the court through any form of postdecree court filings.

There is also a requirement in Ohio to report any suspected abuse of a child, a dependent adult, or someone with a disability, whether sexual or physical in nature. It is up to the therapist to determine if information revealed by any party of therapy warrants suspicion of such abuse. When suspicion occurs, all parties to this Directed Family Counseling/Psychotherapy understand that the authorities may be notified by the therapist in a timely fashion.

It is also understood by all parties to this Directed Family Therapy that Ohio law requires notations in the clinical records of domestic violence. Further, because of the goal of Directed Family Therapy, any reported domestic violence may cause the therapist to notify the court, attorneys for all parties, and/or the Guardian Ad Litem about such abuse since exposure to domestic violence increases the likelihood of the children developing behavioral and/or emotional disorders.

It is also understood by all parties to this Directed Family Therapy that if the therapist determines that there is risk of harm coming to someone at the hands of any of the parties, the therapist may take steps to notify the potential victim or to notify the authorities in order to prevent harm. Further, if the therapist determines that one or more of the parties to this Directed Family Therapy is at risk of harming himself/herself, the therapist may notify any person or agency about such risk and relevant confidential information that would, in the therapist's opinion, be able to decrease the risk of harm coming to that party at his/her own hand. Further, if the therapist concludes that there is a risk of imminent harm occurring to unnamed individuals at large by any party to this Directed Family Therapy, then the therapist may take steps to protect society at large by revealing confidential information to agencies, courts, or other persons who might prevent such harm from occurring, including but not necessarily requiring the therapist to seek involuntary hospitalization of the threatening party.

Because sessions of Directed Family Therapy can include more than one client, there is a risk of other persons in the sessions revealing information about the content of sessions. Therefore, each party understands this limit to confidentiality, and will hold the therapist harmless should any other party in the sessions reveal confidential information to others.

5. Financial Reimbursement

Each party agrees to pay one-half of the cost of the Directed Family Therapy. Insurance may be used, but if insurance or any other third-party payment source declines payment, each party agrees to be solely and personally responsible for payment of his/her portion of the costs of therapy. Each party is directed to the [Insert Your Practice's Fee Statement] for an explanation of fees. No diagnostic code or medical service code will be used except those that are true and honest regarding the parties and the services provided.

____
initial

6. Agreement to Participate in Directed Family Therapy

I have read and understand the contents of this Informed Consent form, and have asked any questions I might have and now sign to state my agreement with its contents, including granting the therapist permission to exchange with the court, all involved attorneys, and/or the Guardian Ad Litem any information about the treatment or the parties to Directed Family Therapy that would, in the therapist's opinion, serve the best interest of the child.

____

SIGNATURE and DATE

____

PRINT NAME

PARENT OF (NAME CHILDREN):

____

____

I gave this person an opportunity to ask questions, and reviewed the contents of this form, determining that it was signed knowingly and willingly.

____

SIGNATURE OF THERAPIST and DATE

CONTRIBUTORS

Kevin D. Arnold, PhD, ABPP, is a psychologist and the Director of the Center for Cognitive and Behavioral Therapy of Greater Columbus. He is also trained as a divorce mediator and is listed with the Franklin County (Ohio) Domestic Relations Court's mediation service. He is a Diplomate in Behavioral Psychology of the American Board of Professional Psychology, a Fellow of the American Academy of Behavioral Psychology, and a board member of the American Board of Behavioral Psychology. He also is the worksample coordinator for the American Board of Behavioral Psychology. Dr. Arnold will serve as president of the Ohio Psychological Association in 2000-2001. Dr. Arnold may be contacted at CCBT, 2121 Bethel Road, Suite D, Columbus, OH 43220.

Jeff D. Sherrill, PhD, is a psychologist in private practice at Meers Inc. in Northwest Columbus. He has been a certified mediator in the Franklin County (Ohio) Domestic Relations Court since 1991. Dr. Sherrill is a past board member of the Ohio Psychological Association and currently serves on the Ohio State Board of Psychology. Dr. Sherrill can be reached at 3246 Henderson Road, Columbus, OH 43220.

RESOURCES

Anderson Publishing Co. (1998). *Anderson's 1999 Ohio Family Law Handbook* (10th ed.). Cincinnati: Author.

Benedek, E. P., Derdeyn, A. P., Effron, E. J., Guyer, M. J., Hayden, K. S., Jurow, G. L., Kemper, K. D., Lazar, R. M., Levy, A. M., Nordhaus, B. F., Ravitz, A., Sacks, H. S., Schetky, D. H., Skoloff, G. N., & Weintrob, A. (1998). *Legal and Mental Health Perspectives on Child Custody Law: A Deskbook for Judges*. Eagen, MN: West Group.

Buchanan, C. M., Maccoby, E. E., & Dornbusch, S. M. (1996). *Adolescents After Divorce*. Cambridge: Harvard University Press.

Cummings, E. M., & Davies, P. T. (1994). *Children and Marital Conflict: The Impact of Family Dispute and Resolution*. New York: Guilford.

Cummings, E. M., & Wilson, A. (1999). Contexts of marital conflict and children's emotional security: Exploring the distinction between constructive and destructive conflict from the children's perspective. In M. J. Cox & J. Brooks-Gunn (Eds.), *Conflict and Cohesion in Families: Causes and Consequences* (pp. 105-129). Mahwah, NJ: Lawrence Erlbaum.

Davies, P. T., & Cummings, E. M. (1994). Marital conflict and child adjustment: An emotional security hypothesis. *Psychological Bulletin, 116,* 387-411.

Dutton, D. G. (1995). *The Domestic Assault of Women: Psychological and Criminal Justice Perspectives*. Vancouver: UBC Press.

Emery, R. E. (1994). *Renegotiating Family Relationships: Divorce, Child Custody, and Mediation*. New York: Guilford.

Garrity, C. B., & Baris, M. A. (1994). *Caught in the Middle: Protecting the Children of High-Conflict Divorce*. San Francisco: Jossey-Bass.

Gottman, J., Notarius, C., Gonso, J., & Markman, H. (1976). *A Couple's Guide to Communication*. Champaign, IL: Research Press.

Greenberg, S. A., & Shuman, D. W. (1997). Irreconcilable conflict between therapeutic and forensic roles. *Professional Psychology: Research and Practice, 28,* 50-57.

Hetherington, E. M. (1999). Should we stay together for the sake of the children? In E. M. Hetherington (Ed.), *Coping With Divorce, Single Parenting, and Remarriage: A Risk and Resiliency Perspective* (pp. 93-116). Mahwah, NJ: Lawrence Erlbaum.

Hetherington, E. M., Bridges, M., & Insabella, G. M. (1998). What matters? What does not? Five perspectives on the association between marital transitions and children's adjustment. *American Psychologist, 53,* 167-184.

Jacobson, N. S., & Christensen, A. (1996). *Integrative Couple Therapy: Promoting Acceptance and Change*. New York: Norton.

Johnston, J. R., & Roseby, V. (1997). *In the Name of the Child: A Developmental Approach to Understanding and Helping Children of Conflicted and Violent Divorce*. New York: Free Press.

Linehan, M. M. (1993). *Cognitive-Behavioral Treatment of Borderline Personality Disorder*. New York: Guilford.

Lyster, M. E. (1996). *Child Custody: Building Parenting Agreements That Work* (2nd ed.). Berkeley, CA: Nolo Press.

Maccoby, E. E., & Mnookin, R. H. (1992). *Dividing the Child: Social and Legal Dilemmas of Custody*. Cambridge: Harvard University Press.

Mahoney, M. J. (1991). *Human Change Processes: The Scientific Foundation of Psychotherapy*. New York: Basic Books.

Stuart, R. B. (1980). *Helping Couples Change: A Social Learning Approach to Marital Therapy*. New York: Guilford.

Walen, S. R., DiGiuseppe, R., & Dryden, W. (1992). *A Practitioner's Guide to Rational-Emotive Therapy* (2nd ed.). New York: Oxford.

Young, J. E. (1994). *Cognitive Therapy for Personality Disorders: A Schema-Focused Approach* (rev. ed.). Sarasota, FL: Professional Resource Press.

Young, J. E., & Gluhoski, V. L. (1996). Schema-focused diagnosis for personality disorders. In F. W. Kaslow (Ed.), *Handbook of Relational Diagnosis and Dysfunctional Family Patterns* (pp. 300-321). New York: Wiley.

Collaborative Divorce: An Interdisciplinary Approach For Resolving Divorce Conflicts*

A. Rodney Nurse and Peggy Thompson

It is difficult to imagine a psychologist, social worker, or (especially) a marital counselor who has not had significant exposure to divorce and its aftermath. For most of us doing psychotherapy, our experience is often with the worst of the "custody battles" over children. What is a difficult process within the family, with direct fallout for the children, has been brought to the attention of the public particularly by the research and writings of Wallerstein and Kelly (1980) and Wallerstein and Blakeslee (1989). Schwartz and Kaslow (1997) in their recent scholarly yet clinical book *Painful Partings,* state: "The anguish may continue to be acute for two to five years after the divorce is final or, for a number of reasons, may persist many years at a chronic, if lowered level" (p. 3). This conclusion suggests the suffering of a large body of our population. This is a group with which we have committed ourselves to work.

Although we have no doubt that the changing family relationships through divorce will continue to be painful for many adults and their children, we hold the strong opinion, shared with an increasing number of mental health and legal professionals, that our present societal/legal system for effecting a divorce is a major contributor to the anguish. Weinstein (1997), for example, points out to her fellow attorneys that the adversarial process polarizes the parents and in practice focuses on their rights as parents, not on the child's welfare. Somebody (a parent) "wins" and somebody (another parent) "loses." And lawyers must make a case for and fight for their client's (one parent) wishes against another lawyer representing the other parent. They must do this vigorously, following the legal ethical principal of zealous representation. The legal process, often litigation driven, is not dynamic. It focuses on specific issues, with little or no reference to the entire family context. In particular the traditional process ignores the child's needs. Although perhaps useful in various civil actions, the adversarial process is ill suited to furthering a humane process of family restructuring that is required in a divorce.

As with law professor Weinstein, many psychologists, sociologists, social workers, and others decry our present system (Johnston & Roseby, 1997). For many years, a part of our practice of family psychology has included conducting child custody evaluations and doing high-conflict and divorce counseling. We came to the same conclusion voiced by many others that "there must be a better way." We have been developing Collaborative Divorce[sm]** as a "better way" which is designed to result in a more humane divorce.

---

* We wish to express appreciation for the collaborative group effort over several years that has made possible the development of Collaborative Divorce. Present colleagues include Karen Fagerstrom, PhD, Nancy J. Ross, LCSW, Pauline Tesler, JD, Diana A. Wilde, Certified Divorce Planner, and Thomas Wolfrum, JD. Earlier contributors were William Anderson, JD, Karlotta Bartholomew, PhD, Faith Janson, JD, Milton Kalish, LCSW, and Grace Orenstein, PhD.

** Collaborative Divorce is a registered servicemark of Collaborative Divorce Training.

WHAT IS COLLABORATIVE DIVORCE?

First, a caveat. Collaborative Divorce is not Collaborative Law. Although Collaborative Law is an integral aspect of Collaborative Divorce, Collaborative Law does not have to involve Collaborative Divorce. These statements will take on additional meaning with the reading of this section.

Collaborative Divorce is an integrated interdisciplinary team system for solving the problems that arise in divorce. Collaborative Divorce in action requires that mental health professionals working with the divorcing family articulate their work with other collaborative professionals specialized in addressing the legal and financial problems of divorce. All collaborative professionals work together to psychologically hold the family while they create a guidance system to further a positive change in a family system. Within the context of a free flow of information while working together as a team, they seek to manage conflict and to help the family restructure from a nuclear family system to a binuclear family system. This team system allows for a diversity of families at various levels of serious conflict to use the collaborative process. The team forms a safety net that helps the parties through difficult situations, putting out wildfires and generally damping down minor conflicts threatening to generate the heat that could easily lead to major conflict.

Because each professional hears other professionals' views of the family undergoing divorce, all members of the team gain a more balanced view of the problems faced and the family dynamics involved. In this way each professional involved, whether trained in mental health, legal, or financial specialties, better understands the whole family system. Gaining this new knowledge and broadened view can be essential for finding creative solutions and working out strategies to solve problems. As the adage goes, two heads are better than one. When this knowledge comes from heads representing several different disciplinary approaches, the ensuing synchrony can result in vastly enriched patterns of problem solving. We believe that we can solve more problems as a team more often because working together we can create more possibilities.

A major intent of Collaborative Divorce is to conserve both the emotional and the financial resources of the family. When each professional is working in his or her area of speciality, the quality and effectiveness of the work is increased significantly. When the emotional forces that drive the conflict are addressed by mental health experts, the power of the emotional forces can be lessened significantly. Lessening the power means more effective use of the disciplinary skills of all involved professionals. Additionally, when the emotional forces of the divorce are contained and controlled, clients are better able to make more efficient use of specific legal services. A financial specialist can focus on the monetary aspects more effectively when the emotional meanings of those aspects are processed by the mental health specialists on the team. Collaborative lawyers spend more time lawyering and less time having to manage the psychological aspects of divorce. Even though there are more professionals involved, the final cost of the process is considerably less than any adversarial process. Most important, the long-term outcome in terms of the well-being of all family members, especially the children, is greatly enhanced. In many cases the overall functioning of the family is improved over the predivorce state by the work and education provided by the process.

THE COLLABORATIVE DIVORCE TEAM

In Collaborative Divorce the couple work with a male/female coaching team comprised of two licensed mental health professionals (usually psychologists, licensed clinical social workers, or marital counselors) who work with the clients initially individually and subsequently jointly. A child specialist (a licensed mental health professional with child training) assesses the children's needs. The coaches and the child specialist work with the emotional issues that drive the divorce process. The child specialist assists children in being heard above the static of the conflict. One member of the team, usually one of the coaches, acts as a case coordinator to keep all team members abreast of situations that arise and to keep the process on track. The team also includes a practical financial counselor who works with both parties. Both parties also work with lawyers who are trained in Collaborative Law (Webb, 1996), integral to Collaborative Divorce.

This core team also has access to other professionals whom the family may need to provide highly specialized team functions. These may include Certified Divorce Planners, Certified Public Accountants (CPAs), Business Evaluators, and other adjunct team members. In addition, the core team may make use of consultants to provide highly selective inputs to the core team, such as psychotherapists, physicians, and real estate evaluators. Figure 1 (below) provides a pictorial presentation of the collaborative coalition, consisting of the core team (at the center of the figure), as described in this contribution, plus adjunct team members used occasionally, plus consultants, also used occasionally.

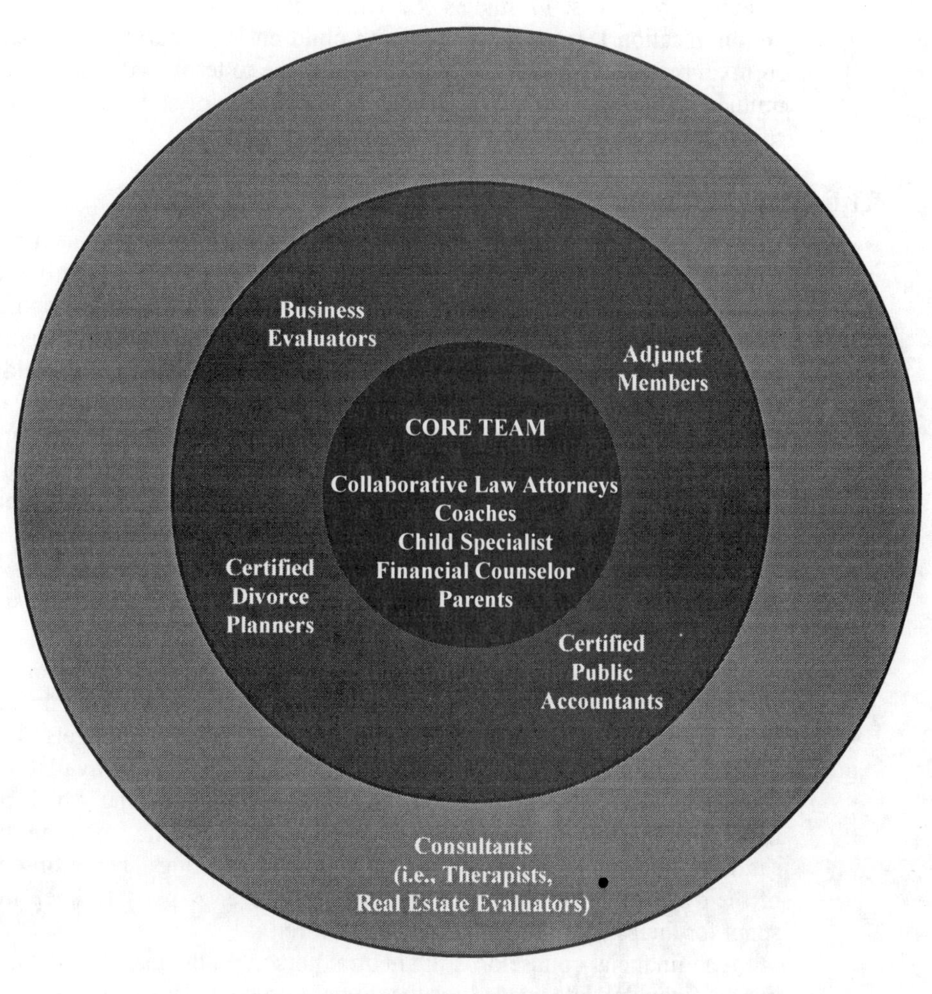

Figure 1. Collaborative Coalition.

The Gender-Balanced Coaching Duo

The coaches, licensed mental health professionals, meet initially individually with the spouse of the same gender. We have found that having a same-sex coach makes gaining the new client's trust in the process faster and easier, because their anger toward and suspicion about their spouse tends in divorce to generalize to all people of the opposite gender. A gender-balanced team increases the potential for effective communication. As Deborah Tannen points out in *You Just Don't Understand* (1990), the different socialization of males and females makes for difficulties in understanding each other. This problem becomes heightened at the time of divorce. A gender-balanced approach helps bridge this difficulty.

What do the coaches do? They assess the personality dynamics of the adults and their relationship through evaluative interviews and screening inventories. They identify and prioritize the concerns of each person. They try to separate psychological facts from fantasy. They work with the individuals to reduce their personal stress and teach them good stress-reduction techniques. They provide information about normal child development and coach positive parenting skills, especially for the less skilled parent. In this process each adult gets to tell a same-gendered person his or her personal marriage story. With some lessened pressure within each partner, the coaches then teach communication skills using a structured communication pattern, originally developed under a National Institute of Mental Health grant and verified as effective by at least 17 studies (S. Miller & P. A. Miller, 1997). The content focus of the communication learning for those with children is primarily on co-parenting. Coaches thus form an active safety net for the clients to come to terms with the emotional issues and communication needs, and facilitate the couple's change of communication patterns through joint four-way meetings.

The Child Specialist

The child specialist assesses children individually and with each parent. Concern is with children's development and temperament, their relationship to family members, including extended family, and their interests, emotional attachments, and supports beyond the family. The specialist assesses children's reaction to the family changes and their worries, hopes, fears, and expressed needs. Our experience is that it is helpful for children to have their own special "outside" person, the child specialist, to talk to about their view of the family changes. The parents appreciate having the opportunity to express their fears and concerns about the children with an expert in the field. It is an opportunity for both parents to focus their attention on the needs of their children. Feedback about the children and their needs is focused on a presentation by the child specialist to the parents and a discussion at one of their four-way meetings with the coaches.

The Financial Specialist

At a very basic level, a practical financial counselor is someone who understands the fundamentals of household financial matters, has good interpersonal skills, can help gather information about assets and debts, and can develop realistic budgets. This counselor can help the couple thoughtfully set priorities for the use of the dollars available, including estimating how much money to spend on the divorce and in considering which professionals are most needed in their situation. As noted previously, it may be the first time that some couples have sat down together to talk about money in a neutral setting. This setting of priorities for the use of their money is an ongoing process that helps each party to keep in mind how money is spent for their benefit and that of their children.

The financial counselor is the neutral person on the team, assisting the couple in collecting the financial data needed for the divorce process. This is a situation in which both parties have an opportunity to see all of their assets and liabilities and look at the living expenses of a divided household. The financial counselor encourages the couple to see the process as information gathering. At this stage the financial counselor actively discourages either party from making claims or trying to negotiate any division of property. The focus is on gathering information, identifying levels of understanding, and identifying issues that appear problematic. When needed, the counselor assists one or both parties to develop realistic individualized budgets. Both parties are free to ask each other factual questions about financial matters. For some couples this is the first time they have actually talked together about their finances. This conferencing with the financial counselor is an opportunity for both parties to agree on their joint financial position - that is, to agree on what's in the pie of assets.

If one party is less sophisticated in financial matters, time may be spent helping that person understand even such simple activities as keeping a checkbook. Knowledge builds confidence and makes an unknown future less fearful. Fear often underlies anger, so, as this process lessens fear, anger tends to diminish. This process allows clients to consider a realistic perspective and fight against the paralyzing fears that, for example, she is bound to end up as a bag lady or he as a man who works only to support his ex-wife. It reduces the tendency on the part of one spouse to think that there are resources hidden by the other spouse.

The information developed by the financial specialist is utilized not only by the attorneys but also by higher level financial specialists, such as CPAs, financial planners, or other business consultants whose expertise may be needed in a specific case. Our experience suggests that it is important that these experts know and understand the goals of the collaborative process and have contact with the team during their work.

Lawyers

Each parent has an attorney trained in Collaborative Law (Webb, 1996). It is a basic tenet of Collaborative Law that attorneys sign an agreement not to go to court. If the parties decide that they must fight their problems out in court, they must end the relationships with the collaborative attorneys and engage other attorneys to represent them. The Collaborative Law attorneys work collaboratively with each other and all team members as well as with their clients. Information is distributed freely among all professionals and the parties. The openness underlines an ethic of working to satisfy the differing interests of the parties. For example, if finances permit, it may be more important for one of the parties, often the wife, to live in the home, at least for a period of time. For the husband, it may be that his interests lie more in having more immediate cash to invest and having the expensive car. In considering their responsibilities as parents, having had input from the child specialist about their children and having problem solved about their children with their coaches, they may reevaluate their priorities in light of their children's needs. This might include joint planning for college education or for allocation of resources to address the special needs of a child. Divorce often poses difficult financial choices.

The Power of the Team

By virtue of the professionals on the team collaborating, information flows freely within the team. Having all professionally relevant information (at least in summary form) available to all team members provides a greatly expanded view of a family's present and possible future problems and positive potentials. This is true, first, because different disciplines (law, mental health, and finance) tend appropriately to seek information relevant to concerns within their area of expertise. Second, this process is reinforced by clients coming to each discipline with different expectations. For example, they would expect to talk budgets with a practical financial person, express their own anxieties or concern for an upset child with a mental health person, and ask questions of an attorney about child support issues and community property worries. Hearing other professionals' information, disciplinary knowledge, and perspective of a family helps all team members gain a more balanced view of the problems faced and the family dynamics involved in the process.

Keeping in mind this shared knowledge and utilizing this enriched perspectival understanding of the family can be essential for finding creative solutions and crafting strategies to solve problems. When team members agree on priorities and strategies for working with a family, they can impact the family in consistent ways even as they exercise skills unique to their own discipline. We believe that it takes a carefully orchestrated system to change the family system in an effective way. Even defective and changing family systems can be very powerful. It takes a strong system to change a strong system.

Team Collaboration Encourages Client Collaboration

Clients get support from different perspectives. They know they are represented by their attorneys. They have the support of their coaches, whose focus is guiding them through the emotional roller coaster of divorce and teaching them ways of dealing with the frustrations of learning to communicate on important matters with each other. This process of talking with and listening to different people often loosens the tyranny of set ideas, softens the seemingly fixed positions of both parties, and allows for the possibility of more creative solutions. As possible solutions to problems appear, fear diminishes and anger subsides. This makes way for better communication between the parties and the possibility of understanding the other's needs. The focus for those with children is on their children's needs and on finding ways to minimize the impact of the divorce on them through positive co-parenting.

HOW CLIENTS ENTER THE SYSTEM

Clients may enter the Collaborative Law/Collaborative Divorce system through any one of three doors: legal, mental health, or financial. Some clients enter the expected way by contacting an attorney trained in Collaborative Law who explains the options available so that they may make a judgment together as to whether this new process might fit the circumstances of their case. If a client is interested, that client may call a coach directly for more information. The client may also suggest to the spouse that he or she call a coach to get information independently. Attorneys cannot be in contact directly with the spouse of their client. Because of this restriction, and because using a collaborative team is a new concept, not yet widely known, lawyers sometimes have difficulty with establishing the collaborative process. Lawyers who are unaware of mental health professionals' ability to work with "normal" populations have understandable difficulty in organizing the team process.

Clients may also begin the Collaborative Law/Collaborative Divorce process by making an initial contact by phone with mental health professionals trained to work as Collaborative Divorce coaches. If the potential case seems appropriate, the coach is able to suggest that the prospective client ask his or her spouse to call a same-gender coach to obtain information about Collaborative Law/Collaborative Divorce. If that step is successful, the divorcing couple might then come for a personal discussion of the process either together or, if they are too antagonistic, separately. This way of engaging the other spouse is preferable to asking that the collaborative process be conveyed through the spouse making the initial contact. (If they could communicate accurately and well, they might not be getting a divorce!)

Sometimes an attempt to refer to an attorney meets resistance. Discussing on the phone and in person the collaborative principal and way of working allows a person who fears attorneys to be reassured that the engagement of an attorney will not escalate the fight. The discussion is helpful not only to clients who fear attorneys, but also to those wary of lawyers because of past experiences in other areas of disputes when the process and the costs did get out of hand (from their standpoint). We find, incidentally, that in our San Francisco Bay area, some independent entrepreneurs who locate us on our website are likely to fit this category or are bent on maintaining control of their divorce. Sometimes it takes firmness and a sense of timing to make a successful referral to an attorney.

Some clients come to the process via the financial door. Clients coming to the financial specialist may see that they need help financially in dividing their assets and liabilities, yet resist or be unaware of the importance of the legal and psychological aspects. The financial specialist must be aware of the legal ramifications so these can be explained to the clients. They also must be sensitive to the interpersonal relationships within the family so that they can describe the usefulness of the child assessment and the need to improve the adults' communication in order to learn to co-parent effectively.

Couples do come with varying needs for service. Those with no children obviously do not need the child specialist. Couples with few financial assets may need little financial assistance. Occasionally couples have already reached a point of co-parenting effectively and need minimal contact with coaches. For some couples, attorneys become consultants whom the couples simply ask to insure that they have not overlooked anything. In the following section, we describe a model that fits the majority of clients but has the flexibility to fit the special circumstances and wishes of other clients.

THE THREE PHASES OF COLLABORATIVE DIVORCE

Keeping in mind the different roles of the coaches, the child specialist, the financial specialist, and the attorneys will be helpful in viewing Table 1 (p. 176), which presents the Three Phases of Collaborative Divorce. Although the table displays the process from the standpoint of the mental health specialist, it is important to remember that the Collaborative Divorce process may be initiated by any member of the team. As noted previously, clients may enter by going first through the door of the financial specialist's office or through that of the attorney's, the most traditional way. As may be seen in Table 1, the three phases of the Collaborative Divorce process are as follows: Phase A, Contracting and Starting; Phase B, Family Appraisal, Learning Co-Parenting Communication; and Phase C, Negotiating and Settling Issues.

Phase A - Contracting and Starting

In Step 1 of the first phase, Contracting and Starting, the couple are oriented to the process, engage in discussions of what to expect, and sign the working agreement. The agreement includes the provision that the mental health professionals will withdraw should the couple decide to leave the system and follow an adversarial process. (Clients sign a similar agreement with the financial specialist and the collaborative attorneys.) Free flow of information between all team members is underlined as a basis for trusting work. Appointments for Step 2 and the first steps of Phase B are made to insure that the process gets underway. Appointment scheduling and planning helps clients feel more secure in the process and offers an immediate sense that "something is being done" to help get them through this usually stressful time.

Completion of Step 1 permits moving to Step 2, which may occur on the same day as Step 1, or a subsequent day. Step 2 consists of the first individual interview with a same-sex coach/mental health professional. Each tells his or her own story to the coach, who also collects background information that we have found essential in identifying parenting strengths and weaknesses.

Each spouse fills out forms describing the marriage history and his or her own history, as well as developmental information about their children. To find out in a systematic way how they view their children, we ask each spouse to fill out a parent form of the Behavior Assessment Inventory for Children (BASC; Reynolds & Kamphaus, 1992). This provides a comparison with a national sample of parents of normal children surveying dimensions of personality strengths, problems, and potential red flags. We also administer a child BASC to children 8 or older later in the process and to adolescents. We also typically ask the children's teachers to fill out the teacher form.

To obtain a sense of parenting style, we administer the Parent-Child Relationship Inventory (PCRI; Gerard, 1994). The PCRI provides information on the degree of practical and emotional support available for the parents, satisfaction in parenting, involvement with their child, how well they communicate with their child, their limit-setting behavior, how much age-appropriate autonomy they can allow their child, and an estimate of whether they lean toward a more traditional view of differentiated father and mother roles or toward more androgynous roles. The inventory author, Anthony B. Gerard (1994, p. 1), recommends the use of this inventory in divorcing contexts.

For personality style, we use the Millon Clinical Multiaxial Inventory-III (MCMI-III). We like this personality inventory because a major section of the MCMI-III reveals something of a client's personality style, screens for personality disorders, and provides for measures of specific symptoms or mood patterns. In the inventory manual the author (Millon, 1994, p. 5) indicates that using the MCMI-III in the context of child custody study is "appropriate, owing to the presence of many such cases in the MCMI-III normative sample." For

TABLE 1: Three Phases of Collaborative Divorce

Phase A - Contracting and Starting		
Step 1. Couple orientation, signing agreement, scheduling		
Step 2. Individual interview 1, by a coach for each spouse, inventories	► ► ►	Coaches provide initial information to child and financial specialists, attorneys.
Phase B - Family Appraisal, Learning Co-Parenting Communication		Child specialist assesses children.
Step 3. Individual interview 2, self and family appraisal for each spouse		Financial specialist meets the couple and helps with information organization.
Step 4. Individual interview 3, learning a communication process		Attorneys meet parents individually to contract and establish working relationships, assisted by receiving information from the financial specialist.
Step 5. Four-way session 1, practice with the communication process		Attorneys may begin four-way sessions with parents to confirm and begin collaborative law process.
Phase C - Negotiating and Settling Issues		Financial specialist concludes organization of finances and conveys to attorneys.
Step 6. Four-way session 2, about major issues		
Step 7. Four-way session 3, child specialist provides feedback	◄ ◄ ◄	Child specialist provides information to parents and coaches regarding the children.
Step 8. Four-way session 4, child issue resolving, plans drafted		
Step 9. Four-way session 5, co-parenting plan concluded	► ► ►	Coaches confer with lawyers about co-parenting plan.
		Lawyers hold four-way sessions to reach settlement.
Step 10. Coaches on call to assist parents as needed.		Lawyers on call postdivorce.

more in-depth understanding of the personality inventories that we use in the Collaborative Divorce process, the reader may wish to consult *Family Assessment: Effective Uses of Personality Tests With Couples and Families* (Nurse, 1999).

Information from the forms and inventories establishes a data-based platform for the coaches as they make an initial assessment of the spouses and their relationship to each other and their children; this assessment will form a basis for professional work in Phase B, as well as being summarized in (usually, brief, telephone) conferences with the child specialist, the attorney, and the financial specialist.

Phase B - Family Appraisal, Learning Co-Parenting Communication

With the completion of Phase A, Contracting and Starting, the coaches move to Phase B, Family Appraisal, Learning Co-Parenting Communication. In Step 3, the initial step of Phase B, each parent is given information synthesized from the information-gathering process in Phase A. Thus parents are provided with a mirror in which to look at themselves as a basis for drawing on their better selves in the forthcoming negotiation process. The focus is on how to further effective parenting, manage feelings toward a spouse, and establish priorities for possible outcomes of the divorce process that each spouse needs or wants most (e.g., having the home, private schooling for one of the children, emotional stabilization of a child, effective co-parenting approaches, etc.).

In Step 4, the middle step in Phase B, the coaches teach the specific communication process that will be used in the negotiation of Phase C. Use of this new process is intended to carry over to assist problem solving for the parents when they no longer have professional assistance. If the groundwork has been laid carefully, the newly organized self-knowledge gained in the previous step can help focus the learning required in the structured communication process. Step 4 is a crucial step because the parents need preparation to embark on a different relationship, that of co-parenting. In the co-parenting relationship they must learn to collaborate in parenting their children, with all of the intimate feelings, hopes, and fears that involves, yet do this in a relationship in which both have chosen not to have intimacy as a couple goal. The change from parenting to co-parenting means each has sole responsibility for a particular child at any specific time period; they must make medical, school, and other decisions jointly for many years with the person with whom they have chosen not to share their life and whom, in these early times of the divorce, they are likely to view ambivalently, at best.

The final step in Phase B is Step 5, wherein the coaches and the clients get together for the first four-way meeting. This session is designed so that the communication pattern learned individually with each coach can be adopted for use by the couple. They begin by practicing on the easier immediate issues.

Meanwhile, as Table 1 (p. 176) shows, during Phase B, while the coaches are doing the family appraisal and teaching a pattern for co-parent communication, the child specialist sees the child alone and with each parent separately. The financial specialist meets with the couple to focus on information organization. The attorneys, by the end of Phase B, may be holding an initial meeting with the couple, if they have not already done so.

Phase C - Negotiating and Settling Issues

In the first step of this phase, Step 6, the coaches and clients hold a four-way meeting to begin work on settling major issues. The focus is usually on co-parenting issues or other issues that also involve strong emotions, such as gifts from one set of parents. Frequently it is important for one spouse, or sometimes both, to come to an understanding of the reasons for wanting the divorce. Although the focus is on negotiating and settling specific issues, or beginning to, this step also is intended to improve the clients' ability to use the communication process, which will form a basis for success in their postdivorce co-parenting process.

In Step 7 the child specialist meets with the coaches and the parents to provide feedback about observations of the children, how they appear to be faring in the divorce, their psychological state, and what they are most likely to need from their parents and in their school, play, and other environments. This step provides a neutral, objective voice speaking for the child and, at the same time, a professional opinion appraising the child.

When the parents and the coaches meet in the four-way format in Step 8, they work to integrate the very important feedback obtained in the previous session about the child. A co-parenting plan begins to be drafted.

In Step 9 the coaches and parents conclude their work on the co-parenting plan. It is then forwarded to the attorneys and the other specialists for discussion among all the professionals. In particular the information and the interdisciplinary discussion process informs the attorneys in their negotiations with the couple. Step 10 indicates the availability of the team after the divorce has been legally granted.

Although we break our process down into the nine steps, in the real-life difficulties of divorcing families, any of these steps can take more than one session. For each family we vary the model to best match the family's situation and problems. One size does not fit all.

It is sometimes important to either slow down or speed up the process. The slowing down is necessary for those couples who are rushing to negotiate without having the knowledge or interpersonal tools with which to negotiate. For other couples needing to be pushed ahead, assets may be dwindling at a rapid rate, there may be deadlines for getting children placed in new schools, or other real-world pressures. In our experience, the most usual action is that the team needs to slow down the divorce train so that the couple can reflect sufficiently to make informed decisions and develop tools that will be of help once they are past the planned services of the team. We do also make ourselves available for follow-up help to the couple and their children as needed, such as to mediate specific issues or recommend appropriate therapists. Because of team roles and because they might need the team in the future, we do not take on families or individuals in families as psychotherapy clients.

A CASE EXAMPLE OF COLLABORATIVE DIVORCE

The following case example* will illustrate how the Collaborative Divorce process can proceed. The family consists of Jill, 45, Jon, 45, and their two children Julie, 5, and Jake, 13. Jon works at a computer firm and Jill is an elementary school teacher. Jon found us on our website. He had moved out of home 2 months before and lives with a friend.

In his first meeting with the divorce coach, following the couple meeting with both coaches to review and sign the Collaborative Divorce agreement, Jon explains that the marriage has been "going downhill for years." Jill has been angry about his working so hard for the family that he doesn't spend much time with the children. He says he does what he can, but his job is demanding. Not only that, he and Jill have been distant in recent years, and Jill withheld sex for several years. That was when their relationship "just died," he believes. He adds, "I don't tolerate people who don't live up to their obligations. She did that to punish me. I'll never let anyone do that to me again."

He tells the counselor, as a very proud former "West Pointer" with a good service record, that he will do whatever he can to make sure that Jill and the children are provided for. He's willing to "give up everything" to make that happen, "because it's the right thing to do." He explains that 2 months ago, he "had it up to here" with the bickering and complaining at home and "just had to move out." He is staying with a friend while he looks for an apartment. When asked about Jill, he says that she is passive but controlling, seems to wind up "the victim, that's the main reason we're divorcing." "I can't take her whining anymore. I will not put up with it, and it's affecting our son, too." Jon makes clear statements about wanting the divorce. He does not want to put out any more money than necessary, although he understands that he will need to see an attorney to "finalize the divorce."

When Jill talks to her counselor, she is adamant about not wanting the divorce. Alternately crying and blaming, Jill states her belief that Jon is suffering from a midlife crisis. He behaves like he's "crazy." "I've always done things his way; he has no reason to leave." His leaving came "out of the blue." "He never said he was unhappy." Jill indicates that Jon had been "more quiet recently" and even, uncharacteristically, "blew up" at her when she was "just

*Names and identifying characteristics have been changed to protect confidentiality.

trying to encourage him to spend more time with their son." She's worried about Jake, who has recently been diagnosed as Attention-Deficit/Hyperactivity Disorder (ADHD) and seems extremely oppositional to her ways of trying to help him be more organized and less forgetful.

Jill says to her coach, "Jon is not the most understanding dad, but he is their dad, and I'm really scared to be a single mom." If she can't get him to change his mind, her one desire is to keep the house. "I can't imagine life without our home." Jill appears defeated by the situation, alternately crying and expressing fears that she won't survive.

Coaches Conference

Combining their interview impressions and results of the inventory information, the coaches hypothesize that Jon is somewhat compulsive and organized in personality style and rather self-focused (narcissistic), but not unreasonably so; he has concerns for his family, although his guilt about leaving may interfere with his good judgment. Jill they see as dependent in personality style but as having demonstrated competencies that could be built upon. Thus if the relationship becomes even more polarized, Jon could become too rigidly "principled," not being able to empathize with Jill's and the children's feelings. Jill could panic and become more disorganized and depressed, resulting in problems of taking hold becoming even more prominent.

Systemically it appears that Jon's expressing his anger through "righteous" behavior results in his overtly dominating her. She responds by retreating to a victim-martyr position, to which he responds with guilt and feelings of being controlled by her. Sometimes she initiates taking the victim-martyr position, to which, because of his guilt (especially over leaving his duty as husband), he feels more guilt, obligation, and is ready to give her what she wants, yet his fury with her increases, only to be let out in subsequent, "principled," minilectures.

Both parents have strengths that can be built upon. They are intelligent and well educated, have stabilized careers, and want to avoid conflict. They are both united in a belief that they do not want the costs to escalate, nor do they want negative emotional fallout with their children. Both are concerned about Jake.

In considering the family relationship problems, although both parents worry about Jake, it may be that Jake's reaching adolescence has kindled problems already present within the family. Coaches also have a concern that the parents seem to regard 5-year-old Julie as "mom's" and Jake more as "dad's," a somewhat flawed basis for beginning to learn to co-parent.

Anticipating the next step in the process, the coaches pass on the information to the finance specialist and the lawyers that Jill is set on having the house. The coaches raise the question as to whether their financial structure could allow either to have the house. The lawyers are informed that the coaches will work with Jon to have him at least "touch base" with his lawyer. With Jill's dependence, she can easily be referred to an attorney, but the attorney is warned against taking over too much for her.

In this planning stage, coaches suggest to the child specialist, in addition to her appraisal of Jake, that useful information might be obtained from whomever diagnosed Jake as ADHD. Coaches indicate that it would be very helpful to get some sense of the developmental level of Jake, with particular regard for his need for time with his father. The child specialist is alerted to evaluate Jill's possible overidentification and possible overprotection of Julie. Concern is expressed over how neglected and angry the children are, because their parents appear to be so involved in their own fight and worries that their sensitivity to the children's needs is likely lessened. Thus, working on the case is underway.

The Course of the Case - What Happened

In their next meetings with their clients, the coaches discussed the apparent individual and couple dynamics. They stressed the need to establish a fair process wherein Jon and Jill would be treated with equal respect and consideration. Jon's coach persuaded him that the process would need to be slowed down to let his wife "catch up," because she was still clinging to the idea that the marriage "could be saved." Jill's coach worked with Jill's fears of letting go of the marriage and needing to hang on. In line with helping both partners look at the financial and legal realities, they were encouraged to meet together with the finance specialist and, subsequently, each with his or her own attorney.

Some individual issues were handled by the coaches. Jon's father had been "taken to the cleaners" by his mother. His father had been an alcoholic at the time, though sober now. Jon noted that his father has been "advising" him recently. That Jon was actually afraid that Jill would win out in this situation was acknowledged by Jon. His own tendency to "give away the store" out of guilt was pointed out. Facing these issues and experiencing some relaxation of his tension, coupled with discussion about his concern for helping his son in a more active way, paved the way for four-way meetings among Jon, Jill, and the coaches.

Jill's coach in the meantime was able to actualize Jill's more independent aspects. Using assertion and cognitive-training techniques, Jill gained more conscious control over how she dealt with her son and how she might view the finances. She could even admit that perhaps staying in the house may not prove realistic.

In their four-way meetings with the coaches, following individualized communication training (S. Miller & P. A. Miller, 1997), Jon and Jill worked on their priorities: (a) maintaining current family support levels from Jon to make house payments and pay bills until final agreements could be reached; (b) working out co-parenting scheduling; and (c) piecing together what had happened in the marriage to lead to initiation of the divorce.

As they began talking through their priorities, they obtained input from the child specialist. She provided some more practical advice regarding Jake's need for help in organization and some compensations at school. Although Jon was reluctant to follow her advice suggesting a referral for medication evaluation for Jake, he did so, and Jake's taking medication improved his attention and task tracking at home. Julie seemed to be doing quite well after some regressive behavior immediately following the separation of the parents. The regularized co-parenting schedule apparently was emotionally settling for her.

During a time when Jon and Jill were working out these issues, including absorbing an analysis from the financial specialist, Jon, in a grand gesture, told Jill that he would forgo getting his fair share of the house so she and the children could stay in it. Both coaches cautioned against premature actions such as this, in all fairness, before all aspects of agreements were considered.

Subsequently, the first four-way meeting with the attorneys was delayed a week when Jon visited his home back east for a family gathering. During that time, he visited with his father, who, it later turned out, told him that far from being "noble," he was just being a "wimp" in letting his wife "take advantage" of him by staying in the house.

On his return, the initial part of this first legal four-way went well. Near the end, when Jill noted that Jon had indicated his willingness to allow her to stay in the house, he reacted strongly and said that he had changed his mind and that the house would need to be sold as soon as possible - a nonnegotiable position. Jill dissolved in tears and ran from the room. The attorneys called a recess that became the end of the meeting. Jill and her attorney took a walk. Jon's attorney talked to Jon and let him know that his abrupt message didn't further the collaborative process. Furthermore, on such a major issue, he should have forewarned his attorney. Jill's attorney worked with her and said that the process would continue, but not that day.

Individual sessions with the coaches led to Jill increasing her ability to manage her feelings under pressure and Jon's reflecting on the sequence of events leading from his family events, his father's message, and his angry, rigid behavior. Both returned to go over finances, particularly including the house, with the financial specialist. They had a four-way session with the coaches that enabled them to resume negotiating. By this time more aspects of their individual lives had fallen into place and more information was available about possible living arrangement choices. Jill understood that for Jon to co-parent effectively, he needed a reasonable apartment of his own. Jon could verbalize how important the sense of "home" was for Jill. They both talked through their disappointment that they would need to sell the house for which they had both worked. Coaches and attorneys recognized that both parents were now less fearful about the future. She had become more assertive. He had become less defensive.

They now had skills for co-parenting that meant that they kept their distance while still being able to communicate and negotiate about co-parenting issues. Their divorce process concluded. Both were aware that in the future they could return to any of the team to work on specific divorce issues as needed.

HOW GROUPS ARE FORMED FOR TEAMWORK

Several considerations are involved in developing a Collaborative Divorce team. The selection must be carefully calculated to obtain professionals with a discipline-related background of education, training, and experience in divorce. Professionals must understand that a paradigm shift will need to occur so that they may use both collaborative thinking and collaborative attitudes in working with colleagues and clients. To successfully make the shift requires a decision to do so, the motivation to follow through, and a willingness to understand that it may take a while for the emotional shift to take place and for some of the original patterns of behavior to be extinguished. This means being willing to accept and own mistakes, make corrections, and move forward. The shift is somewhat different for each discipline, as noted in the following section.

Selecting Team Members

The *collaborative attorneys* on the team need to have the experience of specializing in the practice of family law, preferably having qualified with the Bar in that specialty. These attorneys need to have experience working with mental health professionals in a cooperative way and with respect for what they contribute to the divorce process. The particular paradigm shift for attorneys is from an adversarial to a collaborative stance. The principle of zealous advocacy must somehow be transformed into a commitment to a positive outcome for the entire family, and this requires thinking and responding in a cooperative, collaborative way. This cognitive set means the attorney must be as concerned for finding ways to meet the needs of the other spouse as for his or her own client. Attorneys need to be able to make a paradigm shift within themselves that allows them to take on the new role as collaborator. This shift facilitates their learning to communicate with each other in a nonadversarial way and represent their own client while, at the same time, considering the family as a whole as their client.

Although the role of the collaborative lawyer is different from being a mediator, having some background training in mediation skills is helpful. The good collaborative attorney is very often experienced in negotiating and can make use of a background in reaching settlements on an interest basis, even if the attorney's background is in litigation-driven bargaining. Finally, the collaborative lawyer must be flexible enough to broaden his or her view of the family divorce process as beginning before the first attorney-client contact, involving the entire family changing, and continuing well past the formal divorce decree itself. A forthcoming manual on Collaborative Law by Pauline Tesler (Tesler, in press), to be published by the American Bar Association, will serve as an excellent reference for attorneys. Some family law groups organized under the Bar require continuing education courses in Collaborative Law and Collaborative Divorce.

As with attorneys, *mental health professionals (coaches and the child specialist)* need to possess a knowledge of the divorce process and experience in working with divorcing families. They need some experience with the legal system for divorce. Therapists who have a background in family therapy and who have done couple and family therapy are likely to make the best coaches; others would have to add family training in order to build in skills working with families. Coaches need to have experience working with attorneys in a cooperative way and with respect for the role they play in the divorce process. An additional quality needed by the child specialist, in addition to the above, is a broad perspective of children, normal to disturbed. The specialist needs expertise in diagnosis and therapy with children and adolescents. We have found that the speciality area of early childhood - birth to 5 years - tends to call for a different professional than one who is skilled with children, preteens, and teens. The child specialist needs the skills to work with parents, even though sometimes they will not agree with the specialist's ideas. Sometimes a child therapist can be very good with children but find it difficult to deal with adults; the collaborative process requires that the child specialist have the expertise to manage both children and their parents. The specialist also needs to be able to state his or her understandings and opinions about the children clearly in case consultations. The richness of the teamwork comes from working through the perspectives that different team members have on a case. The child specialist is the voice for the child. Thus, it is important that he or she be able to keep that voice present as the team works.

The mental health professional's paradigm shift is from independent responsibility for helping the individual client and the family to collaborative working in a very focused, action-oriented way. The shift is most pronounced for psychoanalytically/psychodynamically oriented therapists and client centered therapists and is least pronounced with structured, cognitive therapists, who are more accustomed to dealing with specific, narrow, psychological issues within a relatively brief time frame. The need to consider the teamwork as important as their individual contact with their clients is the major shift for most therapists. They need to be open to learning to consider both the legal and financial realities that confront the family. Mental health professional coaches must be able to shift from a therapy oriented model to a coaching stance that, while incorporating therapeutic techniques as well as mediation skills, provides a supportive emotional position for the person with whom they work. They need to be able to demonstrate and model communication and listening skills for the parents. As co-coaches, independent mental health professionals need to be open to learning co-coaching skills in order to collaborate with each other.

In addition to good basic, down-to-earth financial skills, the *financial specialist* needs to already have developed good people skills, including the ability to teach and tutor others. This specialist needs the skill to maintain an overall attitude that is nonjudgmental and neutral. The financial specialist is the neutral who can help the parents gather all the information about their financial state, helping each of them as necessary to understand it. He or she needs to come to the team with sufficient personal awareness and stability to not fall prey to inadvertently taking one or the other parent's side. The specialist must be able to manage the level of feelings that may be present, inasmuch as sometimes this is the only time that the parents have sat together to go over finances. The financial area generates much fear and anxiety in people going through divorce, so the financial specialist must be able to learn to understand the various manifestation of this fear and anxiety (such as overt anger, need to dominate, need to be submissive, etc.). The financial specialist needs to have developed the verbal ability to accurately provide feedback to the team about the observed attitudes and knowledge of the parties. Such feedback can add richly to the team's understanding of the family dynamics when faced with a very specific task (finances) in a way not readily available to other team members. It is a good opportunity in a neutral setting for the parents to understand and agree on what is available to divide, so tutoring skills mentioned previously are important.

The financial person needs to have developed the interpersonal skill to support the parent who is less skilled in financial matters and at the same time not alienate the other parent. Smoothing the transition to financial independence for a dependent partner can be vital to the well-being of the whole family. The financial specialist needs to have the ability and assertiveness to serve the team by helping them keep in mind the financial limits, priorities, and concerns of the family.

Developing Teamwork

In our experience, teamwork takes place when four conditions are met. First, all members of the team have made (or are in the process of making) the needed paradigm shift. Second, they share the common goals and objectives of the collaborative process. Third, all members understand and respect the boundaries of each other's discipline. Finally, team members possess a basic level of professional and personal trust. When these four conditions become operative in working relationships, a strong team is possible.

In order to reach the level where the four elements are sufficiently in place, a team needs to engage in regular discussions on how these specific team members might work together, sharing knowledge about each other's ways of working, professional demands, and ethics. Training together facilitates team development when the training is interdisciplinary, and not simply increasing knowledge and skills in one's discipline, as important as that is.

The team needs to clarify gender attitudes and related potential issues so that they are not split into two camps by their respective alliances with the parents, and so that they are able to maintain a commitment to the welfare of the entire family. All team members, in developing a clarity about professional boundary issues, must trust other team members as they respond. Lawyers and financial team members must rely on the child specialist and the co-coaches for in-depth understanding of the child, adult, and family system dynamics, and be open to ways to put this knowledge into action. Mental health professionals need to appreciate the legal consequences down the road for decisions regarding property and taxes. They also need to appreciate the lawyers' application of collaborative negotiating skills within this "real-world" context.

In beginning cases a consultant to the team may further the development of the team's effectiveness. Should there be two teams in the same geographical region they might consult as teams with each other around specific cases.

The most effective team development requires interdisciplinary training focused on how the disciplines may work together collaboratively. The training needs to focus on how a specific team may work out their particular working relationships. This individualization of the process for a specific team optimizes team effectiveness in working toward the same goals and objectives in a given case.

A Caveat

Not all professionals can work within the collaborative team environment. Some individuals have become attorneys, psychiatric social workers, and financial specialists in order to work primarily autonomously in independent practice. Of these, some maintain a strong preference for the independence and freedom from the need to relate more or less continually in a team fashion as is required within an organization. The need to take responsibility and be in control as a professional may be very strong. Some attorneys have a personality predilection for adversarial situations. Some therapists are only satisfied when they work in-depth aiming at reconstruction personality over a lengthy period of time. Probably many of these people would not be comfortable in the shift to the collaborative mode.

We invite those with cooperative, affiliative wishes to seriously consider expanding their professional and personal horizons by attempting a paradigm shift to a collaborative stance and joining with others and ourselves in working in an interdisciplinary, collaborative team with families going through divorce.

SUMMARY

Collaborative Divorce may be thought of as a systematic, interdisciplinary team approach that involves specific steps and emotionally supportive patterns of interactions that facilitate a cooperative, nonadversarial divorce process. The team consists of a gender-balanced duo of mental health professionals serving as coaches for the parents, a mental health child specialist for the children, and a financial specialist who works with the parents to organize their finances. Attorneys, one for each parent, are equal members of the team. Their legal work is predicated on a commitment to Collaborative Law. All professionals work toward settlement of divorce issues and furthering the well-being of all family members, and sign an agreement not to be involved with this couple's litigation should the couple withdraw from the Collaborative Divorce/Collaborative Law process and enter into an adversarial process. Not going to court and avoiding a "child custody evaluation" reduces potential costs. Having collaborating specialists working together while concentrating their expertise on major family areas improves the odds that all aspects of the family divorce process - psychological, financial, and legal - are managed successfully. A divorce well done, with sensitivity for all family members, can set the stage for less rancor, positively meaningful family relationships, and effective problem solving.

CONTRIBUTORS

A. Rodney Nurse, PhD, ABPP, a clinical and family psychologist, is a founder of Collaborative Divorce. He currently serves as Co-Director of Family Psychological Services, Orinda, California, and also is Director of Family Services for the Boyer Institute, San Rafael, California. A former President and Dean of the California Graduate School of Family Psychology, he is a Life Fellow in the Society for Personality Assessment. Dr. Nurse has written a number of chapters and articles on divorce, personality disorders, and psychological testing and is the author of *Family Assessment: Effective Uses of Personality Tests With Couples and Families.* He can be reached at P.O. Box 175, Orinda, CA 94563.

Peggy Thompson, PhD, is a founder and Co-Director of both Collaborative Divorce and Family Psychological Services in Santa Rosa and Orinda, California. She is also a founder and Co-Director of American Institute of Collaborative Professions. Dr. Thompson has specialized in treating children and families for over 25 years, and for 10 years she has been involved in the divorce process as a custody evaluator, special master, and high-conflict counselor. She is a co-author of *Divorce: A Problem to Be Solved, Not a Battle to Be Fought.* She may be reached at P.O. Box 175, Orinda, CA 94563. E-mail: DRPTCD@aol.com

RESOURCES

Gerard, A. (1994). *Parent-Child Relationship Inventory (PCRI).* Los Angeles: Western Psychological Services.

Johnston, J., & Roseby, V. (1997). *In the Name of the Child.* New York: Free Press.

Miller, S., & Miller, P. A. (1997). *Core Communication: Skills and Processes.* Littleton, CO: Interpersonal Communications.

Millon, T. (1994). *Millon Clinical Multiaxial Inventory-III Manual.* Minneapolis: National Computer Systems.

Nurse, A. R. (1999). *Family Assessment: Effective Uses of Personality Tests With Couples and Families.* New York: Wiley.

Reynolds, D., & Kamphaus, F. (1992). *Manual for Behavior Assessment System for Children (BASC).* Circle Pines, MN: American Guidance Service.

Schwartz, L., & Kaslow, F. (1997). *Painful Partings: Divorce and Its Aftermath.* New York: Wiley.

Tannen, D. (1990). *You Just Don't Understand: Women and Men in Conversation.* New York: Ballantine Books.

Tesler, P. H. (in press). *Collaborative Law: A Manual for Family Law Attorneys.* Chicago, IL: American Bar Association.

Wallerstein, J., & Blakeslee, S. (1989). *Second Chances: Men, Women, and Children a Decade After Divorce.* New York: Ticknor & Fields.

Wallerstein, J., & Kelly, J. (1980). *Surviving the Breakup: How Children and Parents Cope With Divorce.* New York: Basic Books.

Webb, S. (1996, July-August). Collaborative law - A conversation: Why aren't those divorce lawyers going to court? *The Hennepin Lawyer,* pp. 30-32.

Weinstein, J. (1997). And never the twain shall meet: The best interests of children and the adversary system. *University of Miami Law Review, 52,* 79-175.

Evaluation and Treatment of Sexual Disorders: Frottage

Richard B. Krueger and Meg S. Kaplan

Frotteurism is a paraphilia which is defined in the fourth edition of the *Diagnostic and Statistical Manual of Mental Disorders* (*DSM-IV*; American Psychiatric Association, 1994, p. 527). Diagnostic criteria include: "A. Over a period of at least 6 months, recurrent, intense sexually arousing fantasies, sexual urges, or behaviors involving touching and rubbing against a nonconsenting person"; and "B. The fantasies, sexual urges, or behaviors cause clinically significant distress or impairment in social, occupational, or other important areas of functioning."

The first mention that we can find of frotteurism occurs in Krafft-Ebing's *Psychopathia Sexualis* (1886/1965). He presented the cases of four frotteurs and writes: "The simplest explanation seems to be that 'frottage' is a masturbatorial act of a hypersexual individual who is uncertain about his virility in the presence of women. This would also explain the motive of the assault being made not anteriorly but posteriorly. . . ." (p. 351).

The *Oxford English Dictionary* (Burchfield, 1972) notes that the word "frottage" is adopted from the French word "frottage" meaning "rubbing" or "friction" and goes on to state: "The special perversion of frottage . . . consists in a desire to bring the clothed body, and usually though not exclusively the genital region, into close contact with the clothed body of a woman. . . . Like fetishism, too, frottage is evidently a morbid development of the normal sexual excitatory effects of touching or contact with the opposite sex" (p. 1168).

Frotteurism is among the more common paraphilias and has been viewed by prosecutors and judges as a "nuisance" paraphilia (Krueger & Kaplan, 1997). It is difficult to apprehend and prosecute individuals engaging in frotteurism, because it is usually committed in large cities against anonymous individuals where it is difficult to obtain witnesses. It has only rarely been the occasion for an initial presentation for treatment (most of our practice and referrals have been for individuals involved with other deviancies, such as exhibitionism, voyeurism, or pedophilia). Nevertheless, it occurs either by itself or in conjunction with other paraphilias and can be treated.

What follows is a presentation of several features of this disorder, a discussion of the methods of assessment of this disorder, treatment recommendations, several case studies, and a resource list containing bibliographic and other information, with annotations. It should be said at the outset that there is little available literature on frotteurism and that much of what can be said about its treatment derives from more general principles of assessment and treatment of the other paraphilias. We will use the masculine pronoun in discussing frotteurism. Although it is certainly conceivable that frotteurism could exist in a female, we have not seen this in our experience or in the literature.

CHARACTERISTICS AND EPIDEMIOLOGY

Freund, Seto, and Kuban (1997) suggest that frotteurism is a distortion of a hypothesized normal sequence of human sexual interactions. Freund and Kolarsky (1965) set forth such a sequence as consisting of four phases: "(1) a finding phase, consisting of locating and appraising a potential partner; (2) an affiliative phase, characterized by nonverbal and verbal overtures such as looking, smiling, and talking to a potential partner; (3) a tactile phase, in which physical contact is made; and (4) a copulatory phase, in which sexual intercourse occurs" (p. 113).

They hypothesize that a paraphilia involves the omission or distortion of one of these phases, and that a paraphilia would reflect the preference of the patient for a virtually instant conversion of sexual arousal into orgasm. Thus the absence, for instance, of a finding, affiliative, and/or copulatory phase would leave an individual fixated on the tactile phase and could explain his preference for strangers as targets (with no necessity for finding an affiliation) and with an indiscriminate choice of target with regard to attractiveness and age. In our experience, however, frotteurs, or others engaged in paraphilic activity such as exhibitionism or voyeurism, will have specific features that describe their preferred target, for instance desiring a large, middle-aged, well-dressed woman; this behavior does not usually involve contact with an individual known to the frotteur.

The epidemiology of the paraphilias is unknown. The very nature of this activity, that it is sexual and covert, and that it is illegal, would dissuade individuals from being willing to speak about it; there is thus no data that epidemiologists and sexologists have collected in randomized population surveys about the occurrence of any of the paraphilias.

Some data relevant to the incidence of the paraphilias may be gathered from data concerning childhood sexual abuse. Although not all child sexual abusers are necessarily paraphiles, such behavior reflects deviant sexual activity. Russell (1983) reported on the incidence and prevalence of sexual abuse of female children in San Francisco, finding that in a random sample of 930 adult women, 12% reported that they had been abused by a relative and 20% by a nonrelative before age 14. A national sample of 2,000 men and women in Great Britain reported that 12% of females and 8% of males reported some sort of "sexual abuse" before age 16, although intercourse was reported in only 5% of the abusive experiences (Baker, 1985).

If one then focuses on the occurrence of frotteurism within the universe of paraphilias, one discovers that it is relatively common. Abel et al. (1988) reported on a group of 561 nonincarcerated paraphiliacs who responded to advertising in the local paper. These researchers interviewed appropriate respondents under a federal certificate of confidentiality which guaranteed complete confidentiality. They identified 17 categories of paraphilic behavior; frottage was sixth in terms of frequency as was voyeurism, as far as the number of individuals who reported at least one paraphilia (most individuals in this sample reported multiple paraphilias). Of 516 individuals interviewed, 62, or 10%, of this sample received a diagnosis of frotteurism. Similarly, Bradford, Boulet, and Pawlak (1992) reported on a sample of 443 adult males who were consecutively admitted to the Sexual Behaviours Clinic at the Royal Ottawa Hospital; 58, or roughly 14%, of these individuals admitted to frotteurism.

It is also notable that frotteurism very frequently occurs in conjunction with other paraphilias. Abel et al. (1988) reported that of the 62 subjects diagnosed with frotteurism, only 21% had frotteurism as a sole diagnosis, and that there was an average number of paraphilias of 3.8 per frotteur. Bradford et al. (1992) reported that of the individuals reporting frottage, 24% also reported heterosexual pedophilia; 35% heterosexual hebephilia (defined as a sexual preference for peri- and postpubertal victims, 12 to 16 years of age); 21% homosexual pedophilia; 17% homosexual hebephilia; 17% cross-dressing; 65% voyeurism; 29% scatologica (lewdness); 31% attempted rape; 16% rape; and 31% exhibitionism.

ASSESSMENT

Informed Consent and Forensic Considerations

It is recommended that any assessment begin by informing clients that we are mandated reporters of ongoing child sexual abuse, and that if the individual reveals any information that allows us to identify a child who is at risk for being or is being abused, then we have to notify the respective child welfare authorities. With frotteurs, because their targets usually involve adults in subways who are not identifiable, a notification is not mandated unless the individual admits to some other paraphilia with an identifiable child as a target. Informed consent should be obtained and explained prior to doing an assessment. The elements of the information given involve an explanation of the nature and purpose of the interview, and what will be done with the information (i.e., a report will be issued to an attorney, judge, or licensing authority, or no report will be issued). Furthermore, if there are specific tests or instruments, such as the Abel Assessment (Abel, 1994), or the Adult Sexual Interest Cardsort (Abel, 1984), then information regarding the risks and benefits of this assessment or test should be given and consent obtained.

There is no duty that we are aware of to report past crimes. We would add that laws vary according to the state and country that an individual is practicing in, and that clinicians should familiarize themselves with local laws.

Following the initial consultation, if it is determined that the frotteur is out of control, then it seems to us that the clinician would have some duty to protect, and that this in some fashion would require actions to protect both the patient and the public, which might include emergency initiation of antiandrogen medications; hospitalization; or the establishment of a contract with the patient to avoid public places and not to engage in such actions until the next meeting. It would devolve to the clinician to use whatever clinical judgment and skill he or she has to treat the frotteur and choose the appropriate course of action among these alternatives.

It is also important to discuss confidentiality of medical records. In our experience there is no absolute confidentiality of medical records. An evaluation requested by an attorney in writing adds attorney-client privilege to the doctor-patient privilege. However, records can be obtained by medical licensing authorities (only with the patient's consent, but this consent could be insisted upon as a condition of licensure or regaining one's license), or by other parties (such as in child custody disputes or otherwise).

Initial Clinical Interview

It is important to establish the source of the referral and the referral question. If an individual were to come with some fear of arrest, then the clinician might at the outset suggest that this individual engage an attorney. If the person has been arrested and/or prosecuted, it is important to request all available written information concerning this individual and his history, including victims' statements, arrest reports, psychological or psychiatric evaluations, and records of treatment. It is particularly important to obtain information regarding the individual's frotteurism from sources other than the patient, because paraphiliacs are notoriously unreliable historians.

Regardless of whether the individual has been arrested or not, it is important to begin with a very thorough and detailed clinical history and mental status examination. It is also important to establish whether there are any comorbid diagnoses such as major psychiatric syndromes, personality disorders, or medical problems.

A detailed history of the patient's sexual functioning and any paraphilic sexual interests or behaviors follows. Given the reported occurrence of multiple paraphilias in the same individual, when one interviews a frotteur, one should inquire carefully about other paraphilias.

We also do a thorough nondeviant, as well as deviant, sexual history and inquire about the occurrence of any history of sexual or physical abuse. We routinely use the two forms on pages 194 and 195 as an aid in obtaining a sexual history in an ordered way and to survey for a variety of deviant sexual behaviors.

It is important to obtain as detailed a picture of the individual's pattern of behavior as possible. This would include the age of onset; the frequency of occurrence (oftentimes, frotteurism is a high frequency deviant behavior, occurring several times per day); the usual place or places that the frotteur chooses (e.g., subways, buses, dance floors, crowds); the usual targets (male or female, age, appearance); the cognitions that accompany the act ("She is frightened, but can't move"; "She is really enjoying it"; "I don't even think she was aware of anything"; "She knew just what I was doing"); the time of day and the circumstances of the frottage (in the morning on the way to work, or in the evening on the way from work); what is worn; and whether a change of clothes is brought. Discovering the cognitions could offer the clinician some therapeutic advantage because removing or correcting them could increase the frotteur's awareness and motivation for change. If he can be convinced that, contrary to what he thinks, the woman might be frozen in surprise or fear, or find such activity almost unbelievable and disgusting, then he might become much less ready to engage in such activity. In the back of the assessing clinician's mind is always the possibility that in some fashion the information acquired could be used to intervene in a therapeutic way.

Antecedents to the behavior are particularly important to assess, as these offer possible areas that the clinician or a family member might be able to use to help the individual control his behavior. Is the behavior more likely to occur if the individual is angry? Intoxicated? Has had a bad day? How calculated is the behavior? How impulsive?

It is important to assess the individual's sense of control over himself. To assess this we ask "How much in control of your behavior are you?" We present a line indicating 0% control on one end and 100% control on the other and ask an individual to put a mark on the line that represents the percent of control that they think they have, from 0%, or no control at all, to 100%, or absolute control. We pose a hypothetical situation in which there is a high likelihood of not being apprehended for the act. For example, for a pedophile, one might ask what might he do if a young child were to approach him in a park with no one around. How much control would he have over any impulses or thoughts of abusing this child? For a frotteur, one might ask: "In a large crowd, with no police around, with several women in front of you focused on a parade and many people pressing forward, how much control might you have over any impulse to engage in frotteurism?"

Subjective and Objective Instruments

Several instruments are available to assess sexual functioning. One routinely used in addition to the preceding interview is the Derogatis Sexual Functioning Inventory (Derogatis, 1980; Derogatis & Melisaratos, 1979). This is a 258-item, self-administered instrument which presents questions in 10 areas of sexual functioning: information, experience, drive, attitudes, psychological symptoms, affects, gender role definition, fantasy, body image, and satisfaction. Scores are then derived for each of these categories and for overall sexual functioning. A major advantage is its comprehensiveness; a major disadvantage is its complexity. A computerized version is available.

The Clarke Sexual History Questionnaire for Males (Paitich et al., 1977) is another available instrument. This is a 190-item sexual history questionnaire which presents questions regarding a variety of deviant sexual behaviors in males, inquiring about the frequency and age of occurrence of a broad range of sexual behaviors, including the paraphilias. A computerized version is currently under development.

Another instrument routinely used is the Adult Sexual Interest Cardsort (Abel, 1984). It presents 75 items which are statements depicting various sorts of sexual activity. An individual is asked to rate whether each item seems to him extremely sexually repulsive, neutral, or extremely sexually arousing. This offers some indication of the individual's sexual preferences.

Sex offenders are notorious for being poor at self-report (Kaplan et al., 1990), and this has given rise to attempts to assess an individual's sexual preference objectively. One such measure is penile plethysmography (Abel, Blanchard, & Barlow, 1981; Pithers & Laws, 1988). This involves measuring penile tumescence as various stimuli are presented to the patient by having the patient put a mercury strain gauge around his penis as he sits in a separate room or behind a partition, and then presenting various stimuli to him. The Association for the Treatment of Sexual Abusers (ATSA, 1993) has a set of audiotapes for sale, as do other vendors. A problem that exists is that there is no generally accepted set of standardized stimuli. It should be noted that plethysmographic assessment should only be used as an aid in treatment, such as for pre- and postassessment, and not to establish guilt or innocence.

Another way of trying to objectively assess sexual interest relies on visual reaction time, and is marketed as The Abel Assessment (Abel, 1994). This consists of two parts. The first presents a very detailed set of questions which explore an individual's sexual history and interests. The second presents several series of slides which use models to depict images that a paraphile might find arousing. Although there is support to the use of reaction time in assessing sexual interest patterns, and Dr. Abel has data to support his instrument, the validation of this assessment by other objective sources has yet to be done (Krueger, Bradford, & Glancy, 1998).

In our experience there is great utility to presenting questionnaires and to making an objective assessment of sexual interest patterns, as well as relying on clinical interviewing, as individuals frequently are more honest and complete in answering questions provided by questionnaires or computers than they are in face-to-face interviews.

TREATMENT RECOMMENDATIONS

Cognitive and Behavioral Interventions

At the outset, it is important to establish what resources and supports a frotteur or paraphile might have which could aid in his treatment. If he has a significant other or wife or parent, has he informed that individual of his problem? It might be advantageous to have the patient inform this individual, in order to recruit that individual to aid in the patient's treatment, as well as to inform that individual of the nature of the treatment (family members or significant others oftentimes have many questions). We would, if indicated, then have a meeting with the patient and with his family member or significant other to identify ourselves as his caregiver, to introduce ourselves, to explain something of the nature of the disorder and the nature of the treatments available, including risks and benefits, and to try and recruit the parent or significant other into being a treatment ally and a part of the treatment. This is for several reasons. First, it helps to have someone who would have some day-to-day contact with the patient to be able to report if that individual may have relapsed (for instance, that the individual cannot account for the time from which he left work until he came home, or if he has in fact admitted a relapse to the significant other). Second, the presence of an observing family member can itself have a dissuading effect on aberrant behavior. Third, frequently there are dynamic issues that emerge between the offender and his significant other that can be helped by therapeutic intervention.

Cognitive-behavioral techniques have been widely used in the treatment of the paraphilias and have been described in several reviews (Abel et al., 1992; Abel, Rouleau, & Cunningham-Rathner, 1986; Hawton, 1983). Such treatment usually involves group therapy and a number of behavioral techniques. One of these is masturbatory satiation, which has the goal of trying to decrease an individual's arousal to deviant fantasy and stimuli. Typically, an individual is instructed to, in the privacy of his home, masturbate to a nondeviant scenario, achieving ejaculation within a brief period of time, usually 5 to 10 minutes. Then he is asked to continue to masturbate to fantasies of his deviant behavior for an additional 50 minutes. This with time becomes boring and aversive. Patients are asked to record the verbalizations of their fantasies on a tape recorder for review by their therapist at a later date and also to rate their experience of the session as to how aversive or boring they found it. Typically patients finish a specified number of sessions, usually 20, in a course of therapy. With time many subjects report a decrease in the strength and attraction of their deviant fantasies. This is a technique, once learned, which a patient can use again and again in the future should he experience an emergence of his deviant interests or impulses.

Another behavioral technique is covert sensitization, which attempts to associate negative consequences with the individual's deviant behavior and with antecedents to that behavior. Typically, an individual is asked to initially write out what a typical episode of behavior might be and to look carefully for any recurrent antecedents to this behavior. For instance, a frotteur might have a hard day at work, then have a drink or two at a bar before getting on a subway and engaging in such behavior. We would have the frotteur verbalize over a period of 5 minutes or so his feelings about frustrations at work, perhaps his preparation for frottage, such as putting on extra underwear at work, his walking to the subway, and his movements in the subway toward a victim, and his beginning to be aroused. We would then ask him to interrupt this narration and to verbalize the negative consequences of his actions, preferably those that have already been experienced or, if not, imagined consequences. For instance, if a frotteur has been arrested as a negative consequence, we would have him verbalize the detailed process of the arrest, including being apprehended by police, being led away in handcuffs, having his employer or family members find out, being in a jail cell and identified as a sex offender, and/or being threatened by other inmates, and his feelings during this. We would then have him verbalize a brief "escape scene" such as lying on a beach, in order to get out of the set of negative experiences and emotions. All of these verbalizations are done on a tape, which the therapist then listens to and offers feedback about.

Olfactory aversion (Laws, Meyer, & Holmen, 1978) is another technique in which the subject verbalizes the antecedents to and progression of his deviant behavior and then pairs this with the periodic wafting of a noxious olfactory stimulant, such as ammonia. We have found that individuals who can successfully learn this technique can then carry ampules of ammonia (smelling salts) with them which they can step aside and break and waft should they catch themselves in a progression toward offending.

Biological Therapies

Biological therapies of the paraphilias have consisted mainly of the use of antidepressant agents and antiandrogen agents. Stein et al. (1992) have suggested a possible relationship between the paraphilias and obsessive-compulsive disorder. Indeed, particularly with some of the high-frequency behaviors such as exhibitionism or frotteurism, there are many similarities. Patients report obsessions with sexual thoughts and behaviors and a compulsion to engage in them. However, these sexual thoughts and compulsions for the most part are experienced as ego-syntonic (willful, pleasurable, and agreeable) rather than ego-dystonic or alien, as in the obsessive-compulsive disorders.

A number of case reports and some smaller, more controlled trials have suggested that antidepressants, and in particular the serotonin-reuptake inhibitors (SRIs), have efficacy in the paraphilias (Gijs & Gooren, 1996). Whether this is because of the efficacy of these agents against obsessive-compulsive disorder, or because of the sexual side effects of these medications, which include a decrease in libido, retardation of orgasm or ejaculation, and/or a diminution in the deviant sexual interest or activity itself, is unknown.

Antiandrogen agents, with more profound effects on libido, sexual functioning, and side effects, have probably been studied more. Most work on the paraphilias has involved the use of depot or oral Provera in the United States or cyproterone acetate in Canada (Cooper, 1986). These appear to be highly effective. Recently attention has shifted to the use of luteinizing-hormone releasing hormone agonists, such as triptorelin outside of the United States or leuprolide in the United States. These agents work by lowering the secretion of the gonadotropic hormones, luteinizing hormone and follicle-stimulating hormone, which act on the testes to produce testosterone (Bradford, 1998; Rosler & Witztum, 1998). Because these agents result in an initial increase in these gonadotropic hormones, and thus testosterone, it is important to also treat the patient with a testosterone antagonist, such as Flutamide, for several weeks at the inception of treatment until testosterone levels drop. These agents have been highly effective at decreasing deviant arousal and behavior. Because these agents have such a profound effect on sexual functioning, and because they have substantial side effects, such as weight gain, gynecomastia, and osteoporosis, to name some of them, a careful medical evaluation prior to the initiation of treatment, which would include a physical examination and laboratory screen, including chemistries, white count, and sexual hormones (testosterone, luteinizing hormone, and follicle-stimulating hormone), and bone density studies is recommended. It is important to point out that the effects of these agents are reversible, with sexual functioning returning when these agents are stopped. Furthermore, these agents are available in depot form, in which an individual may take an injection once a month or once every 3 months rather than daily. These agents also have many fewer side effects than Provera or cyproterone acetate.

Typically an assessment is conducted to establish how much control the frotteur or paraphile has. This might also include an assessment of other behaviors or fantasies which the frotteur might disclose, such as rape fantasies or an interest in children. If the patient is felt to be dangerous or to have poor control, then antiandrogen medication might be recommended initially. If, however, an individual had some degree of control and could contract not to engage in such acts, then behavioral treatments or SRI medications might be used. In our experience, individuals can use the antiandrogen medications to obtain control and a respite from their struggle, so to speak, and during this time learn behavioral or other techniques or otherwise engage in therapeutic changes that afford them more control until control is established, and then, when these agents are discontinued, experience a continued sense of control.

Relapse Prevention Therapies

Relapse prevention strategies, developed first for individuals with substance abuse problems, have been employed for years for paraphiliacs (Freeman-Longo & Pithers, 1992; Pithers, 1990). This therapeutic modality helps an individual to identify a chain of precursors or a cycle to his deviant behavior and gives him a strategy to interrupt this chain before actually engaging in the offending behavior. For instance, a frotteur might disclose that "early warning signs" of prior relapses have involved feelings of depression, use of alcohol, fatigue, and exhaustion, and would know to seek help from his clinician before relapsing. Other treatments, such as the use of 12-step meetings to abstain from alcohol, or the use of antidepressants, could be used to prevent relapse.

CASE STUDIES

The number of case reports that we have been able to find in the literature is small. These include the four cases described earlier by Krafft-Ebing (1886/1965) and a case of a man who engaged in obscene telephone calls and practiced frotteurism and was treated successfully with psychoanalysis (Myers, 1991). The treatment method of psychoanalysis is not considered to be the current standard for the treatment of the paraphilias; rather cognitive-behavioral therapy, medication therapy, and/or relapse prevention therapy are. However, psychotherapy, couples therapy, and even psychoanalysis, in addition to a whole plethora of other therapies, may be concurrently indicated for treatment of comorbid problems, such as depression, personality disorders, or couples problems.

Case Study A

Mr. A* at the time of our initial evaluation was a 58-year-old male, never married, referred as a condition of probation after he had pled guilty to misdemeanor charges of assault. He gave a history of, at the age of 15 while attending a Fourth of July picnic with his parents, rubbing up behind an adult female with his erect penis, as everyone was watching an event. He reported becoming very sexually excited by this. The patient recalled that rapidly his frotteuristic activity escalated in his later teens to include activities sometimes three or four times per day, usually on the way to or from school or, later, work, where he would rub up against unsuspecting females in subways or buses. He estimated he engaged in this behavior 200 days out of 365 days per year. He also engaged at night in "dirty dancing" at various discos where he would rub up against women who he asked to dance with him. He estimated that he did this perhaps 100 nights out of the year. He also described anticipating holidays in which there would be large crowds of people and parades, such as on St. Patrick's day or other holidays, in which he would engage in such activity. Interestingly, he reported that over the years, particularly on holidays, he witnessed other men who he would recognize through the years as also engaging in frotteuristic activity. He continued this activity throughout his adulthood with only two arrests and no convictions until the episode that mandated him to obtain treatment. By calculation he had, over a 40-year career, engaged in approximately 20,000 acts of frotteurism. He had no other paraphilias. He had a history of being both physically and sexually abused and of being socially phobic at his workplace. He had more than a thousand

*Names and identifying characteristics in all case examples have been disguised thoroughly to protect privacy.

female sexual partners. He had had in the 1980s treatment from two therapists, a social worker and a psychologist, with the treatment focus being his difficulties in heterosexual relationships. He reported that he had not revealed his history of frotteurism to either of these therapists. He had throughout his history maintained an excellent work history and had had no other major *DSM-IV* psychiatric syndromes. He acknowledged problems with intimacy and was distressed that he had been unable to marry and have children.

Treatment consisted of the imparting of masturbatory satiation to decrease his deviant arousal and covert sensitization to associate negative consequences with engaging in such acts. It also included insight-oriented therapy to help him examine his pattern of relationships with women and issues of intimacy and commitment. He did not agree to take antidepressant medication to treat his social phobia, which was suggested. In treatment, following his arrest, his engagement in frotteuristic activity dramatically decreased and he reported no episodes in the year that he was in treatment. After a year of therapy, he reported absolute control over his frotteurism but would not agree to continue in relapse prevention. Had his probation so mandated it, he undoubtedly would have.

This case illustrates the high frequency of frotteuristic activity and the necessity to have some hold over an individual, such as therapy being mandated by probation, in order to treat him; the tendency that such individuals might have to conceal such activity from a therapist who might not know or ask specifically about a paraphilic history; and the existence of other personality issues.

Case Study B

Mr. B. was a 34-year-old physician who was single and in private practice. He ultimately pled guilty to felony counts of sexual assault involving over 30 women over a several-year period for charges that he engaged in the rubbing and manipulation of patients' clitoris during unchaperoned pelvic examinations. His license was withdrawn and, following a prison term, he joined a group of professionals who had engaged in professional sexual misconduct of some form. He initially denied that he had engaged in anything inappropriate, but with the confrontation and support of the group admitted to wrongdoing. He had no other paraphilic or psychiatric history, and by all appearances his relationships and sexual life were normal during this activity.

This case indicates a different form of frotteurism, that propagated by a professional in the course of his professional duties which consisted of the inappropriate and nonconsensual touching of an unsuspecting female for purposes of sexual gratification. This touching did not involve the perpetrator's penis but rather consisted of manipulation by his hands and occurred during the course of professional activity. It was treated with a suspension of his practice.

Case Study C

Mr. C. was a 30-year-old Caucasian male with a history of pedophilic arousal to both prepubescent males and females, but with no attempts at sexual touching of children or solicitation of them. He also had a history of exhibitionism, consisting of exposing himself in convenience stores, around his apartment building, and in public at night. He had a history of manic-depressive disease and was on therapeutic doses of lithium and sertraline. Despite these, and despite intensive cognitive-behavioral treatment which included 2 months of inpatient treatment and intensive weekly outpatient treatment over the course of a year, he still reported high deviant arousal, in particular to the fantasies of touching children around his neighborhood on their arms or legs with his fingers or rubbing up against them in crowds with his clothed penis. He finally agreed to a course of antiandrogens and was given depot leuprolide acetate and flutamide, with a dramatic decrease in his sexual interest and behavior. He continued on this for an 8-month period, then stopped, and had a recurrence of his deviant interest. He then availed himself of 12-step groups for addictive sexual behavior on a frequent basis, but, when he was still not able to control himself, requested and was given another course of depot leuprolide acetate, with similar beneficial results.

This case illustrates the occurrence of frotteurism and pedophilia, and the great difficulty in control that can be experienced by an individual with these disorders. It also indicates the dramatic effects that antiandrogen medications can have on sexual arousal and behavior.

Case Study D

Mr. D. was a 26-year-old male, single at the time of his initial evaluation. He had a history of profound social phobia and obsessive-compulsive disorder and had managed to slowly progress toward leaving his parents' home, living by himself, and attending classes through a variety of treatments including cognitive-behavioral and supportive treatment for his social phobia, and a variety of antidepressant medications including monoamine oxidase inhibitors, tricyclics, and buproprion (which he was on at the time of his evaluation). He was evaluated for what he had self-identified as frotteuristic activity and he also indicated that he had never revealed this activity to any of his therapists. He reported that for the 4 years prior to his evaluation he would periodically travel in subways and would target an adult female in the same subway car. He would then sit next to her without touching her. If she did not move away (and sometimes the subway car would be empty), he would deliberately drop something on the floor in front of the woman. He would then, with his fingers, appear to inadvertently brush against her hip or leg, and apologize. He would in his mind find such activity highly sexually exciting; this behavior was accompanied by an erection. He did not ejaculate at this time and he never tried to press his penis against a female in the usual fashion of a frotteur. He would masturbate several times per evening with his masturbatory fantasies including memories or thoughts of the most recent episode of touching or prior episodes of touching. He said that medications had had no effect on this behavior. He had no other paraphilias. He had had one brief sexual experience with a woman who lived in his building, but otherwise was sexually naïve. Following our initial evaluation, he decided not to accept the recommended treatment for this condition, which was cognitive-behavioral therapy to try and decrease his deviant arousal and supportive and informational therapy to try and help him develop a relationship with a woman.

This case illustrates a somewhat atypical presentation of a frotteur, in which an individual intensely sexualizes what appears to be an innocent and accidental contact with a woman; it also indicates the difficulty that some individuals have in agreeing to therapy for this disorder and comorbid personality issues and other syndromes.

Overall, it may be said that frotteurism is one of the more common paraphilias, and that with current cognitive-behavioral and medical treatments there is much reason to be optimistic that such behavior can be successfully controlled. However, research is needed on the incidence and prevalence not only of frotteurism but of all of the paraphilias, along more scientific assessments of treatment efficacy and outcome.

Nondeviant Sexual History

1. Age reached puberty ______
2. Age 1st ejaculation occurred ______
3. By what means? ______
4. Age of 1st crush ______
5. Age of 1st date ______
6. Age of 1st nongenital touching (petting) ______
7. Age of 1st genital experience ______
8. Age of 1st masturbation ______
9. Masturbation frequency ______
10. Number of sexual partners (female) ______

    (male) ______
11. Sexual orientation ______
12. Sexual imagery ______
13. Masturbation fantasy ______
14. History of physical abuse ______
15. History of sexual abuse ______
16. Sexual dysfunction ______

Paraphilic History

For each reported fantasy, ask age when fantasy first began, number of lifetime acts, and percent of current control over acting on the fantasies.

Paraphilia	Fantasies	Age of Occurrence	Number of Acts
Exhibitionism			
Public Masturbation			
Fetishism			
Frotteurism			
Pedophilia			
Rape			
Sexual Masochism			
Sexual Sadism			
Transvestic Fetishism			
Transexualism			
Voyeurism			
Necrophilia (corpses)			
Zoophilia (animals)			
Coprophilia (feces)			
Urophilia (urine)			
Klismaphilia (enemas)			
Scatalogia (telephone)			
Partialism			

0% Control Over Deviant Urges —————————————— **100% Control Over Deviant Urges**

CONTRIBUTORS

Richard B. Krueger, MD, is a psychiatrist at the New York State Psychiatric Institute, Medical Director of the Sexual Behavior Clinic there, and is in private practice in New York City. He is an Associate Clinical Professor of Psychiatry at Columbia University, College of Physicians and Surgeons, and is active in the teaching of medical students and residents. He received his MD from Harvard Medical School in 1977 and has treated sex offenders since 1985. He was a psychiatric consultant for 3 years to the Sexual Treatment Center in Bridgewater, Massachusetts. He is a board-certified forensic psychiatrist and addiction psychiatrist. He has an expertise in psychopharmacology and has over 16 publications in the area of biological psychiatry. Dr. Krueger may be contacted at the New York State Psychiatric Institute, 1051 Riverside Drive, Unit 45, New York, NY 10032. E-mail: RBK1721305@aol.com

Meg S. Kaplan, PhD, a clinical psychologist, is currently the Director of the Sexual Behavior Clinic at the New York State Psychiatric Institute, and is an Associate Professor of Clinical Psychology in Psychiatry at Columbia University, College of Physicians and Surgeons. She received her PhD in human sexuality from New York University in 1979 and has conducted clinical research in psychosexual disorders since then. Dr. Kaplan is on the Board of the Association for the Treatment of Sexual Abusers and the current Acting Director of the Special Classification Review Board at Avenyl Correctional Facility in New Jersey. She reviews for numerous publications and has over 35 publications in the sexual disorders field. Dr. Kaplan can be reached at the New York State Psychiatric Institute, 1051 Riverside Drive, Unit 45, New York, NY 10032. E-mail: RBK1721305@aol.com

RESOURCES

Abel, G. G. (Producer). (1987a). *Covert Sensitization* [Videotape]. (Available from G. G. Abel, Behavioral Medicine Institute of Atlanta, 3280 Howell Mill Road, Atlanta, GA 30327-4101; 404-872-7929. This is a roughly half-hour videotape in which Dr. Abel provides the rationale for and means to do covert sensitization.)

Abel, G. G. (Producer). (1987b). *Masturbatory Satiation Training for Paraphiliacs* [Videotape]. (Available from G. G. Abel, Behavioral Medicine Institute of Atlanta, 3280 Howell Mill Road, Atlanta, GA 30327-4101; 404-872-7929. This is an excellent half-hour videotape in which Dr. Abel provides detailed instructions on the rationale for and how to do masturbatory satiation.)

Abel, G. G. (1984). *The Adult Sexual Interest Cardsort.* Atlanta, GA: Behavioral Medicine Institute of Atlanta. (Available from G. G. Abel, Behavioral Medicine Institute of Atlanta, 3280 Howell Mill Road, Atlanta, GA 30327-4101; 404-872-7929)

Abel, G. G. (1994). *Abel Assessment for Interest in the Paraphilias.* Atlanta, GA: Abel Screening, Inc. (Available for purchase from Abel Screening, Inc. in Atlanta, Georgia; 404-872-7929)

Abel, G. G., Becker, J. V., Cunningham-Rathner, J., Mittelman, M., & Rouleau, J. L. (1988). Multiple paraphilic diagnoses among sex offenders. *Bulletin of the American Academy of Psychiatry and the Law, 2,* 153-168.

Abel, G. G., Becker, J. V., Cunningham-Rathner, J., Rouleau, J. L., Kaplan, M., & Reich, J. (1984). *Treatment Manual: The Treatment of Child Molesters.* Atlanta, GA: Behavioral Medicine Institute of Atlanta. (This is a very detailed and comprehensive manual which was written by Dr. Abel et al. as part of a grant from the National Institute of Mental Health, and is available from G. G. Abel, Behavioral Medicine Institute of Atlanta, 3280 Howell Mill Road, Atlanta, GA 30327-4101; 404-872-7929)

Abel, G. G., Blanchard, E. B., & Barlow, D. H. (1981). The effects of stimulus modality, instructional set and stimulus content on the objective measurement of sexual arousal in several paraphilias. *Behaviour Research and Therapy, 19,* 25-33.

Abel, G. G. (Producer), & Harlow. N. (Producer) (1987). *Ammonia Aversion for Deviant Sexual Behavior* [Videotape]. (Available from G. G. Abel, Behavioral Medicine Institute of Atlanta, 3280 Howell Mill Road, Atlanta, GA 30327-4101; 404-872-7929. This is an excellent half-hour videotape in which Dr. Abel provides detailed instructions on the rationale for and how to do ammonia aversion.)

Abel, G. G., Osborn, C. A., Anthony, D., & Gardos, P. (1992). Current treatments of paraphiliacs. *Annual Review of Sex Research, 3,* 255-290.

Abel, G. G., Rouleau, J. L., & Cunningham-Rathner, J. (1986). Sexually aggressive behavior. In W. J. Curran, A. L. McGarry, & S. Shah (Eds.), *Forensic Psychiatry and Psychology* (pp. 289-313). Philadelphia: Davis.

American Psychiatric Association. (1994). *Diagnostic and Statistical Manual of Mental Disorders* (4th ed.). Washington, DC: Author.

The Association for the Treatment of Sexual Abusers (Speaker). (1993). *Auditory Audio Stimuli for Penile Plethysmograph.* Beaverton, OR: Author. (Available from the Association for the Treatment of Sexual Abusers, 10700 W.W. Beaverton, Hillsdale Highway, Suite 26, Beaverton, OR 97005-3035; 503-643-1023)

Baker, A. (1985). Child sexual abuse: A study of prevalence in Great Britain. *Child Abuse and Neglect, 7,* 133-146.

Bradford, J. M. (1998). Treatment of men with paraphilia. *The New England Journal of Medicine, 338,* 464-465.

Bradford, J. M., Boulet, J., & Pawlak, A. (1992). The paraphilias: A multiplicity of deviant behaviours. *Canadian Journal of Psychiatry, 37,* 104-108.

Burchfield, R. W. (Ed.). (1972). *A Supplement to the Oxford English Dictionary.* Oxford, England: Oxford University Press.

Cooper, A. J. (1986). Progestogens in the treatment of male sex offenders: A review. *Canadian Journal of Psychiatry, 31,* 73-79.

Derogatis, L. R. (1980). Psychological assessment of psychosexual functioning. *Psychiatric Clinics of North America, 5,* 244-281. (The Derogatis Sexual Functioning Inventory is available from Clinical Psychometric Research, Inc., P.O. Box 619, Riderwood, MD 21139; 800-245-0277)

Derogatis, L. R., & Melisaratos, N. (1979). The DSFI: A multidimensional measure of sexual functioning. *Journal of Sexual and Marital Therapy, 5,* 244-281.

Freeman-Longo, R., & Pithers, W. D. (1992). *Client's Manual. A Structured Approach to Preventing Relapse: A Guide for Sex Offenders.* Brandon, VT: Safer Society Press.

Freund, K., & Kolarsky, A. (1965). A simple reference system for the analysis of sexual dysfunctions. *Psychiatrie, Neurologie, Und Medizinische Psychologie, 17,* 221-225.

Freund, K., Seto, M. C., & Kuban, M. (1997). Frotteurism: Frotteurism and the theory of courtship disorder. In D. R. Laws & W. O'Donohue (Eds.), *Sexual Deviance: Theory, Assessment and Treatment* (pp. 111-130). New York: Guilford.

Gijs, L., & Gooren, L. (1996). Hormonal and psychopharmacological interventions in the treatment of paraphilias: An update. *The Journal of Sex Research, 33,* 273-290. (This is an excellent overall review and compendium of studies in this area)

Hawton, K. (1983). Behavioural approaches to the management of sexual deviations. *British Journal of Psychiatry, 143,* 248-255.

Kaplan, M. S., Abel, G. G., Rathner, J., & Mittelman, M. (1990). The impact of parolees' perceptions of confidentiality on self-reported sex crimes. *Annals of Sex Research, 3,* 293-305.

Krafft-Ebing, R. (1965). *Psychopathia Sexualis.* New York: Arcade Publishing. (Original work published in 1886)

Krueger, R. B., Bradford, J. M., & Glancy, G. (1998). Report from the committee on sex offenders: The Abel assessment for sexual interest - A brief description. *Journal of the American Academy of Psychiatry and the Law, 26*(2), 277-280.

Krueger, R. B., & Kaplan, M. S. (1997). Frotteurism assessment and treatment. In R. D. Laws & W. O'Donohue (Eds.), *Sexual Deviance: Theory, Assessment and Treatment* (pp. 131-151). New York: Guilford. (This book, we feel, is the best compendium of information regarding the theory, assessment, and treatment of sexual deviance)

Laws, D. R., Meyer, J., & Holmen, M. I. (1978). Reduction of sadistic sexual arousal by olfactory aversion: A case study. *Behaviour Research and Therapy, 16,* 281-285.

Myers, W. A. (1991). A case history of a man who made obscene telephone calls and practiced frotteurism. In G. Fogel & W. Myers (Eds.), *Perversions and Near Perversions in Clinical Practice* (pp. 109-123). New Haven: Yale University Press.

Paitich, D., Langevin, R., Freeman, R., Mann, K., & Handy, L. (1977). The Clarke SHQ: A clinical sex history questionnaire for males. *Archives of Sexual Behavior, 6,* 421-436. (The Clarke SHQ is available from Multi-Health Systems, Inc., 908 Niagara Falls Boulevard, North Tonawanda, NY 14120-2060; 800-456-3003)

Pithers, W. D. (1990). Relapse prevention with sexual aggressors. A method for maintaining therapeutic gain and enhancing external supervision. In W. L. Marshall, D. R. Laws, & H. E. Barbaree (Eds.), *Handbook of Sexual Assault* (pp. 343-361). New York: Plenum.

Pithers, W. D., & Laws, D. R. (1988). The penile plethysmograph. In B. K. Schwartz & H. R. Cellini (Eds.), *A Practitioner's Guide to Treating the Incarcerated Male Sex Offender* (pp. 85-94). Washington, DC: U.S. Government Printing Office.

Rosler, A., & Witztum, E. (1998). Treatment of men with paraphilia with a long-acting analogue of gonadotropin-releasing hormone. *The New England Journal of Medicine, 338,* 416-422.

Russell, D. (1983). Incidence and prevalence of intrafamilial and extrafamilial sexual abuse of female children. *Child Abuse and Neglect, 7,* 133-146.

Stein, D. J., Hollander, E., Anthony, D. T., Schneier, F. R., Fallon, B. A., Liebowitz, M. R., & Klein, D. F. (1992). Serotonergic medications for sexual obsessions, sexual addictions, and paraphilias. *Journal of Clinical Psychiatry, 53,* 267-271.

Assessment of Dementia

Martin D. Zehr

As we enter the 21st century, clinicians working with geriatric patients will increasingly confront a distinctly 20th-century malady: specifically, various forms of dementing conditions whose primary impact is on older individuals. The epidemic in dementing conditions during the last half of this century has been well documented. With projections that the proportion of the population aged 85 years and older will be as high as 18% by the year 2040 (Taeuber, 1990), a concomitant rise in the prevalence of dementing conditions will affect 14 million baby boomers and their families in this country alone in the next 50 years (Alzheimer's Disease and Related Disorders Association, 1999). Clinicians and other health care professionals who work routinely with a geriatric population and even those whose work only occasionally involves older adults will, and should, be expected to know rudimentary procedures for addressing questions of possible dementia conditions which will invariably arise in their practice. Recognition of these observations is already widespread among health care professionals and has served as the impetus for recent statements of general principles to assist clinicians dealing with these questions (see, e.g., *Guidelines for the Evaluation of Dementia and Age-Related Cognitive Decline*, American Psychological Association, 1998). For the specialist, typically a neurologist or neuropsychologist who regularly confronts questions regarding the type and extent of a dementia process, there exists a wealth of readily available research-based texts upon which a comprehensive formal evaluation can be based (see, e.g., Parks, Zec, & Wilson, 1993). The average practitioner, who has neither sufficient time nor the resources to devote to such an intensive formal assessment, will nonetheless be expected to be familiar with basic principles of screening for dementia-based cognitive impairment, if for no other reason than to justify referral for a more comprehensive and definitive assessment.

In this age of increasing progress toward the goal of discovering reliable laboratory-based markers for such dementing conditions as Alzheimer's disease (Reiman et al., 1996), psychological testing and trained clinical observation are recognized by the medical community as important facets of the diagnosis and evaluation of dementia (Corey-Bloom et al., 1995). It is certain, moreover, that even when reliable biochemical markers for dementing conditions supplant present exclusionary criteria for diagnosis, and thus, from a histological standpoint, we replace Dr. Alzheimer's 1907 postmortem observations of the neurofibrillary tangles that characterize the disease process with a marker that has direct treatment implications for the living patient, psychological assessment will not diminish in importance. Detailed assessments of cognitive status, which include psychological testing, will retain their importance, if not their purpose, because it is unlikely that an isomorphic relationship will obtain between such biochemical markers and degrees, if not types, of observed patterns of impairment. Psychological assessments will also provide the data upon which conclusions regarding the efficacy of any future treatment must be based.

Finally, in the clinical context, it should be noted that the professional who incidentally becomes involved in questions regarding the cognitive status of the older patient will inevitably be asked at one time or another to provide opinions that have direct implications for possible restrictions of an individual's freedom. This raises important ethical and legal issues (Zehr, 1998). The use of psychological testing data to address what are essentially legal questions and determinations - for example, the capacity to make informed decisions or to consent to treatment - has been explicitly investigated in both research (High et al., 1994) and legal capacity contexts (Marson et al., 1995). The growth of interest in this area where psychological and legal questions intersect has resulted in the adoption of formal institutional guidelines for psychologists addressing these issues (National Center for Cost Containment, Department of Veterans Affairs, 1997) and the recent development of instruments that the practicing clinician can include in a formal evaluation (Grisso & Appelbaum, 1998). The growth of interest in this area is not accidental, of course, but is a direct outgrowth of the changing population demographics which ultimately have a direct impact on the type of questions the practitioner of the new century must be equipped to answer.

For all of these reasons, it is imperative that psychologists who work with older adults in any type of clinical setting have more than a cursory knowledge of methods by which they can properly address questions regarding possible dementia processes, whether these questions are the focus of an explicit referral or whether they arise incidentally, as in, for example, the course of psychotherapy with an older individual. It is not within the scope and purpose of this contribution to provide an exhaustive discussion of assessments for the purpose of obtaining data relevant to such questions; as noted, such references are readily available. Rather, what follows is an attempt, based on my own experience and interests, to provide the practicing clinician with sufficient guidelines for conducting an evaluation upon which an initial competent determination can be based, one which can reasonably be relied on when deciding to advise a patient to pursue a more intensive assessment or to consider practical issues such as possible changes in living circumstances and needs for assistance.

INITIAL CONSIDERATIONS

Definitions

Although it is likely that most health care professionals having any experience working with an older adult population have a heuristic notion of the term dementia, it is nevertheless worthwhile to present a brief review derived from the most commonly relied-upon sources. The fourth edition of the *Diagnostic and Statistical Manual of Mental Disorders* of the American Psychiatric Association (1994), in its discussion of dementia, states:

> The essential feature of a dementia is the development of multiple cognitive deficits that include memory impairment and at least one of the following cognitive disturbances: aphasia, apraxia, agnosia, or a disturbance in executive functioning. The cognitive deficits must be sufficiently severe to cause impairment in occupational or social functioning and must represent a decline from a previously higher level of functioning. (p. 134)

In 1984, representatives of the National Institute of Neurological and Communicative Disorders and Stroke (NINCDS) and the Alzheimer's Disease and Related Disorders Association (ADRDA), in the context of their efforts to provide clinical criteria for the diagnosis of Alzheimer's disease, stated that dementia could be "determined by a history of decline in performance and by abnormalities noted from clinical examination and neuropsychological tests. . . . Dementia is a diagnosis based on behavior and cannot be determined by computerized tomography, electroencephalography, or other laboratory instruments, although specific causes of dementia may be identified by these means" (McKhann et al., 1984, p. 940). For our purposes, it is important to note that a determination of dementia is appropriately based on a combination of history, clinical observations, and objective data derived from formal testing, whereas the diagnosis of a specific source of dementia, for example, Alzheimer's disease, is a medical determination which is also dependent on medical and laboratory tests that serve to either exclude specific causes or, in some cases, to provide a specific and definitive diagnosis. Thus, it is imperative that the clinician who routinely addresses such questions work in conjunction with a physician, usually a neurologist, who is qualified to analyze medical and laboratory data in an attempt to make a definitive diagnosis. This is particularly critical because there are a number of medical conditions, for example, hypothyroidism, that can result in dementia and which are potentially reversible with treatment. Although there are a number of medical conditions that can be associated with a dementia process (discussed briefly later in this contribution), for our purposes most of the present discussion will have as its focus the clinical and neuropsychological correlates of Alzheimer's disease. This is because Alzheimer's disease constitutes by far the most prevalent cause of dementia, accounting for at least 60% of dementing conditions. Vascular conditions are believed to comprise 20% of dementias, and a variety of causes account for the remaining 20% of detected dementias (Breitner & Welsh, 1995). It is also convenient to maintain a primary focus on Alzheimer's disease in this discussion of dementia because most available research-based conclusions are derived from work with Alzheimer's disease patients and because, to a large extent, Alzheimer's disease is, from a clinical perspective, the model for dementing conditions generally, sharing most of its cognitive and behavioral correlates with other known causes of dementia.

Referral Sources and the Basis for Evaluation

For most clinicians, especially psychologists who regularly conduct assessments of older adults for the explicit purpose of addressing questions regarding a dementia process, the initial referral is likely made through another health care professional, usually the patient's primary care physician or a neurologist conducting an evaluation on behalf of the primary care physician. This is, in fact, my own vantage point, as a psychologist working in a large metropolitan medical center. In this setting, it is typically a family member accompanying the patient for medical evaluation or treatment who raises a question of gradually increasing concerns regarding the patient's cognitive abilities, especially memory difficulties, which have increased to an extent such that assistance is often required to ensure reliable completion of such activities as management of a medication regimen or handling finances. In a hospital setting, an older patient admitted for treatment of a medical condition, for instance, a broken hip suffered as a result of a fall, may be observed to demonstrate persistent problems with orientation and short-term memory functions. This raises suspicions regarding a possible dementia and, ultimately, questions regarding the individual's capacity to function independently subsequent to discharge, especially if the patient lives alone. Older inpatients undergoing rehabilitation for various medical conditions may be observed to have pronounced difficulty following instructions or recalling prior discussions of important treatment-related information which may form the basis for physician referral for evaluation of a suspected dementia. Examples of other settings where contact with older adults may provide sufficient observations of behavioral anomalies to raise questions of a dementing condition include (a) contact with social workers for the purpose of obtaining assistance in obtaining Medicare benefits, (b) admission to a mental health facility for treatment of a condition other than depression in an older adult with no prior psychiatric history, and (c) outpatient individual or group psychotherapy following various life crises. As a general rule, aside from situations in which the clinician has the opportunity to make direct observations that form the basis for a recommendation to have the patient evaluated formally, it is the observations of third parties, usually significant others, that provide the requisite data which is the impetus for diagnostic assessment.

It is rare, in my own experience, for an older individual to initiate a medical or psychological evaluation based on his or her own perception of conspicuous cognitive deficits. In those few cases that do occur, it often becomes apparent, during the initial interview, that the individual has developed an obsessive preoccupation with suspected cognitive impairment, sometimes reinforced by published information regarding Alzheimer's disease readily available to the public, that is belied by obvious inconsistent behavior (for instance, driving from a distance, unaccompanied, to my office, without apparent difficulty, at the scheduled appointment time, with full awareness of the purpose of the evaluation). It is much more typical for responses to direct questions regarding cognitive deficits to be characterized by minimization, denial or unawareness of impairment, or a combination thereof. Evidence exists that supports the conclusion that unawareness of cognitive impairment may be associated with a subtype of Alzheimer's disease in which patients demonstrate conspicuous visuoconstructive deficits (Auchus et al., 1994). For these reasons, the clinician must necessarily rely upon significant others, typically a spouse or children, to act as primary informants when gathering historical information that may provide important clues regarding the existence of a progressive dementia condition. The clinician uses any disparity between these reports and the patient's self-report as a possible gauge regarding the extent and impact of a dementing illness, assuming that other sources of relevant data, such as behavioral observations and testing results, reinforce the resulting diagnostic impression.

Clinicians who routinely conduct assessments of older adults will occasionally be asked by physicians, attorneys, or family members to evaluate an individual for the purpose of rendering an opinion regarding an individual's competency (e.g., the ability to make informed decisions regarding health care or management of personal affairs). Although data from a formal evaluation can serve as valuable evidence in addressing such questions, clinicians who respond to such requests must be acutely cognizant of the pitfalls of their involvement. As in all clinical situations, the professional must ask the question "Who is the client?" and must be sensitive to the issues of confidentiality and informed consent with respect to the examinee. If the individual who is the focus of the referral does in fact consent to evaluation and the disclosure of results to specified parties, the clinician must be cautious in drawing conclusions regarding the relationship between evaluation data and possible resultant restriction of liberty interests, keeping in mind that these questions are, ultimately, *legal questions*, not medical determinations (Zehr, 1995). Finally, the clinician who conducts an assessment for these purposes must, unfortunately, maintain a cautious awareness of possible less-than-altruistic motives of interested parties, particularly when questions regarding management of significant financial or property interests are at issue.

SETTING AND PROCEDURAL CONSIDERATIONS

In working with older adults in a formal evaluation, most of the guidelines applicable to assessment generally are relevant (e.g., conducting the interview and testing in a setting relatively free from distractions and conducive to a relaxed discussion of important personal information and elicitation of testing responses representative of the patient's current optimal level of function). Nevertheless, clinicians who do not routinely work with an elderly population must be cognizant of special considerations necessary to ensure that the assessment provides the optimal opportunity for eliciting the data required to address the question of a dementia process. The increased probability of at least mild hearing and visual impairments, for example, may necessitate adjustments in the examiner's behavior or physical accommodations in the setting which increase the likelihood that the patient will respond at an optimal level. Although most older adults can cope with the rigors of formal testing, accommodation to possible effects of fatigue may become necessary, including mandated breaks, especially if the patient appears to be tiring while simultaneously being reluctant to admit fatigue. At the very least, the patient should be advised at the onset regarding the option for breaks; even if none are taken, this advance notice can serve to make the patient more comfortable in the evaluation setting, providing the patient with a measure of control in what is quite likely an entirely novel and perhaps intimidating situation. In summary, most of the considerations applicable to assessments with older adults should appear to be commonsense notions to the clinician. Nevertheless, it has been my experience that professionals who have no experience with this population often demonstrate persistent adherence to commonly held myths about older adults which can influence the outcome of an evaluation (e.g., the notion that most elderly individuals are in failing health, frail, and entirely dependent on others). For novitiates in the field of older adult assessment, I highly recommend a primer prepared by the American Psychological Association for the explicit purpose of addressing these concerns: *What Practitioners Should Know About Working With Older Adults* (1997).

THE INITIAL INTERVIEW

The initial interview with an older individual in the context of an evaluation whose primary purpose is addressing the question of possible dementia generally resembles other clinical interviews, with two notable exceptions. First, and most obvious, is the subject matter that is the focus of the interview: obtaining historical and observational data that is directly relevant to the referral question. Secondly, in this assessment situation, it is always advisable, whenever possible, to have a spouse, child, family member, or close friend present during the interview, preferably someone with frequent opportunities to interact with the patient and observe behavior for an extended period of time. Again, it should be noted, the patient's consent is usually required, but, in my experience, this is rarely a problem. The primary advantage of the presence of the third party is the opportunity it provides the clinician to obtain an independent report regarding the patient's everyday functioning and the nature and length of time associated with observed changes which may or may not be consistent with the patient's own report. Also, the interaction between the patient and third party, particularly if that party is a spouse, can provide invaluable observational data. For example, when a patient continuously defers to the spouse for answers to routine questions, it may be determined that (a) this deference is out of necessity (i.e., the patient is incapable of providing the requested information), and (b) this deferential response pattern represents a conspicuous change on the part of the patient during a specified period of time (i.e., is "out of character"). Because, by definition, a dementia represents a decline in cognitive functioning, the focus of the interview will be on observed changes in behavior which may be affected by concomitant cognitive deficits, usually with gradual onset.

Once the issues of consent and the purpose of the evaluation are explained to the patient, a good starting point is the determination of the patient's perception, through open-ended questioning, of the course of events that were the impetus for the evaluation. Any observed disparity between the patient's self-report, the test results, and the information provided by others may be directly relevant, not only to indications of awareness cited earlier as possible evidence of a dementia process, but also to later recommendations regarding the patient's capacity to compensate for established deficits and consequent need to rely on others for assistance.

In my own practice, the focus of the interview is deliberately concrete; that is, I ask the parties to cite and describe, as specifically as possible, events or behaviors that illustrate the types of problems that precipitated the referral. The ability to execute routine activities of daily living (ADLs) - for example, paying bills, managing a medication regimen, driving, using the telephone, cooking, and reading the newspaper - can provide strong evidence of possible problems attributable to underlying cognitive impairment associated with a dementia process, although alternative explanations must be kept in mind, such as physical restrictions associated with a medical condition or clinically significant depression. The clinician whose goal is to obtain as comprehensive a base of relevant information as possible can avail himself or herself of the structured interview protocols readily available that specifically address these questions (e.g., that presented by R. A. Kane and R. L. Kane [1981], which is useful as a basis for assessment of ADLs). Other available forms of structured interviews are designed in part as a screening device for detection of dementia (e.g., the Geriatric Mental State [Copeland et al., 1976]); however, the examiner should avoid exclusive reliance on such interviews as a basis for conclusions regarding the existence of a dementia process.

Although the vast majority of patients seen for evaluation of possible dementia are in an age category normally associated with retirement status in this society, it is nevertheless important to question the individual to ascertain vocational and educational background, especially because many formal tests and measures of estimated premorbid status require this information. In addition, it is important to question the individual regarding current outside interests and activities and to verify, if possible, the patient's continued enjoyment of these activities. It is often the case that reduced participation in hitherto enjoyed pursuits provides clues implicating possible cognitive decline; for example, a lifelong bridge player may have ceased playing during the previous year while former partners have observed an accompanying inability to recall rules, cards dealt, scores, and so on. Of course, such observations, by themselves, beg the question whether they are possibly attributable to other conditions, such as withdrawal associated with depression. This is a diagnostic question that must be addressed, in any event, when dementia is at issue. To this end, the examiner should always attempt to ascertain whether there are in fact identifiable circumstances in the patient's life that may be the source of a clinical depression, such as the recent loss of a spouse or friends. Other changes in emotional state or personality functioning are also worth noting, such as changes in irritability or increases in aggressive behavior. In some cases, these may implicate other forms of dementia, for instance, Pick's disease, a relatively rare neurodegenerative process whose victims are typically younger than patients with Alzheimer's disease; behavioral problems in the form of lack of impulse control and uncharacteristic aggression are prominent symptoms of this disease (Heston, White, & Mastri, 1987). The clinician should also keep in mind that affective disorders and dementias are not mutually exclusive entities; they can and often do coexist, particularly, for example, in the early stages of Alzheimer's disease, when the patient may be acutely aware of the progression of cognitive deficits and their impact on everyday functioning, including the necessity for increasing dependence on others. Clinical depression can, in fact, exacerbate the impairments primarily attributable to a dementia process (Fields et al., 1998).

In most cases the patient will have had prior medical and laboratory examinations that may exclude readily detectable sources of dementia such as hypothyroidism and thiamine deficiencies. The examiner should nevertheless be attuned to reports of sensorimotor problems that can be associated with dementia, such as prominent motor symptoms which, in conjunction with evidence of dementia, may suggest a neurologic disorder such as Parkinson disease (Aarsland et al., 1996), or reports of diminution of taste and smell, which, while common in older adults, is also associated with Alzheimer's disease (Schiffman, 1997).

TESTING FOR DEMENTIA

An exhaustive review of available test instruments designed to assess cognitive deficits associated with a dementia process is beyond the scope of this contribution, although such comprehensive reviews do exist, particularly in the neuropsychological literature (see, e.g., Spreen & Strauss, 1998). Instead, I will discuss some of the important aspects of functioning that must be assessed in a formal test instrument designed for the purpose of evaluating possible dementia and illustrate these principles as incorporated in some of the more commonly used tests.

Any assessment for purposes of addressing questions of dementia must necessarily include test items that can provide indices of ability in the following areas:

1. Memory (immediate, short-term, and remote).
2. Orientation.
3. Attention/Concentration.
4. Expressive and receptive language functions.
5. General intelligence.
6. Visuospatial abilities.
7. Abstract reasoning and problem solving.
8. Initiation and perseveration of response set.

This is not meant to be an exhaustive listing, and most tasks incorporated in formal testing will likely assess many of these faculties simultaneously. In addition, it is common to find references to constructs that are comprised of various combinations of the preceding factors (e.g., so-called executive functions, which, in common parlance, likely include aspects of Items 7 and 8 above). No tests available to assess these functions in an elderly population are sufficiently comprehensive to provide an adequate evaluation of all these cognitive functions, and it is therefore common practice for the specialist in this area to utilize a battery of tests designed to address as many of these areas as possible.

A critical consideration when testing older adults is the availability of sufficient normative data to render a particular test useful for an individual in a particular age group. This may appear to be such an obvious requirement in test construction and validation that it need not be mentioned; it is, however, the rule rather than the exception that tests are used for the assessment of dementia without attention paid to the adequacy or even existence of age-based normative data. As a striking example of this practice, consider the fact that one of the most commonly used screening instruments for the assessment of dementia, the Mini-Mental State Exam (MMSE; M. F. Folstein, S. E. Folstein, & McHugh, 1975), did not have available age and education-based normative scoring data for many years (Crum et al., 1993). The availability of this data rendered the single cutoff score, previously relied on as an index of dementia, obsolete. Awareness of the necessity to provide relevant normative data for older populations has had a salutory impact on test construction and research in the last few years, as seen in the work of Heaton, Grant, and Matthews (1991). This work has made the Halstead-Reitan battery (Reitan & Wolfson, 1993) and its individual components applicable to the assessment of older adults, and new versions of the Wechsler Adult Intelligence Scale (WAIS-III) and Wechsler Memory Scale (WMS-III; The Psychological Corporation, 1997) can be used for testing of adults through age 89.

Although it is not advisable to rely on a single instrument as a basis for conclusions, where time constraints preclude the use of an extensive battery, tests such as the Mattis Dementia Rating Scale (DRS; Mattis, 1988) have proven to be quite useful in providing a standardized description of cognitive strengths and weaknesses for patients with suspected dementia. The DRS yields separate scale scores for attention, initiation and perseveration, construction, conceptualization, and verbal and nonverbal short-term memory. Normative data for the separate scales and for the total score are now available through age 95 (Vangel & Lichtenberg, 1995). It can be administered in less than 45 minutes, depending on the degree of dementia present. Available data indicate some usefulness in distinguishing mild, moderate, and severe degrees of dementia (Shay et al., 1991) and in differentiating dementia associated with Alzheimer's disease and Huntington's chorea (Salmon et al., 1989).

Although receptive language functions such as comprehension are implicitly assessed in any task requiring adherence to written or spoken instructions, certain language impairments, such as word-finding difficulty, as assessed in a confrontational naming task, are common to Alzheimer's disease and other forms of dementia (e.g., dementia associated with vascular conditions and chronic alcoholism). The Boston Naming Test (Kaplan, Goodglass, & Weintraub, 1983) is an easily administered and reliable test of the ability to name common objects, either without cues or, if necessary, with subsequent stimulus and phonemic cues to ascertain the degree of impairment.

A measure of level of general intelligence is not, by itself, particularly useful in testing for a suspected dementia, except in those cases where there exists a significant perceived disparity between present level of assessed intelligence and estimates of premorbid intellectual abilities based on such information as level of formal education and vocational background. Thus, for example, an assessed overall IQ of 100, which, by definition, is exactly average, has no diagnostic value in a dementia evaluation, but if, in addition, we know that the patient had obtained a doctorate in particle physics and had a successful teaching and research career, the same figure becomes a valuable indicator of probable significant decline in intellectual functions possibly associated with a progressive dementia. The WAIS-III is the current gold standard for assessment of intelligence. It contains subtests such as the Digit Span task, which assesses auditory attention span, and Block Design, which measures nonverbal abstract reasoning ability, both of which are sensitive to dementing conditions. The time required for administration, however, often precludes its use in a dementia assessment, although a shortened version, the Wechsler Abbreviated Scale of Intelligence (WASI; The Psychological Corporation, 1999), can be administered in less than 30 minutes; like the WAIS-III, it has normative data extending to age 89. Other brief intelligence tests suitable for dementia evaluation purposes include the Kaufman Brief Intelligence Test (K-BIT; A. Kaufman & N. Kaufman, 1990) and the General Ability Measure for Adults (GAMA; Naglieri & Bardos, 1997). Both are suitable for use with older adults; the GAMA may be useful when evaluating people who speak English as a second language.

Tasks that assess visuoconstructive abilities are incorporated in the DRS, WAIS-III, MMSE, and GAMA protocols, among others, but two tests particularly worthy of mention in this regard are the Rey Complex Figure Test and Recognition Trial (RCFT; J. Meyers & K. Meyers, 1995) and the Clock Test (Tuokko et al., 1995). These tests represent significantly revised versions of instruments that have been used for years, and both are particularly suited to an older population and have been shown to be useful in assessment of dementia of the Alzheimer's type.

The RCFT, which requires the patient to copy a complex geometric figure, also incorporates immediate and delayed (30-minute) recall tasks and a subsequent recognition memory task, thus providing an excellent assessment of nonverbal memory in combination with an assessment of two-dimensional constructional abilities. The Clock Test provides an assessment of visuospatial construction abilities and nonverbal abstract reasoning abilities in the context of a presumably overlearned ability: reading time from a printed clock face.

The *sine qua non* of dementia conditions generally is the presence of impairments of memory, particularly for immediate and recent (short-term) memory, while memory for remote events remains relatively intact during the early stages of most progressive dementias. For this reason, questions regarding changes in memory functions should comprise a significant proportion of the initial interview; likewise, assessment of memory functions should be a major focus of the formal testing. Whenever possible, the WMS-III should be administered in an assessment of memory, because, like its predecessors, it represents the state of the art in objective assessment of memory functions. In addition, the WMS-III yields eight separate memory scores, including immediate recall for auditory verbal and visual memory and delayed (30-minute) recall for these same stimuli. As previously noted, the normative database for the WMS-III includes adults to age 89, and the manual for the WMS-III includes normative data for all indices in separate dementia sample populations including Alzheimer's disease, Parkinson's disease, Huntington's disease, and multiple sclerosis. Despite the comprehensive assessment of memory functions provided by the WMS-III, it has not been generally adopted for inclusion in dementia assessment batteries at this time, likely due to the time required to administer the entire protocol. The literature on formal memory assessment is, in fact, replete with attempts to devise a brief, reliable assessment of memory impairment associated with dementing conditions (see, e.g., Buschke et al., 1999). For the practitioner interested in a comprehensive review of theoretical and practical issues associated with memory assessment in this context, I would recommend review of the text *Clinical Memory Assessment of Older Adults* (Poon, 1986).

Measures of orientation and attention are incorporated in most single-instrument assessments of cognitive status, whether used for evaluations of suspected dementias or for other purposes, with little variation in orientation questions from the 10 items included in the MMSE. With respect to the latter, it should be noted that each of the 10 orientation items from the MMSE are given the same weighting in the total score as each of the three recall tasks contained in the same protocol, a disproportionate emphasis for purposes of dementia assessment. The most common form of assessment of attention consists of some variation of the Digit Span subtest of the WAIS-III: tasks that measure auditory attention span. Attentional tasks incorporating a visual component, however, should be included in the armamentarium of every clinician involved in the assessment of older adults, if for no other reason than the fact that impaired hearing will preclude the use of Digit Span-type tests of attention. The Visual Search and Attention Test (VSAT; Trenerry et al., 1990) is a timed task that assesses visual scanning ability and sustained attention simultaneously. The most commonly used neuropsychological tests of attention in a visual tracking context, however, are the Trail Making Tests included in the Halstead-Reitan Neuropsychological Test Battery (Reitan & Wolfson, 1993). The Trail Making Tests provide an assessment of visual tracking ability, sustained attention (Trails A), and ability to switch attentional or response set (Trails B), the latter task being particularly affected in dementia conditions. The Heaton et al. (1991) normative data allow interpretation of Trails performance for older adults, but the examiner should also note that the Trail Making Tests incorporate a significant motor component, thus, coexistent medical conditions such as arthritis or Parkinson's disease will render interpretation of results problematic.

As noted earlier, the differential diagnosis of dementia should always include a consideration of the effects of depression. A detailed discussion of this subject is beyond the scope of this contribution, but excellent analyses of this problem in the context of dementia assessment are readily available (see, e.g., Storandt & VandenBos, 1994). For the clinician addressing this issue in the context of formal testing, however, the Geriatric Depression Scale (GDS; Yesavage et al., 1983) is an instrument that should be strongly considered. The GDS is a widely used and well-researched self-report depression inventory which was developed specifically for use with older adults and is easy to administer.

CONCLUSIONS AND RECOMMENDATIONS

Having interviewed the patient and available family members, reviewed available medical, vocational, and social history, and administered formal testing, how does one go about drawing conclusions regarding the existence of a dementia process? The simple answer to this question is that the clinician must judge whether the objective test results and the available observational and historical data are all more consistent with the conclusion of a progressive dementia than with such alternatives as clinical depression or delirium, otherwise referred to as acute confusional state (Pompei et al., 1995). This problem is compounded by the fact that other factors, such as medications with sedative effects, or motivational variables, may render interpretation of test results problematic, in which case the clinician has a duty to note these factors and their potential impact on the evaluation. Should the clinician conclude, after consideration of these variables, that the patient is suffering from a dementia process, the next question to be addressed is the degree or severity of the dementia, because this determination has direct implications for possible required changes in the patient's living circumstances. To assist the clinician in addressing the question of severity, widely used instruments such as the Clinical Dementia Rating (Berg, 1988) can make use of both reported observations and test data as a basis for reliable assessments of degree of dementia, ranging from none to severe.

The question of the cause of a particular case of dementia is, of course, a medical issue, but the nonphysician who is involved in the evaluation of dementia should develop at least a cursory knowledge of the variety of conditions that can result in dementia, some of which can be ruled out through routine medical and laboratory tests. Other causes, such as chronic alcoholism, can be suggested in the course of gathering history and interview data, while others, such as Alzheimer's disease, remain primarily diagnoses by exclusion.

Regardless of the conclusions concerning the ultimate cause of the observed dementia, the clinician who is involved in this type of assessment has an obligation to make recommendations, based on the obtained results, regarding possible changes in living circumstances or needs for assistance that are evident as a direct result of the degree of dementia. These recommendations might range from statements regarding need for supervision of medication regimen or assistance with management of finances to consideration of nursing home placement when it is evident that existing family support is insufficient to meet the patient's basic care needs. In cases where the degree of dementia is judged to be mild or even questionable, the patient may be capable of deriving benefit from available resources designed to assist in the amelioration of mild memory problems (Scogin & Prohaska, 1993). To the extent possible, family members should be present when the conclusion of a dementia process is communicated to the patient, not only for obvious reasons - for example, to insure that family members will retain information regarding recommendations that a patient is, by virtue of his or her dementia, incapable of recalling - but also to use the opportunity to encourage the family to become actively involved in the patient's adaptation to dementia. In the case of Alzheimer's disease, involvement and early counseling with caregivers has been shown to result in an average delay of nearly 1 year in necessity for nursing home placement (Mittelman et al., 1996). Family members and other caregivers should be apprised of available resources specifically designed to assist in education for the purpose of meeting the needs of both patient and caregiver (see, e.g., Tappen, 1997), including the support and valuable information provided by such organizations as the Alzheimer's Association.

In clinical practice, any professional who works with older adults, regardless of specialty, will invariably and with increasing frequency, as a direct result of changing population demographics, which are themselves the product of improved medical care, encounter questions of possible dementias distinguishable from normal aging effects. Because these questions will inevitably arise in clinical practice, it is incumbent on the clinician to acquire at least a rudimentary knowledge of the principles of assessment for dementia so that, at the very least, the need for referral for further investigation can readily be ascertained. For the clinician who works primarily with a geriatric population, a working knowledge of dementia assessment should be considered a critical component of preparatory or ongoing education.

CONTRIBUTOR

Martin D. Zehr, PhD, JD, is currently Director of Neuropsychology at Research Medical Center in Kansas City, Missouri, and an adjunct assistant professor in the Department of Psychiatry at the University of Kansas Medical Center. His training is in clinical psychology and neuropsychology and his special interest is in the area of geropsychology and the law, the subject of numerous articles and presentations. He is a member of the Missouri Bar and the Board of Directors of the Heartland chapter of the Alzheimer's Association. Dr. Zehr can be contacted at Research Medical Center, 2316 East Meyer Boulevard, Kansas City, MO 64132.

RESOURCES

Aarsland, D., Tandberg, E., Larsen, J., & Cummings, J. (1996). Frequency of dementia in Parkinson disease. *Archives of Neurology, 53,* 538-542.

Alzheimer's Disease and Related Disorders Association. (1999). *The Time Is Now: 1999 National Public Policy Program to Conquer Alzheimer's Disease*. Chicago: Author.

American Psychiatric Association. (1994). *Diagnostic and Statistical Manual of Mental Disorders* (4th ed.). Washington, DC: Author.

American Psychological Association. (1997). *What Practitioners Should Know About Working With Older Adults.* Washington, DC: Author.

American Psychological Association. (1998). *Guidelines for the Evaluation of Dementia and Age-Related Cognitive Decline*. Washington, DC: Author.

Auchus, A. P., Goldstein, F. C., Green, J., & Green, R. C. (1994). Unawareness of cognitive impairments in Alzheimer's disease. *Neuropsychiatry, Neuropsychology, and Behavioral Neurology, 7*(1), 25-29.

Berg, L. (1988). Mild senile dementia of the Alzheimer type: Diagnostic criteria and natural history. *Mount Sinai Journal of Medicine, 55,* 87-96.

Breitner, J. C., & Welsh, K. (1995). An approach to diagnosis and management of memory loss and other cognitive syndromes of aging. *Psychiatric Services: A Journal of the American Psychiatric Association, 46,* 29-35.

Buschke, H., Kuslansky, G., Katz, M., Stewart, W., Sliwinski, M., Eckholdt, H., & Lipton, R. (1999). Screening for dementia with the Memory Impairment Screen. *Neurology, 52,* 231-238.

Copeland, J. R., Kelleher, M. J., Kellett, J., Gourlay, A., Gurland, B., Fleiss, J., & Sharpe, L. (1976). A semi-structured clinical interview for the assessment of diagnosis and mental state in the elderly: The Geriatric Mental State Schedule. *Psychological Medicine, 6,* 439-449.

Corey-Bloom, J., Thal, L. J., Galasko, D., Folstein, M., Drachman, D., Raskind, M., & Lanska, D. (1995). Diagnosis and evaluation of dementia. *Neurology, 45,* 211-218.

Crum, R., Anthony, J., Bassett, S., & Folstein, M. (1993). Population-based norms for the Mini-Mental State Examination by age and educational level. *Journal of the American Medical Association, 269,* 2386-2391.

Fields, J., Norman, S., Straits-Troster, K., & Troster, A. (1998). The impact of depression on memory in neurodegenerative disease. In A. Troster (Ed.), *Memory in Neurodegenerative Disease: Biological, Cognitive and Clinical Perspectives* (pp. 314-337). Cambridge, England: Cambridge University Press.

Folstein, M. F., Folstein, S. E., & McHugh, P. R. (1975). "Mini-Mental State." A practical method for grading the cognitive state of patients for the clinician. *Journal of Psychiatric Research, 12,* 189-198.

Grisso, T., & Appelbaum, P. S. (1998). *MacArthur Competence Assessment Tool for Treatment (MacCAT-T).* Sarasota, FL: Professional Resource Press.

Heaton, R., Grant, I., & Matthews, C. (1991). *Comprehensive Norms for an Expanded Halstead-Reitan Battery: Demographic Corrections, Research Findings, and Clinical Applications.* Odessa, FL: Psychological Assessment Resources.

Heston, L., White, J., & Mastri, A. (1987). Pick's disease - Clinical genetics and natural history. *Archives of General Psychiatry, 44,* 409-411.

High, D. M., Whitehouse, P. J., Post, S. G., & Berg, L. (1994). Guidelines for addressing ethical and legal issues in Alzheimer disease research. *Alzheimer Disease and Associated Disorders, 8*(Suppl. 4), 66-74.

Kane, R. A., & Kane, R. L. (1981). *Assessing the Elderly: A Practical Guide to Measurement.* Lexington, MA: Lexington.

Kaplan, E., Goodglass, H., & Weintraub, S. (1983). *Boston Naming Test.* Philadelphia: Lea & Febiger.

Kaufman, A., & Kaufman, N. (1990). *Kaufman Brief Intelligence Test.* Circle Pines, MN: American Guidance Service.

La Rue, A. (1992). *Aging and Neuropsychological Assessment.* New York: Plenum.

Marson, D., Ingram, K., Cody, H., & Harrell, L. (1995). Assessing the competency of patients with Alzheimer's disease under different legal standards. *Archives of Neurology, 52,* 949-954.

Mattis, S. (1988). *Dementia Rating Scale: Professional Manual.* Odessa, FL: Psychological Assessment Resources.

McKhann, G., Drachman, D., Folstein, M., Katzman, R., Price, D., & Stadlan, E. (1984). Clinical diagnosis of Alzheimer's disease: Report of the NINCDS-ADRDA work group under the auspices of Department of Health and Human Services Task Force on Alzheimer's Disease. *Neurology, 34,* 939-944.

Meyers, J., & Meyers, K. (1995). *Rey Complex Figure Test and Recognition Trial.* Odessa, FL: Psychological Assessment Resources.

Mittelman, M., Ferris, S., Shulman, E., Steinberg, G., & Levin, B. (1996). A family intervention to delay nursing home placement of patients with Alzheimer's disease. *Journal of the American Medical Association, 276,* 1725-1731.

Naglieri, J., & Bardos, A. (1997). *General Ability Measure for Adults.* Minnetonka, MN: National Computer Systems.

National Center for Cost Containment, Department of Veterans Affairs. (1997). *Assessment of Competency and Capacity of the Older Adult: A Practice Guideline for Psychologists.* Milwaukee, WI: Author.

Parks, R., Zec, R., & Wilson, R. (Eds.). (1993). *Neuropsychology of Alzheimer's Disease and Other Dementias.* New York: Oxford University Press.

Pompei, P., Foreman, M., Cassel, C., Alessi, C., & Cox, D. (1995). Detecting delirium among hospitalized older patients. *Archives of Internal Medicine, 155,* 301-307.

Poon, L. (Ed.). (1986). *Handbook for Clinical Memory Assessment of Older Adults.* Washington, DC: American Psychological Association.

The Psychological Corporation. (1997). *Wechsler Adult Intelligence Scale-III* and *Wechsler Memory Scale-III.* San Antonio: Author.

The Psychological Corporation. (1999). *Wechsler Abbreviated Scale of Intelligence.* San Antonio: Author.

Reiman, E. M., Caselli, R. J., Yun, L. S., Chen, K., Bandy, D., Minoshima, S., Thibodeau, S. N., & Osborne, D. (1996). Preclinical evidence of Alzheimer's disease in persons homozygous for the *e*4 allele for apolipoprotein E. *New England Journal of Medicine, 334,* 752-758.

Reitan, R., & Wolfson, D. (1993). *The Halstead-Reitan Neuropsychological Test Battery: Theory and Clinical Interpretation* (2nd ed.). Tucson, AZ: Neuropsychology Press.

Salmon, D., Kwo-on-Yuen, P., Heindel, W., Butters, N., & Thal, L. (1989). Differentiation of Alzheimer's disease and Huntington's disease with the Dementia Rating Scale. *Archives of Neurology, 46,* 1204-1208.

Schiffman, S. (1997). Taste and smell losses in normal aging and disease. *Journal of the American Medical Association, 278,* 1357-1362.

Scogin, F., & Prohaska, M. (1993). *Aiding Older Adults With Memory Complaints.* Sarasota, FL: Professional Resource Press.

Shay, K., Duke, L., Conboy, T., Harrell, L., Callaway, R., & Folks, D. (1991). The clinical validity of the Mattis Dementia Rating Scale in staging Alzheimer's dementia. *Journal of Geriatric Psychiatry and Neurology, 4,* 18-25.

Spreen, O., & Strauss, E. (1998). *A Compendium of Neuropsychological Tests* (2nd ed.). New York: Oxford University Press.

Storandt, M., & VandenBos, G. R. (Eds.). (1994). *Neuropsychological Assessment of Dementia and Depression in Older Adults: A Clinician's Guide.* Washington, DC: American Psychological Association.

Taeuber, C. (1990). Diversity: The dramatic reality. In S. Bass, E. Kutza, & F. Torres-Gill (Eds.), *Diversity in Aging: Challenges Facing Planners and Policymakers in the 1990s* (pp. 1-45). Glenview, IL: Scott, Foresman and Co.

Tappen, R. (1997). *Interventions for Alzheimer's Disease: A Caregiver's Complete Reference.* Baltimore, MD: Health Professions Press.

Trenerry, M., Crosson, B., DeBoe, J., & Leber, W. (1990). *Visual Search and Attention Test.* Odessa, FL: Psychological Assessment Resources.

Tuokko, H., Hadjistavropoulos, T., Miller, J., Horton, A., & Beattie, B. (1995). *The Clock Test: Administration and Scoring Manual.* North Tonawanda, NY: Multi-Health Systems.

Vangel, S., Jr., & Lichtenberg, P. (1995). Mattis Dementia Rating Scale: Clinical utility and relationship with demographic variables. *The Clinical Neuropsychologist, 9,* 209-213.

Yesavage, J., Brink, T., Rose, T., Lum, O., Huang, V., Adey, M., & Leirer, V. (1983). Development and validation of a geriatric screening scale: A preliminary report. *Journal of Psychiatric Research, 17,* 37-49.

Zehr, M. (1995, November). *Determinations of Changing Capacity: Sources of Evidence.* Paper presented at the annual meeting of the Gerontological Society of America, Los Angeles, CA.

Zehr, M. (1998). Memory dysfunction in neurodegenerative disease: Ethical and legal issues. In A. I. Troster (Ed.), *Memory in Neurodegenerative Disease: Biological, Cognitive and Clinical Perspectives* (pp. 377-389). Cambridge, England: Cambridge University Press.

Introduction to Section II: Practice Management and Professional Development

This section of *Innovations in Clinical Practice* includes contributions that address practice management and professional development. Successful practice management requires careful consideration of many important issues. Over the years, we have recognized the need for careful planning and practice management. The contributions included in this section address several pertinent issues.

Over the past two decades, there has been an increase in ethical, licensure board, and malpractice complaints against mental health practitioners. Clinicians are often not knowledgeable about how to respond when a complaint is received, and being ill prepared creates a special vulnerability, both psychologically and legally. Robert Henley Woody's contribution provides knowledge and strategies for effective responses to complaints.

Termination of psychotherapy may occur in a variety of ways. It may be initiated by the patient or by the therapist or in response to external forces. It may be planned or it may come as a surprise. In the next contribution, Jeffrey Barnett, Sherry MacGlashan, and Alicia Clarke describe the issues surrounding termination and abandonment.

Leonard Jason, Susan Jahn, and Meredith Miller examine several case studies and how they relate to guidelines that have been developed for mental health professionals who interact with the media. Readers are introduced to the legal, ethical, and professional issues that may arise.

In the fourth contribution of this section, Jeffrey Barnett and Nicole Polakoff address the issues of maintaining clinical competence in general and as it applies to two patient populations, namely those from diverse cultural backgrounds and the elderly. The contribution reviews clinical, ethical, and legal issues pertaining to professional competence and makes recommendations to assist clinicians to competently assess and treat patients.

In the final contribution, John Rudisill suggests that the best marketing that clinicians can do is to create satisfied clients. This contribution deals with marketing as it relates to providing quality services rather than through advertising activities. He describes how to provide services to the three main stakeholders in the service delivery process: the client, the referral source, and the community.

What To Do When You Receive An Ethics, Legal (Malpractice), or Licensing Complaint

Robert Henley Woody

With the new millennium, most mental health practitioners recognize that clinical services are provided under a cloud of legal liability. Living in a litigious society, professionals, regardless of context, discipline, or credentials, face a substantial risk of ethical, regulatory (licensing), or legal (malpractice) complaints.

Over the past two decades, there has been an increase in ethical, regulatory, and legal (malpractice) actions against mental health practitioners. The increase has occurred for all three types of complaints. The reason, in general, is exemplified by regulatory complaints: "With increased public awareness and increased willingness by aggrieved individuals to face the ordeal of bringing charges, licensing boards in many professions have many more cases to adjudicate" (Sinclair, Simon, & Pettifor, 1996, p. 12). Although true for all of the mental health disciplines, consider the example of psychologists. Peterson (1996) estimates an increase of regulatory actions of 500% over the past 10 years and states: "Available data clearly indicate that there has been a significant increase in disciplinary and legal actions against psychologists for unprofessional and unethical conduct" (p. 71). The incidence of ethics complaints is unclear, due to professional associations' being reluctant to adjudicate ethics cases because of the financial expense, the risk of a lawsuit from a respondent, and a willingness to turn the responsibility over to licensing boards. Besides regulatory complaints, legal complaints, such as for alleged malpractice, have also increased dramatically (Besharov, 1985; Woody, 1998a, 1999b). No mental health profession has escaped from an escalation of complaints.

From the outset, it is acknowledged that the complaint process may vary according to the particular jurisdiction. That is, some boards (clearly the minority) maintain a somewhat educative approach, preferring to safeguard the public by establishing control over the alleged wrongdoer by prescribing ways that will improve his or her professional functioning and decision making. Other boards (clearly the majority) maintain a definite prosecutorial approach, giving primary emphasis to safeguarding the public by imposing disciplinary measures on the alleged wrongdoer. With the growing disenchantment with health care providers and increased commitment to consumer protection, there is reason to believe that the modern trend is toward the prosecutorial model, as well as stronger disciplinary actions.

Also as a preface to this contribution, there are noteworthy differences between the procedural aspects of complaints to ethics committees, regulatory agencies, and courts of law. Due to the possibility of being sued by a respondent, professional associations (especially at the state level) have moved away from adjudicating cases. At this point in time, ethics committees generally tend toward being educative. Although an ethics committee may profess to be collegial, there is often a power differential. For example, the ethics committee may invoke rules that preclude the respondent's having legal representation or deny the respondent a face-to-face meeting with the committee. Because having an ethics complaint upheld impacts negatively on the respondent's professional reputation and could lead to a complaint to the state licensing board or connect into a malpractice legal action, a complaint to an ethics committee must be taken seriously. It is advisable for the respondent to be appropriately defensive and to obtain the behind-the-scenes help of an attorney in fashioning responses to the ethics committee. Complaints to regulatory agencies and lawsuits are clearly legal actions, and the respondent should rely on representation by an attorney and demand procedural rights. These matters will be addressed in much greater detail throughout this contribution.

Practitioners are often unknowledgeable about how to respond or behave when a complaint is received, and being ill prepared creates a special vulnerability, both legally and psychologically. This contribution is intended to provide knowledge and strategies for effective responses to complaints.

A significant adverse effect is that a legal complaint evokes considerable anxiety in the practitioner (i.e., the respondent). Koocher and Keith-Spiegel (1998) state: "Receiving a formal inquiry or complaint letter from a licensing board or professional association's ethics committee can be one of the most stressful events in a psychologist's career" (p. 434). The possibility of adverse emotional, behavioral, and physical health problems from licensing and ethics complaints certainly extends to lawsuits or legal actions as well. As a result, even the most seasoned professional will likely experience stress-related disorders such as sleep loss, decreased motivation, psychosomatic illnesses, family conflicts, and disillusionment with his or her career (Charles, Wilbert, & Kennedy, 1984).

THE UNLEVEL PLAYING FIELD

As mentioned, there are basically three types of complaints, namely complaints based on the ethics code of a professional association, a regulatory complaint relevant to licensure, and a lawsuit, usually alleging professional negligence or malpractice. There are similarities and differences among the three types of complaints.

A major commonality is that each of these types of complaints is processed by "triers of fact" who are dedicated to consumer protection. The investigative and decision-making processes aim to provide protection to consumers of mental health services. Stated differently, the interests of the client (or consumer) are of foremost importance, and the practitioner is left to his or her own advocacy and can expect nothing more than rights provided by law (Woody, 1997a).

Mental health professionals often misunderstand this matter, especially when the complaint is to an ethics committee in a professional association of which the practitioner is a member or to a licensing board composed (in part) by members of the practitioner's professional discipline. The erroneous belief is twofold: first, that being a professional allows one a substantial respect or benefit of the doubt; and second, that those processing the complaint will be totally impartial. Neither of these beliefs is assured.

In any complaint arena, consumer protection means that the interests of the service user, the client, are primary. By legal definition, there is "prosecution"of the respondent. When political correctness (doing what will win favor with empowered persons in government) is mixed with egotism and self-righteousness, apostolic zeal, group think, and persecutory inclinations emerge with some triers of fact (i.e., those who make the decisions in complaint cases).

With both ethics and regulatory complaints, many respondents have reported, "I was treated like I was guilty until proven innocent." Elsewhere, this issue has been elaborated on (Woody, 1993), with examples of the flaws in the investigative and decision-making processes and advocacy for equality for consumers and professionals (see also Woody, 1997a, 1997c, 1998).

In reality, there is reason to believe that the nature of all complaints creates bias in favor of the consumer. So professionals should be aware of the following possible (likely?) outcomes: (a) The administrative procedures are sometimes skewed in favor of the complainant; (b) only a modicum of colleagiality is present in hearings; and (c) the triers of fact may succumb to self-serving decision making to the detriment of the respondent. Incidentally, professional concern about the unequal and unfair treatment of mental health professionals, as well as the proliferation of false accusations, has led to a national organization that advocates the interests of practitioners (for additional information, contact: The Professional Advocacy Network, 6230 Wilshire Boulevard, Suite 110, Los Angeles, CA 90048).

ETHICS COMPLAINTS

An ethics complaint is processed by a professional association. It is applicable to only the dues-paying members of the particular association. Therefore, practitioners who are not in the association are not subject to ethics complaints. Innumerable practitioners have reported that the possibility of an ethics complaint led them to terminate membership in certain professional associations. When an ethics committee takes disciplinary action, it is generally in terms of an impact on membership (e.g., suspension or termination) or professional development (e.g., requiring additional training or supervision in an effort to safeguard consumers from further harm from the practitioner).

A finding by an ethics committee that a member has transgressed has two horrifying penalties that can have lifelong impact on the practitioner. First, at least in some professional associations, there are notifications. That is, upon a finding of an ethical violation, the ethics committee may contact a variety of sources, such as other professional associations of which the respondent is a member, organizations or boards (public or private) that have issued certifications or licensures, and employers. Second, the disciplinary finding is commonly published for all members of the particular association to be aware.

Obviously, the notifications and publication of discipline can, and likely will, result in other investigations. For example, if the professional association reported discipline to a licensing board, it is highly probable that a regulatory investigation would be triggered.

REGULATORY COMPLAINTS

A regulatory complaint comes from a government agency, most commonly (for the purposes of this contribution) the licensing board that issued the license that authorizes the professional to practice. In the past, many mental health professionals championed licensing laws, believing that the results would be greater professional opportunities (i.e., elevated status among mental health care providers, higher incomes, and ability to receive payment from third-party insurance sources). The campaign message was that licensing will assure the consumer of qualified practitioners. To the surprise of the mental health professions, licensure was transformed into regulatory laws with a clear-cut prosecutorial bent.

Although some jurisdictions may vary, disciplinary actions by a licensing board are often referred to as being "quasicriminal proceedings," which are spearheaded by prosecuting attorneys. Also, regulatory laws are under political influence. For example, members of a licensing board are commonly appointed by the governor of the state. It is common sense that no governor would appoint a mental health practitioner to a licensing board who sought to protect practitioners from state-regulatory or legal actions, as opposed to wanting to safeguard consumers from the alleged wrongdoing of practitioners. Stated bluntly, the board members, attorneys, and support staff are rewarded, both internally and externally, by forceful prosecution of respondents alleged to have violated the standards promulgated by the regulators.

Regulatory complaints are sometimes referred to euphemistically as "ethics complaints." This usage of the term is only partially correct. The regulatory complaint will consider standards that may have a connection to an ethics code. Some state legislatures have adopted ethics codes from professional associations for statutory purposes. More commonly, statutes contain vaguely worded standards that the practitioner is supposed to interpret. Stated differently, the regulators have considerable flexibility in asserting after-the-fact standards for practice.

A disciplinary action has profound consequences for a licensee. If a violation is found, various disciplinary measures are possible, such as placing the respondent on probation; rescinding or suspending the license; issuing a censure or reprimand; imposing a fine; restricting the types of services or clients; requiring the respondent to receive supervision or treatment, with progress reports to be sent to the agency; mandating additional continuing education; and the list goes on.

In some jurisdictions, certain kinds of regulatory actions can also lead to criminal charges. For example, if the regulatory investigation finds fraudulent billing for services or sexual misconduct with a client, criminal charges may also be filed: "Although there are more professionals sued civilly, criminal and license-related cases are far more serious" (Reaves & Ogloff, 1996, p. 117).

Incidentally, for some disciplines, adverse actions by licensing boards or other governmental agencies are published, which can lead to a *sua sponte* (i.e., self-initiated) investigation by an ethics committee. For example, the Association of State and Provincial Psychology Boards (ASPPB; 1996) has developed the Disciplinary Data System (DDS), a computerized national registry, which provides information about a regulatory action against a psychologist in one state to other states; among others, this information is also made available to the American Psychological Association. Second, the disciplinary finding is commonly published for all members of the particular association to be aware.

As with a negative action by an ethics committee, a disciplinary action by a licensing board has a long-lasting spillover effect. In addition to potentially triggering other *sua sponte* investigations, opportunities for hospital privileges, managed care approved-provider lists, additional certifications and licensures, and continuation of malpractice coverage (at least at the previous rate) may be placed in jeopardy. Of course, there is also the penalty of awareness of the disciplinary action resulting in diminished professional reputation and a decrease in referrals.

LEGAL COMPLAINTS

This category of complaints is characterized by lawsuits based on alleged failure of a mental health practitioner to fulfill the prevailing standards for the profession. The failure can occur by omission or commission. The prevailing standards are not confined to what the profession is actually doing or supporting; there is an extension to what the profession should be doing, with consideration being given to invasiveness (e.g., the jeopardy of rights or interests that would be created for the consumer) and the expense of the treatment (e.g., what is reasonably feasible when cost is considered).

Litigation in general and against mental health practitioners specifically has increased dramatically over the past two decades or so. Due to unreported settlements, dismissed complaints, and the like, it is impossible to arrive at a precise incidence of complaints against mental health practitioners. Suffice it to say that for psychologists:

> The amount of ongoing litigation in the United States has reached appalling proportions, and although the growth in litigation has not been as severe in Canada, often the response to problems or differences among people is the initiation of a lawsuit. Although many people seem to abhor this growing trend, the fact remains unaltered. (Reaves & Ogloff, 1996, p. 117)

Also, recall the comments made earlier about the escalation of complaints against practitioners regardless of mental health discipline.

The most common legal action against a practitioner involves alleged malpractice, which is predicated on professional liability. That is, the service provider is alleged to have damaged a consumer through failing to provide services within the prevailing standard of care for the profession, and thereby failing to satisfy a legal duty.

A legal complaint is based on a so-called "cause of action," that is, the reason for filing the lawsuit that has support from legal theory, as well as from statutory and/or common law. Most lawsuits set forth several causes of action: "Currently, the most visible of these problems is the sexual exploitation of clients, although other violations also exist: inappropriate crossing of social boundaries, involvement in multiple roles with clients, working outside of established areas of competence, or providing treatment under conditions of impaired judgment" (Maddock, 1993, p. 118).

No finite list of causes of action is possible. The attorney for the plaintiff or complainant can construct a cause of action by matching the presumed facts of the case of legal theory and statutory and common law. Generally, the concept of malpractice is present in some form, albeit that the word choice may vary. Virtually all causes of action focus on, as stated previously, the practitioner's alleged failure, by omission or commission, to appropriately fulfill a legal duty, such as regarding standard of care, to the client or consumer. Another way of saying it is that, in his or her professional role, the practitioner has been negligent and the client has suffered injury or damages. Professional negligence includes failure to warn and/or protect; failure to properly supervise hospitalized patients; negligent release of dangerous patients; negligent prescription of contraindicated drugs and negligence of auxiliaries; sexual relations with clients; faulty recordkeeping; inappropriate or negligent release of records; lack of informed consent; failure to satisfy the duty to inform (e.g., to notify a subsequent care provider of a patient's history of suicide attempts); assault and battery; and employer-employee relations (e.g., sexual harassment and age and gender discrimination) (Reaves & Ogloff, 1996).

Although a malpractice insurance policy provides some financial solace (few plaintiffs' judgments result in collection of damages beyond the limits of coverage), there are other devastating effects for the respondent. Much like the previously discussed spillover of negative consequences from ethics and regulatory complaints, a lawsuit, even if it does not result in a judgment for the plaintiff, can inflict long-term damage to the practitioner's health, reputation, and income.

Public awareness of a lawsuit against a practitioner tends to be viewed as proof of incompetence or wrongdoing. Inevitably, publicity of a lawsuit, again regardless of outcome, seems to result in diminished professional reputation and fewer referrals from other professional sources or past clients.

A special effect occurs when the practitioner is later called upon to provide expert testimony in a legal case, say on behalf of a client who is involved in a civil suit (e.g., personal injury, child custody, etc.). It is fundamental that the attorney who believes that the expert's testimony will not further the preferences of his or her client will attempt to impeach the credibility of the expert witness. This is done by asking questions that probe for aspects of the expert's professional credentials (or even personal life) that will potentially diminish the effectiveness of the expert's testimony. It is commonplace to ask questions about any complaints, disciplinary actions, judgments, or settlements that have been levied against the potential expert witness. Therefore, the value of the testimony from a mental health practitioner who has had a negative outcome from an ethics, regulatory, or legal complaint will be lessened. This loss of status means that the practitioner will probably not be used for expert testimony in other cases by the same or (once the negative outcome gets known around the legal community) other attorneys.

It is not unusual for a lawsuit against a mental health professional by one plaintiff to provoke another lawsuit from another plaintiff, such as another past client. This "copycat" phenomenon also seems true for ethics and regulatory complaints.

Of course, an adverse judgment (or sometimes a settlement) will result in other *sua sponte* investigations, with all of the negatives that they would portend, such as loss of license due to the malpractice action. Sometimes even a settlement of a legal action, without an admission or finding of wrongdoing, will also result in other *sua sponte* investigations. Finally, as with disciplinary actions by a licensing board, an adverse legal judgment will likely impact negatively on opportunities for hospital privileges, managed care approved-provider lists, additional certifications and licensures, and continuation of malpractice coverage (at least at the previous rate).

This contribution offers information on the defensive strategies that a respondent should employ once a complaint has been received. A series of 20 psycholegal defensive strategies guides the reader toward healthy and legally safe practice.

TWENTY PSYCHOLEGAL DEFENSIVE STRATEGIES

Strategy 1: Maintain a Healthy Mindset

A motivation for writing this contribution came from my being aware that the aftermath of an ethical, regulatory, or legal complaint often leads the professional to experience ongoing emotional distress over possibly facing another complaint, that is, litigaphobia (Brodsky, 1983). Often the respondent, battle-weary from the litigation, will settle into unhealthy behavioral and personality maladaptations, such as exaggerated defensiveness and decreased career satisfaction. Numerous examples of early retirements or termination of practice in favor of other employment have come to my attention.

The respondent should assiduously avoid succumbing to adverse emotions and maintain a staunch commitment to a healthy mindset. If the respondent allows anxiety, uncertainty, self-doubt, and stress to prevail, there will be irreparable damage to personality or self-esteem, which will likely lead to faulty professional judgments and decreased motivation. A negative mindset contributes to the risk of other complaints and financial consequences. On the other hand, a healthy mindset will preserve the essential support that is available from friends, colleagues, and family members. Without their social and emotional buttressing, the respondent will be much more vulnerable to the onslaught of accusations and prosecutorial events.

This initial defensive strategy, a starting point, is closely related to the final defensive strategy that will be offered, namely to develop a healthy personal-professional life. This continuity underscores the importance of personal fortitude throughout the defense against ethical, regulatory, and legal complaints.

Strategy 2: Accept the Adversarial Nature of the Complaint

As mentioned earlier, many mental health practitioners harbor the misimpression that complaint cases give deference to the professional and that collegiality will be present. It merits restating that such a view is wrong. If anything, the complaint process will be skewed in favor of the complainant, due to the political correctness of protecting the consumer and the disrespect directed at health care providers in this "reform" era (Starr, 1994).

The primary nature of a complaint case is that it is a legal matter. Whether it is the quasi-criminal filter applied to regulatory actions or the adversarial framework for civil lawsuits or criminal charges, the proceeding is governed by, among other sources, the rules of civil/criminal procedure and evidence for the given jurisdiction. Melton et al. (1997) issue the wise caveat: "Nowhere are the differences in training, philosophy, and objectives between lawyers and mental health professionals more clearly on display than in an adversarial proceeding" (p. 526).

Although an ethics committee is not operating in the legal arena per se, the possibility (probability?) that the outcome of an ethics committee will lead to legal considerations (e.g., an adverse outcome for an ethics committee may be referenced in a lawsuit against the practitioner) means that this nonlegal complaint within a professional association should be viewed as a quasilegal proceeding. As an aside, on one ethics committee for a national-level mental health profession upon which I served, about one-third of the members of the ethics committee held a law degree in addition to a doctorate in a mental health discipline; and one or more attorneys for the professional association were almost always present.

Strategy 3: Recognize the Adversaries

Regardless of the past nature or duration of a relationship, the minute a person, such as a client, utters a word about filing a complaint, that person should be thought of solely as a potential party opponent. The complainant has chosen to malign the practitioner and must not be given any leeway thereafter. Stated bluntly, the person has relinquished any legitimate claim to further service or responsibility from the practitioner, beyond common courtesy.

From both the ethical and legal perspectives, the clear-cut view is that once a person has become a party opponent, any and all claim to present or future professional responsibility or legal duty has been eliminated. Indeed, it is common for ethics committee policies or legal statutes or board rules to declare that, for example, filing the ethical, regulatory, or legal complaint removes the complainant's right to confidentiality vis-à-vis the respondent's defense.

Likewise, from the instant that the practitioner receives a letter or telephone call from an attorney who represents a past/present client or any other person who may be thinking about filing a complaint, the attorney should be recognized as an advocate for the legal interests of the potential complainant. In this scenario, it is common for an attorney to indicate something like, "If I can meet with you, it is possible that we can resolve the problem." It would be foolhardy to think that the attorney intends to be open to persuasion; the commitment is to learn as much as possible to use against the naïve practitioner and often to obtain a settlement (that is, a payment) for not filing the complaint. Incidentally, when a legal matter is involved, the attorney approaching the (nonattorney) mental health practitioner is obligated to encourage the practitioner to obtain legal counsel.

Because mental health professionals are not trained academically or prepared psychologically for legal confrontations, they often foolishly believe that, if there is an explanation and apology, the adversary will "forgive and forget." To the contrary, any details or expressions of regret will most likely to be transformed into what attorneys call "admissions against interest." That is, anything communicated to an adversary will be subject to manipulation into a negative: "Whatever you say, can and will be used against you."

Strategy 4: Become Defensive

When the gauntlet has been cast, the mental health professional should be on the defensive immediately. Thinking that a disgruntled past/present client can be talked out of a complaint can later be described by the client as "threatening coercion and an attempt to use undue influence to keep me from exercising my legal rights." In one case, when the owners of a clinical practice suggested a refund of all of the fees that a couple had paid in exchange for their not filing a legal action, this offer was included in later pleadings as a reflection of guilt.

Mental health professionals "should be careful to respond in an appropriate manner from the first moment they are notified" (Chauvin & Remley, 1996, p. 567); that is, they should clearly state than an attorney will handle all future communications (Stampelos & Jones, 1990). More will be said about this matter later.

To summarize, the mental health practitioner should not consider anyone connected with bringing a complaint to be a potential ally. There is no reason to believe that those persons can be cajoled, persuaded, or browbeaten by learned statements or "psychobabble." The only thing that will be of value to the mental health professional is conveying information that is compatible with a legal defense, such as demonstrating that the respondent can produce evidence that will contradict and surpass any admissible evidence that the opposition can produce.

Strategy 5: Be a Warrior

Mental health professionals are trained and conditioned to be nurturant, demonstrate altruism, communicate empathy, and convey unconditional positive regard. Facilitative conditions are fine and dandy (and perhaps even essential) for a treatment relationship. When there is a complaint, however, the relationship with adversaries is oppositional; this fact justifies (and perhaps necessitates) being defensive, assertive, and aggressive.

Part of the benefit of having an attorney is that he or she will be trained for the adversarial nature of legal proceedings. As opposed to being "sweet and lovable" like mental health professionals, attorneys are prepared for combat in the legal arena. The attorney-client relationship will help the mental health professional acquire the attitudes, thought processes, and communications that will maximize the possibility of a positive outcome for the complaint proceedings.

Strategy 6: Adopt a Long-Range Perspective

With awareness of the possibility of filing a complaint, the mental health professional should sight the adversaries and assume a defensive posture. Then it is appropriate to create a temporal framework for the situation.

Many mental health practitioners are prone to believe that a complaint spells the ruin of career and total demise of professional status. Even under the most horrendous of conditions, total career destruction is rare. Far more likely is that there will be a "price to pay" in terms of legal costs, judgments or fines, subjugation to supervision and probation, acquiring additional training, tarnished reputation, and - yes - decreased income.

Creating a temporal framework involves several steps. It is appropriate to accept that the complaint situation is bad and unfortunate, and it would have been, of course, preferable to have been spared the experience. In this litigious era, however, a significant number of complaints come from unavoidable scenarios or situations. That is, after a complaint is made, it is easy to look back and think, "I should have done things differently." Of course, it would be an admission against interest to ever admit poor judgment to other than one's own attorney (because the admission would be protected by attorney-client privilege). In representing mental health practitioners, I always remind them and the triers of fact, such as members of a licensing board, that "hindsight is always 20/20" and that "everyone has made professional judgments that were recognized later as being less that perfect."

A long-range perspective allows the mental health practitioner to accept that "to err is human," take steps to avoid the pitfall in the future, commit to a vigorous defense, and recognize that the complaint does not spell the end of one's career. Although it is said somewhat humorously, I often advise practitioners, "Sure you should take this matter seriously and make corrections, but I'll bet 10 years from now you will look back and wonder why you suffered the severe reaction that you are experiencing."

Strategy 7: Obtain Legal Counsel

Regardless of the facts of the matter, the nature of the allegations, or the seriousness of the possible consequences, only a foolish mental health practitioner would attempt to defend against a complaint without an attorney. Remember the old adage, "Being your own attorney means you have a fool for a client."

There are two reasons that lead a mental health practitioner to rely on self-defense instead of an attorney. The first is psychological, and the second is financial.

Psychologically, the mental health professional, as a therapist, is highly educated and schooled in verbal persuasion, and may incorrectly think that the same verbal skills used in therapeutic interventions will be useful in dealing with a complaint. The opposite can be true. The transparency that is the hallmark of therapeutic responses can lead to a "foot in the mouth" in a complaint situation. Those who do not obtain an attorney are often in denial of the legal consequences present.

When it comes to finances, some mental health professionals may harbor dysfunctional attitudes about expenditures relevant to their business practices. They are often annoyed that they do not command the professional fees commensurate with their training, and they strongly believe that consumers or clients should accept and give high priority to fees for valuable clinical services that help them through the dilemmas of life. Yet some mental health practitioners facing the possibility of an ethical, regulatory, or legal complaint discount the value of the services of an attorney and try to avoid the expense of legal fees.

The necessity of having an attorney knowledgeable about the particular types of law applicable to the jurisdiction of the complaint cannot be overstated. Especially in this highly litigious era, the rational and wise mental health professional will recognize from the outset of practice that certain allies will be necessary throughout his or her career, notably an attorney and an accountant. Just like Diogenes' futile search for an honest person, it would be futile to search for a graduate training program in mental health services that provides adequate knowledge and skills that will eliminate the need for an attorney and an accountant. The most logical approach is to allocate financial resources for the business aspects of the mental health practice and thus be assured of professional allies when the need arises. Certainly the need arises when an ethical, regulatory, or legal complaint is threatened or filed. More will be said about financial expenditures later.

Strategy 8: Trust and Rely on an Attorney

Attorneys often recognize that professionals, because they are highly educated, are difficult to manage and are prone to defeat themselves in the legal arena. Mental health professionals may be their own worst enemies in defending against a complaint.

The problem is simple. Being (presumably) above average in intelligence and highly educated, the professional who becomes a respondent may try to second-guess the attorney, often to the point that it is detrimental to the defense strategies. On attorney is quoted as saying:

> Heaven protect me from intelligent, sophisticated clients. While they're "helping" me win my case, they can find ways I never dreamed of to mess things up. The smarter they are the more ways they can find to botch it. (Wright, 1981, p. 1535)

For examples of how professors suffer from trying to dictate the handling of legal cases in which they were a party, see LaNoue and Lee (1987).

Given the foregoing psychological and financial characteristics, the mental health professional often finds it difficult to trust that the attorney will make wise judgments about defense strategies. Yet this wariness is not predicated on knowledge of legal procedure and evidence, which are virtually unknown to the mental health professional. A related problem emerges when the practitioner has forensic experience and mistakenly assumes that this provides adequate knowledge to make judgments about legal procedures and evidence.

Failing to trust one's attorney leads to unwise fault finding with how the defense is being handled. The mental health practitioner may talk to other professionals who have faced complaints and distort their situations (or selective memories) to justify a belief that his or her attorney is doing a poor job. Needless to say, distrust erodes the quality of the attorney-client relationship. Thus, it is not unusual for professionals of any ilk to decide to change attorneys or to create a set of conditions that leads the attorney to withdraw from the case. Disruption of legal representation is most often detrimental to the respondent.

Strategy 9: Do Not Allow Financial Considerations to Dominate Decision Making

This strategy involves far more than a reluctance to pay for the services of an attorney. Some mental health professionals are overly conservative about spending money for matters pertaining to their business practices. They may be more willing to pay for, say, an upscale office, before paying for risk management services. Although an upscale office may enhance professional image and bring in business, unattended risks can diminish or destroy the best of practices.

Typically, mental health practitioners believe that their own fees are reasonable. In fact, organizational research supports that most workers believe they are entitled to more money than they receive. Thus, it is ironic to hear a mental health professional claim that fees for professional services that would assist with risk management, such as from an attorney or accountant, are too high - especially when often the fees from these other sources are no higher, and sometimes lower, than the fee for mental health services.

This professional characteristic probably connects back to training. The "Ivory Tower" does not prepare the trainee for the realities of practice in the modern mental health marketplace, hence the tendency toward an overly conservative view about spending money for risk management services.

When dealing with a complaint, some mental health practitioners erroneously believe that their malpractice insurance will assuredly protect their best interests. From some carriers, it is possible to also purchase an option for covering the cost of legal defense against a regulatory complaint. Many practitioners do not realize, however, that the contract, particularly for malpractice insurance, allows the carrier to select the attorney. As a result, the practitioner is faced with having an attorney who is being paid by and under the monitoring of the carrier.

As litigation moves forward, the carrier, as a financial investment firm, wishes to minimize expenditures. Even if the attorney wants to litigate the matter fully, as would protect the interests of the practitioner, the carrier can issue a mandate to settle the case. If the practitioner opposes the settlement idea, the policy usually calls for financial liability to shift to the practitioner, at least to some extent.

The current trend is for settlements to be reported to a regulatory source. Consequently, the spillover effect can occur, such as the initiation of a licensing investigation, and perhaps even on to an ethics investigation. In addition to the spillover effect of complaints in other investigative arenas, news of a settlement can circulate among other professionals, referral sources, and potential clients in the community, resulting in damaged reputation and decreased income. The spillover effect will be discussed further in later strategies.

The mental health practitioner cannot assume that his or her legal interests will be fully protected by malpractice insurance. Several insurance sources have acknowledged that obtaining a settlement protects their financial interests but does not protect the reputation or other legal interests of the practitioner. This dilemma leads some practitioners to hire a personal attorney, at their own expense, to deal with the attorney who is being paid by the insurance company and with the insurance sources that are pushing for a settlement.

Having a personal attorney does involve an expense. In keeping with the long-range perspective, the cost may, however, be a small price to pay. In other words, perhaps the personal attorney will be able to ward off or at least reduce the negative consequences of a settlement.

The principle, stated bluntly, is that the insurance company is not about to place the practitioner's preferences above its financial objectives. The practitioner must be ready to aggressively pursue optimal support from the insurance carrier, while at the same time being prepared to enlist other allies, such as a personal attorney, as needed.

Strategy 10: Formulate a Factual and Defensible Explanation

Research on perception and communication makes it clear that the "eye of the beholder" leads to distortion of reality. Just as the complainant will have a subjective version of the bases for the allegations, the respondent too will be vulnerable to inaccurate perception or memory of the relevant events.

Although talking to colleagues about the situation could be helpful for clarification purposes, the practitioner should be mindful of not creating potential witnesses for the opposition. This will be discussed subsequently.

Careful study of the laws, published ethics, and position statements will assist the practitioner in best understanding the issues that underlie the complaint. Although the adversarial proceedings are alarming, the practitioner must work through the emotionality in order to obtain the clear legal and professional understanding that is necessary for a meaningful defense.

Without such a clear understanding, the mental health professional will probably not provide the best testimony and will handicap his or her attorney. There are many ways to acquire a factual and defensible explanation for what has triggered the complaint. Careful study of laws and positions statements, including ethics codes and guidelines promulgated by professional associations, can help the practitioner consider how his or her practices may or may not be appropriate. A particular shortcoming is that mental health professionals are prone to rely on the ethics or standards to which they were exposed in graduate school, which could, with the passage of years, be outdated. Therefore, the information being considered should be applicable to current standards.

Although expensive, consultation with an expert on pertinent issues may be helpful. If this is done, the practitioner, along with his or her attorney, should keep the discussion on an academic level, as opposed to exposing the facts of the complaint per se (later strategies will deal with unwise discussions about a complaint with other people).

Finally, a position statement or the opinion of an expert may not necessarily prove useful in a legal defense or mandated for all situations. Professional information and opinions must pass through a legal filter for applicability to the complaint case at hand. Therefore, the attorney should advise what aspects should be included/eliminated or emphasized/downplayed.

Strategy 11: Trust No One But Your Attorney

It is important to know that an attorney is governed by strict regulations (e.g., bar rules) and statutory law. Contrary to popular misconception (reflected in jokes about lawyers), no other profession surpasses the practice of law for strict regulation, namely from the state bar and other governmental sources.

An attorney must, among other things, unrelentingly advocate the legal interests of the client. Just as a mental health professional provides services without endorsing a client's pathology, the attorney too defends, without endorsing the allegedly wrongful conduct of the mental health practitioner who is facing a complaint. Stated differently, the attorney will be devoted to setting forth the best possible defense and achieving the most desirable outcome possible for the mental health professional who is a respondent in complaint proceedings.

This advocacy framework protects the communications between the attorney and mental health practitioner via attorney-client privilege. As any mental health practitioner knows, the principle of psychotherapist-client privileged communication has eroded considerably (Woody, 1999a). At this time in the evolution of society, there is no doubt that attorney-client privilege is the most sacrosanct of legal principles relevant to privileged communication.

With that statement, it can be asserted that no one will be more committed to the mental health practitioner's legal interest than the attorney. Also, no one will have communications from the mental health practitioner that are protected from discovery for the legal proceedings more so than the attorney. For example, a client can write material to help that attorney prepare for a trial, which would be highly damaging if the statements or documents could be obtained by the prosecution. The preparation of this kind of document is potentially protected from discovery by so-called "attorney work product" privilege.

Strategy 12: Avoid Creating Witnesses for the Other Side

Given the perplexing and emotional nature of responding to a complaint, most respondents would like to talk about the situation with others. Their motive may be quite logical, such as to resolve anxiety and gain better understanding of the situation.

Although a spouse potentially has privilege from testifying against his or her spouse in legal proceedings, the nature of the allegation could result in the spouse's deciding to testify anyway. For example, if the mental health practitioner is accused of sexual misconduct with a client, and confesses to the spouse that the allegation is true, and the spouse decides "enough is enough" and seeks a divorce, the practitioner has created a witness for the prosecution who can be highly damaging.

Innumerable complaints have involved situations comparable to the preceding marital scenario, except that the confessions were made to long-time friends, business partners, significant others, and the like. Often the other person who received the confession in confidence would like to avoid testifying against the mental health practitioner, but the legal process can require it, such as by a subpoena or court order.

The only prudent approach is to not talk about the complaint to any other person, except one's own attorney. If the stress of the situation leads the respondent to seek therapy for himself or herself, note that the psychotherapeutic relationship is not assuredly protected from legal discovery methods. The solution is simple and suggested by the headings for this and the preceding section: Trust no one but your attorney, and avoid creating witnesses for the other side.

Strategy 13: Learn to Respond Properly to Discovery Methods and During Testimony

There is ample reason to assert that mental health professionals are prone to say too much and the wrong thing in a legal proceeding (Wright, 1981). This attribution is understandable, in that mental health practitioners are trained in meticulous and extensive verbalizations for therapeutic purposes. Nonetheless, adapting verbal and written communications to be effective for the legal context is a challenge for anyone, and mental health practitioners are no exception. Considerable self-control enters into the picture. Academic knowledge of how to respond and testify in a legal proceeding is needed; this is another area that is neglected during graduate training. Fortunately, there are excellent treatises available on this subject (e.g., Brodsky, 1991; Chapter 18 of Melton et al., 1997; and Wright, 1981).

The distinctive characteristic of legal proceedings is that they are controlled by procedural rules; these do not always accommodate the story being told in the way that the mental health practitioner might prefer. As Melton et al. (1997) put it: "The clinician as scientist-practitioner is accustomed to the pursuit of truth through dispassionate examination of data; the attorneys on both sides are instead committed primarily to persuasion, and the 'truth' as the clinician sees it is but one more piece of information subject to manipulation in service of the greater goal of achieving the desired verdict" (p. 526). After emerging from a legal proceeding pertaining to a defense against a complaint, numerous mental health practitioners have commented about how information was manipulated and the procedural and evidence rules allowed or disallowed information in a manner that the practitioners thought was incorrect or unfair.

To be unable to communicate in the manner defined by the legal situation is a distinct disadvantage. When faced with a complaint, the mental health practitioner must invest time and energy to honing communication skills as necessitated by the context and situation. If this matter is left unattended, be it by the mental health professional or the attorney, the outcome will likely be less than desired.

Strategy 14: Be Modest in Professional Representations

It is a misconception to believe that "tough talk" is the best way to approach a complaint. Regrettably, there are a few attorneys who follow this misguided notion, probably because they lack refined skills as a lawyer.

Certainly one must maintain a solid defense and launch a strong offensive. However, a wise warricr chooses the battleground and avoids unnecessary risk and negative fallout. Attempting to intimidate the opposition is foolish. Emphasis should be on persuading the opposition that the evidence will support the mental health practitioner. In some instances, it is strategically wise to indicate that a countersuit may be filed, such as motion for legal fees or other sanctions.

Attempts at intimidation or one-upmanship do not represent astute legal maneuvers. To complement legal research and analysis, which provides the substance for the defense, the best approach is to practice defensive modesty in professional representations.

Among other things, care should be taken to avoid any self-aggrandizement that might be interpreted as a form of narcissism. For example, factual and modest professional credentials should be presented. Attempts to set forth minutiae or dubious qualifications (Woody, 1997b) will likely backfire, as they will be reframed as misrepresentation or a lack of bona fide professionalism. One's résumé or vitae should include only certifications that meet national standards and are endorsed by a substantial (and conservative) portion of the mental health profession; for example, any "diplomate" that did not involve an examination (beyond a "paper review") might be better omitted.

Often the respondent will blurt out, "I've been in practice for many years, and it is outrageous that I would be accused of any wrongdoing." Prosecutors and members of ethics committees have been known to chortle at this retort, considering it to be pompous or narcissistic blathering. Years of experience do not matter. What matters is what can or cannot be proven in accord with legal procedures relevant to the allegations. Another self-impeding response is for the respondent to say, "Everyone else does this sort of thing." Obviously two wrongs do not make a right.

Blaming the complainant without justifying the conduct of the mental health practitioner is potentially destructive. A respondent's remark such as, "The complainant is a psychopath" (without addressing the respondent's conduct) has led several prosecutors or opposing counsels to retort, "Tell your client that I don't care if the complainant is an ax murderer, I want to be convinced that your client did not commit malpractice."

As one final ineffective response, claiming to be innocent in the face of clear and convincing evidence of wrongdoing and issuing a plea for forgiveness or minimal penalty usually falls on deaf ears. The prosecutor or finder of fact (e.g., a judge, jury, licensing board, or ethics committee) will say, sometimes with a tone of sadness, "He (or she) just doesn't get it." This means that there is so little professional understanding or self-responsibility demonstrated by the respondent that there is little or no basis for other than bringing the legal hammer down firmly.

On the positive route, the mental health professional should set forth being competent, reasonable, prudent, honest, and dedicated to positive social values, high professional standards, and the well-being of clients. This message should be tempered with a balance of confidence but without a sociopathic or narcissistic bent. By one-downmanship, the practitioner is maximizing the potential for creditability: "The implicit goal of witnesses is to be credible and believed" (Brodsky, 1998, p. 484).

Strategy 15: Implement a Risk Management System

Comments were made earlier about exercising risk management. When a complaint is pending, it is a time to reevaluate the effectiveness of the overall risk management system. During this period, there is elevated risk of other complaints (which will be discussed later) and the last thing wanted would be having to defend on two fronts, especially because emotional and financial resources are already diminished and the opposition would benefit from having more than one complaint underway.

Risk management goes beyond simply having an attorney and accountant as professional allies. There are innumerable policies and practices that can be implemented to insulate the mental health professional from legal risks (detailed materials are available in Woody, 1988a, 1988b, 1989, 1991, 1997b). Suffice it to say, risk management is an essential part of modern mental health practice, and the approach must be carefully planned and tailored to the particular mental health practice, constantly monitored for effectiveness and weak spots, and enhanced to ward off unnecessary or avoidable risks.

Strategy 16: Define an Appropriate Standard of Care

From one point of view, waiting until there is a legal complaint to define an appropriate standard of care for one's mental health practice fits the old adage of, "closing the barn door after the horses have gotten out." However (and keeping with old adages), "better late than never."

There is no surefire list of issues or conditions to embrace in an appropriate standard of care. Likewise, there is no compendium of authoritative statements that would allow for assured decision making about what standards are applicable to a particular practitioner. Nonetheless, the best documents to consult are position statements from professional associations (including the relevant ethics code) and the laws pertaining to the jurisdiction in which the mental health services are provided.

At one time, the standard of care that was demonstrated in the locale generally could be a valid and reliable criterion for legally safe mental health practice. In the modern age, however, local practices have minimal, if any, influence on defining the standard of care. Nowadays, although there may be some legal fine points that govern expert testimony about the standard of care that consider local practices, the standard of care is commonly defined by what the reasonable and prudent practitioner in the same profession would do in a particular clinical case. Knapp and VandeCreek (1997) offer two important guidelines: "In determining appropriate standards of care, judges will assume that a deviation from a professional code of conduct constitutes a deviation from the acceptable standards of care" (p. 11); and "The standard of care is not to be thought of as the level of care of the average among all practitioners ranging from the worst to the best, but rather as the reasonable average level of care among ordinarily good practitioners" (p. 11). Nonetheless, a caveat is in order: there is legal debate about how to establish the standard of care, and some triers of fact (opinion: especially licensing boards) are prone to elevate the standard to more than "the reasonable average level of care among ordinarily good practitioners"; in other words, to what hindsight suggests as a foolproof way of dealing with the situation.

When a legal complaint is underway, the mental health professional should think through the standards that have relevance to or are appropriate for his or her competencies and clientele, and state them in writing. This document should be made available to all clients and significant others from the outset of treatment. In fact, this sort of information and more should have been made available to clients (and significant others) upon entering treatment.

If a clear-cut standard is set forth by the mental health practitioner, a would-be complainant would have the burden of proving that he or she had reason to believe that other or higher standards would apply. This is not to say that a mental health professional can state low-level standards or extract an implicit or explicit disclaimer of liability from clients. The standard of care must always be compatible with the previously mentioned test of the "reasonable and prudent" practitioner (albeit that this test is subject to legal debate, but for purposes herein, it is a useful viewpoint); and it should be appropriate to the unique set of circumstances of the practice.

Once an appropriate standard of care has been set forth by the mental health professional, it is wise to seek peer review and endorsement. These review sources should be asked to confirm or disconfirm that the standard of care decided upon by the mental health professional is consonant with published standards, ethics, and laws, and appropriate for the unique circumstances of the practice. Also, the standard of care should be continually evaluated for effectiveness and propriety and modified as necessary (note that standards can be expected to vary to some degree depending upon the clinical aspects of the particular case [i.e., for appropriateness]).

Why set forth a standard of care after the complaint is filed? Doing so will lessen the possibility of other complaints, give the practitioner some degree of solace in knowing the standards, and afford the defense attorney with critical information for justifying that the alleged wrongful conduct (cited in the complaint) was, in fact, what would have been done by a reasonable and prudent practitioner and that the complaint should be dismissed.

Incidentally, a legal principle precludes using a remedial effort as evidence of earlier negligence. Just as a landlord's repairing a stairway cannot be used as evidence of previous negligence in a lawsuit filed by a tenant who fell and was injured on the stairway (i.e., premise liability), a mental health practitioner's defining a supportive after-the-complaint standard of care cannot be used as evidence of previous failure to meet an appropriate standard of care.

Strategy 17: Buttress Your Professional Credentials

The mental health professional dealing with a complaint should make an effort to strengthen his or her professional credentials. Much like the earlier comments about remedial measures not being admissible evidence to prove a previous condition, the fact that the practitioner obtains additional professional training in an area (even directly) relevant to the alleged wrongful conduct cannot be used as evidence of earlier incompetence. To the contrary, the astute defense attorney will present these efforts to acquire additional training as proof of the practitioner's dedication to advancing competency to assure quality care for clients.

Strategy 18: Screen Clients to Eliminate Undue Risks

All potential clients should be evaluated carefully before being accepted for ongoing mental health services. The evaluation will confirm that the mental health practitioner is competent to offer quality care and maintain a treatment plan for the particular person seeking treatment. By screening for clients who test or exceed the practitioner's competence, the practitioner is able to (a) minimize the possibility of a second complaint being filed, as would likely compound the problems in defending against the first complaint; and (b) gain additional training in the particular area, as would allow for improved competence. Screening clients provides both the potential client and the practitioner with benefit, namely by the client's being assured of quality care and the professional's gaining risk management.

When a complaint has been filed, care should be taken to avoid other complaints following suit. In service to this goal, the mental health professional should, if anything, assume a rather narrow scope of service. That is, it is prudent to define competency in a cautious way and accept only clients who seem to have positive treatment potential, as determined by the practitioner's competencies. On one hand, this caution may lessen income, but on the other hand, it will minimize legal and financial risk.

A common question is: What types of clients file legal complaints? There is no definitive answer to this question. It should be recognized that, as Brock and Barnard (1999) put it: "Risk-free therapy simply does not exist; we only can minimize and manage the risk we create" (p. 199). One legal colleague often starts and ends his seminars with the cry, "Remember, don't trust *any* of your clients!"

My experience in defending mental health professionals faced with complaints suggests that clients with even a trace of narcissism are perhaps the most likely to file an ethics, regulatory, or legal complaint. That is, the nature of the pathology leads the narcissist to avoid self-responsibility for his or her lot in life, and when something goes wrong, to point a finger of blame at someone else.

Because narcissism is part of numerous diagnoses, concern is justified about the potential litigiousness of clients with hysterical, psychopathic, sociopathic, and paranoid features, among others. Also, Knapp and VandeCreek (1997) highlight the legal liability of working with clients who have multiple personality disorders and recovered memories of abuse (of course, these conditions likely have a link to narcissism and other pathologies cited earlier).

On hearing such ideas, mental health practitioners are likely to respond, "That's almost everyone in my clientele." This point cannot be disputed, and it means the practitioner should exercise caution about every client.

Of special concern, there is reason to believe that when the client has an unpaid bill and the mental health practitioner attempts to collect, even if the services and the delayed payment have been for the client's benefit, there is a tendency for clients to consider filing a complaint, especially if the aforementioned narcissistic set is present (Brock & Barnard, 1999; Woody, 1988a, 1988b, 1997b; Wright, 1981). Therefore, it is important to screen clients for ability to pay for the psychological services. Accepting a client who is likely to accrue a deficit in payment (even a co-pay portion), regardless of the reason, is ill advised.

A risk also arises from inept case management. The mental health practitioner who lets his or her own egotistical needs enter into the treatment context exacerbates the risk for a legal complaint. Knapp and VandeCreek (1997) say:

> If patients suspect that their psychotherapists did not respect them or placed other concerns above helping them, then patients can become militant about seeking redress for any perceived ethical or professional error, however trivial. Obviously, ill feelings toward psychotherapists and negative outcomes in therapy, such as failure to improve or worsening symptoms, are intertwined. (p. 7)

To counter the possibility of a disenchanted client's filing a complaint, Brock and Barnard (1999) urge defusing the anger, helping the client face the source of the adverse emotion, and communicating "empathic responding in a most Rogerian manner while simultaneously maintaining one's personal integrity" (p. 204).

Strategy 19: Guard Against a Copycat Complainant

Our society has produced many examples of "copycat" faulty behaviors. The same underlying pathological ego gratification that leads a person to commit, say, a horrible crime in the same manner that another person committed a like crime, can produce copycat complaints against mental health practitioners.

There is no database for estimating or describing this phenomenon, but attorneys working in professional liability know that it occurs. Thus, the prudent mental health practitioner should safeguard against a complaint triggering one or more other complaints.

Previous strategies have provided guidance for avoiding copycat complainants, such as not talking unnecessarily about the complaint. In general, the best approach is, as reflected in most of the strategies, to act cautiously, conservatively, and with impeccable professionalism, and minimize revealing anything about an existing complaint. For example, requests for interviews from, say, newspaper and television reporters should be politely refused, even though it might be tempting to tell your side of the story. Also, the mental health professional should be alert for any inquiries by other clients, past or present, about the complaint;

sometimes these inquires are presented as, "I want to support you," only to be turned later into, "I want to sue you."

Strategy 20: Develop a Healthy Personal-Professional Life

Certainly ethical, regulatory, and legal complaints can potentially penetrate the sense of confidence and self-esteem of any mental health professional. When a complaint is being processed, the practitioner needs, more than ever, a strong sense of self-identity and value. Otherwise, gnawing doubts will feed insecurity, professional competence will lessen, and personal health and relationships will suffer.

The self-analysis and reconstruction must, of course, be rooted in reality. The possible adverse effects of the complaint should not be denied; rather, they should be realistically appraised, considered for learning how to avoid other negative consequences in the future, and integrated into a modern view of mental health practice. The latter "modern view" means accepting that, to repeat an earlier quotation: "Risk-free therapy simply does not exist; we only can minimize and manage the risk we create" (Brock & Barnard, 1999, p. 199). In other words, reality dictates that the respondent's future mental health practice may well bring one or more additional complaints, and "forewarned is forearmed."

A concomitant of a healthy self-concept is maintaining and developing a social-emotional support system. It is common for the respondent to tend toward obsession about the complaint, which is detrimental to relations with family and friends.

When an ethical, regulatory, or legal complaint disrupts interpersonal relations, it seems probable that the professional has taken his or her career too seriously; that is, he or she has attributed too much importance to the work being the defining point for life. With or without a legal complaint, this idea is obviously unwise and unhealthy; there must be a reasonable balance between career and life in general. The protection of relationships with family and friends will yield ego strength that will be essential for effective defense against the complaint.

Finally, as devastating as the complaint may seem at the time it is underway, the mental health professional should realize that it will eventually become part of his or her career history. Rather than simply viewing the complaint as an eternal blemish, it can be reframed appropriately as a valuable learning experience.

From living though the complaint process, the mental health practitioner will gain priceless insight into the true nature of professionalism in today's litigious society. With this enriched understanding of the profession that used up so many precious moments and afforded incalculable benefits, the mental health practitioner will be able to move on though life as a better person.

CONTRIBUTOR

Robert Henley Woody, PhD, ScD, JD, is Professor of Psychology at the University of Nebraska at Omaha, and in private practice as an attorney at law in Omaha, NE. He teaches ethics and law for psychologists and family therapy. In his law practice, he defends mental health professionals in ethics, licensing, and malpractice proceedings. Dr. Woody may be contacted at Department of Psychology, University of Nebraska at Omaha, 60th and Dodge, Omaha, NE 68182; or the Woody Law Office, Post Office Box 34880, Omaha, NE 68134-0880.

RESOURCES

Association of State and Provincial Psychology Boards (ASPPB). (1996). Disciplinary data system pilot project kicks off. *ASPPB Newsletter, 17*(1), 1 & 4.

Besharov, D. J. (1985). *The Vulnerable Social Worker*. Silver Spring, MD: National Association of Social Workers.

Brock, G. W., & Barnard, C. P. (1999). *Procedures in Marriage and Family Therapy* (3rd ed.). Boston: Allyn and Bacon.

Brodsky, S. L. (1983). Litigaphobia: The professionals' disease [Review of B. Schutz, *Legal Liability in Psychotherapy*]. *Contemporary Psychology, 28,* 204-205.

Brodsky, S. L. (1991). *Testifying in Court: Guidelines and Maxims for the Expert Witness*. Washington, DC: American Psychological Association.

Brodsky, S. L. (1998). Forensic evaluations and testimony. In G. P. Koocher, J. C. Norcross, & S. S. Hill, III (Eds.), *Psychologists' Desk Reference* (pp. 483-485). New York: Oxford University Press.

Charles, S. C., Wilbert, J. R., & Kennedy, E. C. (1984). Physicians' self reports of reactions to malpractice litigation. *American Journal of Psychiatry, 141,* 563-565.

Chauvin, J. C., & Remley, T. P., Jr. (1996). Responding to allegations of unethical conduct. *Journal of Counseling & Development, 74*(6), 563-568.

Knapp, S. J., & VandeCreek, L. (1997). *Treating Patients With Memories of Abuse: Legal Risk Management*. Washington, DC: American Psychological Association.

Koocher, G. P., & Keith-Spiegel, P. (1998). Guide to dealing with licensing board and ethics complaints. In G. P. Koocher, J. C. Norcross, & S. S. Hill, III (Eds.), *Psychologists' Desk Reference* (pp. 434-436). New York: Oxford University Press.

LaNoue, G. R., & Lee, B. A. (1987). *Academics in Court: The Consequences of Faculty Discrimination Litigation*. Ann Arbor, MI: University of Michigan Press.

Maddock, J. W. (1993). Ecology, ethics, and responsibility in family therapy. *Family Relations, 42*(1), 116-123.

Melton, G. B., Petrila, J., Poythress, N. G., & Slobogin, C. (1997). *Psychological Evaluations for the Courts* (2nd ed.). New York: Guilford.

Peterson, C. (1996). Common problem areas and their causes resulting in disciplinary actions. In L. J. Bass, S. T. DeMers, J. R. P. Ogloff, C. Peterson, J. L. Pettifor, R. P. Reaves, T. Rtfalvi, N. P. Simon, C. Sinclair, & R. M. Tipton (Eds.), *Professional Conduct and Discipline in Psychology* (pp. 71-89). Washington, DC: American Psychological Association; and Montgomery, AL: Association of State and Provincial Psychology Boards.

Reaves, R. P., & Ogloff, J. R. P. (1996). Liability for professional misconduct. In L. J. Bass, S. T. DeMers, J. R. P. Ogloff, C. Peterson, J. L. Pettifor, R. P. Reaves, T. Rtfalvi, N. P. Simon, C. Sinclair, & R. M. Tipton (Eds.), *Professional Conduct and Discipline in Psychology* (pp. 117-142). Washington, DC: American Psychological Association; and Montgomery, AL: Association of State and Provincial Psychology Boards.

Sinclair, C., Simon, N. P., & Pettifor, J. L. (1996). The history of ethical codes and licensure. In L. J. Bass, S. T. DeMers, J. R. P. Ogloff, C. Peterson, J. L. Pettifor, R. P. Reaves, T. Rtfalvi, N. P. Simon, C. Sinclair, & R. M. Tipton (Eds.), *Professional Conduct and Discipline in Psychology* (pp. 1-16). Washington, DC: American Psychological Association; and Montgomery, AL: Association of State and Provincial Psychology Boards.

Stampelos, C. A., & Jones, D. P. (1990). What your client should do when the Department of Professional Regulation investigates him. *Florida Bar Journal, 64*(4), 68-70.

Starr, P. (1994). *The Logic of Health Care Reform*. New York: Whittle Books (Penguin).

Woody, R. H. (1988a). *Fifty Ways to Avoid Malpractice: A Guidebook for Mental Health Professionals*. Sarasota, FL: Professional Resource Exchange.

Woody, R. H. (1988b). *Protecting Your Mental Health Practice: How to Minimize Legal and Financial Risk*. San Francisco: Jossey-Bass.

Woody, R. H. (1989). *Business Success in Mental Health Practice: Modern Marketing, Management and Legal Strategies*. San Francisco: Jossey-Bass.

Woody, R. H. (1991). *Quality Care in Mental Health Services: Assuring the Best Clinical Services*. San Francisco: Jossey-Bass.

Woody, R. H. (1993). Regulatory equality for clients and psychotherapists. *Voices: The Art and Science of Psychotherapy, 29*(2), 87-92.

Woody, R. H. (1997a). Disenchantment with psychology: Termination or perseverance? *Voices: The Art and Science of Psychotherapy, 33*(3), 37-43.

Woody, R. H. (1997b). Dubious and bogus credentials in mental health practice. *Ethics & Behavior, 7*(4), 337-345.

Woody, R. H. (1997c). *Legally Safe Mental Health Practice: Psycholegal Questions and Answers*. Madison, CT: Psychosocial Press (International Universities Press).

Woody, R. H. (1998). Defending against legal complaints. In G. P. Koocher, J. C. Norcross, & S. S. Hill, III (Eds.), *Psychologists' Desk Reference* (pp. 437-442). New York: Oxford University Press.

Woody, R. H. (1999a). *Psychological Information: Protecting the Right of Privacy*. Madison, CT: Psychosocial Press (International Universities Press).

Woody, R. H. (1999b). Professional ethics, regulatory licensing, and malpractice complaints. In F. W. Kaslow (Ed.), *Handbook of Couple and Family Forensics* (pp. 461-474). New York: John Wiley.

Wright, R. H. (1981). What to do until the malpractice lawyer comes: A survivor's manual. *American Psychologist, 36*(12), 1535-1541.

Risk Management and Ethical Issues Regarding Termination And Abandonment

Jeffrey E. Barnett, Sherry G. MacGlashan, and Alicia J. Clarke

CASE EXAMPLES*

Case Example A

For several months, you have been providing treatment to a patient for depression. In addition to outpatient psychotherapy with you, she has been treated with antidepressant medication by a colleague, a psychiatrist. The patient cancels and reschedules several appointments and then fails to show up for two consecutive sessions. When you are only able to reach her answering machine, you leave messages to which she makes no response. Several weeks pass and you have no contact with this patient. You are quite concerned because of the difficulties she has experienced with depression, and you have concerns regarding her appropriate use of the medication.

Case Example B

A patient who has been in treatment with you for many months decides that treatment is no longer needed. Toward the end of a session with you, he informs you that he believes he has achieved all of his goals and, therefore, this will be his last session. Although it is clear that he has improved significantly since entering treatment and is no longer in distress, you feel caught off guard and are unsure how to respond.

Case Example C

You and a patient have been working together in outpatient psychotherapy for several months. Despite your best efforts, it is clear that she is not improving. You question if she is actually benefiting from the treatment you are providing. You discuss this with her, and the two of you decide to keep working toward the agreed-upon treatment goals. Additional months pass without any progress being achieved. You become concerned because she is becoming increasingly dependent on you and her condition is worsening.

Case Example D

A patient of yours regularly leaves your office without paying. When you raise the issue for discussion, he makes excuses and promises prompt payment. Despite several small payments, this pattern persists and his outstanding balance continues to grow. When you confront him, he states that he cannot afford to pay his bill. He tells you that he has lost several jobs because of his depression and states that because it has been so serious lately he has been unable to work. Although concerned about him clinically, you are unsure if you should provide any further treatment because of his stated inability to pay for it.

*All case examples are fictitious and do not represent actual patients known to the authors.

Case Example E

Your patient with a significant anxiety disorder is beginning to achieve some benefits after eight sessions of outpatient treatment. In keeping with her insurer's requirements, you complete and submit the required treatment plan and request for further authorization. You are quite hopeful due to the progress made thus far and her clear motivation and commitment to treatment. You are alarmed to learn that the utilization review personnel have denied authorization for any further treatment, stating that it is not found to be medically necessary. You are left feeling frustrated, upset, and unsure of what to do.

Case Example F

After many years of clinical practice, you find yourself becoming increasingly distressed by changes in the mental health field. After experiencing mounting frustrations and symptoms of burnout, you decide to close your practice and retire. Having made this difficult decision, you feel relieved and decide to move forward with your plans immediately. You give your patients 2 weeks' notice and begin moving forward with your life.

INTRODUCTION

As illustrated by the preceding case examples, termination of the psychotherapy relationship has the potential to occur in a variety of ways. It may be initiated by either patient or psychotherapist, by mutual agreement, or in response to external forces or pressures. It may be planned and well thought out or it may come as a surprise. It may leave the patient hurt and abandoned, or may be a solidifying process that facilitates integration of gains made in treatment while serving as the culmination of a successful course of treatment.

Seen in this way, it is evident that how psychotherapists address and conduct the termination process can have far-reaching effects on those they serve. Thus, termination is an important component for the psychotherapy process. Many authors have consistently emphasized its importance for clients and psychotherapists alike for clinical (e.g., Basch, 1980; Goodyear, 1981; Wolberg, 1977), ethical (e.g., Gutheil & Appelbaum, 1982; Simon 1987; Stromberg et al., 1988), and legal (e.g., Ewing, 1990; Macbeth et al., 1994; B. A. Weiner & Wettstein, 1993) reasons.

CLINICAL ISSUES

The appropriate handling of psychotherapy patients' termination was addressed early by Freud (as cited in Chang, 1977), who stated:

> An analysis is ended when analyst and patient cease to meet for the analytic session. . . . There are two criteria . . . that the client is no longer suffering from his former symptoms and that the analyst is satisfied that no repetition of the patient's specific pathology . . . is to be feared. (p. 18)

These words imply the need for a systematic and orderly manner of appropriately addressing each patient's treatment needs when ending the psychotherapy relationship. They also suggest that termination is an important part of the psychotherapy process, not an afterthought or surprise. I. B. Weiner (1975) conceptualized termination as one of three phases of each client's psychotherapy: the initial assessment phase, the middle phase of ongoing psychotherapy, and the final phase of psychotherapy - termination. He states that this final phase of psychotherapy "is exceeded only by the initial phase in its importance for determining the amount of help a patient receives" (p. 263). Most importantly, termination should be considered a mandatory and vital component of the psychotherapy process and, thus, should be given the appropriate level of attention by psychotherapists.

Unfortunately, this final phase of treatment has historically been relatively neglected in training programs and in the professional literature (Bostic, Shadid, & Blotcky, 1996; Brady et al., 1996; Maholick & Turner, 1979; Penn, 1990). It is fortunate that it has received growing attention in recent years, as the manner that psychotherapy is terminated can determine whether or not self-learning during the middle phase of treatment will continue as a life-enriching resource or fade into a nonmeaningful experience (I. B. Weiner, 1975). To effectively bring psychotherapy to a close, the clinician needs to be able to judge when termination is appropriate and how it should best be approached and implemented.

[illegible] the initial phase of psychotherapy is critical in building rapport, a carefully planned and implemented termination is also critical in securing trust in the comprehensive treatment process while minimizing premature, inappropriate termination, symptom return, and/or feelings of exploitation (Barnett & Sanzone, 1997). Termination should be addressed from the outset of the psychotherapy relationship (Kramer, 1986; Quintana & Holahan, 1992; Strupp & Binder, 1984) and, when relevant, should be included in the informed consent process that is so important for establishing the agreed-upon parameters of the treatment process. When treatment is time limited or when interruptions to the treatment process may be anticipated, addressing these issues from the outset will help to ensure that each patient's treatment needs are adequately met.

In conceptualizing termination as a discrete phase of each patient's treatment, it should be pointed out that appropriate termination of psychotherapy involves several important issues and activities. This phase can be viewed as having three distinct purposes: assessment, resolution, and generalization. First, the psychotherapist should conduct an assessment of any ongoing treatment needs and the patient's readiness for terminating treatment. Secondly, time must be spent working through and hopefully resolving the remaining affective issues and bringing closure to the relationship. Finally, maximizing the generalization of learning and increasing the patient's self-reliance and confidence are necessary.

Working through termination themes, guided by the needs of each patient, brings about an effective termination process. Some of these major themes include closure, sadness, increased self-efficacy and personal power, ending, growing up, autonomy, individuation, summarizing, consolidating, and saying good-bye (Ward, 1984). At times, patients may experience the perceived end of treatment as a significant loss. Because loss is believed to be inherent in termination, a state of crisis may be expected for some patients. Patients may be expected to react to termination with affective, cognitive, interpersonal, and defense reactions similar to grief reactions (Ward, 1982). Yet, when this phase of treatment is appropriately addressed, termination may be seen as a phase of growth and development (Maholick & Turner, 1979; Quintana, 1993; Ward, 1984). It provides the clinician and patient the opportunity to transform the relationship to incorporate the patient's growth, reflect on the patient's involvement and activities in treatment, and show how the patient has learned and contributed. Thus, it may be seen as an opportunity for growth, solidifying the gains made in treatment and helping the patient to move forward independently.

TERMINATION AND BRIEF PSYCHOTHERAPY

In the present age of brief psychotherapy and the influence of managed care, many clinicians do not provide the more long-term treatments described previously. Empirical findings validate the use of specific time-limited treatment protocols for patients with a variety of presenting problems (see Sanderson & Woody, 1995, for a comprehensive review of empirically validated treatments).

Very often, after an initial assessment of a patient's treatment needs has been completed, a specific course of treatment, which has a clear ending date, can be agreed upon. This approach, when applicable, provides the patient with a very clear expectation of when treatment will end. With such time-limited treatment approaches, the termination phase of psychotherapy is, of necessity, much briefer as well. Typically, this more short-term relationship does not bring with it the previously described issues to be worked through and resolved. Additionally, when patients are aware of the predetermined termination date, they may be preparing themselves for termination throughout the course of treatment. As Shectman (1986) points out, having a predetermined length of treatment set from the outset provides a certain structure which may make separation much less traumatic. Clearly, patient expectations in briefer psychotherapies are different from those in long-term and more open-ended treatments.

Research concerning the termination of short-term psychodynamic psychotherapy has found that many successful psychotherapists tend to spend very short periods of time discussing termination with their patients (Budman & Gurman, 1996). Additionally, Marx and Gelso (1987) reported that the majority of the brief psychodynamic psychotherapy patients they studied tended to report generally positive reactions to the ending of their psychotherapy relationships. Budman and Gurman (1996) further emphasize the importance of assessing each brief psychotherapy patient's termination needs. For some patients, this phase of treatment will accentuate insecurities and separation and loss issues; for others, these issues are not relevant and a significant focus on and exploration of such issues is unwarranted.

These issues are especially relevant when taking the view of psychotherapy as being an intermittent lifelong endeavor. Kaslow (1992) describes a model in which psychotherapy is returned to at different difficult times in a person's life. Patients view psychotherapy as a resource to return to when life-cycle issues and stressors arise. When viewed in such a way, brief treatment is provided and then returned to at later dates when needed. Thus, the finality of termination assumed in more traditional psychotherapies typically does not exist for either the patient or psychotherapist. In fact, numerous studies (e.g., Grunebaum, 1983; Hartlaub, Martin, & Rhine, 1986; Kovacs et al., 1981) have found that a majority of psychotherapy patients who successfully complete treatment return later for additional psychotherapy.

Authors such as Pinkerton and Rockwell (1990) recommend that brief psychotherapists take a flexible approach to termination. As previously stated, and articulated further by Wolberg (1980), psychotherapists must assess each patient's termination needs and respond based upon the patient's psychodynamics, the nature of presenting problem(s) and the course of treatment, and the quality of the therapy relationship. For some, termination may trigger significant reactions; for others, it creates no significant problems. Pinkerton and Rockwell (1990) describe this later group as including

> (1) patients adequately prepared for ending,
> (2) those characterologically not too dependent,
> (3) people seen for a limited number of sessions and concluding before a strong relationship has been developed, and finally,
> (4) patients sufficiently detached emotionally that they avoid a close encounter with the therapist. (p. 364)

VOLUNTARY TERMINATION

Voluntary termination occurs when the patient and psychotherapist mutually agree that it is appropriate for the treatment relationship to end. The initial suggestion for termination may come from either the patient or the psychotherapist.

As illustrated in Case Example B provided previously, a client may propose termination. The psychotherapist's first response to this expression is to consider whether it reflects an accurate assessment of progress instead of resistance to further work in treatment. If the desire for termination is found to be reflective of significant progress made toward treatment goals, then, in keeping with the initial treatment contract, it is appropriate to move forward through this final phase of treatment. If found to be a reflection of resistance, the psychotherapist can identify that there is unfinished business to address without pressuring or seducing the patient to stay. The psychotherapist should present the information realistically, stating that there may be more to accomplish in terms of meeting the treatment goals with the patient, hopefully agreeing to continue working to achieve them. However, it should be kept in mind that the patient's stated desire for termination may actually reflect an indication of a readiness for treatment to end.

Termination may also be proposed by the clinician. Some patients may ignore evidence of their progress or avoid calling attention to it. Others may not be improving in treatment. This may be due to resistance to change, some secondary gain being derived from being in psychotherapy, characterologic issues, or psychotherapist inadequacies. As highlighted by Case Example C, the psychotherapist must determine if continued treatment is in the client's best interest. If not, the psychotherapist is obligated to discuss the discontinuation of treatment in a thoughtful and sensitive manner. Additionally, as treatment goals still remain, the clinician should follow through on the issue of referral to an appropriately trained clinician. It is hoped that termination can be discussed with patients in a supportive manner, avoiding any criticism or comments that may be perceived as signs of failure or rejection. Hopefully, the clinician's focus is always on the patient's needs and best interests. Thus, the clinician should be cautious in his or her timing and be alert to countertransference feelings that may be affecting the decision to discuss termination.

The issue of the timing of termination is an important one. It will hopefully be based on the achievement of specific objective criteria such as reaching predetermined treatment goals. The termination phase of treatment may also be initiated when the patient's coping abilities have improved, maladaptive or dysfunctional behaviors have been reduced, and the ability to apply treatment gains to life situations has been learned. At times, termination may be initiated because of patient noncompliance with treatment requirements or because the patient may be so dysfunctional or disordered that referral to another provider or hospitalization may be appropriate. Additionally, if treatment does not prove to be beneficial, if the patient has progressed as far as possible, or if increases in dysfunctional behavior are seen, the clinician is called upon to address the appropriateness of initiating termination (Maholick & Turner, 1979). As illustrated in Case Example C, a clinician may need to initiate termination when it is clear that a patient is not benefiting from treatment. Continued treatment under such circumstances may not be in the patient's best interest. Other examples of clinician-initiated termination include a patient being threatening to the clinician or, in group therapy, a patient acting in ways that are consistently destructive to the group.

It is important to note that if the opportunity for considering or initiating termination is ignored, the psychotherapist runs the risk of harming the patient. One possibility is that by ignoring termination indicators the psychotherapist may be encouraging the patient to use the treatment as a "substitute for real living" and blocking the chance for the patient to engage in realistic, effective life experience (Maholick & Turner, 1979, p. 586). In other words, permitting maladaptive behavior to continue is inconsistent with the intent, and an inappropriate use, of psychotherapy. An inappropriate extension of treatment may falsely imply that the clinician condones or supports the patient's behavior, running the risk of reinforcing or encouraging it. If the psychotherapist cannot act in the best interests of each patient with honesty and appropriate support by modeling real-life consequences and limit setting, the therapist may actually be harming the patient in the long run.

An additional example to consider is when the patient has not made an actual commitment to treatment. Once again, even if the patient does not see a need to end treatment, the psychotherapist may recognize the presence of criteria that imply the need to consider termination. Maholick and Turner (1979) further proposed that "perhaps a successful good-bye would be the most therapeutic thing for a person at that particular nodal point in his living" (p. 587). The next step then becomes the appropriate implementation of termination.

IMPLEMENTING TERMINATION

In working toward closure, the psychotherapist and patient should be cognizant of and avoid pitfalls, allowing enough time for reacting, anticipating, reminiscing, and planning (Penn, 1990). Patient and therapist should have an open discussion of termination issues. As Bennett et al. (1990) recommend, the following points should be discussed and agreed upon:

1. How many sessions should remain.
2. The goals for those sessions.
3. The nature of the formal follow-up that might be required.
4. Plans for any techniques the client might use to enhance the continued benefits of the therapy.
5. Whether you (the therapist) will be available for consultation. (p. 57)

From the previous discussion, it can be seen that it would not be appropriate to discontinue psychotherapy during the session when termination first comes up for discussion, as was addressed in Case Example B. Clinicians will be well served by adhering to this guideline no matter how appropriate the termination might seem to be. I. B. Weiner (1975) listed the following reasons for this guideline:

1. The patient or the therapist may be mistaken in their initial impression of the patient's readiness to terminate.
2. Transference and countertransference attitudes are both capable of influencing this kind of decision.
3. Unless the patient has already passed an extended period of sustained improvement, special care must be taken to assure that his apparent improvement of the moment will not succumb to the next life problem he faces.
4. The pain of such separations tends to be eased by opportunities to prepare for them. . . . Valuable opportunities for a closing burst of activity in the therapy will be lost if it is ended abruptly. (pp. 280-281)

Two types of termination are available for the psychotherapist and patient to consider. Time-limited termination involves a fixed duration of time during which treatment sessions continue at their usual frequency and then stop completely. Spaced termination occurs when the time between treatment sessions is gradually extended so that the date of the final session is not set in advance but is approached in measured steps (I. B. Weiner, 1975). Choosing between the two depends upon the nature and goals of the treatment contract. However, as I. B. Weiner (1975) further points out, "Generally speaking, time-limited termination works most effectively in uncovering psychotherapy, whereas spaced termination becomes increasingly appropriate the more supportive the treatment has been" (p. 284).

Additionally, the psychotherapist should work to assist the patient to build on gains made in treatment through a continued process of self-observation (Quintana, 1993). The clinician should reinforce patient self-observational abilities when the client acts as his or her own therapist. The psychotherapist may also help the patient resolve transference feelings by promoting the real relationship between them. This may be accomplished by engaging in increasing amounts of appropriate self-disclosure as the termination nears.

PREMATURE OR FORCED TERMINATION

At times termination must occur before the agreed-upon treatment goals have been achieved. This may occur because external circumstances force the termination of treatment. I. B. Weiner (1975) described the following possibilities: The client or psychotherapist moves out of town; the psychotherapist becomes ill, disabled, or retires; the client can no longer afford treatment or has no more insurance coverage; or psychotherapist rotation or termination of position occurs.

As discussed by Greenspan and Kulish (1985), premature termination can be assumed to be a function of any combination of psychotherapist, patient, and interactional variables within the therapeutic relationship. Patient attributes that can lead to a higher dropout rate include lower socioeconomic class, low motivation, the perception of problems as internal to oneself and not as situational, lack of perseverance, poor social integration, less suggestibility, impulsivity, and the presence of antisocial and authoritarian attitudes. As cited by Greenspan and

Kulish (1985), Brandt and Pope (1965) report that psychotherapist variables found to be commonly associated with premature patient termination are interviewer anger, incompetence, inexperience, male gender, and the therapist's dislike for his or her client.

If events occur that necessitate a forced termination, this does not mean that there are no benefits of treatment and that the termination process should be abrupt, angry, or ignored. A closing phase of psychotherapy should still occur so that patient autonomy and independence may be promoted, gains made in treatment reinforced, reactions to termination processed and worked through, and posttermination recommendations made and implemented.

How much time should be taken to address these issues in the termination phase and when the patient should be informed of a forced termination are not entirely clear. However, in one study of the views of psychologists and psychiatrists (Chang, 1977), 42% of the respondents stated that they would inform their patients 2 weeks before the date of forced termination, 19% 3 weeks before, and 12% 4 weeks before. Interestingly, these clinicians reportedly could not give concrete reasons for their estimates; instead, their responses were intuitive guesses, because they had not received much training on this issue.

Penn (1990) recommended an individualized approach based upon each patient's personality and treatment needs. Six weeks' advance notice is recommended for patients who have been in psychotherapy for over 6 months, but this is a flexible guideline dependent on the patient's presenting difficulties, personality factors, abandonment or loss history, and the length and type of treatment being provided. The dynamic nature of this process is further illustrated by Penn (1990), who stated: "If the topic is broached too early, it may cut off the work in progress; if it is broached too late, there will not be time to work through the feelings and consolidate the gains made" (p. 382). Finally, Brady et al. (1996) suggest that psychotherapists be alert to a variety of both patient and therapist factors that may impact how patients respond to the end of treatment. Therapist attention to their own needs, experiences, attitudes, and feelings is important to promote successful termination.

ETHICAL AND LEGAL GUIDELINES

Ethical standards that address these issues and provide guidance for mental health professionals include the National Association of Social Workers (NASW) Code of Ethics (NASW, 1996), which states:

> Social workers should take reasonable steps to avoid abandoning clients who are still in need of services. Social workers should withdraw services precipitously only under unusual circumstances, giving careful consideration to all factors in the situation and taking care to minimize possible adverse effects. Social workers should assist in making appropriate arrangements for continuation of services when necessary. (p.15)

As was illustrated in Case Examples D, E, and F, the clinician has an obligation to ensure that all treatment needs are appropriately addressed regardless of the reason for a termination. These obligations are mandatory, regardless of whether termination is initiated by the patient or therapist, or in response to some external factors. Once a formal treatment relationship has begun, the clinician maintains responsibility for the patient's welfare, either until treatment is successfully completed, the clinician is discharged of his or her duty by the patient, or other treatment arrangements are made that appropriately address the patient's treatment needs. Stated succinctly in the Ethical Principles of Psychologists and Code of Conduct (American Psychological Association, 1992) is the clear guidance that "Psychologists do not abandon patients or clients" (p. 1606). Similar guidance is provided in the ethics codes of marriage and family therapists, counselors, and psychiatrists (American Association for Marriage and Family Therapy, 1991; American Counseling Association, 1995; American Psychiatric Association, 1993). It is important to note that even if a patient drops out of treatment as was illustrated in Case Example A, the clinician's responsibility for, and obligation to, the patient has not necessarily ended. As stated by Ewing (1990), "Although patients have an absolute right to terminate treatment unilaterally, their exercising this right does not necessarily relieve the psychotherapist of his or her duty or care" (p. 722). The landmark legal ruling in *Collins v. Meeker* (1967) illustrates these points well:

> It is the settled rule that one who engages a physician . . . to treat his case implicitly engages him to attend throughout the illness or until his services are dispensed with. In other words, once initiated, the relationship of physician and patient continues until it is ended by the consent of the parties, revoked by the dismissal of the physician, and until his services are no longer needed. A physician has a right to withdraw from the case, but if he discontinues his services before the need for them is at an end, he is bound first to give notice to the patient and afford the latter ample opportunity to secure other medical attendance of his own choice. If a physician abandons a case without giving his patient such notice and opportunity to procure the services of another physician, his conduct may subject him to the consequences and liability resulting from abandonment of the case. (p. 493)

Thus, in Case Example A, when the patient discontinues treatment and will not come back to discuss termination, the clinician maintains an obligation to ensure that this patient's treatment needs are adequately addressed, an obligation that has been repeatedly emphasized in court rulings (e.g., *Brandt v. Grubin,* 1974; *Miller v. Greater Southeast Community Hospital,* 1986). Ewing (1990) recommended that clinicians "make a good faith effort to contact the patient, determine the patient's reasons for terminating, and take appropriate therapeutic steps to deal with the termination" (p. 723). At a minimum, authors (e.g., Macbeth et al., 1994) generally recommend the use of a letter to the patient that communicates the psychotherapist's concerns about the patient, any recommendations deemed appropriate to include the scheduling of termination sessions, and the offer to be of assistance in arranging for referrals to other health care providers if needed. Sample letters are provided on pages 242 to 243 which may be used as models by clinicians who have had a patient drop out of treatment (Case Example A), when a patient is initiating termination (Case Example B), when treatment must be terminated because of lack of benefit to the patient (Case Example C), or when treatment must be terminated because of other factors (Case Examples D, E, and F). It should be emphasized, however, that these sample letters are general models and will need to be modified based on each patient's particular circumstances.

One special termination circumstance of importance to consider is that of the patient who is not benefiting from treatment and may possibly be harmed by its continuation. This was illustrated in Case Example C. In keeping with the ethical tenets of beneficence and nonmalfeasance (Thompson, 1990), continuing treatment under these circumstances would be unethical and not in keeping with the commitment to each patient's welfare. The Code of Ethics of Marriage and Family Therapists (American Association for Marriage and Family Therapy, 1991) states, "marriage and family therapists continue therapeutic relationships only so long as it is reasonably clear that clients are benefiting from the relationship" (p. 2). Similar guidance is provided in the other mental health professions' ethics codes and is codified into law (Annotated Code of Maryland, 1992) as illustrated for psychologists:

> Psychologists shall: (1) make or recommend referral to other professional, technical, or administrative resources when the referral is clearly in the best interest of the client; (2) Terminate the professional relationship in an appropriate manner, notify the client in writing of this termination, and assist the client in obtaining services from another professional: (a) When it is reasonably clear the client is not benefiting from the relationship. (pp. 2-3)

An additional special termination circumstance is the need to terminate treatment because of financial reasons, as illustrated in Case Example D. The NASW Code of Ethics (NASW, 1996) provides clear guidance, stating:

> Social workers in fee-for-service settings may terminate services to clients who are not paying an overdue balance if the financial contractual arrangements have been made clear to the client, if the client does not pose an imminent danger to self or others, and if the clinical and other consequences of the current nonpayment have been addressed with the client. (p. 15)

Although it is clear that psychotherapists need not provide treatment indefinitely to patients who cannot or do not pay their bills, certain ethical obligations exist. Advance financial and billing arrangements should be made from the outset of the professional relationship; the psychologists' ethics code (American Psychological Association, 1992) recommends: "If limitations to services can be anticipated because of limitations in financing, this is discussed with the patient, client, or other appropriate recipient of services as early as is feasible" (pp. 1602-1603). Again, even if the patient can no longer pay for services, one must not abandon him or her. Gutheil and Appelbaum (1982) cite relevant case law stating, "Courts are likely to look less favorably upon therapists who have stopped seeing patients for failure to pay their bills than those who have been terminated for any other cause" (p. 155). Thus, the patient's treatment needs should be addressed and alternative arrangements made if clinically indicated. If treatment is to be terminated, at least a few sessions should be offered to assist the patient in working through termination issues. When financial hardship exists, this can be done at a reduced rate by using a payment plan, or pro bono. Simultaneously, arrangements can be made for the referral of the patient to an appropriate treatment professional who can meet both the patient's clinical and financial needs. The use of community clinics, professionals who utilize a sliding fee scale, and pro bono resources may all be helpful.

Although clinicians cannot force patients to follow through with referrals, steps may be taken to help facilitate the transfer to another psychotherapist and to follow-up to encourage the patient's compliance. Again, follow-up letters such as those provided on pages 242 to 243 may effectively serve such a purpose by communicating the clinician's recommendations and concerns clearly in a manner that leaves a tangible record of the clinician's attempts to meet a reasonable standard of care. This final point is important both clinically and as a risk management strategy should questions arise later about how the clinician handled the termination process.

Case Example A illustrates a situation in which treatment is to be terminated because of patient noncompliance. Some courts have ruled that noncooperation in treatment, threats against a psychotherapist, and other conditions can justify clinician-initiated termination (see *Eyrich v. Dam,* 1989; *Herold v. State,* 1982). Although it may be appropriate to officially terminate such a patient's treatment, it must be done according to the legal and ethical guidelines discussed previously. The patient should be contacted in writing and informed of the termination, the reasons it is occurring, and what alternatives exist for the patient's treatment. If the clinician deems that ongoing treatment is needed, this must be stated clearly, and specific recommendations for continued treatment should be made. The clinician should also suggest possible referral sources and offer to assist in the referral process. It is crucial that the clinician not tacitly condone a patient dropping out of treatment if in his or her professional judgment treatment services are still needed.

When the clinician must initiate termination because of personal reasons as illustrated in Case Example F, procedures used should be sensitive to patient needs as illustrated in psychology's ethics code (American Psychological Association, 1992), which states: "Psychologists make reasonable efforts to plan for facilitating care in the event that psychological services are interrupted by factors such as the psychologist's illness, death, unavailability, or relocation" (p. 1606). Similarly, social workers' ethics code (NASW, 1996) states: "Social workers who anticipate termination or interruption of services of clients should notify clients promptly and seek the transfer, referral, or continuation of services in relation to the client's needs and preferences" (p. 15). It can be seen that all possible steps should be taken to avoid abandoning patients and to ensure that their treatment needs are adequately addressed. Also implied in these two guidelines is the need to ensure appropriate coverage for patients during periods of therapist absence, whether anticipated or not. Stromberg et al. (1988) emphasized this point, stating: "Claims of abandonment sometimes arise when therapists fail to provide adequate coverage during nights, weekends, or other absences" (p. 495). As Barnett and Sanzone (1997) further pointed out: "Since patients at times experience crises and emergencies between sessions, it is important to ensure accessibility to them and to make appropriate arrangements for coverage by another qualified health care provider during episodes of absence or inaccessibility" (p. 11). But care must be taken to select a colleague who is appropriately trained and qualified to meet the patient's treatment needs. Utilizing lesser trained personnel such as supervisees or students is clearly not appropriate and leaves the clinician open for charges of negligence (Gutheil & Appelbaum, 1982). These points are emphasized as well in legal rulings such as *Johnson v. Ward* (1986).

A final termination dilemma of importance concerns the role of managed care and other third-party payors, as illustrated in Case Example E. Clinicians may be tempted to unilaterally terminate treatment because of an adverse utilization review decision. Yet the clinician maintains an ongoing responsibility for the patient's welfare, even in such situations. The landmark legal decision in *Wickline v. State of California* (1986) provides guidance for the clinician in such situations:

> Patient who requires treatment and is harmed when care which should have been provided is not provided should recover for injuries suffered from all those responsible for deprivation of care, including when appropriate, health care payors.
>
> Third party payors of health care services can be held legally accountable when medically inappropriate decisions result from defects in the design or implementation of cost containment mechanisms, such as when appeals made on behalf of a patient for medical or hospital care are arbitrarily ignored or unreasonably disregarded or overridden.
>
> Physician who complies without protest with limitations on treatment imposed by a third-party payor when physician's medical judgement dictates otherwise cannot avoid his ultimate responsibility for his patient's care. (p. 810)

The guidance provided by this and other cases (e.g., *Wilson v. Blue Cross of Southern California,* 1990) addresses the clinician's ongoing responsibility for the patient's welfare, regardless of third-party payor decisions. Terminating treatment because of an adverse utilization review decision would be inappropriate. At a minimum, the clinician must formally appeal this decision in an effort to obtain continued authorization. But clinicians must bear in mind that third-party payors may deny authorization only for payment for treatment. They cannot deny authorization for providing treatment. Only the clinician can make this decision. This highlights the distinction between insurers' possibly being fiscally motivated in their utilization review decisions and clinicians' ethical and legal responsibility to make clinically motivated treatment decisions. Thus, should an appeal be denied and the patient be unable to afford treatment that the clinician's judgment deems necessary, steps should be taken to make alternative financial and/or treatment arrangements as needed. The clinician maintains responsibility for the patient's welfare and should make sure that the patient is not abandoned.

CONCLUSIONS

Termination is an integral component of the psychotherapy process and can contribute greatly to the patient's overall success in treatment when handled appropriately. It should be anticipated and planned for as well as discussed actively with the patient over time. Circumstances do arise when treatment must end for reasons other than the patient's treatment goals being successfully achieved. During these situations it is important to take appropriate care to ensure that any remaining treatment needs are adequately met. A failure to do so may result in harm to the patient and possibly lead to claims of abandonment and malpractice suits. Taking adequate time to work through patient reactions and remaining treatment needs, making referrals to suitable treatment resources if clinically indicated, and assisting in the transition to another health care provider are all important steps to take. Adhering to the underlying ethical tenets of beneficence and nonmalfeasance, along with compliance with the general ethical principle of striving to ensure the welfare of those we serve, will all assist in the decision-making process that leads us to handle each patient's termination in an ethical and appropriate manner.

Barnett (1998) makes the following specific recommendations for clinicians:

1. Clarify expectations and obligations from the outset. The use of a written contract which is discussed and agreed to as treatment begins is helpful.
2. Review with patients their insurance coverage, limits to managed care contracts, and how utilization review may impact on treatment. Set up arrangements for addressing patient treatment needs if continued authorization is denied.
3. Make adequate arrangements for coverage during any periods of planned or reasonably anticipated absences.
4. Provide patients with other treatment resources if needed and work to assist them in their transition to other health care providers.
5. Do not terminate the treatment of patients who are in crisis regardless of payment issues. Provide needed treatment or help them find it elsewhere.
6. Do not tacitly condone patients dropping out of treatment when your clinical judgment indicates continued care is needed. Notify patients of your assessment and recommendations.
7. Carefully document all discussions of termination issues, agreements reached, decisions made and their rationale, and patient follow through with recommendations.
8. Termination is a phase of each patient's treatment. Plan for it, prepare for it, process it.

Sample Letters From Clinician to Patient For Use in the Termination Process

SAMPLE LETTER A: A patient in need of ongoing care drops out of treatment.

Date

Name
Address

Dear ____________________:

I was sorry to learn that you canceled our most recent scheduled appointments. I have been unable to reach you by telephone and am quite concerned about you. As you know, it is very important that your use of medication be actively monitored by a physician. Dr. _________ informs me that the two of you have not met recently either.

Although you have received some benefit from treatment thus far, it is clear that additional treatment will be needed for you to be able to reach the treatment goals we discussed. If for some reason you decide not to continue your needed treatment with me and Dr. ________, I am hoping you will consider following up elsewhere. Should you need a referral to another health care provider please contact my office and I will be pleased to help you. At a minimum, please keep in mind that the community hotline number is _______. It may be contacted in times of crisis or emergency or you can go to your local hospital's emergency room.

Again, I am hoping you will follow through with your needed treatment. Please let me know if I can be of further assistance.

Sincerely,

____

SAMPLE LETTER B: A patient making progress initiates termination.

Date

Name
Address

Dear ____________________:

As we discussed at your most recent session, it is my understanding that you have decided to discontinue our work together. As we reviewed during that session, you have made significant progress toward your stated treatment goals. Although not all goals have been fully achieved, I respect your desire to continue this important work on your own. However, I believe it is in your best interest for us to have at least one final meeting to discuss your plans and to review treatment to date. Experience has shown me that individuals who discuss their plans prior to ending treatment tend to be more successful in their posttreatment endeavors. I am hoping that you will contact my office so that these final appointments may be scheduled.

Should you decide not to follow through on this recommendation, I am hoping you will feel free to contact me if any additional difficulties are experienced or if I can be of any additional help in the future. I am also hoping you will give serious consideration to the use of the community support groups on the list of resources I provided you with.

Best wishes for success in your ongoing endeavors.

Sincerely,

____

SAMPLE LETTER C: Treatment being terminated due to lack of benefit to the patient.

Date

Name
Address

Dear ____________________:

As we discussed the last several times we met, it is clear to me that our ongoing work together has not been beneficial to you. Although I understand your desire for your treatment under my care to continue, I strongly believe it to be in your best interest for us to end our work together.

As we reviewed when we met, I am providing you with the names, addresses, and telephone numbers of the following four psychotherapists (____________). Each of these professionals is licensed, has training and experience in _________, and are located in your local area. I am hoping you will contact them and make arrangements to begin treatment. If any difficulties are experienced I will be happy to assist in this transition.

Again, as we agreed I will meet with you up to four more times to assist you during this time of transition. Once arrangements are made with a new psychotherapist, with your written consent, I will be happy to share any information I can to assist in the transfer of your care. Please discuss these or any other issues that concern you during our upcoming meetings.

Sincerely,

____

SAMPLE LETTER D: Therapist initiated termination because of an adverse utilization review decision.

Date

Name
Address

Dear ____________________:

As we discussed during your most recent appointment, your managed care company, ABC, Inc., has rejected the treatment plan we submitted stating that your treatment needs are not found to be medically necessary according to their utilization review criteria. As I explained when we met, this means that ABC, Inc. will not reimburse any additional treatment expenses at this time. This does not mean, however, that additional treatment is not needed or that you would not benefit from it.

To review, this is the plan of action we agreed on: I will file a written appeal of the utilization review decision immediately. While we await the outcome of the appeal process, we will continue your treatment with you paying me the reduced ABC, Inc. rate. If authorization is granted, treatment will continue and any fees due you will be reimbursed. If the appeal is denied, I will provide you with up to four additional sessions at one-half my usual rate and assist you to obtain more economically priced services elsewhere. Or, if desired, we can work out a payment plan so you may continue treatment under my care.

Please rest assured that I am committed to ensuring that your ongoing treatment needs are met regardless of utilization review decisions made by ABC, Inc. I look forward to continuing our work together at our next appointment on ____________.

Sincerely,

____

CONTRIBUTORS

Jeffrey E. Barnett, PsyD, is a licensed psychologist in private practice in Maryland. He is also an Adjunct Associate Professor in the Department of Psychology at Loyola College in Baltimore, Maryland, where he trains masters and doctoral students in clinical and counseling psychology. Dr. Barnett is a frequent lecturer and author on legal and ethical issues in mental health. He is a past ethics committee chair for the Maryland Psychological Association and a past president of that organization. Dr. Barnett may be contacted at 1511 Ritchie Highway, Suite 201, Arnold, MD 21012.

Sherry G. MacGlashan, MA, is a student in the PsyD program in clinical psychology at Loyola College in Baltimore, Maryland. Her interests in ethics is a product of her active involvement as a parent, educator, and community leader in Maryland. Ms. MacGlashan is a member of Psi Chi and Alpha Sigma Nu, and a student member of the Maryland Psychological Association. She is also the student representative from Loyola College to the Committee on Graduate Studies. Ms. MacGlashan resides with her husband, daughter, and son in Timonium, Maryland.

Alicia J. Clarke, MS, is a student in the PsyD program at Loyola College in Baltimore. She is an active student affiliate of the Maryland Psychological Association, serving as co-chair of this organization's Graduate Student Committee. Her work with graduate students further extends to her involvement in Psi Chi and in the American Psychological Association for Graduate Students where she acts as campus representative for Loyola College. Her work and interest in ethical issues also include the changing roles of state and provincial psychological association's ethics committees. Ms. Clarke currently resides in Sparks, Maryland, with her husband and daughter.

RESOURCES

American Association for Marriage and Family Therapy. (1991). *Code of Ethics*. Washington, DC: Author.

American Counseling Association. (1995). *Code of Ethics and Standards of Practice*. Alexandria, VA: Author.

American Psychiatric Association. (1993). *The Principles of Medical Ethics With Annotations Especially Applicable to Psychiatry*. Washington, DC: Author.

American Psychological Association. (1992). Ethical principles of psychologists and code of conduct. *American Psychologist, 47,* 1597-1611.

Annotated Code of Maryland. (1992). Health Occupations Article, Title 10, Chapter 36.05: *Code of Ethics and Professional Conduct.*

Barnett, J. E. (1998). Termination without trepidation. *Psychotherapy Bulletin, 33*(2), 20-22.

Barnett, J. E., & Sanzone, M. M. (1997). Termination: Ethical and legal issues. *The Clinical Psychologist, 50,* 9-13.

Basch, M. F. (1980). *Doing Psychotherapy*. New York: Basic Books.

Bennett, B. E., Bryant, B. K., Vanden Bos, G. R., & Greenwood, A. (1990). *Professional Liability and Risk Management.* Washington, DC: American Psychological Association.

Bostic, J. Q., Shadid, L. G., & Blotcky, M. J. (1996). Our time is up: Forced terminations during psychotherapy training. *American Journal of Psychotherapy, 50,* 347-359.

Brady, J. L., Guy, J. D., Poelstra, P. L., & Brown, C. K. (1996). Difficult good-byes: A national survey of therapists' hindrances to successful termination. *Psychotherapy in Private Practice, 14,* 65-76.

Brandt v. Grubin, 329 A.2d 82 (N.J. Super Ct. Law Div. 1974).

Budman, S. H., & Gurman, A. S. (1996). Theory and practice of brief psychotherapy. In J. E. Groves (Ed.), *Essential Paper on Short-Term Dynamic Therapy* (pp. 43-65). New York: New York University Press.

Chang, A. F. (1977). The handling of therapist's premature termination in psychotherapy. *Psychology, 14,* 18-23.

Collins v. Meeker, 424 P.2d 488, 489, 493 (Kan. 1967).

Ewing, C. P. (1990). Legal issues in terminating treatment. In E. A. Morgenson (Ed.), *The Encyclopedic Handbook of Private Practice* (pp. 720-726). New York: Gardner Press.

Eyrich v. Dam, 473 A.2d 539 (N.J. 1984).

Goodyear, R. K. (1981). Termination as a loss experience for the counselor. *Personnel and Guidance Journal, 59,* 347-350.

Greenspan, M., & Kulish, N. M. (1985). Factors in premature termination in long term psychotherapy. *Psychotherapy, 22,* 75-82.

Grunebaum, H. (1983). A study of therapists' choice of therapist. *American Journal of Psychiatry, 140,* 1336-1339.

Gutheil, T., & Appelbaum, P. (1982). *Clinical Handbook of Psychiatry and the Law.* New York: McGraw-Hill.

Hartlaub, G. H., Martin, G. L., & Rhine, M. W. (1986). Recontract with the analyst following termination: A survey of seventy-one cases. *Journal of the American Psychoanalytic Association, 34,* 895-910.

Herold v. State, 499 A.2d 429 (Md. App. 1982).

Johnson v. Ward, 344 S.E. 2d 166 (S.C. Ct. App. 1986).

Kaslow, F. W. (1992). Legal issues of psychotherapy practice. *The Independent Practitioner, 12*(3), 131-135.

Kovacs, M., Rush, A. J., Beck, A. J., & Hollon, S. (1981). Depressed outpatients treated with cognitive therapy or pharmacotherapy. *Archives of General Psychiatry, 38,* 33-39.

Kramer, S. A. (1986). The termination process in open-ended psychotherapy: Guidelines for clinical practice. *Psychotherapy, 23,* 526-531.

Macbeth, J. E., Wheeler, A. M., Sither, J. W., & Onek, J. N. (1994). *Legal and Risk Management Issues in the Practice of Psychiatry.* Washington, DC: Psychiatrists' Purchasing Group.

Maholick, L. T., & Turner, D. W. (1979). Termination: That difficult farewell. *American Journal of Psychotherapy, 33,* 583-592.

Marx, J. A., & Gelso, C. J. (1987). Termination of individual counseling in a university counseling center. *Journal of Counseling Psychology, 34,* 3-9.

Miller v. Greater Southeast Community Hospital, 508 A.2d 927 (D.C. App. 1986).

National Association of Social Workers. (1996). *Code of Ethics of the National Association of Social Workers.* Washington, DC: Author.

Penn, L. S. (1990). When the therapist must leave: Forced termination of psychodynamic therapy. *Professional Psychology: Research and Practice, 21,* 379-384.

Pinkerton, R. S., & Rockwell, W. J. K. (1990). Termination in brief psychotherapy: The case for an eclectic approach. *Psychotherapy, 27,* 362-365.

Quintana, S. M. (1993). Toward an expanded and updated conceptualization of termination: Implications for short-term, individual psychotherapy. *Professional Psychology: Research and Practice, 24,* 426-432.

Quintana, S. M., & Holahan, W. (1992). Termination in short-term counseling: Comparison of successful and unsuccessful cases. *Journal of Counseling Psychology, 39,* 299-305.

Sanderson, W. C., & Woody, S. (1995). Manuals for empirically validated treatments. *The Clinical Psychologist, 48*(4), 7-11.

Shectman, F. (1986). Time and the practice of psychotherapy. *Psychotherapy, 23,* 521-525.

Simon, R. I. (1987). *Clinical Psychiatry and the Law.* Washington, DC: American Psychiatric Press.

Stromberg, C. D., Haggarty, D. F., Leibenluft, R. F., McMillian, M. H., Mishkin, B., Rubin, B. L., & Trilling, H. R. (1988). *The Psychologist's Legal Handbook.* Washington, DC: The Council for the National Register of Health Service Providers in Psychology.

Strupp, H. H., & Binder, J. L. (1984). *A Guide to Time-Limited Dynamic Psychotherapy.* New York: Basic Books.

Thompson, A. (1990). *Guide to Ethical Practice in Psychotherapy.* New York: Wiley.

Ward, D. E. (1982). A model for the more effective use of theory in group work. *Journal for Specialists in Group Work, 7,* 224-230.

Ward, D. E. (1984). Termination of individual counseling: Concepts and strategies. *Journal of Counseling and Development, 63,* 21-25.

Weiner, I. B. (1975). *Principles of Psychotherapy.* New York: Wiley.

Weiner, B. A., & Wettstein, R. M. (1993). *Legal Issues in Mental Health Care.* New York: Plenum Press.

Wickline v. State of California, 192 Cal. App. 3d 1630 (1986).

Wilson v. Blue Cross of Southern California, No. B040697 (July 27, 1990).

Wolberg, L. R. (1977). *The Techniques of Psychotherapy.* New York: Grune & Stratton.

Wolberg, L. R. (1980). *Handbook of Short-Term Psychotherapy.* New York: Grune & Stratton.

Ethical Dilemmas In Interactions With the Media*

Leonard A. Jason, Susan C. Jahn, and Meredith S. Miller

The mass media are ideal for conveying positive, health promotion messages (Winett, 1993). Each year, Americans watch 1,550 hours of television and spend an average of 1,160 hours listening to radio (Pratkanis & Aronson, 1992). Television broadcasts, in particular, provide an additional benefit - the opportunity to see attractive, esteemed persons model desired behaviors. Visually observing others employing adaptive coping patterns reinforces the verbal message and increases the chance that viewers will try the new behavior (Winett, 1986). These messages can be broadcast into the homes of millions of Americans; mental health practitioners have incorporated health promotion activities on some popular shows and on the news (Pratkanis, 1997; Schanie & Sundel, 1978).

There are many ways that mental health practitioners can work with the media, including advocating for empirically based practices, policies, and programs (Biglan, 1995) and providing the public with information about new clinical research findings (Winett, 1986). Practitioners have also profitably worked with media professionals on many types of collaborative interventions directed toward health promotion initiatives (Jason, 1998). One of the most common situations in which mental health practitioners interact with the media is when they are called by reporters to comment on a particular issue or study.

Several authors have made suggestions on how best to handle personal interactions with the mass media (D. Canter & Breakwell, 1986; Koocher & Keith-Spiegel, 1998; Martin, 1996; McCall & Stocking, 1982; Sleek, 1997). McCall and Stocking (1982), for example, suggest that when contacted by newspaper, magazine, and television journalists, clinicians first need to decide whether to cooperate. It is often useful to request basic information about the story or topic before agreeing to be interviewed. Once they have a good sense of what the main points are, mental health professionals need to decide whether they are the most qualified or whether someone with different credentials would make a more competent source. When the interview begins, according to McCall and Stocking (1982), mental health professionals should talk only about topics that they know well. In addition, it is important to know that journalists sometimes feel apprehensive about interviewing researchers, as they sense that mental health professionals might distrust them and their profession.

Before 1981, psychologists were actually forbidden to engage in media psychology. This changed with the guidelines and recommendations in the 1981 *Ethical Principles of Psychologists and Code of Conduct* (American Psychological Association [APA], 1981), which allowed psychologists to give personal advice through the media (Wachs, 1998a). These APA guidelines have frequently been used by other mental health professionals (e.g., social workers, psychiatrists, and counselors). According to Wachs (1998a), by 1990, there was one published document involving guidelines for psychology working with the media (McCall, 1990), and three documents were unpublished (APA, 1986-1987, 1987, 1989). Unfortunately, a major objection emerged when efforts were made to consolidate these documents. The objection was that the end product could possibly be used against psychologists in court cases

*We would like to thank Guy Fricano and Renee Taylor for their expert editorial assistance.

(Wachs, 1998a). To address this concern, these guidelines have now become suggestions. Recently, Wachs (1998b) has written a useful document that addresses general issues that psychologists need to consider when interacting with the mass media to educate a wide audience. General suggestions include issues of competence, integrity, professional and scientific responsibility, respect for people's rights and dignity, concern for others' welfare, deception, testimonials, social responsibility, and advertising and endorsements.

In addition to Wachs' (1998b) document, Standard 3.04 of the APA *Ethical Principles of Psychologists and Code of Conduct* (1992) provides some useful recommendations for when psychologists interact with the media. First, psychologists must be sure that "statements are based on appropriate psychological literature and practice" (p. 1604). This applies to, for example, the temptation to exaggerate findings. M. B. Canter and colleagues (1994) suggest that psychologists can best comply with this standard by discussing the topic with the interviewer beforehand. The second requirement within Standard 3.04 states: "Statements are otherwise consistent with this Ethics Code" (p. 1604). Thus, psychologists are required to adhere to any other standards within the Ethics Code that relate in any way to working with the media. For example, Standard 1.04, which states that psychologists cannot give advice in an area in which he or she is not competent, must always be taken into consideration. Lastly, Standard 3.04 also states: "The recipients of the information are not encouraged to infer that a relationship has been established with them personally" (p. 1604). In other words, psychologists cannot suggest to anyone in the public, through their media presentations, that they are engaging with anyone in a therapeutic relationship. These guidelines sometimes do not provide enough specific guidance for the myriad of ethical questions that occur when psychologists interact with the media.

Fortunately, the APA Public Affairs Office also offers several resources to psychologists working with the media. For example, "How to Work With the Media: Interview Preparation for the Psychologist" is a 24-page booklet designed to help the mental health professional become a better spokesperson throughout the interview process, whether it be with the print, radio, or television media (APA, 1998a). A shorter brochure, "Some Questions and Answers about Dealing With the Media: A Guide for Psychologists" (APA, 1998b), is also informative. The APA Public Affairs Office also makes available to the news media a computerized database of psychologists with expertise on a variety of topics.

Ethical issues also need to be considered when mental health professionals deliver online counseling services on the Internet, which is another type of media-based intervention (Duncan, 1997; Sampson, Kolodinsky, & Greeno, 1997). A survey of 3,764 counseling-related home pages conducted between April 1996 and August 1996 revealed that there were at least 275 practitioners offering counseling services over the Internet. Sampson et al. (1997) projected that this activity may be increasing at a rate of between 55% and 72% per year. Issues that have arisen for online counseling include determining how to license practitioners (Bloom, 1998; Sampson et al., 1997), resolving the problem of not being able to see nonverbal behavior (Bloom, 1998; Duncan, 1997), and figuring out how to guarantee confidentiality (Duncan, 1997; Sampson et al., 1997). Because of this increasing use of online counseling, the APA has appointed an Internet Task Force (Task Force on New Technologies) which is currently studying issues involving online counseling.

There are considerable legal, ethical, and professional issues in interacting with the media. Because there are still few formal guidelines, many ethical issues can arise that might be difficult for mental health professionals to deal with. In this contribution, we examine several case studies and how they relate to the guidelines that have been developed for mental health professionals who interact with the media.

CASE STUDIES

I have frequently been asked to comment on issues by reporters and other media professionals. During a 1-month period in the spring of 1998, several interesting exchanges occurred between reporters and myself (Leonard Jason), and they highlight the type of ethical issues that can occur when interacting with the media. These case studies are presented below.

I was asked by a local television producer to appear on a show that would discuss the effects of TV violence on adolescents and children. As I had written a book on the topic of television and kids called *Remote Control: A Sensible Approach to Kids, TV, and the New Electronic Media* (Jason & Hanaway, 1997), I thought this might be an opportunity to present some of the literature on the effects of media violence on children's behavior and attitudes. For example, by the time our children graduate from high school, they have been exposed to over 200,000 violent acts on television.

When I arrived at the television station, I was met by the producer, who escorted me to a conference room, where I waited for about 15 minutes, hoping for an opportunity to review the proposed content of the show prior to broadcast. However, this opportunity never came. Hurried, the producer then returned and brought me to the studio where the live show would occur. I sat down on a chair and a technician put a microphone on my tie. I was now securely tethered to the seat, and I proceeded to wait for the host to appear. The host walked on to the set, said hello, and mentioned that there would be several pieces aired before I would be asked for opinions about the topic. There was no time for further exchange. She then walked to a different location and her live piece began. In her 1-minute introduction, she stated that the show would be on the topic of children who are stolen or kidnapped, emphasizing recent grisly episodes of people killing pregnant mothers and cutting out the fetuses. (After the introduction piece, the host walked back to the set where I was sitting, and she sat down next to me.)

As I listened to this introduction, I realized that I was not an expert on this topic. It had little to do with the TV violence literature that I was familiar with. My first impulse was to get up and walk off the set. However, my name and university had already been mentioned on air, and I was concerned about the social and political implications of an unannounced departure. I also wondered how representatives from my university would feel about this matter. My mind flashed to another episode about 12 years ago, when a TV interviewer incorrectly introduced me as the "Chairperson of the Psychology Department" on live television. At that time, I corrected the interviewer and said that I was not the Chairperson, but the Director of Clinical Training. That episode seemed relatively easy compared to the ethical dilemma I was now faced with. Should I discreetly leave the set, remain, or publicly announce that I am not an expert on the designated topic of the program?

As I pondered what to do, I heard the host mention that there were two other experts on the show: a representative from the Center for Missing Children in Washington, who would be interviewed first through a long-distance feed from Washington, and another interviewer from another location who would also be brought in by satellite feed. I figured that I could listen to their opinions and defer to those experts when questions arose. I became a bit more reassured and decided to remain at the station.

What occurred next was an unfortunate stroke of bad luck. The expert from Washington was being interviewed, and after she began giving some of the characteristics of people who commit these types of offenses, her voice was cut off so that I could only see the visual feed. The host had an earplug, so she could hear the entire conversation, and the audience at home continued to have the audio piece: I was the only participant without access to this vital information. Once again, it seemed that it would be exceedingly difficult to comment on the issues without hearing input from the other experts. At this point, I decided to discreetly leave the television studio, and I began to try to take the microphone off my tie, but then a viewer telephone call came in, and the host designated me to comment on it.

As I listened to the caller, the voice began breaking up and I could hear only about 70% of what was being asked, while the host and audience were able to fully hear the question without any difficulty. The question from the caller referred to a person in Texas who was in the military, whose wife feigned a pregnancy but, in reality, had stolen a baby. The question was, "Why could a husband who was intelligent not realize what was going on with this faked pregnancy?" The host then looked at me and said: "Is this the action of an evil person?"

At this point, I was looking at one of four TV monitors positioned about 15 feet in front of me. I had been fidgeting with the microphone trying to get it off and had not been successful. As I looked at the monitor, I realized that I appeared to be staring off into space because I was looking at the monitor and not the host. I then felt several kicks to my leg, which I realized were attempts by the host to get me to look at her. I then turned my confused gaze to her and tried to figure out what to do.

Now I had several choices. I could have mentioned that I had difficulty hearing what had transpired. I could have also said that I was not an expert on this topic, and then leave the studio. Pressurized situations and awkward moments like these probably happen more frequently than we would like to admit. In these situations, it is not often that we have the luxury of thinking through all the issues before an action is required.

The host, by this time, was looking at me expectantly. Because this was live television, she was subtly pleading with me to say something. I began by saying that I had not been able to hear the entire question. I then responded to the question of whether this was an "evil person" by stating that the term "evil" is probably not an appropriate term for understanding behavior, even if we think the action is reprehensible. Regarding the husband who was not aware of the faked pregnancy, I stated that sometimes, if we need to believe something strongly enough, it is possible to engage in denial in order to attain a desirable outcome. Both the host and the two experts reacted positively to these statements. Fortunately, as the show developed, the topic did change to the issue of violence and children. I represented the problem as a complex one that involved the easy availability of guns, breakdowns in family supervision and monitoring, and excessive violence on the media (by the end of elementary school, children have seen 8,000 murders on television). The host was pleased with my comments and, at the conclusion of the show, the News and Programming Director approached me, having remembered some of my previous televised health promotion series on smoking and stress, and asked if I would develop another series for the station.

What began as an ethical crisis turned out to be a relatively positive experience with some possibly desirable second-order outcomes. However, the ethical issue still remains: Should I have declined to comment or discreetly left the studio once I realized that I was not an expert on the topic that was to be discussed? General Principle C - Professional and Scientific Responsibility indicates that a particular psychologist cannot be an expert on every topic. If a topic arises in which the psychologist has little or no information, discussion on that topic might be terminated or the consumer might be referred to an appropriate source of information (Wachs, 1998b). I initially attempted to leave the studio, but found myself in a compromising situation with the host asking me to comment on a question from a viewer that I had not fully heard. By stating that I had not completely heard the question, I was at least sharing with the host and viewers that I would be able to comment only briefly on a few issues that I had heard and was comfortable discussing. If we examine APA Ethical Standard 1.04a - Boundaries of Competence, we are required to provide services "only within the boundaries of" our competence or experience (APA, 1992, p. 1600). I was not an expert on the initial topic, but, as a trained clinical psychologist, I could briefly comment on an inappropriate and stigmatizing word used by the interviewer: "evil." In addition, I made general comments about defenses that people use and how they can help explain behaviors that might seem unusual. Moreover, I waited until the topic changed to my area of expertise, and then commented more fully to the reporter.

One week after the preceding episode, I was called by a reporter from a large metropolitan newspaper to discuss the withdrawal of the tobacco companies in a proposed tobacco settlement. I was asked to comment on whether or not the courts would agree with the tobacco companies' claim that restrictions on advertising imposed by Congress would be ruled unconstitutional. Clearly, this was a question of extreme importance. Additionally, it was argued that if the tobacco companies did not voluntarily agree to cease advertisements to our youth, it would be difficult if not impossible for the legislators to impose these restrictions on them. In a sense, one of the primary reasons for including the tobacco companies in these negotiations was to obtain their voluntary agreements to terminate marketing efforts aimed at our youth.

Although I might have strong feelings about this particular issue, was I the most appropriate person to give an opinion on a legal issue such as this? Should I have referred the reporter to a lawyer or other legal authority? As an antismoking researcher, I used the occasion to express my opinion that, regardless of the decision whether Congress could impose restrictions on advertising, or if the tobacco companies did voluntarily restrict advertising to youth, there would still be billions of dollars aimed at solicitation for those 18 and over, and much of that advertising would continue to have some influence on our youth. Pairing smoking with images of being slender and reducing weight has an enormous appeal to teenage girls. I then stated that what was really needed is the banning of all tobacco ads, as was done in Canada. Even if the tobacco companies did withdraw from the negotiations, the money from higher taxes on cigarettes could be used for a countering antismoking campaign, and antismoking ads are actually more effective than smoking ads. In this case, the ethical issue is whether I had the right to take this occasion to express my opinions when the original question posed to me was one in which I was not an expert.

I contemplated whether it was appropriate to comment upon a legal issue when I was not a legal expert. I could have deferred the reporter's questions to someone who was a legal expert or commented on areas in which I had expertise. I chose to do the latter, and with the intention to "serve the best interests" of society by communicating my knowledge about effective vehicles to stop the sale of cigarettes (General Principle C - Professional and Scientific Responsibility; APA, 1992). In doing so, I had to decide if my belief systems were interfering with my judgment in making a statement to the reporter (General Principle B - Integrity; APA, 1992: "Psychologists strive to be aware of their own belief systems, values, needs, and limitations and the effect of these on their work," p. 1599). I decided that, even though I am not a legal expert, I would comment on research findings that I was familiar with and give an informed opinion on the original topic, in accordance with APA Ethical Standard 1.04a - Boundaries of Competence (APA, 1992).

A week after that episode, I encountered another ethical issue. A reporter from a major Chicago metropolitan newspaper called me and described a recent study, which found that suburban youngsters were smoking more than urban youngsters. Although I am familiar with research in this area, I was not familiar with the study the reporter was referring to. I asked the reporter several questions concerning where the study had been completed and the ethnic composition of the sample. However, the reporter was not able to answer all of my questions as fully as I would have preferred. I then asked the reporter to send me the study so that I could read it before I commented on it. However, because the reporter had a deadline to meet, he communicated that he would not be able to get me the study in time for his editorial deadline. In this situation, I could have declined to comment on the story because I had insufficient knowledge about the methodology of the study I would be commenting on. However, because I was familiar with other research in this area, and I felt that there were important policy implications of these studies, I decided to comment more generally on what was known in this research area. I communicated that if, in fact, there are lower rates of smoking in urban areas, it is critical to identify protective factors that deter urban youth from smoking. It is possible that norms, values, and practices in urban communities might have effective messages that could be harnessed in order to reduce the prevalence of teen smoking. This perspective points to a positive way of thinking about solutions to social problems, with more community-based participation and involvement. Again, the unanswered ethical question is whether I should not have even begun this interview due to not knowing the facts about this particular study, or if it was appropriate to use this opportunity to contribute potentially important issues to the public debate.

In this case example, I initially tried to glean information about the study in question from the reporter so that I could ascertain whether or not I was familiar enough with the topic to make a comment. In failing to obtain adequate information about the study, I then decided to comment on studies I was familiar with. One could argue that this action was in accordance with General Principle B - Integrity (APA, 1992). I cited familiar studies in discussing what other researchers have found regarding lower rates of smoking among some inner-city minority groups. One might argue that it would have been more prudent to terminate the interview, but if I only commented on what I knew had been validated, then I was upholding General Principle C - Professional and Scientific Responsibility (APA, 1992).

A final example involves an interview between myself and a reporter from the *Congressional Quarterly* occurring shortly after the previously described episodes. The reporter was most interested by what occurred in Woodridge, Illinois over the past 10 years in the town's successful effort to reduce merchants' tobacco sales to minors. During the course of the interview, she asked about what was happening at state and local levels, and I mentioned that a fierce battle was raging, with some agencies supported by merchants who advocated ineffective educational campaigns (i.e., educate rather than fine merchants who sell minors cigarettes), whereas others were endorsing more effective enforcement efforts (fining merchants using stings). In an effort to share with her the seriousness of the struggle, I described an event that occurred at a press conference with the mayor of a nearby city. At that event, the mayor was addressing the press, and just as he reached the section in his written remarks about a study which I had been conducting with the city, I noticed the mayor discard those pages describing my study and substituting other pages from an agency which was urging the mayor to adopt ineffective educational approaches to reduce cigarette sales to minors. I learned that officials at the agency had made a deal with the mayor to endorse less effective educational measures. Not wanting to go public with this episode, I told the reporter that this anecdote was strictly off the record and explained that I did not want to cause conflict with the mayor. However, when talking to a reporter on a sensitive subject such as this, is it ever appropriate to describe a politically sensitive incident and then say that it is "off the record"? Can we become personally liable for these types of situations?

If one examines the *Ethical Principles of Psychologists and Code of Conduct* (APA, 1992), it is unclear whether or not psychologists should ever make statements that are "off the record." The reality is that once a statement has been made, the reporter decides whether or not to use it. Therefore, the best decision is not to say "off the record," as anything that is said might be used in a story. The key issue is that whatever is being discussed, the psychologist needs to act in accordance with General Principle B - Integrity (APA, 1992) and General Principle C - Professional and Scientific Responsibility (APA, 1992).

DISCUSSION

When mental health professionals collaborate with the media, ethical issues often emerge. Although recommendations have been made to assist clinicians in their interactions with the media, there remains a need for more comprehensive guidelines. Frequently, there are few easy answers to the types of ethical issues that we regularly confront when working with the media.

When entering a studio of a television show or beginning an interview with a reporter, spending an adequate amount of time determining the nature of the topic to be discussed is critical. However, even when this has occurred, there will be times when practitioners will be placed in uncomfortable and compromising situations, such as being asked to comment on issues that are beyond one's expertise. Although, in principle, it is always best to avoid these situations, mental health practitioners often have to make quick, value-laden decisions that incorporate ethics, politics, and professional obligations, as illustrated in the case studies herein.

Many of the case studies described in this contribution addressed having incomplete information and needing to decide whether to terminate an interview or use the opportunity to provide an audience with potentially useful information. A conservative approach would have been to not offer any information to the reporters. Perhaps because I considered myself an advocate for different validated practices, I was more willing to use these opportunities to provide the public with important scientific information that might provide a foundation or context for better understanding a social problem or a possible community solution.

Mental health professionals have an important role to play in helping influence the way the media interprets issues involving health and mental health. For example, viewers of television are bombarded with messages to use products that sometimes have minimal nutrient value or are hazardous to one's health, and omnipresent advertisements on the roadsides encourage viewers to try unhealthy products. These influences need to be recognized because they undoubtedly exert a negative impact on our nation's health (Jason & Hanaway, 1997). When we interact with the media, either by commenting on a study or by collaborating on a health promotion initiative, we have the opportunity to provide alternative health promotion messages.

Some mental health professionals might want to adopt more proactive positions in dealing with the media. Rather than waiting for the media to approach us, we can work with them on initiating and implementing large-scale, media-based interventions (Jason & Salina, 1993). No large-scale intervention can be implemented by one person. As a first step in designing a program, a group of interested sponsors could be invited to an organizational meeting. If you have a personal contact within an organization, that person could be called to discuss the projected project. The contact person might be able to identify the organization's level of interest in the intervention, as well as identify appropriate people who might be interested in participating. At the organizational meeting, it would be important to focus on a current, serious, unmet need in the community. At such a meeting, it also would be important to encourage all invited guests to participate in brainstorming and problem-solving sessions to better meet the problem. When people help design their own program components, they tend to be more enthused and active in implementing the intervention. After a series of core group meetings, additional sponsors might be invited to contribute to the intervention.

We have worked with these types of planning groups to develop and implement community-owned, large-scale media interventions (Jason, 1998). We have found that the media represents an excellent forum to alert thousands of community residents to health promotion initiatives. Once alerted to these programs, participants can pick up materials and resources that reinforce the concepts broadcast and encourage opportunities for practice. Perhaps the most exciting possibilities lie in more interactive interventions. Groups can be assembled to watch the programs together, or participants can receive additional support by actually being put in contact with helpers, self-help groups, or other community agencies.

Mental health professionals today are frequently asked to comment on media stories. Some are even more ambitious in their efforts to work collaboratively with the media on health promotion programs. When ethical issues arise during these interactions, mental health professionals can examine guidelines within the American Psychological Association's ethical statements, but the principle recommendations of such statements are somewhat general and broad. The division of media psychology has been more explicit in providing suggestions to guide practitioners, but unfortunately these have only recently been developed (Wachs, 1998a). Even when such suggestions are better known, psychologists will need to have access to individuals or expert groups for advice when confronting the types of ethical challenges illustrated by the case studies. We strongly recommend that organizations involving mental health practitioners consider developing a more stable infrastructure of support to aid a growing number of our colleagues who might need consultation in resolving these types of ethical issues.

We endorse efforts made by mental heath organizations such as the American Psychological Association to regularly provide workshops on these issues at national and regional conventions, and to publish case studies of psychologists' experiences (Bersoff, 1995; M. B. Canter et al., 1994). In addition, in conjunction with Division 46 and the Public Information Committee, the APA Public Affairs Office conducts a day of training at the APA annual convention.

CONCLUSION

In summary, the authors have examined guidelines and suggestions that have been disseminated over the past decade concerning practitioners' interactions with the media. Our personal experiences suggest that these guidelines are helpful and need to be more widely distributed and used by practitioners working with the media. The case studies provided, however, suggest that even more work needs to be done to help mental health professionals deal with the multiple ethical issues that arise when interacting with the media.

CONTRIBUTORS

Leonard A. Jason, PhD, is a professor of psychology at DePaul University. Dr. Jason is a former president of the Division of Community Psychology of the American Psychological Association (APA) and past editor of *The Community Psychologist.* He received the 1997 Distinguished Contributions to Theory and Research Award from the Society for Community Research and Action (Division 27 of the APA). Dr. Jason may be contacted at DePaul University, Department of Psychology, 2219 North Kenmore Avenue, Chicago, IL 60614-3504.

Susan C. Jahn is currently Grant Administrator for the Chronic Fatigue Syndrome Epidemiology Project at DePaul University in Chicago, Illinois. She has recently published several articles in the areas of health psychology. Prior to assuming this position, she received her Bachelor of Science in Psychology with minor in Biology from DePaul University. Ms. Jahn can be contacted at DePaul University, Department of Psychology, 2219 North Kenmore Avenue, Chicago, IL 60614-3504.

Meredith S. Miller is currently a doctoral candidate in community/clinical psychology at DePaul University. She received her Bachelor of Arts in Psychology from Brandeis University. Formerly she served as Senior Research Assistant for the Case Management of Substance Abusers with HIV Project at the University of California, San Francisco. Her current research focuses on homeless youth and high-risk sexual behaviors. Ms. Miller may be contacted at DePaul University, Department of Psychology, 2219 North Kenmore Avenue, Chicago, IL 60614-3504.

RESOURCES

American Psychological Association. (1981). *Ethical Principles of Psychologists and Code of Conduct.* Washington, DC: Author.

American Psychological Association. (1986-1987). Ethics Committee Task Force. In T. Nagy (Chair), *Media Guidelines for the Psychologist.* Washington, DC: Author.

American Psychological Association. (1987). *Ethical Guidelines for Media Psychologists.* Washington, DC: Public Information Committee Subcommittee on Ethical Guidelines.

American Psychological Association. (1989). Division 46 Guidelines Committee. In K. Wachs (Chair), *Suggestions for Media Mental Health Professionals.* Washington, DC: Author.

American Psychological Association. (1992). Ethical Principles of Psychologists and Code of Conduct. *American Psychologist, 47,* 1597-1611.

American Psychological Association. (1998a). *How to Work With the Media: Interview Preparation for the Psychologist.* Washington, DC: Author.

American Psychological Association. (1998b). *Some Questions and Answers about Dealing With the Media: A Guide for Psychologists* [Brochure]. Washington, DC: Author.

Bersoff, D. N. (1995). *Ethical Conflicts in Psychology.* Washington, DC: American Psychological Association.

Biglan, A. (1995). *Changing Cultural Practices: A Contextualist Framework for Intervention Research.* Reno, NV: Context Press.

Bloom, J. W. (1998). The ethical practice of WebCounseling. *British Journal of Guidance and Counseling, 26*(1), 53-59.

Canter, D., & Breakwell, G. (1986). Psychologists and "the media." *The British Psychological Society, 39,* 281-286.

Canter, M. B., Bennett, B. E., Jones, S. E., & Nagy, T. F. (1994). *Ethics for Psychologists: A Commentary on the APA Ethics Code.* Washington, DC: American Psychological Association.

Duncan, D. M. (1997, April). *Counseling Over the Internet: Ethical and Legal Considerations.* Presentation at the American Counseling Association's 1997 World Conference, Orlando, FL.

Jason, L. A. (1998). Tobacco, drug, and HIV preventive media interventions. *American Journal of Community Psychology, 26*(2), 151-173.

Jason, L. A., & Hanaway, L. K. (1997). *Remote Control: A Sensible Approach to Kids, TV, and the New Electronic Media.* Sarasota, FL: Professional Resource Press.

Jason, L. A., & Salina, D. (1993). Quality media connections. Another look at successful interventions. *Prevention Forum, 13,* 2-8.

Koocher, G. P., & Keith-Spiegel, P. (1998). *Ethics in Psychology: Professional Standards and Cases.* New York: Oxford University Press.

Martin, S. (1996, October). Do's and don'ts for interviewing with the media. *APA Monitor* [Newspaper, selected stories online]. Retrieved June 30, 1998 from the World Wide Web: http://www.apa.org/monitor/oct96/media.html

McCall, R. B. (1990). Ethical considerations of psychologists working in the media. In C. Fisher & W. Tryon (Eds.), *Ethics in Applied Developmental Psychology: Emerging Issues in an Emerging Field. Annual Advances in Applied Developmental Psychology* (pp. 163-185). Norwood, NJ: Ablex Publishing.

McCall, R. B., & Stocking, S. H. (1982). Between scientists and public: Communicating psychological research through the mass media. *American Psychologist, 37*(9), 985-995.

Pratkanis, A. R. (1997). The social psychology of mass communications: An American perspective. In D. F. Halpern & A. E. Voiskounsky (Eds.), *States of Mind: American and Post-Soviet Perspectives on Contemporary Issues in Psychology* (pp. 127-159). New York: Oxford University Press.

Pratkanis, A. R., & Aronson, E. (1992). *Age of Propaganda: The Everyday Use and Abuse of Persuasion.* New York: W. H. Freeman.

Sampson, J. P., Jr., Kolodinsky, R. W., & Greeno, B. P. (1997). Counseling on the information highway: Future possibilities and potential problems. *Journal of Counseling and Development, 75,* 203-212.

Schanie, C. F., & Sundel, M. (1978). A community mental health innovation in mass media preventative education: The alternatives project. *American Journal of Community Psychology, 20,* 573-581.

Sleek, S. (1997, September). How to take your message to the media: Media psychologists offer advice on the best strategies for communicating through television, radio, and print. *APA Monitor* [Newspaper, selected stories online]. Retrieved June 30, 1998 from the World Wide Web: http://www.apa.org/monitor/sep97/media/html

Wachs, K. (1998a). *An Informal History of Suggestions for Psychologists Working With the Media.* Unpublished manuscript.

Wachs, K. (1998b). *Suggestions for Working With the Media.* Manuscript in preparation.

Winett, R. A. (1986). *Information and Behavior: Systems of Influence*. Hillsdale, NJ: Erlbaum.

Winett, R. A. (1993). Media based behavior change approaches for prevention. In D. S. Glenwick & L. A. Jason (Eds.), *Promoting Health and Mental Health in Children, Youth, and Families* (pp. 181-204). New York: Springer.

Maintaining Professional Competence for Working With Culturally Diverse And Aging Clients

Jeffrey E. Barnett and Nicole Polakoff

CASE EXAMPLES*

Case Example A

You greet an octogenarian patient who arrives for an initial consultation. This patient struggles to his feet and, with the aid of a walker, slowly and shakily makes his way to your office from the waiting room. Not knowing much about him yet, you find yourself thinking about how feeble and weak he seems. You wonder if there's any point to working with him in psychotherapy. After all, his mind is probably in the same condition as his body, if not worse.

Case Example B

An important referral source refers an elderly patient to you for evaluation. Not wanting to disappoint this referral source, you decide to proceed with the evaluation despite not having any specific training in working with this particular population. You conduct several general psychological tests and prepare your report. In reviewing the results with a colleague, you are surprised when questioned about the impact of impaired eyesight and hearing, age-appropriate memory decline and psychomotor retardation, and the side effects of the patient's various medications. You are even more alarmed when your diagnosis of dementia is challenged and you are told that your evaluation borders on incompetence.

Case Example C

You have begun treatment with a first-generation Japanese-American female who has been experiencing conflicts with her parents since she entered adolescence. Now a college freshman, she describes a worsening situation as her parents complain of how she is rejecting their traditional values and practices. You are concerned by these reports as well as by her lack of eye contact with you, and you decide she would benefit from assertiveness training. You are then surprised to learn that her efforts to be more assertive are causing her greater conflict with her parents and you are confused as she becomes increasingly depressed despite all your efforts to help her.

Case Example D

A Hispanic-appearing patient with a heavy accent enters your office for an initial consultation. It is reported that she has not been eating or sleeping well, her hygiene is poor, she has been isolative and withdrawn, and she spends hours sitting alone in the dark rocking back and

*These case examples are fabrications and do not represent any individuals known to the authors.

forth. When you question her, she tells you, "My soul has left me. I have nothing left." Concerned, you assess for the presence of a thought disorder and, in your mind, begin making plans to have her admitted to a psychiatric hospital, involuntarily if necessary.

Mental health clinicians all receive basic training in assessment and treatment skills that may be utilized with a wide variety of patients. But it is generally understood that this training does not provide us with the necessary knowledge and skills needed to meet all patients' needs. When confronted with patients with specialized needs that fall outside their scope of practice, clinicians typically refer these patients to other professionals who possess the needed training, skills, and experience. It is widely accepted that no clinician can possess the special competencies needed to treat all patients.

This contribution will address the issue of clinical competence first in general and then as it applies to two patient populations: those from diverse cultural backgrounds and the elderly. Although these two groups may be viewed as specialty areas, we will argue that as the demographics of our changing society continue to evolve, so too must the range of mental health clinicians' core competencies. This contribution will first review clinical, ethical, and legal issues pertaining to professional competence. Then, specific dilemmas and the requisite body of knowledge needed for competencies will be provided. Finally, specific recommendations will be made that will assist clinicians to competently assess and treat our patient population in the new millennium.

COMPETENCE

Mental health clinicians are generally well trained and highly skilled professionals. We try to provide much-needed services to a diverse group of individuals in a caring and competent manner. Because of our positions as health care professionals, mental health clinicians hold the public's trust and confidence. So as not to jeopardize this valued professional position, adherence to standards of professional competence are of great importance.

Not actually a unitary concept, competence is generally believed to be a multifaceted construct. Welfel (1998) defines competence as being comprised of three key components: knowledge, skill, and diligence. Knowledge involves receiving education related to the history, theory, and research in the mental health field. Skill is related to the successful application of this knowledge to diagnostic and treatment issues with patients (Meehl, 1997). Implicit in the skill component of competence is the capacity to make appropriate decisions regarding which interventions in one's knowledge base are appropriate for specific clinical situations. Skill may be developed initially through practical or other clinical placements; it continues to develop in professionals through ongoing training and clinical experiences. The final aspect of competence, diligence, is described by Welfel (1998) as a "consistent attentiveness to the client's needs that take priority over other concerns" (p. 65). This may also include engaging in additional reading, consultation, and supervision in order to provide the most effective and appropriate care.

Haas and Malouf (1995) further describe the competent clinician as someone who has the knowledge to understand a clinical issue, the skills to apply the knowledge in an effective way, and the judgment to use both the knowledge and the skills appropriately. Gross and Robinson (1987) additionally separate competence into five basic components. These include accurate representation of professional qualifications, ongoing professional development through continuing education, providing only those services for which one is qualified and trained, maintaining accurate knowledge and expertise in specialty areas, and gaining assistance in solving personal issues that interfere with or decrease one's effectiveness.

Although these definitions of competence vary with regard to some specifics, they are all based on the same underlying virtues or tenets of ethics upon which all standards of mental health practice are based. These tenets include (a) beneficence, the obligation to help others; (b) nonmaleficence, the duty not to cause harm to others; (c) fidelity, the promise to meet certain standards and to provide services in an agreed-upon manner; (d) autonomy, the obligation to help patients toward their effective functioning independent of you; (e) justice, which emphasizes accessibility to appropriate and competent care to all individuals; and (f) self-interest, which directs mental health professionals to take appropriate steps necessary to prevent any impairment of professional competence (Thompson, 1990).

PROFESSIONAL ETHICS AND STANDARDS

These basic tenets of ethics have contributed to the development of each profession's code of ethics, which also include specific guidelines and standards concerning competence. For example, the Ethical Principles of Psychologists and Code of Conduct (American Psychological Association [APA], 1992) provides a standard of competence which is representative of guidelines provided in all mental health ethics codes:

> Psychologists strive to maintain high standards of competence in their work. They recognize the boundaries of their particular competencies and the limitations of their expertise. They provide only those services and use only those techniques for which they are qualified by education, training, or experience. Psychologists are cognizant of the fact that the competencies required in serving, teaching, and/or studying groups of people vary with the distinctive characteristics of those groups. In those areas in which professional standards do not yet exist, psychologists exercise careful judgment and take appropriate precautions to protect the welfare of those with whom they work. They maintain knowledge of relevant scientific and professional information related to the services they render, and they recognize the need for ongoing education. Psychologists make appropriate use of scientific, professional, technical, and administrative resources. (p. 1599)

Although these guidelines on competence are offered as a general principle to guide one's professional conduct, several more standards are included in psychology's ethics code which address specific areas of practice. These include Boundaries of Competence with regard to clinical services, teaching, and research, and maintaining expertise in these areas; Competence and Appropriate Use of Assessments and Interventions; Competence in Teaching, Training, Supervision, Research, and Publishing; and Competence in Forensic Activities (APA, 1992, pp. 1597-1611).

Similar guidelines are provided in other professional codes of ethics. The Code of Ethics of Social Workers (National Association of Social Workers [NASW], 1996), for example, lists competence as one of its six core values. This core value states: "Social workers practice within their areas of competence and develop and enhance their professional expertise. Social workers continually strive to enhance their professional knowledge and skills and to apply them in practice" (p. 4). In addition to specific standards on providing services only after receiving appropriate education, training, and supervised experience, social work's ethics code also provides specific guidelines on cultural competence and social diversity. These guidelines state:

> Social workers should understand culture and its function in human behavior and society, recognizing the strengths that exist in all cultures.
>
> Social workers should have a knowledge base of their clients' cultures and be able to demonstrate competence in the provision of services that are sensitive to the clients' cultures and to differences among people and cultural groups.
>
> Social workers should obtain education about and seek to understand the nature of social diversity and oppression with regard to race, ethnicity, national origin, color, sex, sexual orientation, age, marital status, political belief, religion, and mental or physical disability. (p. 6)

Great consistency is seen in the standards of competence articulated by the various mental health professions. In the Code of Ethics and Standards of Practice of the American

Counseling Association (ACA, 1996), similar guidelines are provided within its section on Professional Responsibility. Specific standards of practice are provided for each aspect of the counseling relationship. Of special interest are requirements for maintaining and increasing competence through continuing education, self-monitoring for impairment, not offering services when distress or impairment may hold the potential for harm to a client, and the use of accurate representation of credentials and advertising.

Each of the mental health professions' ethics codes also provide clear guidance in providing services only within one's defined scope of practice. For example, the code of ethics of the American Association for Marriage and Family Therapy (AAMFT, 1991) cautions: "Marriage and family therapists do not diagnose, treat, or advise on problems outside the recognized boundaries of their competence" (p. 3).

It is clear that all of these standards are based on the underlying ethics tenets of beneficence, nonmaleficence, fidelity, autonomy, justice, and self-interest. However, it is interesting to note that competence refers to a professional's performance or functioning rather than just his or her knowledge or abilities. A mental health professional may be highly knowledgeable and experienced and thus able to provide services appropriately; however, competence refers to the utilization of this knowledge and ability in professional functioning. It is also important to keep in mind that competence refers to the services we provide within a particular area of functioning. One is not necessarily globally competent or incompetent. This may actually vary between and within various areas of endeavor (Overholser & Fine, 1990).

As previously stated, mental health professionals are guided by their respective ethics codes in deciding which behaviors meet their profession's standard of competence in a particular area of functioning. These ethics codes place a great emphasis on knowing one's boundaries and only practicing within one's given areas of competence. In addition to being given these professional standards to aspire to, mental health professionals each have the responsibility to monitor their own competence and examine the boundaries of their competence in determining whether it is appropriate for them to provide services in specific situations. Although this may seem a daunting task, it may best be achieved through self-monitoring and self-evaluation, peer consultation, and supervision. Actively monitoring, maintaining, and improving our competence in relevant areas of our professional roles is a duty we owe the public we serve.

The failure to maintain these high standards may have a negative impact on the welfare of mental health consumers and their perception of mental health professionals. In one study, which investigated patients' perceptions of the ethical practices of their therapists (Claiborn et al., 1994), adults responded to a questionnaire regarding several major areas of practice including competence. An interesting finding of this study is that patients rated their therapists to be appropriately competent less than 50% of the time. Given that a patient's perceptions of the therapist's expertise may affect the therapist's ability to effect change in the patient, competence would seem to be an area that all professionals would want to be aware of and constantly striving to increase.

LICENSURE AND CERTIFICATION

In most jurisdictions, licensure and certification provide assurance to consumers of mental health services that practitioners have achieved certain minimal standards of education, training, experience, and knowledge. To become licensed or certified as a mental health professional, one must first complete an approved course of formal education, the specifics of which are typically codified into statutes. One must then demonstrate having received approved levels and types of clinical training and supervised experience that meet specific standards for entry into the profession. Finally, one must demonstrate possessing the minimal body of knowledge relevant to the profession by successfully completing a required examination. Once clinicians have entered the profession, it is important that they adhere to a code of conduct and ethics as well as ensue ongoing professional development to maintain their skills and abilities.

In keeping with the definitions of competence and the ethical standards reviewed previously, licensure and certification statutes typically incorporate provisions that require practicing mental health professionals to meet minimal requirements for ongoing continuing education. Several authors (e.g., Dubin, 1972; McNamara & Flanders, 1985) point out that 50% of the clinician's knowledge and skills will become obsolete within 10 to 12 years after receiving the training. This assertion is based on the fact that knowledge becomes dated over time as the body of knowledge of one's profession advances and because knowledge can erode from memory over time. Welfel (1998) points out that knowledge is not static and that research is constantly revealing new information. Thus, a graduate degree can serve only as a starting point for competence. One of the most obvious ways to avoid this knowledge erosion is through involvement in ongoing continuing education activities. Mental health professionals will be better able to serve others competently by attending seminars and workshops and by keeping up with professional literature. These steps may assist clinicians to increase competence in an area of ongoing practice, to maintain competence in a developing or changing field, and to expand their scope of practice by developing new competencies.

In addition to professional reading and attending workshops and seminars, the opportunity for the supervised practice of skills is an important component of developing and maintaining competence. Further, continuing education programs that have been shown to produce the most significant increases in professional competence have included the following components: They had an identified target audience, they included participants with a genuine desire to learn, participants had identified a weakness in the specific area that the program addressed, the learning objectives of the program were clear, active participation in discussion and clinical procedures was required, and there was an opportunity for supervision in practice beyond the training (VandeCreek, Knapp, & Brace, 1990). However, mental health clinicians will gain competence only when the program is appropriate for their needs, when they are motivated enough to participate actively, when they take the time necessary to review and study relevant literature, and, in some cases, when they seek additional supervision.

Although licensure does not guarantee what a practitioner will actually do, it does offer some protection to the public from grossly incompetent and unqualified professionals. Limitations of licensure with regard to competence include that it can only specify minimal acceptable standards for continuing education and knowledge; licenses do not typically specify the types of patients or the techniques that a practitioner is competent to work with and utilize. The mental health professions' licensing and certification statutes are typically generic with regard to competence. They tend to specify only that licensed or certified professionals use only those therapeutic tasks in which they are sufficiently trained (G. Corey, M. S. Corey, & Callanan, 1998). Again, the potential problem is that it is the judgment of the clinician that often dictates how this guideline is put into practice. Therefore, when faced with dilemmas such as whether one is competent to provide certain services to a particular population, the use of self-examination, consultation, and supervision is of great importance.

RELEVANT CASE LAW

Failure to meet professional standards of competence holds several potential consequences. In addition to sanctions by licensing and certifying organizations and professional associations, mental health professionals may be sued for malpractice. If they are found guilty, they may be required to pay for damages. Additional costs of a successful malpractice suit include loss of income, professional status, and hospital membership, as well as removal from positions on provider panels. Clinicians may also face an increase in malpractice insurance premiums or an inability to obtain ongoing coverage. Professional incompetence tarnishes not only the individual's reputation, but also that of the mental health profession. Yet despite meeting basic licensure or certification requirements and knowing of these risks, mental health professionals have violated these standards and been found guilty of malpractice through their lack of adequate competence. The following cases are representative of the types of violations of the standard of competence engaged in by mental health professionals.

Several cases highlight the importance of attending to accepted treatment protocols and acting in accordance with an accepted standard of care. In *Michael and Virginia Cobo v. Ernest A. Raba, M.D.* (1994), the plaintiff was treated by a psychiatrist for over 8 years because of chronic depression. Although psychotherapy was provided during this time, often as frequently as four times each week, the plaintiff did not improve and reportedly suffered many losses, including his career and marriage. It was charged that the defendant refused to consider alternative treatments such as medication or a referral to another health care provider despite his patient not improving over a period of 8 years. A judgment was found in favor of the plaintiff and the defendant was required to pay damages of $850,000.

In a similar case, *Osheroff v. Chestnut Lodge Inc. et al.* (1985), a patient was provided with intensive psychodynamic psychotherapy to treat his chronic major depression. Treatment was provided in accordance with a psychodynamic model of understanding and treating depression which excluded biological explanations and treatment alternatives. Despite 7 months of intensive psychotherapy in an inpatient setting, the plaintiff suffered increased symptoms of depression and his condition apparently worsened. His family had him discharged from Chestnut Lodge and placed in another treatment facility. There, his condition improved quickly when he received treatment that included medication. In the suit against Chestnut Lodge, an arbitration panel ruled in favor of the plaintiff and ordered damages of $250,000. Both sides appealed this ruling, but before going to court the case was settled for an undisclosed amount.

Mental health professionals may also be held liable for malpractice if a reasonable standard of care is not met in any of several important areas of clinical practice. In a number of legal rulings, courts have found mental health professionals to be negligent for failing to adequately obtain informed consent prior to providing treatment. In the landmark case of *Canterbury v. Spence* (1972), the court found that in order to meet the standard of care, clinicians must explain to patients any relevant risks that a typical patient would need to consider before deciding on a course of treatment. Further, in *Wiley v. Karem* (1982) the court added that for complicated treatments which hold a risk of significant harm, clinicians must explain these risks as well as alternatives available in a manner that the patient can understand. In more recent cases (e.g., *In re Martin*, 1995; *In re R.A.J.*, 1996), however, courts have consistently ruled that treatments may be imposed on patients without their consent when the risk of serious harm to the patient or others exists when the treatment is not provided.

Courts have also ruled on cases alleging neglect or improper diagnosis. In one important case, *Hedlund v. Superior Court* (1983), the court found that health care practitioners will be held liable for damages if they do not evaluate patients for disorders such as depression or do not appropriately respond to serious symptoms such as suicidal ideation. Similarly, in *L.L. et al. v. J.R., cc Ins. Co., et al.* (1994), the court found against mental health counselors who had evaluated and treated a man but failed to diagnose his homicidal and suicidal tendencies which he acted on shortly thereafter. A $1 million verdict was reached in this case. In *Cantone v. Rosenblum* (1992), a child with severe hearing impairment was misdiagnosed as having childhood psychosis and placed in a residential treatment center for emotionally disturbed children. The court ruled against the evaluating clinician and the facility for both negligent and improper diagnosis and treatment. Alternatively, courts have ruled in favor of mental health professionals, even when a tragic outcome occurs, if the clinician has met the reasonable standard of care of their profession. In *Smith v. King* (1993) a patient committed suicide, but the court found that the counselor had appropriately assessed and diagnosed the patient and that, as a result, the suicide could not have reasonably been anticipated.

Negligent psychotherapy is an area where courts have ruled on standards of care as well. In numerous cases courts have ruled against mental health clinicians for incorporating inappropriate social and sexual relationships into a patient's treatment and for engaging in inappropriate sexual relationships with patients' significant others. For example, in *Wasson v. Westbranch Residential Treatment Center, Inc.* (1992) a verdict of $3.34 million was found against a counselor who had an affair with a patient's mother during the patient's treatment. Further, in *Anonymous v. Dr. Goldberg* (1991) a $1.7 million verdict was reached against a psychiatrist who engaged in a sexual relationship with a patient during the course of treatment. Courts have also ruled against clinicians for failing to consider alternative treatments when patients are not benefiting from ongoing psychotherapy (see *Michael and Virginia Cobo v. Ernest A. Raba, M.D.*, 1994, discussed previously).

Additionally, courts have ruled on negligent use of somatic treatments such as the improper use of medication or electroconvulsive therapy (ECT) by psychiatrists. In *Lojuk v. Quanolt* (1983) the court ruled against a psychiatrist who failed to disclose the risks of ECT prior to its administration. Similarly, in a number of cases courts have ruled against physicians who do not warn patients of the potential side effects of medications they prescribe and who do not adequately monitor for the presence and consequences of such side effects. In *Sugar v. Dr. Levine* (1991) a $240,000 verdict was reached against a psychiatrist for inappropriately prescribing medications and not closely monitoring their impact on the patient, who then suffered significant harm from the resulting toxicity and withdrawal. Also, in *Harrington v. Rush Presbyterian St. Luke's Hospital et al.* (1989) a jury ordered a $4 million verdict for failure to monitor the effects of a medication on a patient who died as a result of taking it.

Finally, courts have ruled against clinicians for failing to appropriately refer patients for needed additional treatment. In *Helen B. Wojtowicz et al. v. Gerald E. Boutin et al.* (1995) the court ruled against a psychologist who did not refer a seriously depressed patient to a psychiatrist or for hospitalization. The patient committed suicide and a $580,000 verdict against the psychologist was reached. Also, in *Kokensparger v. Athens Mental Health Center* (1989) the court ruled that the center and the professionals involved in a patient's care were liable for the patient's death for not referring him for tests that would likely have disclosed the presence of a brain tumor, rather than claiming that the patient's symptoms were caused by schizophrenia. However, in several other cases (e.g., *Frank Chou, Executor v. Eileen McGee, M.D.*, 1996) where an appropriate referral was made, yet the patient still experienced a negative outcome, the referring clinicians were not found liable.

These and similar cases highlight the need to provide treatment which is consistent with the reasonable standard of care of one's profession. Pakman, Cabot, and Bongar (1994) further elucidate this standard in citing *Hood v. Phillips* (1976, p. 291), where it is ruled that treatment provided should be consistent with what a "reasonable and prudent member of the [particular] profession would undertake under . . . similar circumstances" (p. 179). Clearly, to practice competently, the prudent mental health clinician should (a) have a knowledge of relevant standards for assessment, diagnosis, and treatment; (b) be familiar with and consider treatment alternatives; and (c) consult with others.

To meet this reasonable standard of care of one's profession, Woody (1985) recommends that all mental health professionals demonstrate and exercise the level of knowledge and skill common to members of the profession in good standing. He adds further: "The professional has an obligation to keep abreast of scientific advances and to elevate the quality of practice within the bounds of reasonable expenditure of finances and personal effort" (p. 514). Thus, in keeping with the need for continuing education and ongoing professional development discussed previously, practitioners are advised to maintain their current levels of knowledge and skill and to develop their competence through the acquisition of new abilities as dictated by increases in the scientific base of understanding within the mental health professions.

OUR CHANGING SOCIETY

We know that as mental health professionals, we strive to meet the assessment and treatment needs of those we serve in a competent and caring manner. In fact, one way we demonstrate our caring for and valuing of patients is by ensuring our competence. This should include sensitivity to individual differences and needs. As cited previously, "psychologists are cognizant of the fact that the competencies required in serving, teaching, and/or studying groups of people vary with the distinctive characteristics of those groups" (APA, 1992, p. 1599). Additionally, in that we as mental health professionals are licensed or certified (and trained) generically, special competencies may be necessary to competently meet the needs of those we serve.

As we enter this new millennium it is quite evident that our society is in the midst of some significant changes which are already impacting how we define competence. Our society is aging and diversifying at unprecedented rates. Outdated conceptualizations about our patient population, their treatment needs, and how best to meet them may hinder us in meeting a reasonable standard of care. In order to provide assessment and treatment services competently, awareness of individual differences and special needs and providing services consistent with them are of great importance.

Our society is currently diversifying at a rapid rate. It was estimated in 1997 that the United States population was 72.7% Caucasian, 12.1% African-American, 11% Hispanic, 3.6% Pacific Islander, and 0.7% Native American, Eskimo, and Aleut (U.S. Census Bureau, 1997). Yet, by the year 2000, it is predicted that approximately one-third of the population will be made up of people of color (Iijima Hall, 1997). Current immigration trends indicate that of immigrants in the United States, 42% are Hispanic and 41% are Asian. It is predicted that these groups will comprise more than 50% of the U.S. workforce in the 21st century (Ibrahim, 1991).

In addition to cultural diversification trends, our society is aging rapidly. Figures indicate that the number of adults 65 years of age and older has tripled since 1900. It is estimated that our population will move from 16% over age 60 to over 26% in this group by the year 2025 (Department of International Economic and Social Affairs, United Nations, 1990).

These two trends are ongoing and are rapidly changing the society in which we live and, thus, the population that we serve. The following two sections will address issues of competence in working with these two groups.

PROFESSIONAL COMPETENCE AND OLDER ADULTS

The definition of older adults varies, but individuals over the age of 60 are generally considered to be in this category. Given the statistics of our rapidly aging population, and to engage in ethical practice, mental health professionals would benefit from efforts to increase competence in working with older adults. This includes understanding older adults' treatment needs.

According to Erik Erikson's stages of development, each phase is explained in terms of the extremes of successful and unsuccessful solutions (Liptzin, 1985). In this progression, older adults deal with the crisis of integrity versus despair, where individuals have a sense of satisfaction and fulfillment looking back over their lives, or they may have a sense of despair at lost opportunities (Ornstein & Carstensen, 1991). Liptzin (1985) defines integrity as a sense of coherence about one's life and despair as the feeling that life will not last long enough to try new things or to attempt to solve problems. This stage of life brings with it severe social, psychological, and physical factors that the competent professional should be cognizant of when working with older adults (Schulz & Heckhausen, 1996).

Assessment of Older Adults

Given the multitude of changes that occur in older adults' lives, and given the fact that most of the mental health professionals working with older adults will be younger than their patients, the psychological assessment of older adults poses a challenge to the practitioner. Edelstein et al. (1996) outline the most common reasons for conducting evaluations for older adults. These are to determine

(1) whether an individual is cognitively impaired;
(2) what constitutes the best placement for an individual;
(3) the extent and nature of functional capacity;
(4) the capacity to make decisions;
(5) whether an individual is appropriate for nursing home placement;
(6) diagnosis;
(7) a plan for appropriate interventions or care;
(8) the effect of interventions and/or care. (p. 36)

Once the decision has been made to conduct an assessment of older adults, the competent clinician must consider several important issues and make the appropriate adaptations. Redinbaugh (1997) highlights five relevant areas that should be incorporated in the assessment of older adults that provide important information about the individual, especially when interactions between these domains are taken into consideration. The five domains include psychological distress, physical health, cognitive functioning, social relationships, and medication and substance use (Redinbaugh, 1997). It is of great importance that detailed information be gathered in each of these areas and that clinicians understand their impact on the individual being assessed. Additionally, to ensure that the evaluations of older adults are completed in a competent manner, clinicians must be aware of the normal aging process. They must not, as highlighted in Case Example A, assume that all older adults are expected to be depressed, fearful, or senile. Being aware of age-appropriate changes will assist us in knowing when to refer to medical professionals for evaluations of physical symptoms, when presenting symptoms are aspects of mental health disorders, and when they are normal aspects of the aging process. Examples of factors to keep in mind include psychomotor slowing and decreases in strength as well as decreases in hearing and vision, as highlighted in Case Example B. When conducting assessments of older adults, clinicians should also be sure to utilize assessment instruments that are specifically normed with this population and tests developed specifically to assess them. Examples include the Geriatric Depression Scale (Yesavage et al., 1983), which is a self-report measure used to assess the presence of depression in the elderly; the Older Adults Resources and Services Questionnaire (Fillenbaum & Smyer, 1981), which assess health problems and their impact on daily functioning; and the Wechsler Memory Scale - III (Wechsler, 1997), which is an excellent measure of a variety of aspects of memory functioning and is normed for use with individuals up to 89 years of age. The importance of utilizing appropriate assessment tools with older adults cannot be overstated. Without them, we may make errors with profound consequences for the individuals involved such as assuming the presence of dementia when in fact depression may be present or by inappropriately considering the role of typical aspects of the aging process, as illustrated in Case Example B.

Treatment of Older Adults

Therapeutic relationships with older adults may be difficult for some practitioners because they may bring up personal concerns about aging, parental figures, health, and dying (Shmotkin, Eyal, & Lomranz, 1992). Examples may include avoiding addressing certain issues that we have yet to resolve ourselves, such as our parents' impending death or their recently developed dependency on us. Such concerns may contribute to a practitioner's reluctance to work with this population as well as impact our effectiveness. A mental health clinician's personal biases regarding the elderly, as illustrated in Case Example A, may also have an important impact on the effectiveness of our assessment and treatment of this population. Part of becoming competent to work with older adults involves gaining awareness of one's own biases and then working to resolve them. Edelstein et al. (1996) refer to prejudicial beliefs about older adults as "ageism," and they point out that clinicians are not immune to holding such negative beliefs. In contrast to some clinicians' biases and stereotypes, it has been found that older adults may be successful in mental health treatment (Knight, 1996). To assist them in achieving this success, it is recommended that we focus on and utilize older adults' existing strengths, which include a proven ability to overcome and survive many of life's challenges (Hays, 1996) and the individual's accumulated life experience and knowledge (Schulz & Heckhausen, 1996).

Ethnically Diverse Older Adults

Hays (1996) argues that obtaining a rich history from older adults regarding cultural background will increase practitioners' understanding of those individuals and thus will increase their competence in working with such an individual. Therefore, it seems that professionals need to assess the boundaries of their competence with regard not only to the age of their patient, but also to the cultural and ethnic background of patients. In order for the assessment of older adults to be truly complete with regard to both issues of age and ethnicity, information regarding their cultural history should be obtained. Many cultures possess specific beliefs about mental illness, family roles, and the meaning of seeking treatment. One would not want to make treatment recommendations that are in direct conflict with such beliefs and cause even greater distress for the patient, as highlighted in Case Example C.

PROFESSIONAL COMPETENCE AND MULTICULTURAL POPULATIONS

Greenfield (1997) states that culture implies "sharing or agreement, that is, social convention" (p. 115). Culture may also provide a context in which we may see ourselves as separate individuals as well as in relation to others (Shiang et al., 1998). Ethnicity may be a powerful factor in determining how individuals think, feel, and behave (Root, 1985). Pederson (1991) proposes that by defining culture broadly and including in this definition status variables, affiliations, and ethnographic variables, we have a construct that is generic to all therapeutic relationships. These variables are becoming more and more prevalent and researched by the mental health professions. As reported previously, American society is experiencing rapid changes in demographics. As ethnic minorities become a larger part of the total U.S. population there will be an increasing need for mental health services for this population. This requires new perspectives and methods in the training of mental health professionals (Bernal & Castro, 1994). By early in the 21st century, it is predicted that some ethnic groups which are considered minority groups will outnumber the rest of the population (Welfel, 1998). For example, cultural competence will be of particular importance in states such as California, where it is predicted that within 20 years, Caucasians will no longer be the ethnic majority (Del Rio, 1997). Therefore, as the population as a whole changes, so too will the consumers of mental health services. This calls for us as professionals to gain skills and knowledge and to challenge our own beliefs and attitudes to provide the most effective services to culturally diverse clients (K. Enchemendia et al., 1996).

Mental health professionals will need a sensitivity to and general knowledge of cultural differences in the use of language, mannerisms, communication styles, and expressions of distress among different groups and a freedom from stereotyping of racial group psychopathology (Plummer, 1997). Similarly, Ho (1985) stresses the importance of knowledge of, and sensitivity to, the divergent values held by members of different cultures. Examples include placing a different value on independence versus interdependence, conflict versus harmony, assertiveness versus compliance, primacy of the individual versus primacy of the relationship, and nonconformity versus conformity, as illustrated in Case Example C. Mental health professionals will also need specific information about mores and beliefs of different groups. The patient described in Case Example D may be describing *susto*, which means "fright" or "soul loss." Goleman (1995) describes this as an "illness tied to a frightening event that makes the soul leave the body, causing unhappiness and sickness" (p. C3). For many individuals from Central America, this is a reaction to a significant loss such as the death of a loved one, which results in depression. This patient was describing her feelings of depression in a culturally bound way that, if misinterpreted, could easily lead to misdiagnosis and mistreatment.

The need for cultural competence has been posed as an ethical imperative (Bernal & Castro, 1994; Ponterotto & Casas, 1991). Given our changing demographics, it appears that mental health professionals in general will be highly likely to encounter diverse clientele, students, and research participants (K. Enchemendia et al., 1996). Therefore, appropriate training, and knowledge of, and adherence to professional standards for work with ethnic, linguistic, and culturally diverse populations are necessary for ensuring the quality of care that is received. Although many theories and techniques may be applicable to diverse groups, individuals should neither be assessed, diagnosed, nor treated without an understanding of the frame of reference of the client (Gonzalez, 1995). Atkinson, Morten, and D. W. Sue (1993) propose that clinicians without cultural competence who provide services to clients from diverse cultural backgrounds are not only practicing in an unethical manner, but also are potentially harmful and in violation of human rights.

To avoid problems in the field related to serving such a diverse population, one professional organization, the American Psychological Association, has published guidelines consistent with those of other mental health professions which identify general principles of ethical practice that address the population being served, gaining respect and understanding of clients' values, beliefs, and worldview, and gaining either the ability or the resources to interact in the client's language (Bernal & Castro, 1994). The "Guidelines for Providers of Psychological Services to Ethnic, Linguistic, and Culturally Diverse Populations" (APA, 1993) state that psychologists may need to educate and explain the process of psychological intervention to their clients and that such information should be presented in language that is clearly understandable to the client. When limitations in communication become apparent, clinicians must either make an appropriate referral or use a translator with some appropriate psychological background (Atkinson et al., 1993). If a professional translator is not available, in some cultures it may be appropriate to use a family member as a translator.

A second APA guideline (1993) states: "Psychologists are cognizant of relevant research and practice issues related to the population being served" (p. 46). This entails acknowledgment that cultural factors may have an impact on behavior and that these factors need to be accounted for in treatment and assessment. D. R. Sue (1996) recommends that culturally competent mental health professionals receive training that increases awareness of cultural perceptions, the impact of culture on behavior, and an understanding of how culture influences the direct manifestations of behaviors, as illustrated in Case Examples C and D. In order to be competent, the professional must have knowledge of the individual's culture as well as his or her level of acculturation in order to assess the difference between normal and abnormal behavior (Shiang et al., 1998). For example, Chinese-American psychologists rated a sample of Chinese-American clients as alert, honest, ambitious, and friendly, while European-American psychologists rated these same clients as confused, anxious, and nervous (D. R. Sue, D. W. Sue, & S. Sue, 1997). In this example, certain traits were seen as positive and adaptive in one culture, and abnormal and maladaptive in another. When cultural group norms are considered in the assessment process, misdiagnosis and inappropriate treatment plans are less likely to occur (Ramirez et al., 1996).

The APA (1993) guidelines specify in an illustrative statement: "Psychologists respect clients' religious and or spiritual beliefs and values, including attributions and taboos, since they affect world view, psychosocial functioning, and expression of distress" (p. 46). An understanding of the role that religion plays in an individual's life may assist professionals in assessing the nature of the problem as well as helping to determine the most effective intervention for that particular client (Gonzalez, 1995). For many patients, their faith and religious beliefs are a source of strength to draw on which may be utilized in treatment. For others, confusion over religious issues may underlie presenting problems. These issues should all be addressed in the assessment of each patient.

TRAINING AND EDUCATION

Another aspect of being cognizant of important and applicable research and practice issues involves participation in training and education to increase understanding regarding cultural, social, psychological, and economic information relevant to the particular population being served (APA, 1993). Iijima Hall (1997) also recommends that the courses on cultural training should be similar to other courses in that they should "teach mental health professionals how to be good clinicians in terms of analyzing problems, deciding on alternatives, seeking consultation, and minimizing negative consequences" (p. 647).

Speight et al. (1995) further specify that courses must facilitate awareness, include multiculturalism throughout the program, and incorporate discussions of economic, political, and social issues including gender, sexual orientation, race, and class. Additional information regarding the oppression of many groups should be included in this criteria as this may have a strong impact on mental health. Many mainstream professionals do not have an understanding of such oppression (Iijima Hall, 1997). This training process must be ongoing in order for a mental health professional to be competent in working with culturally diverse clients. One may be considered culturally competent only when one is in the process of actively developing appropriate interventions and skills and practicing them with culturally diverse clients (Atkinson et al., 1993).

Another guideline of particular importance to assessment and treatment refers to the appropriateness of utilizing particular assessment instruments with a patient. This APA (1993) guideline states: "Psychologists consider the validity of a given instrument or procedure and interpret resulting data, keeping in mind the cultural and linguistic characteristics of the person being assessed. Psychologists are aware of the test's reference population and possible limitations of such instruments with other populations" (p. 46). Many intelligence and personality measures have been criticized for underrepresenting minority populations in the standardization of the measure, examiner cultural bias, and cultural loading on the content of test items (Dana, 1988; Dana & Whatley, 1991; Plummer, 1997). Examples include the Wechsler Adult Intelligence Scale (WAIS) and the Minnesota Multiphasic Personality Inventory (MMPI), both of which have been revised and renormed on populations that are more inclusive of cultural diversity. The most recent versions of these tests should always be used so that bias issues are minimized. Velasquez et al. (1997) report that the MMPI overpathologizes Chicanos in comparison to the revised version, the MMPI-2. They also emphasize the importance of assessing each patient's level of acculturation when considering assessment results. Canul and Cross (1994) report that Chicanos who are less acculturated tend to have higher L (Lie) scale scores on the MMPI-2. Failure to be cognizant of this finding may lead to misinterpretation of assessment results, which may then result in misdiagnosis. Further, Dana (1988) cautions us in using the MMPI-2 with different cultural groups because its norming included representative samples of Blacks and Native Americans, but other groups are underrepresented, thus limiting our ability to confidently interpret findings for those groups. Finally, many psychological test items may reflect cultural loading with European-American cultural experience and knowledge.

In order to increase the validity of tests, Greenfield (1997) recommends analyzing culture-specific meanings, culture-specific ways of expressing knowledge and problem-solving, and the validity of the assessment tool with regard to cross-cultural ability testing. Clinicians must become well-informed consumers of psychological tests. A careful review of test manuals with a critical eye toward the utility, relevance, and fairness of a particular assessment device for a specific individual or population is crucial.

The effects of invalid assessment procedures may cause great harm to the patient as such procedures may result in misdiagnosis and inappropriate treatment. This is of particular importance for professionals working with diverse populations. Historically, culture has not been emphasized in mental status examinations. Only in the latest revision of the *DSM* (*Diagnostic and Statistical Manual of Mental Disorders*, 4th ed., American Psychiatric Association, 1994) are professionals prompted to take an individual's culture into consideration when making a diagnosis (Plummer, 1997). The inclusion of an appendix describing culture-bound syndromes in the *DSM-IV* may be considered a critical step toward greater understanding of the importance of culture and its impact on mental health (Shiang et al., 1998).

Minority groups have a higher rate of misdiagnosis of mental illness than the majority population (Al-Issa & Tousignant, 1997). For example, studies have consistently found that historically Blacks have been diagnosed as schizophrenic more than Whites (Abe-Kim & Takeuchi, 1996). Many factors may contribute to the misdiagnosis of a minority individual. The results of several studies seem to indicate that cultural differences in communication styles, language use, and the expression of symptoms contribute to misdiagnosis (Velasquez et al., 1997). Ramirez et al. (1996) emphasize the need for clinicians to be trained to determine whether patients' behaviors "reflect personality abnormalities or are normal within their cultural context" (p. 284). Further, a reliance on cultural stereotypes should be avoided. Clinicians should be knowledgeable of empirical findings and use them when interpreting assessment results. The training of multiculturally competent professionals should certainly include information pertaining to the ways in which different groups tend to express symptoms. Mental health professionals may at times operate from an ethnocentric perspective, because research, theories, and techniques based on the majority population are frequently erroneously generalized to minority groups (Shiang et al., 1998). Thus, we should not base culturally diverse individuals' diagnoses solely on the criteria of the majority population, as illustrated in Case Example C. Culturally competent clinicians should seek out information about a given culture. This may not only decrease the likelihood of misdiagnosis, but may also improve a patient's treatment. Such an investigation may reveal possible strengths in the cultural values of an individual which may be built upon in treatment (APA, 1993).

BIAS AND PREJUDICE

Atkinson et al. (1993) suggest that culturally competent professionals are always actively in the process of becoming aware of their own assumptions, biases, and personal limitations. Racial stereotypes, holding a bias that one's own race is superior, and lack of cultural perspective may have deleterious effects in a therapeutic setting (Priest, 1991). It is the ethical responsibility of the practitioner to resolve any tendencies toward diagnosing without first accounting for the cultural context from which the behavior was derived, as what is deemed deviant in one culture may be considered normal in another (Ramirez et al., 1996).

Gonzalez (1995) points out the attitudes, knowledge, and skills that culturally competent clinicians must possess with regard to their own assumptions, biases, and values. The attitudes of culturally competent professionals (a) are sensitive to the effects of their own culture as well as respectful of others, (b) recognize the boundaries of their competence with regards to their own biases, and (c) are comfortable with differences between themselves and their clients (Atkinson et al., 1993). Competent professionals have knowledge about their own heritage and how it affects their definitions of normality and abnormality; they possess knowledge about how racism, oppression, and stereotyping affect them personally as well as how they affect others; and they are knowledgeable about differences in communication styles and the impact that their own styles may have on various individuals (Atkinson et al., 1993). Competent professionals actively seek educational, consultative, and training experiences regarding the myths and stereotypes of various groups, and they are always seeking to understand themselves as cultural beings (Helms, 1990).

WITHIN-GROUP DIFFERENCES

Despite much education and training to become a culturally competent clinician, mental health professionals must be aware of and investigate the possibilities of within-group differences, the effects of other variables such as acculturation, and the possible effects of having many cultural identities on an individual's behavior. It is important that professionals not make the mistake of overemphasizing the culturally unique perspectives of clients and remain attuned to those common-ground universals and within-group differences that are shared across cultures (Pedersen, 1991). The African-American culture is diverse with regard to several variables including level of employment, education, economic status, legal status, family stability, marital status, and many more (Priest, 1991). Asian-American culture is also very diverse, and many different subcultures are included in this category. Family values vary within the Asian-American culture; therefore, understanding a Chinese family does not automatically imply understanding of a Filipino family (Root, 1985). Chinese-Americans are a diverse group with differences in political history, language, geography, and economic structure (Shiang et al., 1998). The role of religion in an individual's life should be assessed on an individual basis to avoid stereotyping. For example, many patients in the Mexican-American culture view their mental illness in a religious context; however, this varies by level of acculturation, age, and other factors (Gonzalez, 1995). Insight into the role of religion, both on an individual level and on a cultural level may help clinicians define their role as well as assist them in deciding on appropriate therapeutic techniques.

LIMITATIONS OF CURRENT GUIDELINES

The recommendations presented in this contribution attempt to sensitize mental health clinicians to issues of competence as they pertain to the elderly and ethnically diverse individuals. No set of guidelines can provide specific guidance for all individuals or all situations. Rather, they provide a framework for understanding these individuals' diverse needs. Attention to these guidelines will hopefully prompt clinicians to develop their competence in working with these patients. Because of the evolving nature of the profession and the populations they serve, mental health clinicians will best serve patients by keeping abreast of current developments in this important area of practice.

It has been emphasized throughout this contribution that, given the changing demographics of the American population, ongoing training and education; increased sensitivity to culture specific issues, needs, and biases; awareness of personal limitations; and increased use of consultation, supervision, and referral when applicable are all necessary to protect the welfare of consumers of mental health services and to maintain professional competence on both a general and a specific level. Finally, as Zayas et al. (1996) recommend, we must be aware of the existence of cultural differences, have adequate knowledge of each patient's culture, be able to distinguish between culture and pathology in our assessment, and ensure that we take culture into account when planning and providing treatment.

CONTRIBUTORS

Jeffrey E. Barnett, PsyD, is a licensed psychologist in private practice in Maryland. He is also an Adjunct Associate Professor on the Core Faculty of the Department of Psychology at Loyola College in Baltimore, Maryland. Dr. Barnett is a frequent lecturer and author on legal and ethical issues in mental health. He is a past ethics committee chair and a past president of the Maryland Psychological Association. Dr. Barnett may be contacted at 1511 Ritchie Highway, Suite 201, Arnold, MD 21012.

Nicole Polakoff, MS, is a 3rd-year student in the Clinical Psychology PsyD program at Loyola College in Baltimore, Maryland. Her professional interests include psychological assessment, the treatment of children, group psychotherapy, and ethics. Ms. Polakoff can be contacted at npolakoff@aol.com

RESOURCES

Abe-Kim, J. S., & Takeuchi, D. T. (1996). Cultural competence and quality of care: Issues for mental health service delivery in managed care. *Clinical Psychology: Research and Practice, 27*, 284-288.

Al-Issa, I., & Tousignant, M. (1997). *Ethnicity, Immigration, and Psychopathology*. New York: Plenum.

American Association for Marriage and Family Therapy. (1991). *Codes of Ethics.* Washington, DC: Author.

American Counseling Association. (1996). American Counseling Association Code of Ethics. In B. Herlihy & G. Corey (Eds.), *ACA Ethical Standards Casebook* (pp. 27-59). Alexandria, VA: Author.

American Psychiatric Association. (1994). *Diagnostic and Statistical Manual of Mental Disorders* (4th ed.). Washington, DC: Author.

American Psychological Association. (1992). Ethical principles of psychologists and code of conduct. *American Psychologist, 47*, 1597-1611.

American Psychological Association. (1993). Guidelines for providers of psychological services to ethnic, linguistic, and culturally diverse populations. *American Psychologist, 48*, 45-48.

American Psychological Association. (1997). *What Practitioners Should Know about Working With Older Adults.* Washington, DC: Author.

Anonymous v. Dr. Goldberg, Norfolk County, Mass., Superior Ct., 1991, Case No. 88-297.

Atkinson, D., Morten, G., & Sue, D. W. (1993). *Counseling American Minorities.* Madison, WI: Brown & Benchmark.

Baker, R., Lichtenberg, P., & Moye, J. (1998). A practice guideline for assessment of competency and capacity of the older adult. *Professional Psychology: Research and Practice, 29*, 149-154.

Bernal, M., & Castro, F. (1994). Are clinical psychologists prepared for services and research with ethnic minorities? *American Psychologist, 49*, 797-805.

Canterbury v. Spence, 464 F.2d 772, 789 (D.C. Cir. 1972).

Cantone v. Rosenblum, 587 N.Y.D.2d 743 (N.Y. App. Div. 1992).

Canul, G. D., & Cross, H. J. (1994). The influence of acculturation and racial identity attitudes on Mexican Americans' MMPI-2 performance. *Journal of Clinical Psychology, 50*, 736-745.

Cartier v. Long Island College Hospital, 490 N.Y.S.2d 602 (App. Div. 1985).

Claiborn, C., Berberoglu, L., Nerison, R., & Somberg, D. (1994). The client's perspective: Ethical judgments and perceptions of therapist practices. *Professional Psychology: Research and Practice, 25*, 268-274.

Corey, G., Corey, M. S., & Callahan, P. (1998). *Issues and Ethics in the Helping Professions*. Pacific Grove, CA: Brooks/Cole.

Dana, R. H. (1988). Culturally diverse groups and MMPI interpretation. *Professional Psychology: Research and Practice, 19*, 490-495.

Dana, R. H., & Whatley, P. R. (1991). When does a difference make a difference? MMPI scores and African Americans. *Journal of Clinical Psychology, 47*, 400-406.

Del Rio, R. (1997, December). A personal approach to cultural competence. *California Psychologist, 30*, 31.

Department of International Economic and Social Affairs, United Nations. (1990). Population growth and structure, population studies No. 113. In *World Population Monitoring* (pp. 27-50). New York: Author.

Dubin, S. S. (1972). Obsolescence or lifelong education: A choice for the professional. *American Psychologist, 27*, 486-497.

Edelstein, B., Staats, N., Kalish, K., & Northrop, N. (1996). Assessment of older adults. In M. Herson & V. B. Van Hasselt (Eds.), *Psychological Treatment of Older Adults* (pp. 35-41). New York: Plenum.

Enchemendia, K., Enchemendia, R., Crawford, L., & Robinson, W. (1996). Predicting critical competence: Implications for practice and training. *Professional Psychology: Research and Practice, 27*, 386-393.

Fillenbaum, G. G., & Smyer, M. A. (1981). The development, validity, and reliability of the OARS Multidimensional Functional Assessment Questionnaire. *Journal of Gerontology, 36*, 428-434.

Frank Chou, Executor v. Eileen McGee, M.D., Cuyahoga County (OH) Court of Common Pleas, 1996, Case No. 268337.

Goleman, D. (1995, December). Psychiatry finds room on couch for patient's cultural background. *New York Times*, C2-4.

Gonzalez, F. (1995). Working with Mexican-American clients. *Psychotherapy, 32*, 696-706.

Greenfield, P. (1997). You can't take it with you: Why ability assessments don't cross cultures. *American Psychologist, 52*, 115-124.

Gross, D. R., & Robinson, S. E. (1987). Ethics in counseling: A multiple role perspective. *Texas Association for Counseling and Development Journal, 15*, 5-15.

Haas, L. J., & Malouf, J. L. (1995). *Keeping Up the Good Work: A Practitioner's Guide to Mental Health Ethics* (2nd ed.). Sarasota, FL: Professional Resource Press.

Harrington v. Rush Presbyterian St. Luke's Hospital et al., Circuit Ct. of Cook County, Ill., 1989, No. 79-L-15578.

Hays, P. (1996). Culturally responsive assessment with diverse older clients. *Professional Psychology: Research and Practice, 27*, 188-193.

Hedlund v. Superior Court, 699 P.2d 41 (Cal. 1983).

Helen B. Wojtowicz, PR of the Estate of Chester Wojtowicz v. Gerald E. Boutin, Ph.D., University Mental Health Center, Robert R. D'Amico, D.O. et al., Pinellas County (FL) Circuit Court, 1995, Case No. 93-3403-CI-15.

Helms, J. (1990). Three perspectives on counseling and psychotherapy with visible racial and ethnic group clients. In F. C. Serafica (Ed.), *Mental Health of Ethnic Minorities* (pp. 171-201). New York: Praeger.

Ho, D. Y. E. (1985). Cultural values and professional issues in clinical psychology: Implications for the Hong Kong experience. *The American Psychologist, 40*, 1212-1218.

Hood v. Phillips, 573 S.W.2d 291 (Tex. Civ. App. 1976).

Ibrahim, F. (1991). Contribution of cultural world view to generic counseling and development. *Journal of Counseling & Development, 70*, 13-19.

Iijima Hall, C. (1997). Cultural malpractice. *American Psychologist, 52*, 642-651.

In re Charles c., 562 N.Y.S.2d 208 (N.Y. App. Div. 1990).

In re Martin., 527 N.W.2d 170 (Minn. Ct. App. 1995).

In re R.A.J., 554 N.W.2d 809 (N.D. Sup. Ct. 1996).

Knight, B. (1996). *Psychotherapy With Older Adults* (2nd ed.). Thousand Oaks, CA: Sage.

Kokensparger v. Athens Mental Health Center, 578 N.E.2d 916 (Ohio Ct. Cl. 1989).

L. L. et al. v. J.R., cc Ins. Co., et al., Milwaukee Co., Wisc., Circuit Ct., Case Nos. 89 CV 02811 and 89 CV 4145., 91-98 (1994).

Liptzin, B. (1985). Psychotherapy with the elderly: An Erikson perspective. *Journal of Geriatric Psychology, 18*, 183-202.

Lojuk v. Quanolt, 706 F.2d 1456 (7th Cir. 1983).

McNamara, R., & Flanders, P. (1985). Continuing education for psychologists: A reexamination. *The Clinical Psychologist, 24*, 31-35.

Meehl, P. (1997). Credentialed persons, credentialed knowledge. *Clinical Psychology: Science and Practice, 4*, 91-98.

Michael and Virginia Cobo v. Ernest A. Raba, M.D., Durham County (NC) Superior Court (1994).

National Association of Social Workers. (1996). *NASW Code of Ethics*. Washington, DC: Author.

Ornstein, R., & Carstensen, L. (1991). *Psychology: The Study of Human Experience*. San Diego, CA: Harcourt Brace.

Osheroff v. Chestnut Lodge Inc. et al., 490 A.2d 720-724 Md. App., April 10, 1985.

Overholser, J. C., & Fine, M. A. (1990). Defining boundaries of professional competence: Managing subtle cases of clinical incompetence. *Professional Psychology: Research and Practice, 21*, 462-469.

Pakman, W. L., Cabot, M. G., & Bongar, B. (1994). Malpractice arising from negligent psychotherapy: Ethical, legal, and clinical implications of *Osheroff v. Chestnut Lodge. Ethics and Behavior, 4,* 175-197.

Pedersen, P. (1991). Multiculturalism as a generic approach to counseling. *Journal of Counseling and Development, 70,* 6-11.

Plummer, D. (1997, November). Diversity issues in the assessment process. *The Ohio Psychologist, 44*(2), 20-22.

Ponterotto, J. G., & Casas, J. N. (1991). *Handbook of Racial/Ethnic Minority Counseling Research.* Springfield, IL: Charles C. Thomas.

Priest, R. (1991). Racism and prejudice as negative impacts on African American clients in therapy. *Journal of Counseling and Development, 70,* 213-215.

Ramirez, S., Wassef, A., Paniagua, F., & Linskey, A. (1996). Mental health providers' perception of cultural variables in evaluating ethnically diverse clients. *Professional Psychology: Research and Practice, 27,* 284-288.

Redinbaugh, E. M. (1997). Psychological assessment of older adults. *The Ohio Psychologist, 44*(2), 23-25.

Root, M. (1985). Guidelines for facilitating therapy with Asian American clients. *Psychotherapy, 22,* 349-355.

Schulz, R., & Heckhausen, J. (1996). A life span model of aging. *American Psychologist, 51,* 702-714.

Shiang, J., Kjellander, C., Huang, K., & Bogumill, S. (1998). Developing cultural competency in clinical practice: Treatment considerations for Chinese cultural groups in the United States. *Clinical Psychology: Science and Practice, 5,* 182-210.

Shmotkin, D., Eyal, N., & Lomranz, W. (1992). Motivations and attitudes of clinical psychologists regarding treatment of the elderly. *Educational Gerontology, 18,* 177-192.

Smith v. King, 615 So.2d 69 (Ala. 1993).

Speight, S., Jones Thomas, A., Anderson, R., & Anderson, M. (1995). Operationalizing multicultural training in doctoral programs and internships. *Professional Psychology: Research and Practice, 26,* 401-406.

Sue, D. R. (1996). Ethical issues in multicultural counseling. In B. Herlihy & G. Corey (Eds.), *ACA Ethical Standards Casebook* (pp. 193-215). Alexandria, VA: American Counseling Association.

Sue, D. R., Sue, D. W., & Sue, S. (1997). *Understanding Abnormal Behavior.* New York: Wiley.

Sugar v. Dr. Levine, Marin County, Calif., Superior Ct., 1991, Case No. 141594.

Thompson, A. (1990). *Guide to Ethical Practice in Psychotherapy.* New York: Wiley.

U.S. Census Bureau. (1997). *National Population Estimates* [On-line]. Available: http://ftp.census.gov/population/estimates/nation/intfile3-lotx

VandeCreek, L., Knapp, S., & Brace, K. (1990). Mandatory continuing education for licensing psychologists: Its rationale and current implementation. *Professional Psychology: Research and Practice, 21,* 135-140.

Velasquez, R., Gonzalez, M., Butcher, J. N., Castillo-Canez, I., Apodaca, J. X., & Chavira, D. (1997). Use of MMPI-2 with Chicanos: Strategies for competence. *Journal of Multicultural Counseling and Development, 25,* 107-120.

Wasson v. Westbranch Residential Treatment Center, Inc., Harris County, Tex., Dist. Ct., 1992, Case No. 90-190.

Wechsler, D. (1997). *Wechsler Memory Scale, 3rd ed.*. San Antonio: The Psychological Corporation.

Welfel, E. (1998). *Ethics in Counseling and Psychotherapy.* Pacific Grove, CA: Brooks/Cole.

Wiley v. Karem, 421 So.2d 294 (La. App. 1982).

Woody, R. H. (1985). Public policy, malpractice law, and the mental health professional: Some legal and clinical guidelines. In C. P. Ewing (Ed.), *Psychology, Psychiatry, and the Law: A Clinical and Forensic Handbook* (pp. 509-525). Sarasota, FL: Professional Resource Exchange.

Yesavage, J. A., Brink, T. L., Rose, T. L., Lum, O., Huang, V., Adey, M., & Leirer, V. O. (1983). Development and validation of a geriatric screening scale: A preliminary report. *Journal of Psychiatric Research, 17,* 37-49.

Zayas, L. H., Torres, L. R., Malcom, J., & DesRosiers, F. S. (1996). Clinicians' definitions of ethnically sensitive therapy. *Professional Psychology: Research and Practice, 27,* 78-82.

Using Quality of Care Indicators As a Marketing Tool

John Rudisill

Increased competition for provision of psychological services has necessitated an emphasis on marketing activities for psychological practitioners. Many practitioners experience role conflict between being a provider of quality clinical services and being businesspersons selling their wares. Providers often regard marketing as something that makes them uncomfortable, either because of its "enterprising" nature (Holland, 1985) or because marketing activities seem self-centered and less virtuous than helping others. Other private practitioners regard marketing as a necessary evil that a provider must reluctantly do to create business when clinical work is unavailable. In short, many practitioners experience an uncomfortable tension associated with the split between marketing and service provision.

One way to bridge the gap between clinician and marketer is for the clinician to focus on marketing activities that arise naturally out of the provision of quality service. The most effective marketing is a job well done. Satisfied clients and their referral sources are likely to let others within their personal networks know of the clinician's helpfulness and will generate future referrals.

This contribution deals with marketing as it relates to providing quality services and does not cover ordinary advertising activities such as how to place a telephone ad or write a brochure, or issues indirectly related to quality such as pricing.

Clinical practices grow by providing quality service to three stakeholders in the service delivery process: the client, the referral source of the client, and the community. The amount of work a practice has grows in two ways: by attracting new clients or by increasing the services provided to existing clients. Quality service increases both areas of growth potential for the practice.

Providers typically show a gradient of comfort level across each of the three primary stakeholders. Providers are most comfortable with working with clients, less comfortable in dealing with referral sources, and least comfortable in community interactions. A focus on quality service in dealing with each of these stakeholders can reduce our anxiety and avoidance. Providing quality service allows us to positively impact human effectiveness while garnering increased market share.

PROVIDING QUALITY SERVICE TO CLIENTS

Service Setting

Can clients easily find your practice in the telephone book? Is your practice easily accessible to the clients you wish to serve? Do you have a sign to help people locate your practice? Is there an attractive symbol or logo to symbolize the practice for clients? Is entry to your practice safe and confidential? From the perspective of the client, are the furnishings comfortable? Does the appearance of the practice communicate what you want in terms of climate? Does the decor fit the population you want to serve? Have you considered having a unique waiting room that adds to the therapeutic impact of the practice? For example, you might consider a client educational area with videotape education, a play area for children, or even an aquarium to encourage relaxation.

Support Services

Are your office staff friendly and supportive when a client calls? Are staff committed to making the client feel comfortable by both reducing the stigma of seeking help and providing instrumental support in understanding and dealing with third-party payers? Do staff do the little extra service-oriented things such as sending out maps and reminders of appointments and explaining the billing process? Quality support service is not only consistent with a therapeutic atmosphere but also encourages business. Staff attitudes that are professional, caring, courteous, and respectful are invaluable in communicating to clients that they are valued.

Efficiency

It is helpful to ask yourself a set of questions in regard to efficiency. Is your practice efficient? Do you have adequate computer and software support to increase the efficiency of routine and repetitive operations? Do you have forms designed and placed in wordprocessing programs for easy modification and use? Has each aspect of your contact with clients been engineered to flow smoothly to reduce the "hassle" factor for clients? For example, are insurance claims filed for your clients within 3 days of their visit?

Client Information Materials

Does your practice have an information guide that the client can read and refer to that clarifies the many issues surrounding services, billing and collections, confidentiality, and practice philosophy? Is bibliotherapy routinely provided to help clients work outside of the session? Are videotapes loaned out or at least assigned at the local library? Is handout material available to clients through the providers, for example, instructional (how to parent a hyperactive child) or resource-oriented (listing of support groups for widows/widowers)? Stamping all materials (e.g., newspapers, magazines, brochures, and pamphlets) "Compliments of [the name and number of your practice]" allows clients to network for you with other people in need within their personal networks. It also communicates a personal touch which adds to the relationship between the client and the practice. Some practices with the resources and space have developed resource centers for self-help and client education. These services can expedite client progress and also serve as value-added marketing tools.

Follow-Up

Telephone or written follow-up of clients who fail to show for appointments communicates caring to the client, adds a valuable mechanism for clinician feedback regarding the reasons for premature termination, and also retains clients within the practice. Whenever I call clients, I make it clear that I am calling to see how they are doing and not to solicit another appointment. If the client wants to make another appointment, I suggest that she or he call the office administrator (so the client will not experience duress in the process). Both short- and long-term follow-up of clients after termination allow the clinician to receive feedback on treatment provision and insure that the client will feel comfortable returning to the practice if additional services are needed.

Evaluation

Practices have successfully implemented a variety of helpful approaches to evaluation. One approach is the suggestion box, which asks clients to make anonymous comments about the practice in any ongoing way. This method provides feedback to the practice and gives direction to change efforts when systemic problems are repeatedly identified. If clients sign suggestions, a communication based on your response to their suggestion should be sent back to the clients. Some practices convene a "Consumer Board" that can comment on how practice changes and developments affect the consumer of services. Another less permanent technique is the focus group, in which clients are brought together (usually clients with at least 15 or more sessions who agree to keep the names of other participants confidential) to ask about their experiences with the practice, covering everything from intake procedures to termination. This is an excellent opportunity to improve the quality of everything from your waiting room to your informed consent policy.

Provider Quality

Ultimately, one of the most important aspects of quality and marketing appeal is the provider. Improving your professional competence through continuing education, supervision, conferences, workshops, reading, and so on provides better care for clients and will eventually earn you a respected reputation in the professional community.

PROVIDING QUALITY SERVICE TO REFERRAL SOURCES

Feedback to Referral Sources

Do you routinely get clients to release information so you can keep referral sources informed about their referrals? It is helpful to find out if your referral sources prefer phone conversations or written material for their charts. You should keep the referring clinician informed regarding whether or not the client called and scheduled an appointment, provide information on your assessment and treatment planning, and suggest follow-up information on the progress and termination of your client. Feedback to referral sources increases the continuity and coherence of care within the delivery system. It also creates additional referrals for you by providing enhanced service to the referral source and by keeping your name in front of the referral source. Sending a letter to referral sources when you refer a case to them is also a helpful professional practice. From a marketing perspective, sending a referral sets up a "norm of reciprocity" with the professional recipient of the referral and may get you referrals back.

Feedback to Third-Party Payers

Since managed care organizations, in many instances, have become an integral part of the health care delivery system, it is important to regard them as any other referral source. Care managers should be kept informed, treated respectfully, and, when necessary, educated regarding the optimal treatment of the client. Required paperwork should be submitted in a timely fashion. Sending in termination reports at the end of a successful therapy is especially likely to win additional referrals.

Service Options

The design of specific treatment programs aimed at solving the problems of your referral sources is especially responsive to referral source needs. Even when a practice does not have a relevant treatment program, augmenting individual therapy with support group referrals can be helpful. By working closely with support groups, new referral networks are opened for the practice. One option is to host or start a support group at your practice location. It is important to offer not only services you prefer offering but also services that clients and referral sources in your area need.

Develop Specialty Areas

Developing and marketing specific specialty areas of interest which will be in demand by managed care and other referral sources can enhance your opportunities to serve that client population. By developing increased knowledge and experience with a specific type of client problem, you not only tend to be referred those clients but also begin to develop special expertise with that population.

Educating Referral Sources

Sending materials to referral sources, such as newsletters, articles published, handouts on specific problems, or announcements of practice capabilities, can be informative to your referral sources as well as remind them of your willingness to help with their client's psychological problems. Some practice newsletters can be purchased and modified to your use.

Acknowledging Referral Source Support

Showing appreciation to your sources of frequent referrals such as sending a holiday gift (e.g., a subscription to a magazine dealing with psychological topics or, better yet, something that won't be thrown away such as an envelope opener) is a good way to express appreciation for your relationship. Much of marketing is related to practicing high quality interpersonal relationships.

Professional Associations and Organizations

Being a part of local professional associations and organizations contributes both to the professional community and to your own professional development. Incidentally, such connections allow networking with professional referral sources. With your active involvement, professionals within your professional organizations, such as universities, hospitals, agencies, and so on, will learn about your services so that you can meet their referral needs. Involvement in professional associations and organizations often means that you will get the referral when another professional needs to refer a case out of his or her practice (e.g., marital therapy for a client seen individually).

Outcome Data

Collecting information about outcomes, even if restricted to simple measures of client satisfaction, provides feedback to improve your own performance. Outcome data can also be used to market the effectiveness and efficiency of the practice to referral sources. Monitoring your success ratios provides data to "sell" your services to managed care organizations and other providers. Developing practice guidelines or clinical protocols and testing their implementation also improves quality. Monitoring the satisfaction of referrers can also help you improve the quality of your practice (speed, quality of care, etc.).

PROVIDING QUALITY SERVICES TO THE COMMUNITY

Listening

Listen and record requests for services made by people who call your practice. Pay attention to needs that are expressed by existing clients. Hold discussions with referral sources or formally survey them regarding their needs. Pay attention to problems in the community. If there are unmet consumer needs in the community you may be able to offer a quality solution through psychological services.

Copying Others

Learn from other practices and even other types of service providers what consumers experience as quality service. Try to find the highest quality approach (benchmark) and try to emulate that standard in your practice.

Prevention Programs

There are many opportunities for practitioners to provide primary or secondary prevention. Examples include prevention speeches and workshops to lay and professional groups and client screening programs (such as National Depression, Anxiety, Eating and Substance

Abuse Disorders Days). These are excellent ways to provide a valuable service while increasing professional visibility and influencing referral sources. Some secondary prevention programs (e.g., step-parenting groups, smoking cessation groups) are excellent niche markets that can expand the service offerings of your practice.

Educational Efforts

Offering free educational lectures and workshops to local social service organizations, civic or cultural groups, churches, synagogues, and even corporations provides education to the public on various psychological health topics while getting your name out to the community. Participating in exhibitions, conventions, and health fairs provides a public service that also gets your name in front of people. Teaching in the local university or adult education center can both educate the community and increase your personal visibility as a provider. Developing your own website with educational features can also be an educational service with marketing value. Public service announcements and press releases can be used for educational or preventive efforts of interest to the public.

Consultation

Developing paid and volunteer consultation in a variety of settings is another way to share your expertise and enhance your visibility for marketing purposes. This activity has increased marketing clout if you consult with gatekeepers.

Community Involvement

The provider who advocates for quality mental health and consumer education through articles, media exposure, and volunteer work not only provides a service to the community but also increases exposure to potential referral sources. Joining organizations or boards in the community not only serves your community but also provides opportunities to meet people and to increase your visibility. The Chamber of Commerce, schools, and civic, fraternal, and religious organizations are possible options. Often the local United Way organization has a board clearinghouse with which you can sign up. If you have expertise in a specific area or disorder (e.g., cardiac rehabilitation), then involvement in a related organization (e.g., the American Heart Association) can allow you to share your expertise while creating referral sources. Your practice can also sponsor individuals, groups, teams, or events that endorse the community emphasis that reflects your beliefs and interests.

Media Involvement

Because media are always looking for quality material to fill newspaper space and air time, your expertise can be helpful. Newspapers and TV news programs often need comments from experts. Business publications have "People on the Move" features that allow you to inform the public about a new provider joining your practice. Writing articles or appearing on TV and radio programs to educate the public can reach large audiences with your information. It has been said that private practice workload is a product of visibility x time. If this maxim is true, increasing your visibility will decrease the time it will take you to have a viable private practice. Whenever one of your colleagues appears in the local newspaper, it can be thoughtful to acknowledge the event by sending to her or him another copy of the article with an accompanying note.

Networking

Keeping track of your network including names, addresses, phone numbers, and important facts about the relationship allows you to expand your resources to help your clients. Building the quality of these relationships with periodic phone calls, lunches, notes, and so forth allows you to use and be used by your network to help clients. Networks are strengthened by your being willing to serve the people in your network and not hesitating to ask for advice or favors from your network. It is also helpful to your clients to be networked with the local social service agencies in your community. Calling or visiting agencies to ask what they do and share what you do will allow you to provide better community access for your clients.

Diversity

Be sensitive to issues of diversity in all aspects of your practice. Do the demographics of your group practice reflect the community in which you live? Have you been sensitive to issues of diversity in each aspect of service delivery?

Responsibility

If something is not going well in the practice, chances are it has something to do with you. Are you responsive to clients and staff requests? Are you timely? Are you credible as a provider? Do you follow through with what you promised? Are you competent? Do you have personnel problems that you are avoiding? Taking responsibility means feeling accountable for everything that affects the quality of your practice.

SUMMARY

A variety of marketing interventions for behavioral health care providers in private practice has been discussed through a focus on quality service provision. Many other marketing interventions are possible, such as advertisement, promotions, pricing adjustments, announcements, sales meetings, open houses, and so forth. It is the contention of this contribution, however, that many psychologists can become better marketers by attending to what they are both comfortable with and committed to: namely, helping others through quality service.

CONTRIBUTOR

John R. Rudisill, PhD, is Director and Professor of the Division of Applied Psychology, Department of Family Medicine, Wright State University School of Medicine. Dr. Rudisill is managing partner of a large private practice and has written published articles on practice management. Dr. Rudisill may be contacted at The Division of Applied Psychology, Department of Family Medicine, One Franciscan Way, Dayton, OH 45408. E-mail: john.rudisill@wright.edu

RESOURCES

American Psychological Association Practice Directorate as part of the APA Practitioner's Toolbox Series. (1996). *Marketing Your Practice.* Washington, DC: American Psychological Association.

Bloom, P. N. (1984, September-October). Effective marketing for professional services. *Harvard Business Review, 62*(51), 102-110.

David, J. (1997). Deciding what services to provide: Behavioral healthcare product planning and market research. *Behavioral Healthcare Tomorrow, 6,* 61-66.

Holland, J. L. (1985). *Making Vocational Choices.* Englewood Cliffs, NJ: Prentice-Hall.

Klein, H. E. (1983). How to improve the marketing of therapy services. In P. A. Keller & L. G. Ritt (Eds.), *Innovations in Clinical Practice: A Source Book* (Vol. 2, pp. 233-241). Sarasota, FL: Professional Resource Exchange.

Kotler, P. (1992). *Marketing Management* (8th ed.). Englewood Cliffs, NJ: Prentice-Hall.

Maister, D. H. (1993). Quality work doesn't mean quality service. In *Managing the Professional Service Firm* (Part II, Chapter 7, pp. 69-75). New York: Free Press; Toronto: Maxwell MacMillan Canada; New York: Maxwell MacMillan International.

Ridgewood Financial Institute. (1997). *Psychotherapy Finances.* Juno Beach, FL: Author.

Yenney, S. L., & American Psychological Association Practice Directorate. (1994). *Business Strategies for a Caring Profession.* Washington, DC: American Psychological Association.

Introduction to Section III: Assessment Instruments and Office Forms

This section of *Innovations in Clinical Practice* includes various instruments, checklists, and forms for practitioners to use in collecting and organizing information. It reflects the goal of our series to share useful assessment materials. Although some of the items included here have been formally developed and normed, others were designed for informal application and should not be used as formal instruments. We have included them here because we believe they can be used effectively by practitioners to collect information from their clients. We also wish to alert readers to the fact that a number of practical instruments and forms are available in other contributions in this volume. Specifically, the contributions in Section I by Kevin Arnold and Jeff Sherrill, and by Richard Krueger and Meg Kaplan, and in Section IV by Bobby Stinson, II, Robert Friedberg, Richard Page, and Michael Cusack, provide useful forms for practitioners.

The value of forms and instruments depends upon their appropriate application by the clinicians who use them. It is important to emphasize that they are not necessarily designed to generate the types of inferences often associated with more formalized tests that have a long history of use. Readers should recognize the potential as well as the stated limitations to these materials and use them in accordance with accepted ethical principles. It is assumed that anyone who uses these instruments will have a general clinical knowledge of the area being evaluated.

Given the limitations noted previously, we have attempted to insure that the materials that follow include sufficient information to allow readers to evaluate their appropriate application. Certain basic information and instructions have been included with each contribution and, when necessary, the resource sections contain references to more detailed studies. Readers who wish to use such material are advised to obtain the additional resources. If there is a desire to use the material for research purposes, most authors would appreciate being contacted so that data may be shared.

In the first contribution, we present a sample psychotherapist-patient contract that has been prepared by Eric Harris and Bruce Bennett of the American Psychological Association Insurance Trust. The contract addresses such issues as nature of services offered, meeting times, fees, insurance reimbursement, record keeping, and confidentiality. Readers may adapt the contract for their own practices.

In the second contribution of this section, Joanne Davis, Rachel Pallen, Christine DeMaio, and Thomas Jackson describe the development and uses of The Emotional, Sexual, and Spiritual Intimacy Scale. Clinicians may use the scale in couples therapy as a comparison for pretherapy estimates of the three levels of intimacy. The scales may also be used as a pre- and posttherapy assessment tool to determine if the typical goals of increased intimacy have been achieved in therapy.

All clinicians struggle with fee collections and many are unhappy with their success rate. Lawrence Ritt presents policies and a pre-authorization form that are designed to increase fee collections.

Finally, Astra Brantley provides a record form for documenting clinical supervision. The form permits the documentation of the supervisee's clinical work as well as documentation of performance of supervisory tasks and functions.

Psychotherapist-Patient Contract*

Eric A. Harris, Bruce E. Bennett, and APA Insurance Trust

This draft psychotherapist-patient contract has been prepared for two reasons. First, it allows one to comply with the requirement that practitioners have the informed consent of their patients (American Psychological Association, 1992, Standard 4.02). Second, it allows a therapist to establish a legally enforceable business relationship with the patient and avoids risks that such business issues will become the basis of a malpractice suit or an ethics or licensing board complaint. Most commentators suggest that full informed consent is both ethically necessary and a good risk management strategy.

This draft was designed for psychotherapy practices. It can and should be modified to include other practice areas such as psychological evaluations, testing, neuropsychological assessment, family therapy, group psychotherapy, and so on, if these are a part of a practitioner's work.

There is a great diversity of business practices among practitioners. You should redraft the contract to fit your business practices, rather than adjusting your practices to fit the contract. Since regulations and laws governing certain institutions are somewhat different than those governing private practitioners, this contract may also need to be modified before it can be used in hospitals, clinics, or other institutional settings.

This document includes some basic, general language about the risks and benefits of psychotherapy, but these should be supplemented, either in writing or orally, by the therapist on a case by case basis. This approach was selected because the risks and benefits of therapy can vary considerably from case to case. Therefore, it is hard to design a single draft which is appropriate for all situations. For example, it is probably important to have a much more thorough discussion of risks and benefits with those patients considered to be either most difficult or most risky. If one is a group or family therapist, there may also be additional issues that need to be included. The psychotherapist may orally provide whatever additional information is required and make a note in the record about what was said. Of course, this will not be as protective as a signed agreement, but in most cases, it makes the most sense clinically.

This model contract was originally developed for Massachusetts psychologists, however, most of it can be used anywhere. There are two exceptions: (a) patient access to their own records, and (b) the laws and regulations governing therapeutic confidentiality and testimonial privilege and exceptions to these protections of the psychotherapist-patient relationship. The model provides sufficient alternative sections to cover almost all variations regarding record access. However, there is too much variation from state to state in laws governing privilege, confidentiality, and exceptions to both that there should be an adaptation made for each state in which a psychotherapist practices.

The reader is strongly advised to have their personal attorney review their informed consent document prior to implementation. The document should be in compliance with local and state statutes regulating the practice of their profession. It should also avoid language that could be interpreted as a guarantee or implied warranty regarding the services rendered.

What follows is specific draft text that you may adapt for your practice or agency. Sections of the draft where you should insert numbers are designated XX and sections you may want to specially modify are bracketed [with some examples of possible alternate language included within the brackets].

[PLACE ON YOUR LETTERHEAD]

Outpatient Services Contract

Welcome to my practice. This document contains important information about my professional services and business policies. Please read it carefully and jot down any questions that you might have so that we can discuss them at our next meeting. Once you sign this, it will constitute a binding agreement between us.

PSYCHOLOGICAL SERVICES

Psychotherapy is not easily described in general statements. It varies depending on the personality of both the therapist and the patient and the particular problems which the patient brings. There are a number of different approaches which can be utilized to address the problems you hope to address. It is not like visiting a medical doctor, in that *psychotherapy* requires a very active effort on your part. In order to be most successful, you will have to work on things we talk about both during our sessions and at home.

Psychotherapy has both benefits and risks. Risks sometimes include experiencing uncomfortable feelings such as sadness, guilt, anxiety, anger and frustration, loneliness, and helplessness. Psychotherapy often requires discussing unpleasant aspects of your life. Psychotherapy has also been shown to have benefits for people who undertake it. Therapy often leads to a significant reduction in feelings of distress, better relationships, and resolutions of specific problems. But there are no guarantees about what will happen.

Our first few sessions will involve an evaluation of your needs. By the end of the evaluation, I will be able to offer you some initial impressions of what our work will include and an initial treatment plan to follow, if you decide to continue. You should evaluate this information along with your own assessment about whether you feel comfortable working with me. Therapy involves a large commitment of time, money, and energy, so you should be very careful about the therapist you select. If you have questions about my procedures, we should discuss them whenever they arise. If your doubts persist, I will be happy to help you to secure an appropriate consultation with another mental health professional.

MEETINGS

My normal practice is to conduct an evaluation which will last from two to four sessions. During this time, we can both decide whether I am the best person to provide the services which you need in order to meet your treatment objectives. If psychotherapy is initiated, I will usually schedule one 50-minute session (one appointment hour of 50 minutes duration) per week at a mutually agreed time, although sometimes sessions will be longer or more frequent. Once this appointment hour is scheduled, you will be expected to pay for it unless you provide XXX hours/days advance notice of cancellation [or unless we both agree that you were unable to attend due to circumstances which were beyond your control]. [If it is possible, I will try to find another time to reschedule the appointment.]

PROFESSIONAL FEES

My hourly fee is $XXX. In addition to weekly appointments, it is my practice to charge this amount on a prorated basis for other professional services you may require such as report writing, telephone conversations which last longer than XX minutes, attendance at meetings or consultations with other professionals which you have authorized, preparation of records or treatment summaries, or the time required to perform any other service which you may request of me. If you become involved in litigation which requires my participation, you will be expected to pay for the professional time required even if I am compelled to testify by another party. [Because of the complexity and difficulty of legal involvement, I charge $XXX per hour for preparation for and attendance at any legal proceeding.]

BILLING AND PAYMENTS

You will be expected to pay for each session at the time it is held, unless we agree otherwise or unless you have insurance coverage which requires another arrangement. Payment schedules for other professional services will be agreed to at the time these services are requested. [In circumstances of unusual financial hardship, I may be willing to negotiate a fee adjustment or installment payment plan.]

If your account is more than 60 days in arrears and suitable arrangements for payment have not been agreed to, I have the option of using legal means to secure payment, including collection agencies or small claims court. [If such legal action is necessary, the costs of bringing that proceeding will be included in the claim.] In most cases, the only information which I release about a patient's treatment would be the patient's name, the nature of the services provided, and the amount due.

INSURANCE REIMBURSEMENT

In order for us to set realistic treatment goals and priorities, it is important to evaluate what resources are available to pay for your treatment. If you have a health insurance policy, it will usually provide some coverage for mental health treatment. I will provide you with whatever assistance I can in facilitating your receipt of the benefits to which you are entitled including filling out forms as appropriate. However, you, and not your insurance company, are responsible for full payment of the fee which we have agreed to. Therefore, it is very important that you find out exactly what mental health services your insurance policy covers.

You should carefully read the section in your insurance coverage booklet which describes mental health services. If you have questions, you should call your plan administrator and inquire. Of course, I will provide you with whatever information I can based on my experience and will be happy to try to assist you in deciphering the information you receive from your carrier. If necessary to resolve confusion, I am willing to call the carrier on your behalf.

The escalation of the cost of health care has resulted in an increasing level of complexity about insurance benefits which sometimes makes it difficult to determine exactly how much mental health coverage is available. "Managed Health Care Plans" such as HMOs and PPOs often require advance authorization before they will provide reimbursement for mental health services. These plans are often oriented towards a short-term treatment approach designed to resolve specific problems that are interfering with one's usual level of functioning. It may be necessary to seek additional approval after a certain number of sessions. In my experience, while quite a lot can be accomplished in short-term therapy, many patients feel that more services are necessary after insurance benefits expire. [Some managed care plans will not allow me to provide services to you once your benefits are no longer available. If this is the case, I will do my best to find you another provider who will help you continue your psychotherapy.]

You should also be aware that most insurance agreements require you to authorize me to provide a clinical diagnosis, and sometimes additional clinical information such as a treatment plan or summary, or in rare cases, a copy of the entire record. This information will become part of the insurance company files, and, in all probability, some of it will be computerized. All insurance companies claim to keep such information confidential, but once it is in their hands, I have no control over what they do with it. In some cases they may share the information with a national medical information data bank. If you request it, I will provide you with a copy of any report which I submit.

Once we have all of the information about your insurance coverage, we will discuss what we can expect to accomplish with the benefits that are available and what will happen if the insurance benefits run out before you feel ready to end our sessions. It is important to remember that you always have the right to pay for my services yourself and avoid the complexities which are described above.

CONTACTING ME

I am often not immediately available by telephone. While I am usually in my office between 9:00 a.m. and 5:00 p.m., I usually will not answer the phone when I am with a patient. I do have call-in hours at XXXXX on XXXXX. When I am unavailable, my telephone [is answered by an automatic answering machine which I monitor frequently] [is answered by my secretary or answering service who usually know where to reach me] [is answered by my voice mail which I monitor frequently]. I will make every effort to return your call on the same day you make it with the exception of weekends and holidays. If you are difficult to reach, please leave some times when you will be available. [In emergencies, you can try me at my home number.] If you cannot reach me, and you feel that you cannot wait for me to return your call, you should call your family physician or the emergency room at the nearest hospital and ask for the [psychologist or psychiatrist] on call. If I am unavailable for an extended time, I will provide you with the name of a trusted colleague whom you can contact if necessary.

MINORS

If you are under 18 years of age, please be aware that the law may provide your parents with the right to examine your treatment records. It is my policy to request an agreement from parents that they consent to give up access to your records. If they agree, I will provide them only with general information about our work together unless I feel that there is a high risk that you will seriously harm yourself or another, in which case I will notify them of my concern. I will also provide them with a summary of your treatment when it is complete. Before giving them any information I will discuss the matter with you, if possible, and will do the best I can to resolve any objections you may have about what I am prepared to discuss.

CONFIDENTIALITY

In general, the confidentiality of all communications between a patient and a [psychologist, social worker, psychotherapist, etc.] is protected by law, and I can only release information about our work to others with your written permission. However, there are a number of exceptions.

In most judicial proceedings, you have the right to prevent me from providing any information about your treatment. However, in some circumstances such as child custody proceedings and proceedings in which your emotional condition is an important element, a judge may require my testimony if he/she determines that resolution of the issues before him/her demands it.

There are some situations in which I am legally required to take action to protect others from harm, even though that requires revealing some information about a patient's treatment. For example, if I believe that a child, an elderly person, or a disabled person is being abused, I must [may be required to] file a report with the appropriate state agency.

If I believe that a patient is threatening serious bodily harm to another, I am [may be] required to take protective actions, which may include notifying the potential victim, notifying the police, or seeking appropriate hospitalization. If a patient threatens to harm himself/herself, I may be required to seek hospitalization for the patient, or to contact family members or others who can help provide protection.

These situations have rarely arisen in my practice. Should such a situation occur, I will make every effort to fully discuss it with you before taking any action.

I may occasionally find it helpful to consult about a case with other professionals. In these consultations, I make every effort to avoid revealing the identity of my patient. The consultant is, of course, also legally bound to keep the information confidential. Unless you object, I will not tell you about these consultations unless I feel that it is important to our work together.

While this written summary of exceptions to confidentiality should prove helpful in informing you about potential problems, it is important that we discuss any questions or concerns which you may have at our next meeting. The laws governing these issues are quite complex and I am not an attorney. While I am happy to discuss these issues with you, should you need specific advice, formal legal consultation may be desirable. If you request, I will provide you with relevant portions or summaries of the applicable state laws governing these issues.

Your signature below indicates that you have read the information in this document and agree to abide by its terms during our professional relationship.

PROFESSIONAL RECORDS [*Option 1:* For therapists who practice in states that do not require the practitioner to provide patients with access to their records.]

As I am sure you are aware, I am required to keep appropriate records of [the professional services I provide] [your treatment] [our work together]. Because these records contain information which can be misinterpreted by someone who is not a mental health professional, it is my general policy that patients may not review them. However, if you request, I will provide you with a treatment summary unless I believe that to do so would be emotionally damaging. If that is the case, I will be happy to forward the summary to another appropriate mental health professional who is working with you. [This service will be provided without any additional charge.] [You should be aware that this will be treated in the same manner as any other professional (clinical) service and you will be billed accordingly.] [There will be an additional charge for this service.]

PROFESSIONAL RECORDS [*Option 2:* For therapists who practice in states that require the practitioner to provide patients with access to their records unless to do so would cause emotional damage, upset, etc.]

Both law and the standards of my profession require that I keep appropriate treatment records. You are entitled to receive a copy of the records, unless I believe that seeing them would be emotionally damaging, in which case, I will be happy to provide them to an appropriate mental health professional of your choice. Because these are professional records, they can be misinterpreted and/or can be upsetting, so I recommend that we review them together so that we can discuss what they contain. [I am sometimes willing to conduct such a meeting without charge.] Patients will be charged an appropriate fee for any preparation time which is required to comply with an information request.

______________________________ ______________________________

PATIENT PSYCHOTHERAPIST

______________________________ ______________________________

DATE DATE

CONTRIBUTORS

Eric A. Harris, EdD, JD, is a licensed psychologist and attorney. Dr. Harris is a consultant to the American Psychological Association Insurance Trust (APAIT) where he provides risk management service to Trust policyholders. Dr. Harris is the legal counsel to the Massachusetts Psychological Association, where he served as the Director of Professional Affairs for 10 years. He is also a faculty member at the Massachusetts School of Professional Psychology. Dr. Harris is currently a member of American Psychological Association's (APA) Committee on Legal Issues (COLI) and served for many years on the Committee for the Advancement of Professional Practice (CAPP). In the 15 years before Dr. Harris became a consultant to APAIT, he conducted a part-time clinical psychology practice. Dr. Harris has written, consulted, and lectured extensively on risk management and on managed care issues.

Bruce E. Bennett, PhD, is the Executive Director of APAIT and a former member of the APA Board of Directors. Dr. Bennett was instrumental in revising the *APA Ethical Principles of Psychologists and Code of Conduct.* His areas of expertise are in professional liability and risk management, marketing and promoting psychological services, ethics, insurance, and malpractice issues. Dr. Bennett may be contacted at the American Psychological Association Insurance Trust, 750 First Street NE, Suite 605, Washington, DC 20002-4242. Telephone: (800) 477-1200.

RESOURCES

American Psychological Association. (1992). Ethical principles of psychologists and code of conduct. *American Psychologist, 47,* 1597-1611.

Bennett, B. E., Bryant, B. K., VandenBos, G. R., & Greenwood, A. (1990). *Professional Liability and Risk Management.* Washington, DC: American Psychological Association.

Berglas, S., & Levendusky, P. G. (1985). The Therapeutic Contract Program: An individual-oriented psychological treatment community. *Psychotherapy, 22,* 36-45.

Greene, G. L. (1989). Using the written contract for evaluating and enhancing practice effectiveness. *Journal of Independent Social Work, 4,* 135-155.

Koocher, G. P., & Keith-Spiegel, P. C. (1998). *Ethics in Psychology: Professional Standards and Cases* (2nd ed.). London: Oxford University Press.

Miller, L. J. (1990). The formal treatment contract in the inpatient management of borderline personality disorder. *Hospital & Community Psychiatry, 41,* 985-987.

Selzer, M. A., Koenigsberg, H. W., & Kernberg, O. F. (1987). The initial contract in the treatment of borderline patients. *American Journal of Psychiatry, 144,* 927-930.

Yoemans, F. E., Selzer, M. A., & Clarkin, J. F. (1992). *Treating the Borderline Patient: A Contract-Based Approach.* New York: Basic Books.

The Emotional, Sexual, and Spiritual Intimacy Scale (ESSI)

Joanne L. Davis, Rachel J. Pallen,
Christine M. DeMaio, and Thomas L. Jackson

INTRODUCTION

According to provisional data, the divorce rate per 1,000 population for the entire United States was 4.2 in 1998 (Centers for Disease Control and Prevention, 1999). Information gathered on the impact of divorce suggests significant negative consequences including increased risk for alcoholism, depression, suicide, and mental and physical health problems for the adults and children involved (Stanton, 1997). In light of the high rates and negative impact of divorce, it has become increasingly important for professionals and the lay public to gain greater understanding of why some relationships fail and others succeed.

Researchers in the social sciences are beginning to investigate inter- and intrapersonal factors that may increase the probability of long, healthy, and happy relationships. Intimacy is one factor that has been explored in attempts to answer this question. One of the primary difficulties in conducting research on intimacy, however, is the multitude of definitions that researchers have used. The various definitions limit one's ability to compare results across studies. A second difficulty has been the limited scope of definitions and the subsequent effect on the assessment instruments developed to measure intimacy. That is, the majority of measures focus on emotional aspects of intimacy, excluding consideration of other, perhaps equally important components of intimate relationships.

Researchers in the fields of social psychology have long debated the definition of intimacy. In the past, a common assumption was that certain types of relationships were equated with certain levels of intimacy. For example, it was believed that a married couple would report greater intimacy than a dating couple. However, society in general and researchers in particular can no longer assume this to be true. The rates of child maltreatment, domestic violence, and divorce suggest that the status of the relationship may in fact have little to do with the level of intimacy within that relationship (Berscheid, Snyder, & Omoto, 1989). Recently, researchers have increased efforts to define intimacy and to identify mechanisms associated with greater or lesser degrees of intimacy within relationships.

The various definitions of intimacy typically incorporate three general themes, although the specific dimensions vary greatly. Perlman and Fehr (1987) state that these themes are "the closeness and interdependence of partners, the extent of self-disclosure, and the warmth or affection experienced" (p. 16). Based on a comprehensive review of the literature, Prager (1995) maintained that intimacy is best to be considered a superordinate concept that is comprised of several subordinate concepts. In particular, she distinguished between intimate interactions and intimate relationships. Intimate interactions are defined by the following characteristics: (a) both partners reveal something personal or private; (b) both partners experience positive feelings about themselves and the other person; and (c) both partners perceive a mutual understanding between them (Prager, 1995). This three-component definition of intimate interactions accounts for the behaviors, experiences, and perceptions that are commonly identified within intimate relationships. These include touching, holding, verbalizing affection, affectionate touching, attentive listening, and genuine validation.

Confusion surrounding the definition of intimacy has led to the development of many different measures purported to be measures of "intimacy," but such measures may be gauging different constructs. The purpose of the studies leading to this contribution was to develop a measure of intimacy that incorporated constructs commonly identified in individuals reporting strong, close, intimate bonds with others, based on Prager's (1995) conceptualization, as well as constructs identified amongst individuals reporting significant dysfunction and dissatisfaction within their relationships. Further, we wanted to broaden the intimate constructs assessed by incorporating emotional, sexual, and spiritual aspects of interpersonal relationships. The initial items (*N* = 94) for The Emotional, Sexual, and Spiritual Intimacy Scale (ESSI) were developed by the authors through an examination of themes of intimacy in the clinical and empirical literature investigating both functional and dysfunctional interpersonal relationships. The items were chosen to represent three aspects of interpersonal relationships: emotional, sexual, and spiritual intimacy. The items were presented on a 6-point, forced-choice continuum scale for which respondents were asked to indicate how strongly they agreed with each statement as it related to their relationship (i.e., 1 = Strongly Disagree, 6 = Strongly Agree). Participants were asked to respond for their current relationship, or if they were not presently in a relationship, their most recent relationship. Following the scale, participants were asked whether they responded for a current or past relationship, as previous research has found significant differences for this variable (Davis, 1996). Because a significant proportion of participants, particularly younger ones were possibly not yet sexually active, we were concerned about the response rates to the sexual items. In an attempt to increase the response frequencies for these items, the terms "sexual activity" and "sexual intimacy" were used and a broad definition of these terms was provided (i.e., "For the purposes of this scale, sexual activity and sexual intimacy include: fondling, oral, genital, or other sexual contact with or by another person"). The participants also had the option of responding "Not Applicable" to individual items. A high total score on the ESSI indicates a high degree of perceived general intimacy. High scores on the individual factors speak to the respective aspects of intimacy.

Two studies on the ESSI were conducted. The purpose of the first study (*N* = 199) was to develop test items. The second study (*N* = 194) was conducted to establish the psychometric properties of the refined scale. The studies eventually resulted in a final 44-item scale (see pp. 292-293), based on a rational-empirical procedure of item analysis. Participant scores on the final 44-item ESSI ranged from 59 to 255 with a mean score of 190.94 (*SD* = 36.22). Internal consistency for the total scale was demonstrated by an alpha coefficient of .94.

Total scale differences were found on the ESSI as a function of relationship status. Single participants reported significantly lower intimacy than all other groups. Further, married participants reported significantly higher intimacy than those dating several people and those in exclusive relationships.

A principal component factor analysis with nonorthogonal rotation was conducted on the data, resulting in three factors. The three factors accounted for approximately 65% of the variance with alphas of .95, .97, and .94 respectively. Clearly, these findings suggest that the ESSI represents a psychometrically sound measure.

THE ESSI FACTORS

The first factor, Emotional Intimacy (EI), is defined by 19 items sampling the degree of closeness and comfort one feels toward her or his partner. The emotional intimacy items include statements such as "I tell my partner my innermost thoughts" and "When I feel upset I want my partner to comfort me." In the combined sample, this factor yielded a mean score of 4.98 (*SD* = 0.89), with women having reported significantly higher mean EI scores (*M* = 5.14, *SD* = .84) than did men (*M* = 4.81, *SD* = .93). Significant differences were also found for relationship status, with single participants (*M* = 4.59, *SD* = .91) and those dating several people (*M* = 4.83, *SD* = .68) having scored significantly lower on the EI factor than did those participants in exclusive relationships (*M* = 5.24, *SD* = .85) or those who were married (*M* = 5.57, *SD* = .67). The single group did not differ from those who reported dating several people.

The second factor, Sexual Intimacy (SXI), is defined by 14 items sampling satisfaction, pleasure, and comfort with the sexual aspect of one's relationship. The SXI items include statements such as "My sexual needs are fulfilled by my partner" and "I communicate to my partner what I like and dislike sexually." The combined sample SXI yielded a mean score of 4.16 (*SD* = 1.61). Significant differences were revealed by relationship status, with the single group (*M* = 3.12, *SD* = 1.87) scoring significantly lower than those dating several people (*M* = 4.74, *SD* = .78), those in exclusive relationships (*M* = 4.58, *SD* = 1.27), and the married group (*M* = 5.36, *SD* = .58).

The third factor, Spiritual Intimacy (SPI) is defined by 11 items assessing both attitudes regarding the importance of spirituality in one's intimate relationships and the degree of spiritual intimacy within one's current relationship. The SPI items include statements such as, "Spirituality is a necessary part of my relationship" and "I feel closer to my partner when we go to church or pray together." In the standardization sample, this factor yielded a mean score of 3.45 (*SD* = 1.35). No differences were found by gender or relationship status.

DISCUSSION AND APPLICATIONS

Analysis of the ESSI yielded three factors of intimate relatedness. The first factor, emotional intimacy, assesses the perceived level of communication and affective expression in the targeted relationship. The second factor, sexual intimacy, provides a measure of the level of sexual satisfaction and perceived physical closeness with partners. The third factor, spiritual intimacy, gauges the level of importance placed on spiritual interconnectedness within the interpersonal relationship, as well as one's general attitude toward spirituality within relationships.

The external validity of the present study is limited due to the college sample, however, a study currently underway using the ESSI with functional and dysfunctional couples from the community is demonstrating identical results to those already found and hypothesized. Although the ESSI is still in development, the items will not change in the future, it is psychometrically sound across samples, and it continues to provide intuitively reasonable results that are consistent with previous research. It is felt that this scale may be added to other extant measures to more comprehensively assess the strengths and weaknesses of relationships in both research and clinical realms.

Clinical Use of the ESSI

A scoring template and scoring instructions are included on pages 294 to 295. Clinicians, while advised to use the ESSI with the caution it deserves as a still-developing device, may wish to utilize this scale in three basic ways. First, in the case of couples therapy, the ESSI may be used as a pretherapy comparison between partners' estimates of the three different areas of intimacy as well as global intimacy in their current relationships. Secondly, the ESSI seems a natural as a pre- and posttherapy assessment tool to determine if the typical goals of increased intimacy have been successfully addressed as a function of the therapeutic process and orientation. Finally, each of the 44 questions can serve as a single discussion item for individuals or couples as clients to further explore areas of agreement, disparity, or an area in need of improvement. In the meantime, the ESSI will continue to be developed on clinical populations, as a measure of change process, and as a discriminator among salient groups and individuals.

The Emotional, Sexual, and Spiritual Intimacy Scale (ESSI)

The following questions concern emotional and sexual behaviors and attitudes. For the purposes of this scale, sexual activity and sexual intimacy include: fondling, oral, genital, or other sexual contact with or by another person. Please indicate your level of agreement/disagreement with each statement (see example below). If you have never been sexually active, *answer as many questions as apply to you* and indicate with a "NA" those that do not apply. If you are not currently in a relationship, please refer to your most recent relationship.

EXAMPLE:

Strongly Disagree 1	2	3	4	5	Strongly Agree 6	Not Applicable NA

3 45. I find my partner attractive.

Strongly Disagree 1	**2**	**3**	**4**	**5**	**Strongly Agree 6**	**Not Applicable NA**

_____ 1. Our religious beliefs are an important topic of discussion.
_____ 2. I feel closer to my partner after sexual activity.
_____ 3. I tell my partner my innermost thoughts.
_____ 4. It is important that my partner and I share the same religious beliefs.
_____ 5. I feel comfortable with my partner.
_____ 6. My sexual needs are fulfilled by my partner.
_____ 7. I enjoy thinking about my partner.
_____ 8. My relationship is healthy because religion and spirituality are involved.
_____ 9. My partner and I are sexually spontaneous.
_____ 10. I feel close to my partner.
_____ 11. Taking time for spiritual meditation increases the tranquility within my relationship.
_____ 12. I feel "oneness" with my partner during sexual activity.
_____ 13. My partner listens to me.
_____ 14. I trust my partner.
_____ 15. My partner understands me.
_____ 16. I feel satisfied when my partner does things to please me sexually.
_____ 17. I feel comfortable expressing my feelings to my partner.
_____ 18. I display affection towards my partner.
_____ 19. I believe I fulfill my partner's sexual needs.
_____ 20. My partner and I are open to sexual exploration.
_____ 21. My relationship with my partner is based on spirituality.
_____ 22. My partner and I hold similar values and goals.
_____ 23. In relationships, I aim toward shared spirituality.

Strongly Disagree					**Strongly Agree**	**Not Applicable**
1	**2**	**3**	**4**	**5**	**6**	**NA**

______ 24. I value the time I spend with my partner.
______ 25. When I feel upset I want my partner to comfort me.
______ 26. I comfort my partner when he or she is upset.
______ 27. When I have a problem I talk about it with my partner.
______ 28. I am able to be myself with my partner.
______ 29. I communicate to my partner what I like and dislike sexually.
______ 30. My partner and I share things about ourselves equally.
______ 31. My spirituality is the most important aspect of my intimate relationship.
______ 32. I enjoy pleasing my partner sexually.
______ 33. Spirituality is a necessary part of my relationship.
______ 34. I believe my partner accepts me for who I am.
______ 35. I accept my partner for who he/she is.
______ 36. I enjoy surprising my partner sexually.
______ 37. I listen to my partner.
______ 38. My partner pleases me sexually.
______ 39. I become sexually aroused when I see my partner.
______ 40. My relationship is sexually satisfying.
______ 41. Religion is not important in my intimate relationship.
______ 42. I am more attracted to my partner when we discuss our spiritual beliefs.
______ 43. I feel closer to my partner when we go to church or pray together.
______ 44. I feel accepted by my partner during sexual activity.

Do Not Write Below This Line

MEAN FACTOR SCORES

EI	[ ]	Rated Range: High / Medium / Low
SXI	[ ]	Rated Range: High / Medium / Low
SPI	[ ]	Rated Range: High / Medium / Low
TOTAL NONMEAN SCORE	[ ]	Rated Range: High / Medium / Low

Scoring Template for ESSI

In order to score the ESSI, it is necessary to calculate three mean factor scores; one each for Emotional, Sexual, and Spiritual intimacy, as well as a total (nonmean) Intimacy score. To calculate the means, the "Agreement-Disagreement" numbers on the individual items are added and then divided by the number of items that were *not* answered "Not Applicable" (NA). In general, assuming that there are no NA answers, there are 19 Emotional items, 14 Sexual items, and 11 Spiritual items. For each NA answer, the number of items to divide into the total factor score decreases by one. The template below will simplify the scoring procedure. Please note that one Spiritual item (#41) must be reverse-scored. Representative male, female, single, and married means and standard deviations are provided in the text.

Means and Standard Deviations for the Standardization Sample*

Emotional Intimacy Overall Mean Score = 4.98 (*SD* = 0.89)
Sexual Intimacy Overall Mean = 4.16 (*SD* = 1.61)
Spiritual Intimacy Overall Mean = 3.45 (*SD* = 1.35)
Mean Overall Total Score (All 44 Intimacy Scale Items) = 190.94 (*SD* = 36.22)

*See text for significant group differences and directions for relative patient comparisons.

FACTOR	ITEM NUMBER	ANSWER (level of agreement-disagreement)
Emotional Intimacy (EI)	3	____
	5	____
	7	____
	10	____
	13	____
	14	____
	15	____
	17	____
	18	____
	22	____
	24	____
	25	____
	26	____
	27	____
	28	____
	30	____
	34	____
	35	____
	37	____

A. Total Nonmean **EI** Score (Sum of item scores above) ________

B. 19 - _____ (Number of items answered *NA*) = _____

TOTAL MEAN **EI** FACTOR SCORE = _____ (A) ÷ _____ (B) = [ ]

FACTOR	ITEM NUMBER	ANSWER (level of agreement-disagreement)
Sexual Intimacy (SXI)	2	___
	6	___
	9	___
	12	___
	16	___
	19	___
	20	___
	29	___
	32	___
	36	___
	38	___
	39	___
	40	___
	44	___

A. Total Nonmean **SXI** Score (Sum of item scores above) ______

B. 14 - ____ (Number of items answered *NA*) = ____

TOTAL MEAN **SXI** FACTOR SCORE = ____ (A) ÷ ____ (B) = [ ]

FACTOR	ITEM NUMBER	ANSWER (level of agreement-disagreement)
Spiritual Intimacy (SPI)	1	___
	4	___
	8	___
	11	___
	21	___
	23	___
	31	___
	33	___
	41-R	___ (#41 is reverse-scored: 1 = 6; 2 = 5; 3 = 4; 4 = 3; 5 = 2; 6 = 1)
	42	___
	43	___

A. Total Nonmean **SPI** Score (Sum of item scores above) ______

B. 11 - ____ (Number of items answered *NA*) = ____

TOTAL MEAN **SPI** FACTOR SCORE = ____ (A) ÷ ____ (B) = [ ]

TOTAL NONMEAN EI SCORE (A) ____
TOTAL NONMEAN SXI SCORE (A) + ____
TOTAL NONMEAN SPI SCORE (A) + ____

OVERALL TOTAL NONMEAN INTIMACY SCORE
(The Sum of All 44 Intimacy Scale Items Except NA Items) [ ]

CONTRIBUTORS

Joanne L. Davis, PhD, is a postdoctoral fellow at the National Crime Victims Research and Treatment Center at the Medical University of South Carolina. Her training is in clinical psychology with special interests in the area of victimization and violence. She has published articles and presented at numerous national conferences on these topics. Dr. Davis may be contacted at 171 Ashley Avenue, National Crime Victims Research and Treatment Center, Medical University of South Carolina, Charleston, SC 29425.

Rachel J. Pallen, MA, is a Psychology Intern at the VA Medical Center in Columbia, Missouri. Her research and clinical interests include intimacy, couples treatment, and issues related to victimization. Ms. Pallen can be reached at the Harry S. Truman VAMC, Psychology Service, Columbia, MO 65201.

Christine M. DeMaio, MA, is an advanced graduate student in the clinical psychology doctoral program at the University of Arkansas. Her research and clinical interests include intrafamilial violence; in particular, treatment of incestuous families and psychopathy. Ms. DeMaio may be reached at the Department of Psychology, 216 Memorial Hall, University of Arkansas, Fayetteville, AR 72701.

Thomas L. Jackson, PhD, is Professor and Director of Clinical Training in the Department of Psychology at the University of Arkansas. His research and clinical interests include the areas of sexual assault and violence and have resulted in over 50 articles, chapters, and books including *Acquantaince Rape: Assessment, Treatment, and Prevention.* He has also consulted and presented papers to over 70 regional, national, and international groups. Dr. Jackson is a Fellow in Division 12 (Clinical) of the American Psychological Association as well as in the American Association of Applied and Preventive Psychology, the Association of State and Provincial Psychology Boards, and is Past Chair of the Committee of Accreditation of the American Psychological Association. Dr. Jackson can be contacted at the Center for Research on Aggression and Violence, 115 Memorial Hall, University of Arkansas, Fayetteville, AR 72701.

RESOURCES

Berscheid, E., Snyder, M., & Omoto, A. M. (1989). Issues in studying close relationships: Conceptualizing and measuring closeness. In C. Hendrick (Ed.), *Close Relationships: Review of Personality and Social Psychology* (Vol. 10, pp. 63-91). Newbury Park, CA: Sage.

Centers for Disease Control and Prevention. (1999). *National Vital Statistics Reports, 47*(21). U.S. Department of Health and Human Services (PHS) 99-1120.

Davis, J. L. (1996). *An Examination of the Interpersonal Functioning of Adult Survivors of Childhood Sexual Abuse.* Unpublished master's thesis, University of Arkansas, Fayetteville, AR.

Perlman, D., & Fehr, B. (1987). The development of intimate relationships. In D. Perlman & S. Duck (Eds.), *Intimate Relationships: Development, Dynamics, and Deterioration* (pp. 13-42). Newbury Park, CA: Sage.

Prager, K. J. (1995). *The Psychology of Intimacy.* New York: Guilford.

Stanton, G. T. (1997). *Why Marriage Matters: Reasons to Believe in Marriage in Post-Modern Society.* Colorado Springs, CO: Pinon Press.

Pre-Authorization Forms And Policies for Increasing Fee Collections

Lawrence G. Ritt

The "Our Financial Policy" form (p. 298) and the "Pre-Authorized Health Care Form" (p. 299) are designed to inform your patients of their financial obligations and increase your chance of receiving full payment even when their insurance company refuses to pay or pays less than your customary fees. These forms are particularly useful for practitioners who are willing to accept insurance reimbursement as a courtesy to their patients but have not signed on as providers in a patient's managed care plan and do not automatically accept the allowable fees and co-payment allowed by the insurer. It also alleviates the problems that sometimes occur when patients do not pay their co-payment.

The "Our Financial Policy" form explains to your patients that, if they have insurance, 20% of your charges will be due at the time of visits and full payment will be due from them or their insurance company within 45 days thereafter.

The "Pre-Authorized Health Care Form" provides written authorization for you to charge the patient's credit card account if payment is not received in a timely fashion. If you do not currently have a credit card merchant account for processing patient charges, your local bank can assist you in setting up such an account.

Be sure to keep the original copy of these forms with patient records and give a copy to your patients for their records.

[PUT ON YOUR OWN LETTERHEAD]

Our Financial Policy

- Full payment or guarantee of payment is due at the time of each visit.
- We accept cash, check, Visa/MasterCard/Discover/American Express

REGARDING INSURANCE*

Your insurance policy is a contract between you and your insurance company and we are not a party to that contract. Please be aware that some (perhaps all) of the services we provide may be noncovered services in your contract with your insurance company.

In order to accept assignment of insurance benefits, we require your authorization to charge your credit card account for the balance of charges not paid by your insurance company. We also require that 20% of your fee be paid at the time of service (100% will be required without your credit card authorization). Our office manager will provide the necessary authorization form for your signature. Any unpaid balance is your responsibility whether your insurance company pays us or not. After we have received payment from your insurance company, you will be mailed a statement in our regular billing cycle for any unpaid balance. If the result is an overpayment, we will immediately reimburse you. If your insurance company unnecessarily delays your claim or you do not respond to your statement before the next billing cycle (approximately 30 days), your credit card will be charged (as per the signed agreement) and a copy of the transaction will be mailed to you.

With your written consent and authorization, we will release a diagnosis, itemized list of services, and charges to your insurance company. If you or your insurance company require reports or information, we will provide such information with your authorization and will charge you for the time required to prepare the reports or otherwise communicate with your insurance company.

USUAL, CUSTOMARY, AND ALLOWABLE CHARGES

Usual, customary, and allowable charges are insurance company terms for the *benefits allowed in your plan.* We are committed to providing the best treatment possible for patients and our fees reflect what is usual and customary for mental health specialists in our area with our level of training and experience. You are responsible for payment of our fees regardless of any insurance company's determination of what they consider to be usual, customary, and allowable charges.

Thank you for understanding and agreeing to abide by these policies. Please let us know if you have questions or concerns.

______________________________ ____________________

Signature of Patient or Responsible Party   Date

*For the purposes of this and other agreements prepared by our office, "Insurance" and "Insurance Company" refer to any third party that might accept responsibility for paying some or all of your health care costs, including but not limited to HMOs, PPOs, other health care plans, employers, current and former spouses, and so forth.

[PUT ON YOUR OWN LETTERHEAD]

Pre-Authorized Health Care Form

As the patient named below (or person responsible for payment of this patient's fees), I hereby authorize (name of provider) to keep my signature on file and to charge my credit card account for the balance of charges not paid by insurance within forty-five (45) working days after the date that a claim is filed.

I assign my insurance benefits to the provider listed above.

I understand that this form is valid for three (3) years unless I cancel the authorization through written notice to the health care provider named above.

____
Patient Name

____
Responsible Party (If Not Patient)

____
Cardholder Name (Name on Credit Card)

____
Cardholder Billing Address

____
City State Zip

______________________________ ______________
Credit Card Account Number Expiration Date

______________________________ ______________
Cardholder Signature Date

CONTRIBUTOR

Lawrence G. Ritt, PhD, is president of Professional Resource Press, publisher of the *Innovations in Clinical Practice: A Source Book* series and other applied resources for mental health practitioners. He is a licensed psychologist who maintained a full-time independent clinical psychology practice in Sarasota, Florida from 1974-1999. Dr. Ritt may be contacted at Professional Resource Press, P.O. Box 15560, Sarasota, FL 34277-1560.

A Clinical Supervision Documentation Form

Astra P. Brantley

The Clinical Supervision Notes Record Form (CSNRF) was designed for documentation during the supervision of psychotherapy work. The CSNRF has been under development since 1989. The purpose of the CSNRF is twofold: it permits the documentation of the Supervisee's clinical work with clients as well as documentation of performance of oversight tasks and functions. The CSNRF facilitates the efforts of the clinical Supervisor to adhere to the ethical standards of many mental health professions and regulatory bodies that delineate clinical Supervisors' accountability for monitoring and evaluating the skill acquisition and professional conduct of therapists-in-training (Barnett, 1991; Bridge & Bascue, 1988; Neufeldt, Iversen, & Juntunen, 1995; Williams, 1995).

The CSNRF is a one-page, two-sided form; the front of the page contains Part I: Therapeutic Intervention Report, and the back of the page contains Part II: Supervision Notes. An optional supplemental second page is provided for instances in which the Supervisee (S-ee) and/or the Supervisor (S-or) identify special concerns.

Part I is completed by the Supervisee prior to the supervision session; it details dates of service, issues discussed in therapy sessions, client's response to interventions, and proposed future actions. During the supervisory session or immediately upon its conclusion, the Supervisor completes Part II on the back of the page. Part II includes recommended supplemental training such as books, films, tapes, videos, and so on, observations of the Supervisee's self-awareness/countertransference issues, and the supervisory focus for the current session. A copy of the completed CSNRF is made available to the Supervisee at the end of the supervisory session. The CSNRF fosters accountability in both the Supervisee and Supervisor, facilitates recall from one session to the next session, and creates a database that can be used in comprehensive overviews for interim and final evaluations of the Supervisee. The CSNRF can be used to record the supervision of individual, marital and family, and group therapy activities.

PART I: THERAPEUTIC INTERVENTION REPORT

Part I of the Therapeutic Intervention Report, which has seven sections, is completed by the Supervisee prior to the supervision session, and begins with basic information about the Supervisee and the client.

In the upper-right-hand corner, the Supervisee enters the **DATE __/__/__** that the form is completed. In addition to the Supervisee's name and basic identifying information about the client, space is available for the Supervisee to enter the specific types of clinical services and dates these services were performed as follows:

SERVICE(S):	**DATES OF SERVICE:**
Initial Diagnostic Interview	**5/2/97**
Psychotherapy	**5/9/97, 5/16/97, 5/23/97, 5/30/97**

The next section to be completed by the Supervisee is called **Special Concerns.** This section provides the opportunity for the Supervisee to "red flag" critical risk-management issues. These "red flag" issues require that some precautionary means be taken and be carefully documented for future reference. For example, if the issue is **Suicide**, the Supervisor needs to insure that the Supervisee assessed suicidal risk (i.e., whether the client has a clearly articulated plan for self-annihilation, has the availability of some lethal means to carry out the proposed plan, has a suicide note planned or crafted, and/or some other preparation such as disposing of personal possessions). The final clinically significant factor that should enter into a determination of suicide risk is the client's willingness to outline a detailed contract for safety. Documentation should clearly distinguish between client suicidal ideation and a person with a serious intent as reflected in a plan for suicide. **Ethical/Sexual Allegations Precautions** might include working in a room with a one-way mirror or leaving the door ajar. **Health** and/or **Psychiatric/Neuropsychological** issues require referrals, and the results of the referrals should be documented.

Under the next heading, the Supervisee has the opportunity to designate information that was the catalyst for the client's seeking therapy. **Reason(s) for Referral, Issues Generated in Session, and Therapeutic Intervention Implemented** are provided for the Supervisee to succinctly identify up to three reasons for referral or therapeutic issues, and to highlight the therapeutic actions taken.

The section that logically follows, **Client's Response to Intervention(s) and Overall Progress** allows for the Supervisee to highlight the client's response to intervention or the client's progress on the previously identified issues in the preceding section.

Additional Information provides space for any other remarkable aspects of the case not allotted for in the preceding five sections.

Finally, in the last section, **Future Plans**, the Supervisee specifies how the Supervisee would go about addressing the unresolved issues from the "Issues Generated . . ." Section, prior to supervisory input.

PART II: SUPERVISION NOTES

In Part II, the Supervisor completes Supervision Notes. It includes six sections, and the last portion is for the Supervisor's signature and date of the supervision session.

The first section, intended for the Supervisor's priority consideration, notes whether any Special Concerns were identified by the Supervisee *or* if, in the Supervisor's opinion, based on the details that were revealed in the Supervisee's case presentation, a special concern exists. If special concerns are present, then the optional **Special Concerns Supplement** is used to document the precautionary measures to be taken by the Supervisee (and Supervisor, if applicable).

The **Special Concerns Supplement** should be a complete documentation of the special concerns, capable of being used independently of Part I and Part II of the CSNRF.

The section immediately following the **Special Concerns** section is labeled **Supporting Data**. This section allows for the identification of some documents related to the case being reviewed by the Supervisor. The Supervisee is expected to use the actual **Case Record** or any part thereof, including progress notes, mental status forms, therapy, and/or termination summaries in order to illustrate the basis for his or her case conceptualization/clinical intervention. The part of the case record used is documented in this section. Space is also available to note if either an **Audiotape or Videotape** was produced and the date of the taping. If any other materials are reviewed during the supervision session, such as psychological or medical test results, records from a hospital admission or a previous therapist or even a genogram, these may be identified under **Other**.

The Supervisor proceeds from **Supporting Data** to the section entitled **General Supervision Comments and Process Observations**. This section is to be utilized for entering information related to the key elements of the supervision relationship - the contract, the phase, or the structure (Holloway, 1995). Some examples of contract issues might be: "Did the Supervisee prepare the CSNRF for the supervision session as agreed upon?" "Is the Supervisor available at the specified time?" Based upon the phase of development of the supervision relationship, either Beginning, Mature, or Terminating, certain issues are more likely to be evinced in the supervisory interaction. Finally, the structure of the supervision relationship primarily refers to the power difference in the relationship and the various types of power exercised, for instance, social, referent, and expert. Some structure issues might be: "Is the Supervisor knowledgeable about the differential diagnostic issues?" "Is the Supervisor able to facilitate referrals?" **Process Observation** issues would include if a Supervisee appears to be uncooperative, or confused, or to convey some other feelings or behaviors that influence the quality of the supervision session. Some Supervisors might use this area to identify process characteristics that are similar to those occurring between the Supervisee and the client.

The **Supervisee Self-Awareness** section is for entering the Supervisor's assessment of the Supervisee's perceptions with regard to his or her own personality characteristics and personal growth issues that might have impact upon the course of treatment. The issues recorded will depend upon the theoretical orientation of the Supervisor, but some examples might include issues related to countertransference themes, defense mechanisms, or elements of family systems theory, based upon whatever is most pertinent in describing the therapist factors (Holloway, 1995) of the Supervisee and their possible influence on the development of a therapeutic alliance, treatment strategies, and criteria for termination.

Three subdivisions are included in the **Supervision Focus** section. The purpose of this is to allow the Supervisor to give a succinct overview of the primary supervision targets for this session. The contents of this section should logically flow from all the previous sections in both Part I and Part II of the CSNRF. The first subdivision of this section requires the Supervisor to indicate the **Skills/Clinical Competence** of the Supervisee targeted for discussion during this supervisory session. Choices Supervisor may select from include **Counseling Skills, Case Conceptualization, Professional Role, Emotional Awareness,** and **Self-Evaluation** (Holloway, 1995). A line before each clinical competence allows the Supervisor to place an "X" when indicating its selection or a numeral (1, 2, 3) indicating the priority given each of the several skills/clinical competencies. If any skill/clinical competence was not significantly discussed, the Supervisor should leave the space blank.

The second subdivision of this section is entitled **Issues**. Here issues central to the skills/clinical competencies identified in the previous subdivision may be enumerated. Parsimony is advised, thus one Supervisor's ideas should be communicated accurately and effectively in a bullet manner. If only one skill/clinical competence was selected in the preceding subdivision, then the issues may be written "Difficulty with empathy (sex/age)." However, if more than one skill/clinical competence was selected, then the number of the skill/clinical competence should be indicated. If the number "1" had been assigned **_1_ Counseling Skills**, then the issue would be designated "(1) Difficulty with empathy (sex/age)."

The third subdivision under **Supervision Focus** is called **Strategies**. Each strategy elaborated should correspond to an issue identified in the previous subdivision. A strategy for the example being used might include exploring cross-cultural competency using a cultural genogram.

The final section of Part II is intended for identifying resources for the Supervisee's training or continuing education; it is entitled **Recommended Supplemental Training Resources**. Resources may include, but are not limited to, items from the print or visual media, workshops, and consulting with special resource persons.

Clinical Supervision Notes Record Form

PART I: THERAPEUTIC INTERVENTION REPORT

(to be completed by Supervisee)

SUPERVISEE________________________________ DATE_____/_____/_____

CLIENT NAME________________________________ CLIENT NUMBER__________

SERVICE(S): DATES OF SERVICE:

____

____

SPECIAL CONCERNS: Suicide/Violence ❐ Ethical/Sexual Allegations Precautions ❐ Psychiatric/Neuropsychological ❐ Health ❐ Other ❐ Specify: __________

REASON(S) FOR REFERRAL, ISSUES GENERATED IN SESSION, AND THERAPEUTIC INTERVENTION IMPLEMENTED:

1) ____

____

2) ____

____

3) ____

____

CLIENT'S RESPONSE TO INTERVENTION(S) AND OVERALL PROGRESS:

1) ____

____

2) ____

____

3) ____

____

ADDITIONAL INFORMATION:

____

FUTURE PLANS:

PART II: SUPERVISION NOTES

(to be completed by Supervisor)

SPECIAL CONCERNS from reverse side (circle one) **YES** **NO**

SUPPORTING DATA from: Case Record ☐ Audio-Visual Record ☐ Date:______ Other ☐ (specify)____________

GENERAL SUPERVISION COMMENTS AND PROCESS OBSERVATIONS:

____

____

____

SUPERVISEE SELF-AWARENESS/COUNTERTRANSFERENCE ISSUES:

____

____

____

____

SUPERVISION FOCUS:

SKILLS/CLINICAL COMPETENCE:

__ **Counseling Skills**
__ **Professional Role**
__ **Self-Evaluation**
__ **Case Conceptualization**
__ **Emotional Awareness**

ISSUES:

____

____

____

STRATEGIES:

____

____

____

RECOMMENDED SUPPLEMENTAL TRAINING RESOURCES:

SIGNED: DATE:

Clinical Supervision Notes Record Form

SPECIAL CONCERNS SUPPLEMENT

(to be completed by Supervisee)

SUPERVISEE________________________________ DATE______/______/______

CLIENT NAME________________________________ CLIENT NUMBER____________

SPECIAL CONCERNS: Suicide/Violence ☐ Ethical/Sexual Allegations Precautions ☐
Psychiatric/Neuropsychological ☐ Health ☐ Other ☐ Specify: ____________

SUPERVISOR: DATE:

CONTRIBUTOR

Astra P. Brantley, PsyD, is a Licensed Clinical Psychologist in Maryland and the District of Columbia, a National Certified Counselor, and a Certified Christian Conciliator by the Institute for Christian Conciliation. Her specialty areas include extended family psychotherapy, Christian/Biblical counseling and care, and the clinical supervision of other practitioners, including clergy. Dr. Brantley received her BA in Psychology from DePaul University, her MSEd degree in Guidance and Counseling from Chicago State University, and her doctoral degree in Clinical Psychology from Central Michigan University. She is a member of the American Psychological Association, the American Association of Christian Counselors, and the Maryland Psychological Association, among others, and is listed in the National Register for Psychologists. Dr. Brantley may be contacted at The Brantley Group, 601 N. Eutaw Street, Suite #111, Baltimore, MD 21201-4527. E-mail: BrantleyGroup@maranatha.net

RESOURCES

Barnett, J. (1991, May/June). Ethical Guidelines for Documentation in Psychotherapy and Supervision. *The Maryland Psychologist, 5*(6), 7-9.

Bridge, P. J., & Bascue, L. O. (1988). A record form for psychotherapy supervisors. In P. A. Keller & S. R. Heyman (Eds.), *Innovations in Clinical Practice: A Source Book* (Vol. 7, pp. 331-336). Sarasota, FL: Professional Resource Exchange.

Holloway, E. (1995). *Clinical Supervision: A Systems Approach.* Thousand Oaks, CA: Sage.

Neufeldt, S. A., Iversen, J. N., & Juntunen, C. L. (1995). *Supervision Strategies for the First Practicum.* Alexandria, VA: The American Counseling Association.

Williams, A. (1995). *Visual and Active Supervision: Roles, Focus, Technique.* New York: W. W. Norton.

Section IV: Community Interventions

Although the primary focus of the *Innovations* series is on clinical interventions, we have always included this section because of our belief that practitioners are at risk for selecting unnecessarily narrow roles that may limit their potential influence on the community. Mental health professionals are, in fact, in excellent positions to address a diversity of problems that are sometimes overlooked by traditional clinicians. We have included five contributions in this realm that take the practitioner out of the typical role in the office.

There is a growing demand to provide clinical services to adolescents who have committed sexual offenses. In the first selection in the section, Garry Perry, Stan Dimnik, Phyllis Ohm, and Brenda Wilks overview a process they use to prepare adolescents for sex offender group treatment.

In the second contribution, William Deardorff reviews procedures for enhancing surgical outcome with psychological preparation. He reviews the literature and the changing medical context within which surgery occurs (e.g., shorter hospital stays, outpatient surgery), and presents a protocol for preparing patients for surgery.

Therapists who work with adolescents know the limitations of traditional practice with this population. Limitations include the confines of an office and the reliance on verbal exchanges. Jennifer Davis-Berman and Dene Berman describe the opportunities of adventure therapy.

Sports and athletic activities appeal to people of all ages. Unfortunately, athletes sometimes drop out of sports activities even though they possess numerous skills that are characteristic of excellent athletes. The next contribution, by Bobby Stinson, II, Robert Friedberg, Richard Page, and Michael Cusack, focuses on why some athletes are more vulnerable to dropping out of athletics than others. The authors discuss the relationship between attributional style and athletic performance, including the decision to drop out of athletics.

In the final contribution of this section, Robert Basil describes the special challenges of providing mental health services to the Deaf community. Mental health professionals require specialized training to work with deaf clients, and this contribution outlines many of the issues involved.

Psychoeducational Groups For Adolescent Sex Offenders*

Garry P. Perry, Stan Dimnik, Phyllis Ohm, and Brenda L. Wilks

There is a growing demand on mental health agencies and private practitioners to provide clinical services to adolescents who commit sexual offenses (Blanchard, 1995; Kahn, 1990; National Task Force on Juvenile Sexual Offending, 1993; Perry & Orchard, 1989, 1992; Perry, Orchard, & Ohm, in press; Ryan & Lane, 1991). This contribution presents an overview of a process the authors utilize to prepare adolescents for sex offender specific treatment. The information in this contribution will be useful to clinicians because it provides a framework for preparing clients for therapy and describes the content of a group designed to prepare adolescents who have committed sex offenses.**

PREPARING CLIENTS FOR THERAPY

A number of authors have stressed the importance of engaging the client in the therapeutic process in order to maximize the impact and long-term effects of therapy (Bowman & Delucia, 1993; Egan, 1994; Ludgate, 1995; Miller & Rollnick, 1991; Paquin & Perry, 1990; Perry & Paquin, 1987). Paquin and Perry (1990) and Perry and Paquin (1987) have emphasized the importance of educating clients about the therapeutic process so they can become active participants in the process of change. We believe that it is essential for youths and their families to be informed about what will happen in therapy, the role of the therapist, how interventions will focus on their specific problems, how treatment will be evaluated, the expected impact therapy may have on youths and their families, the expectations of the youths, and their role in the course of therapy. This approach demystifies the therapeutic process and sets the stage for a collaboration in dealing with youths' and their families' issues.

Youths' understanding of what is expected of them throughout the therapeutic process will help to insure longevity of treatment. Developmentally, adolescents are struggling with gaining a sense of significance and competence in their lives. Therapy needs to work interactively with these developmental struggles to assist youths in learning to deal with problematic behavior (e.g., criminal actions) and to be able to take the information and skills they have learned in therapy and use it to help them deal with a range of other developmental demands they are facing.

Perry and Orchard (1992) have built on the work of Paquin and Perry (1990) and Perry and Paquin (1987) by suggesting that one of the central tasks for therapists working with adolescent sex offenders is to insure that the adolescents and their families learn to *maintain, transfer,* and *generalize* what they learned in therapy to their lives in the community. *Maintenance* refers to the person's ability to retain the information and skills learned during therapy over time. *Transfer* refers to the person's ability to take information learned in therapy and

---

*The authors would like to thank Ms. Pat Perry, Dr. Steve Boechler, Dr. Tim Greenough, Ms. Carol Holub, and Ms. Sharon Childerhose for their comments on an earlier version of this contribution.

**Male pronouns will be used throughout when talking about adolescents who commit sexual offenses because the majority of our clients are male; this in no way implies that women/girls do not commit offenses.

apply it in his or her life. *Generalization* refers to the spread of skills the person has learned in therapy to situations that were not specifically targeted in therapy.

We believe the process of learning to maintain, transfer, and generalize must be consciously initiated by the clinician at the start of therapy. This perspective is especially important for adolescent sex offenders because the focus of treatment must be not only to assist youths in altering offending behaviors but also to help them become safe in the community, develop socially appropriate ways to meet their needs, and make long-term lifestyle changes.

A central premise in providing therapy is to engage the client in the therapeutic process (Egan, 1994; Paquin & Perry, 1990). Hains et al. (1986) and Ross and Loss (1988) have written about the importance of developing psychoeducational interventions to help adolescent sex offenders prepare for the process of sex offender specific therapy.

Ross and Loss (1988) described an educational model to provide information to adolescent sex offenders; a classroomlike setting, in which the youths were referred to as students, was used to present information in a highly structured manner. Information was presented on the following topics: psychology of the offender, the sex offender's history (crime cycle), victimization, sex education, home supervision, expectations of the treatment program, goal setting, and agreement writing. The curriculum was presented over 10 weekly sessions varying in length from 60 to 80 minutes.

The subjects in the Hains et al. (1986) study participated in twice-weekly sessions for 7 weeks, with each session being 50 minutes in length. An educational format was used to convey information on sexual knowledge, improve psychological attitudes related to sex issues (e.g., dating), and train in problem solving and moral judgment. The experimental subjects made significant gains over controls in the domains of sexual knowledge, positive trends in attitudes, and problem solving.

PSYCHOEDUCATION GROUP FOR ADOLESCENT SEX OFFENDERS

Prior to becoming involved in treatment, all adolescents referred to our clinic - and, when possible, their families - are assessed utilizing a procedure outlined by Perry and Orchard (1992) and Perry et al. (in press). The youths referred to our adolescent sex offender program include both adjudicated and nonadjudicated males between the ages of 12 and 18 years who have committed at least one sexual offense. Interventions offered include individual, group, and family therapy (Perry et al., in press).

Adolescents who have committed sex offenses participate first in our Psychoeducation group (Psycho-Ed). This group is designed to prepare the youth for participation in other group interventions and begins the process of the youth talking about his own issues. Factors that guided the development and implementation of our Psycho-Ed group are outlined in Table 1 (p. 313).

Psycho-Ed groups are composed of four to six youths and two facilitators (male and female). We have found groups of this small size to be more productive and ultimately more cost-effective because the participants gain more from involvement in the process. Group sessions are 2 hours long and are held once a week for 15 weeks.

Each group session begins with a sharing of food and juice provided by facilitators and a group check-in. The group is scheduled after school, and the youths are often tired and hungry. The sharing of food is a way of providing energy to the youths and provides a medium for check-ins.

Check-ins occur at the beginning of each group and require each youth and facilitator to discuss his or her past week's activities, citing positive and negative events. If a youth believes he was acting or thinking of acting inappropriately (e.g., experiencing deviant fantasies) or was exposed to situations that may place him at risk for offending (e.g., a neighbor wants him to babysit) he can share it with the group. There is time to discuss concerns and, if

TABLE 1: Factors That Guided the Development of Our Psychoeducational Group for Adolescent Sex Offenders

The group needed to:

1. create a safe and nourishing environment where youths feel comfortable in discussing offending and nonoffending issues.
2. create an atmosphere that assists youths in identifying and altering problematic behaviors.
3. acknowledge and integrate the growth the youths have already undergone with the content of group sessions.
4. provide opportunities to learn experientially and in developmentally appropriate ways.
5. present information in a conceptual way that would enhance the youths to take responsibility for their actions and to develop prosocial ways of meeting their needs.
6. integrate a problem-solving model into a lesson format so youths begin to realize that for every situation there are a number of possible solutions and that they have to choose which is best for them.
7. recognize that learning may be constrained by cultural or subcultural norms but is not automatically indicative of individual pathology.
8. consider community safety to be a primary consideration and interweave it into discussions.
9. recognize that therapy is a process; youths need to be involved in the process of change from the beginning.

more time is needed, arrangements are made to meet with one of the facilitators outside of the group.

The curriculum for our Psycho-Ed group is outlined below.

Session 1 - Introduction

This session is used to introduce group members and facilitators to each other; set the group rules; review the structure of the group, the responsibilities of all group members, and the content of the group; discuss youths' misperceptions and myths about what will happen in treatment; and have the youths disclose their offenses. Youths are encouraged from the outset of the session to become involved in discussions.

Group rules are established by the group members and the facilitators. The purpose of this task is to get the youths actively involved in the group. Group rules have included confidentiality, being on time, developing strategies to manage conflicts within the group, being respectful, breaks, and consumption of food and beverages. The rules are continually assessed and modified; if needed, new ones are developed.

The first session concludes with each youth disclosing the offenses for which he was referred to treatment. Using the metaphor of the "journey" for the first time, youths are challenged to inform their "fellow travelers" where they have come from. Youths are supported and encouraged to describe their offending behaviors in detail. Youths have reported feeling relief at having been able to state, often for the first time, the nature of their offending. They also report that, once having shared their offending safely, they feel amenable to trusting both group members and facilitators.

The facilitators highlight the importance for the youth to understand that his actions (sexual offending) have had significant negative impact on their victims and secondary victims (e.g., victim's family). The concept of empathy is highlighted throughout all the modules and is specifically addressed in Sessions 10 and 11.

Sessions 2 and 3 - Healthy Sexuality

Information in these two sessions was drawn from the work of Bignell (1980), Canera (1981), Denney and Quadongno (1992), Perry and Ohm (1999), Westheimer (1994), and Younger (1992). Sessions 2 and 3 are aimed at exploring healthy sexuality from the perspective of providing information on the "facts of life" and to highlight that healthy sexuality is simply a whole lot more fun than unhealthy sexuality (e.g., sexually abusing others). The facilitators emphasize that the expression of one's sexuality is a necessary part of human experience, but also that this expression can and must occur in ways that do not harm oneself or others.

Session 2 begins with the youths completing a "Sexual Knowledge Questionnaire" (the Sexual Knowledge Questionnaire used by facilitators is a modification of a scale cited by Bignell [1980]). This task stimulates the youths to explore their knowledge of sexuality and to encourage questioning and exploration of their own sexuality both throughout the group and, it is hoped, after the group is completed. After completing the questionnaire, excerpts from literature that encourage the broadest interpretation of human sexuality are read. Youths are invited to peruse a number of resources that focus on human sexuality which have been brought to the group by facilitators (e.g., Canera, 1981; Westheimer, 1994; Younger, 1992).

The youths are then shown excerpts from anatomically explicit videos entitled *Human Sexuality: Values and Choices* (Search Institute, 1986) and *AIDS: The New Facts of Life* (Canadian Public Health Association, 1989). After showing these videos, facilitators lead a discussion about the role of healthy sexuality. Youths and facilitators explore myths surrounding masturbation, consenting sexual activities, and the use of contraception - in particular, condoms. We have condoms on hand, and youths are encouraged to take some condoms.

Most high school students in our area have been introduced to some form of "sex education" within the schools and have been introduced to a value orientation that encourages abstinence while limiting information on how one might develop a more healthy sexual lifestyle. Although abstinence is certainly discussed and posed as an alternative, the primary aim of our interventions is to foster a sense of informed curiosity to investigate and take responsibility for one's own sexuality.

Session 3 begins with a discussion about the impact of the information given the previous week. Youths are asked to review notions of "normality" in human sexual behavior by reflecting on their own introductions to sexuality. As they discuss their introduction to sexuality they are encouraged to explore the values and knowledge imparted by family, friends, and the media.

After this initial discussion, youths watch the video *Degrassi Talks . . . Sexuality* (1992). This video provides information on adolescents' struggles with puberty, masturbation, and sexual orientation. At times humorous, at times poignant, this video normalizes many of the struggles youth in the group have already engaged in. It enforces the notion that they are not alone in their "journey."

After showing the video, facilitators introduce a discussion on gender and sexual orientation. This process allows youths to explore myths associated with human sexuality (e.g., homosexuality). The session ends with a discussion of the role healthy sexuality plays in a person's life and validates healthy sexual fantasizing.

Sessions 4 and 5 - Change

Youths begin Session 4 by identifying times in their lives or in those of someone close to them when a major transition was unexpectedly entered into or imposed against their will. The theme of motivation to change is investigated by having the youths first identify times in their past when they were motivated to change a behavior but failed to alter behavior (e.g., offending behaviors).

The facilitators stress that motivation needs to be paired with a process for altering behaviors. Youths are then introduced to the problem-solving method as a means of translating motivation into action (Goldstein, 1988). This model incorporates the following steps: recognition of problems, definition of problems, alternate ways of solving problems, evaluation of possible solutions, implementation of a strategy, and evaluation of the strategy used. This model stresses skill development in alternate-solution thinking, consequential thinking, causal thinking, interpersonal sensitivity, means-ends thinking, and perspective taking.

After the model has been reviewed, the youths are asked to apply the model to a simulated case. The case model is drawn from the video *The Crown Prince* (National Film Board of Canada, 1989). This video presents a story in which two youths are victims of domestic violence; one of them goes on to become physically abusive of his brother and commits a sexual assault. Youths are shown the first half of the video and then are asked to develop a workable solution to one character's predicament. Youths are then asked to predict outcomes for each of the main characters for the next session.

The first part of Session 5 focuses on reviewing the problem-solving method discussed in Session 4. Youths are asked to reveal their predictions for the character in the video. They are then shown the second half of the video *The Crown Prince.*

After viewing the second half, the group considers what factors led them to correctly/incorrectly guess their outcomes. They are asked to identify the factors that enhanced or detracted from the problem-solving process (e.g., the thoughts, feelings, behaviors of each character that contributed to the abuse) and what moved the family to a workable solution. The theme of being held accountable as a catalyst to change is discussed.

The second half of Session 5 introduces the notion of cyclical behavior. The youths review their understanding of the characters in the video in light of new information regarding cyclical patterns of behavior and are encouraged to explore the repetitive, learned, and at first seemingly impulsive nature of abusive behavior.

Group members are asked to draw parallels between behavior seen in the video and that which they have observed within their own families or those of friends. The youths invariably start to apply problem solving to behaviors they previously held as intractable. Finally, they are asked to consider the optimum conditions needed for change within their present situations.

Session 6 - Denial

Youths are introduced to the notion of "denial" as a typically human behavioral strategy - at times useful, at other times problematic. Youths are encouraged to describe their offenses, detailing as accurately as possible their thoughts, feelings, and actions at critical points in their offending cycle. They themselves wrestle with determining at what juncture denial became essential to avoid detection or negative consequences.

Facilitators provide, and elaborate on, a handout that describes varying types of denial identified by Salter (1988). Salter has developed a system of classifying denial across a continuum from outright denial ("I did not commit the offense") to total acceptance. The stages in Salter's continuum are denial of behavior, minimization of the extent of behavior, denial of seriousness of the behavior, denial of responsibility, and full admission with responsibility and guilt.

Youths and facilitators arrive at a synthesis during a "detective game" in which one youth volunteers to be "questioned" and the other youths take on the role of "detectives." Through a series of probes and prompts, they attempt to explore the youth's denial and try to identify the precise type of denial employed by him. When the group is completed with one youth, another youth volunteers until each member has been questioned.

We have found this process to be a less threatening and more humorous process to explore denial. The youths are allowed to ask a range of questions but are not allowed to be abusive of one another. The youths have indicated that this procedure is a helpful way for them to explore issues they had not wanted to explore in the past.

Armed with their new knowledge of denial, youths become adept at pointing out the instances of denial in their offending patterns and can begin to see how these denial strategies helped protect the perpetrator within them. We have found that the youths are able to transfer their newfound understanding of denial to discussions throughout the rest of the sessions.

Session 7 - Accountability Versus Responsibility

Accountability refers to the action of external agents in uncovering the offending behavior and insuring that the offending behavior is publicly acknowledged and that consequences follow. These external agents (e.g., the victims, the police, and the courts) ensure that the youth is "held accountable."

Responsibility refers to the process in which the youth acknowledges his actions and the harm he has perpetrated on others, agrees to make amends both publicly and privately for the harm, and takes measures to ensure that this does not happen again. The youth "takes responsibility" for his actions.

Youths are challenged to distinguish between the notions of accountability and responsibility and to identify by whom they were held accountable and when, when they first acknowledged responsibility, and what obstacles impeded them from taking responsibility for their actions. This process assists the youths in exploring the interaction between personal and external (e.g., family pressure) factors and how these factors affect their decisions.

Youths are then asked to apply their understanding of these terms by critically analyzing a fictitious story created by facilitators depicting "Jim's" sexual offending history. Youths are asked to take on the role of investigative reporter and interview each other.

As investigative journalists they are given a roughly scripted interview. Youths are broken into pairs and alternate between taking on the persona of the character "Jim" and that of the investigative reporter. The reporter interviews "Jim" to determine what obstacles prevented him from taking responsibility for his offending behavior. Youths then switch roles. Facilitators encourage, discuss, and assist youths in staying focused.

After discussing the fictitious character "Jim," the youths are asked to interview each other with respect to discovering obstacles to taking responsibility or being held accountable in their own offending history. We have found that youths are able to recognize situations in their own lives where they have failed to take responsibility for their offending and other behaviors. As the youths discuss their own needs to take responsibility, facilitators discuss the need for them to take responsibility not only for offending behaviors but also to insure they never reoffend. This perspective is connected to the roles of understanding their crime cycles and developing and following a safety plan.

Session 8 - Crime Cycle

Youths are introduced to a crime cycle model which integrates the work of Kahn (1990) and Lane (1994). This model presents a four-stage approach to conceptualizing the offense/crime cycle: pretend normal, build-up, offending behaviors, and justification. Kahn's (1990) model is integrated into the build-up stage and assists the youths in identifying their motivation to offend and how they overcame internal and external barriers to offending and the victim's resistance.

After discussing this model, the youths are shown a video, *One Hit Leads to Another* (Friday Street Productions/Kinetic Films & Videos, 1991) which explores the cyclical nature of violence. The youths are invited to apply the four-stage cycle of abuse to the characters and situations depicted in the video. They describe behaviorally how each phase was manifested by the characters, then are asked to speculate as to what thoughts and feelings might have been associated with each phase.

Youths are then asked to apply their knowledge of the offense cycle to their own situations. They are divided into pairs and instructed to identify and discuss both internal (thoughts, feelings) and external (e.g., lack of appropriate supports) factors that affected the decisions they made at each step of the model. They are encouraged to use a range of skills (e.g., challenging, supporting) to help each other clearly describe what was happening in their lives.

The session concludes with each member sharing with the group his perceptions of the factors at each stage of his offense cycle. Facilitators and other youths provide feedback and suggestions.

Session 9 - Willpower Not Enough - The Safety Plan

At the beginning of this session youths are presented with information that a number of adolescents have reoffended after being caught because they relied on willpower not to reoffend. The facilitators stress that each youth has to develop and apply a plan to insure his safety in the community. The term "safety plan" is introduced. It is based on the relapse prevention model discussed by Perry and Orchard (1992) and Perry et al. (in press).

Relapse prevention is a process that helps a client explore the factors in his life that lead him to engage in destructive behaviors (e.g., gambling, alcohol consumption, aggressive behaviors, sexual offending behaviors). The premise is that if a youth knows the internal and external factors that lead him to engage in destructive behaviors, he can learn to alter these factors early in the sequence in order to stop the process. The stages for the relapse prevention model generally include teaching the youth to (a) monitor thoughts, feelings, and actions to identify destructive patterns; (b) develop coping strategies; (c) identify high-risk situations which may lead to problematic behaviors; (d) develop ways to alter situations that are risky; and (e) identify and use supports to assist in altering behaviors and identify situations that are directly connected to destructive behaviors.

Perry et al. (in press) have expanded this model to help the youth not only become aware of factors that lead to his sexual offending but also develop a healthy lifestyle. The premise is that if a youth is meeting his needs/wants in healthy ways he is less likely to begin the process that leads him to offend.

After this information has been presented and discussed, the youths are invited to apply their understanding of safety plans to a scenario previously prepared by the facilitators. This scenario describes an offending youth who returns home for the holidays from an open custody community home. The youth in the scenario is presented as being challenged by a number of thoughts, feelings, behaviors, and situations that could conceivably result in a sexual assault. They are asked to assess risk at every stage of the cycle. The youth are then encouraged to determine a means of mitigating risk at each turn, thereby creating a fairly complex safety plan for the youth in the scenario.

A safety plan is specific to each youth's offending pattern and lifestyle and needs to be continually adjusted through their lifespan. For example, a youth who offends against children by isolating them (e.g., babysitting) needs to initially develop a plan where he has no unsupervised access to children. This plan needs to look at all potential situations where the youth may have access to children (e.g., playgrounds). As the youth progresses through therapy, the safety plan is continually revisited, modified, and expanded. We also believe that an important aspect of any safety plan is not just the avoidance of situations but also the ongoing management of needs and wants in healthy ways, because as the youth gets older, his lifestyle and risks will change (e.g., gets married, has children of his own).

The session concludes with the youths developing a basic safety plan for themselves. Each youth presents his plan to the group and the facilitators and other youths provide feedback. Once the plan is accepted it is recorded and revisited in Session 13 when each youth will restate his safety plan, reframing it from the perspective of meeting needs in healthy ways.

It is important to note that the safety plan developed in this group is a rudimentary plan that will continue to be modified and expanded throughout treatment. The plan sets the stage for the youths to work at taking responsibility for being safe in the community rather than relying on willpower.

Sessions 10 and 11 - Empathy

The concept of empathy was first raised during Session 1 in the introduction and is restated during each group. During Session 10, youths are introduced to the distinction between sympathy and empathy. The former depends on emotional and intellectual accord and involves supporting and condoning the other person's feelings; the latter involves understanding the other person's feelings and circumstances without having to take on that person's position (Egan, 1994; Hepworth, Rooney, & Larsen, 1997).

Critical to learning empathy skills is the development of affective words and phrases. Facilitators have developed a game that matches words and phrases to hand-drawn faces. Youths are given 15 faces each and told to, as quickly as possible, pick corresponding affective words from a common pile of words. Youths choose one affect word from the pile and must negotiate each choice with their peers; they have to justify their choice and secure agreement from their peers before taking another word from the list. Correct matches are placed on the head table; the process of negotiation continues until all matches have been completed. The purpose of the exercise is twofold: first, to assist in empathic skill development, and second, to encourage discussion and debate surrounding use of or failure of empathy in the past.

Invariably, youths notice that with increased stress, their ability to match is significantly affected. They further connect this with the observation that their capacity to empathize with their victims diminishes within the context of increased stress.

Session 11 builds on the previous session by having the youths attempt to model a range of emotions through role plays. Youths are randomly assigned affective words and phrases with which they, along with one partner, are to construct a role play that incorporates the words/phrases into a meaningful sequence. Once ready, the youths act out their role play while the other youths observe behind a viewing mirror, listing each feeling they think has been demonstrated. Teams are scored on their ability to discern feelings as well as demonstrating them when their turn to role play arises.

Youths then create a five-column list of affective words from words handed out the previous week, arranging words according to how intense and/or unpleasant the feelings are (e.g., irritation, frustration, anger, rage). Finally, youths explore affective words associated with human sexuality, noting and hypothesizing about the paucity of commonly used words. Youths explore how it is that other feelings (such as anger, frustration, embarrassment, etc.) become so closely correlated with sexual feelings.

Sessions 12 and 13 - Meeting Needs in Healthy Ways

The youths have been introduced to the notion of meeting their needs in healthy ways since Session 2. Sessions 12 and 13 are designed to build on the material discussed throughout the previous sessions by having the youths look at how they will integrate feedback from others into life journeys and begin the process of learning to plan how to meet their needs in healthy ways. As they discuss these features, the facilitators assist the youths in integrating the material they discuss into expanding the safety plans they developed previously in Session 9.

Session 12 explores how the youths integrate their self-perceptions with feedback from others. As they discuss feedback from other members, the facilitators point out that an important aspect of being safe is to find people to whom they can talk about their concerns and issues. Having a support group in the community that can assist each youth to deal with life situations and offending concerns is an important part of therapy with adolescents who commit sexual offenses. This is considered an important part of the youths' safety and lifestyle plans because, in the past, these youths have not tended to utilize supports in their lives in appropriate ways. We stress developing family support networks; if these are not available, we look for other potential sources of support which will be there long term for the youths.

At the start of Session 12, the youths complete a brief questionnaire which, when scored, assigns each youth the characteristics of a particular animal (e.g., fox, owl, bear, shark) that represents attributes the youth may assume in conflict situations (D. Johnson & F. Johnson, 1982). As well, youths are anonymously assigned an animal persona by both their peers and facilitators, thus allowing comparison between the youths' perceptions and those assigned them by others. Youths are then encouraged to challenge attributes they perceive as having been inaccurately assigned to them; to determine which attributes they would preferably like to strive to acquire; and finally, to speculate what combination of attributes would best suit themselves.

This session ends with a discussion of how the youths' self-perceptions may at times differ from how others perceive them. The task for the youths is how to discuss these differences and to integrate feedback into lifestyle changes. This does not mean the youths need to always agree with others, but they need to learn to listen and process information. Facilitators connect this process to the problem-solving model discussed in Session 4. Youths will leave therapy at some point in their lives, and they are encouraged to look for support persons in their lives from whom they can receive feedback.

Session 13 moves beyond the identification of harmful or "at risk" thoughts, feelings, behaviors, and situations to trying to envision a world in 1 year, 2 years, and 3 years hence in which every youth is meeting his needs in healthy ways.

This requires the youths to be able to project their present development into the future, sensing what their family, peers, and community relationships might look like (assuming they were to eschew the pathological view of themselves as being "essentially flawed" and being incapable of fundamental change).

Youths are interviewed by their peers to create this world in writing, pictures, or any other medium chosen by the individual (youths often describe the process of individuation in which they have left home, assumed employment or continued through school, and invariably worked through a number of temporary relationships to assume the goal of a long-term sexual relationship).

Finally, the youths revise their safety plans from Session 9, taking into account their newly acquired longer term views of growth and health and identifying who will be supports in their lives who can help them stay safe in the community. Where possible the youths' families (immediate and extended) are identified as providing long-term sources of support. We have found that some youths struggle with identifying supports in their lives outside the professionals working with them (e.g., social worker, therapists, psychologist). Their families are dysfunctional or nonexistent, they have few adult prosocial role models, and they have few friends or destructive friends. Part of the therapeutic process is to assist these youths in developing supports in their lives (e.g., prosocial friends and adult role models). Initially professional supports will be used, but the youths need to look for and develop community-based supports as well.

The safety plan the youths put together at the end of Session 13 will become the basic plan to assist them in being safe and meeting needs in healthy ways. Thus the youths have a rudimentary safety plan they can build on in other group therapeutic interventions (individual, group, family).

Session 14 - Bringing It Together

After check-ins, the youths and facilitators participate in an exercise entitled "string/web game." This exercise is utilized as a method of putting closure on the group. By this point in the group the youths have developed a sense of camaraderie and have become aware that, as a group, they have only just begun to embark on their journey to a healthy sexuality and lifestyle and not reoffending.

Youths and facilitators sit in a circle. One of the facilitators holds a large ball of string and makes a positive statement about the contributions made to the group by an individual in the group; at the same time the facilitator passes the ball to the individual about whom the statement was made, while holding the end of the string. That youth also holds onto the string and passes the ball to another youth or facilitator while acknowledging a positive contribution that individual has made to the group. This exercise continues until each member of the group is holding onto several strands of string. At a point predetermined by facilitators, the game ends with the strands being cut; each participant takes those strands passed to him home with him.

This exercise, as well as being a fitting end to the metaphor of the journey (as fellow travelers reminisce about high points of their journey), acknowledges the positive contributions of each participant, and allows each youth to anticipate his future role as an architect in building his own healthy lifestyle (as opposed to being merely a target of change). Youths have, on a number of occasions, in following groups,* recalled some of the positive affirmations made in this exercise.

As each session has begun with the sharing of food and camaraderie, so does the final session end with a meal. The sharing of food, as well as the "web game," appear well suited, and are a fitting end, to the metaphor of the journey (as fellow travelers recount the highs and lows of their trip). The game, in particular, acknowledges in a warm, positive, and accepting way the contributions of each participant to the journey.

This final session consolidates the notion of youths who are able to anticipate their future roles as healthy citizens and to see themselves as architects in the building of their own healthy lifestyles. It should be noted that, often months afterwards, youth will refer to the positive attributions made by peers and facilitators during this final session.

---

*After completing the psychoeducational group the youths are referred to other groups at our clinic.

SUMMARY

The task for therapists working with youths is to find ways to involve them in the therapeutic process and motivate them to work on issues. We have found this group process to be a useful method to engage the youths in the process of change. The information is presented in an interactive approach where the youths are respected and not looked at as damaged individuals. They are perceived as youths who come with some strengths in their lives, and the process of therapy is to build on strengths and alter problematic behaviors.

Table 2 (below) presents an overview of the expected outcomes of the youths participating in the Psycho-Ed group.

TABLE 2: The Expected Outcomes for the Youths Participating in Psycho-Ed Group

1. To begin the process of ensuring safety for both the youth and potential victims in the community.
2. To promote the metaphor of youth on a developmental youth journey.
3. To normalize much of the youth's behavior while beginning to tease out the behaviors, feelings, and beliefs that support unhealthy behavior.
4. To model respect and empathy for and with the youth in a world where youths have themselves been vilified, ostracized, and at times attacked.
5. To challenge the hopelessness inherent in a model that assumes lifelong pathology.
6. To prepare youth for the next sequence of treatment by introducing a common conceptual framework, a common language, and a similar group process.
7. To help youths become more open to talking about their own issues.
8. To help youths learn that they are responsible not only for committing their offenses but also for maintaining their safety in the community.
9. To help youths learn about factors that may lead a person to commit an offense and the factors in their own lives that lead them to offend.
10. To encourage youths to begin to assess how they will meet their needs and wants in prosocial ways.
11. To teach empathy, so that youths become aware that sex offenses hurt people in a variety of ways.
12. To provide information on healthy sexuality and to provide a forum for youths to discuss sexuality and the role it plays in their lives and help them learn and hopefully practice safe sex.
13. To teach youths about the difference between consenting and coercive sexual contacts.
14. To help youths develop healthy lifestyles that will reduce risk and assist youths in meeting needs in healthy ways.

Table 2 highlights that the youths have not only learned the central aspects of what they need to change to be safe in the community but also have begun the process of making changes in their lives that will help them develop a healthy, nonabusive lifestyle.

Adolescents who commit sexual offenses and subsequently complete Psycho-Ed are referred on to a range of other services at our clinic. We have found the impact of participating in Psycho-Ed a valuable experience for the youths.

We believe the process outlined above has been successful at preparing youths for sex offender specific therapy and for setting the stage for the youths developing nonabusive, healthy lifestyles. We have not collected systematic outcome data but have clinically followed the youths who have completed this group throughout the rest of their sex offender programming at our clinic. Other clinicians working with them have indicated that these youths are willing to challenge themselves and others, are aware of their safety needs, are less likely to minimize their own offending behaviors and those of others, are working at integrating material presented to them, and are open to feedback.

CONTRIBUTORS

Garry P. Perry, MA, has 16 years clinical experience and training in providing assessment and treatment services to a wide range of clients. Part of his current job duties involve supervising clinical staff in Young Offender Program and providing consultation to community agencies. He has published and presented papers on a variety of topics (e.g., enhancing long-term effects of treatment and training), has conducted numerous workshops for professionals and paraprofessionals, and has taught courses at universities. He has developed a specialization in assessment and treatment of adolescent and adult sex offenders and is co-author of a book entitled *Assessment and Treatment of Adolescent Sex Offenders.* He is a member of the Association for the Treatment of Sexual Abusers, Canadian Guidance and Counselling Association, and Psychological Society of Saskatchewan. Mr. Perry can be reached at Child & Youth Services, 715 Queen Street, Saskatoon, Saskatchewan, Canada, S7K 4X4. E-mail: perryg@sdh.sk.ca

Stan Dimnik, MSW, has worked with adolescents and their families for over 20 years. He has received education and training in both Canada and England. His work experiences include providing services to youth and families in both rural and urban areas in Canada and overseas, as well as in First Nations settings. Influenced by systems and ecological approaches, he has emphasized understanding youth within their own cultural, socioeconomic, and spiritual contexts. He has worked for the Departments of Social Services in a variety of roles and was the manager of an adolescent treatment facility. He is currently employed as a Forensic Social Worker working primarily with adolescent sex offenders and their families. Mr. Dimnik may be contacted at Child & Youth Services, 715 Queen Street, Saskatoon, Saskatchewan, Canada, S7K 4X4.

Phyllis Ohm, PsyD, has worked with children, adolescents, and youths for over 20 years. Her current job duties involve providing assessment and treatment services to adolescents (male and female) who have committed offenses and their families and to street youth involved in prostitution. She also provides consultation to community agencies and has supervised doctoral students. She has published and presented papers on a variety of topics and has conducted workshops for professionals. She has developed a specialization in the assessment and treatment of adolescent and adult sex offenders. Dr. Ohm can be reached at Child & Youth Services, 715 Queen Street, Saskatoon, Saskatchewan, Canada, S7K 4X4.

Brenda L. Wilks, CSW, has extensive experience in working with physically challenged and otherwise vulnerable young adults, victims of sexual assault, and for the last 6 years as a Social Worker in a Young Offender facility that houses both male and female youths. She has extensive experience working with delinquent females. She brings to her work with adolescents who have committed sexual offenses a clear and unambiguous message from the perspective of the victim to equally challenge the objectification of the victim and offender. Ms. Wilks may be contacted at Kilburn Hall, 1302 Kilburn Avenue, Saskatoon, Saskatchewan, Canada, S7M 0J7.

RESOURCES

Cited Resources

Bignell, S. (Ed.). (1980). *Family Life Education Curriculum Guide.* Santa Cruz, CA: Network Publishers.

Blanchard, G. T. (1995). *The Difficult Connection: The Therapeutic Relationship in Sex Offender Treatment.* Brandon, VT: The Safer Society Press.

Bowman, V., & Delucia, J. (1993). Preparation for group therapy: The effects of preparer and modality on group process and individual functioning. *Journal for Specialists in Group Work, 18,* 67-79.

Canera, M. (1981). *Sex: The Acts and Your Feelings.* New York: Crown Publishers.

Denney, N. W., & Quadongno, D. (1992). *Human Sexuality* (2nd ed.). St. Louis: Mosley Year Book.

Digorgio-Miller, J. (1994). Clinical techniques in the treatment of juvenile sex offenders. *Journal of Offender Rehabilitation, 21*(1-2), 117-126.

Egan, G. (1994). *The Skilled Helper: A Problem-Management Approach to Helping* (5th ed.). Pacific Grove, CA: Brooks/Cole.

Goldstein, A. (1988). *The Prepare Curriculum: Teaching Prosocial Competencies.* Champaign, IL: Research Press.

Hains, A. A., Herman, L., Baker, K., & Garber, S. (1986). The development of a psycho-educational group program for adolescent sex offenders. *Journal of Offender Counseling, Services & Rehabilitation, 11,* 63-76.

Hepworth, D. H., Rooney, R. H., & Larsen, J. (1997) *Direct Social Work Practice: Theory and Skills* (5th ed.). Pacific Grove, CA: Brooks/Cole.

Johnson, D., & Johnson, F. (1982). *Joining Together: Group Theory and Group Skills.* Englewood Cliffs, NJ: Prentice Hall.

Kahn, T. J. (1990). *Pathways: A Guided Workbook for Youth Beginning Treatment.* Orwell, VT: The Safer Society Press.

Lane, S. (1994, June). The cycle. *Interchange,* pp. 1-18.

Ludgate, J. W. (1995). *Maximizing Psychotherapeutic Gains and Preventing Relapse in Emotionally Distressed Clients.* Sarasota, FL: Professional Resource Press.

Miller, W. R., & Rollnick, S. (1991). *Motivating Interviewing: Preparing People to Change Addictive Behavior.* New York: Guilford.

National Task Force on Juvenile Sexual Offending. (1993). The revised report from the National Task Force Group on Juvenile Sexual Offending, 1993, of the National Adolescent Perpetrator Network. *Juvenile & Family Court Journal, 44,* 1-121.

Paquin, M. J., & Perry, G. P. (1990). Maintaining successful interventions in social, vocational and community rehabilitation. *The Canadian Journal of Community Mental Health, 9,* 39-49.

Perry, G. P., & Ohm, P. (1999). The role healthy sexuality plays in assisting adolescent sex offenders to maintain safety in the community: Ethical and practical considerations. *Canadian Journal of Counselling, 33,* 157-169.

Perry, G. P., & Orchard, J. M. (1989). Assessment and treatment of adolescent sex offenders. In P. A. Keller & S. R. Heyman (Eds), *Innovations in Clinical Practice: A Source Book* (Vol. 8, pp. 187-211). Sarasota, FL: Professional Resource Exchange.

Perry, G. P., & Orchard, J. M. (1992). *Assessment and Treatment of Adolescent Sex Offenders.* Sarasota, FL: Professional Resource Exchange.

Perry, G. P., Orchard, J., & Ohm, P. (in press). *Assessment and Treatment of Adolescent Sex Offenders* (2nd ed.).

Perry, G. P., & Paquin, M. J. (1987). Practical strategies for maintaining and generalizing improvements from psychotherapy. In P. A. Keller & S. R. Heyman (Eds), *Innovations in Clinical Practice: A Source Book* (Vol. 6, pp. 151-164). Sarasota, FL: Professional Resource Exchange.

Ross, J., & Loss, P. (1988). *Psychoeducational Curriculum for the Adolescent Sex Offender.* Unpublished manuscript. (Jonathan Ross can be contacted at Waypoint New Hope, Summerville, SC.)

Ryan, G. D., & Lane, S. (Eds.). (1991). *Juvenile Sexual Offenders: Causes, Consequences and Correction.* Toronto, Ontario: Lexington Books.

Salter, A. C. (1988). *Treating Child Sex Offenders and Victims: A Practical Guide.* Newbury Park, CA: Sage.

Westheimer, R. K. (1994). *Dr. Ruth's Encyclopedia of Sex.* New York: Continuum.

Younger, F. (1992). *Five Hundred Questions Kids Ask About Sex.* Springfield, IL: Charles C. Thomas.

Audio-Visual Resources

Canadian Public Health Association. (1989). *AIDS: The New Facts of Life* [Videotape]. Ottawa, Ontario: Author.

Degrassi Talks . . . Sexuality [Videotape]. (1992). Santa Monica, CA: Direct Cinema Ltd.

Friday Street Productions/Kinetic Films & Videos. (1991). *One Hit Leads to Another* [Videotape]. (Available from http://www.kineticvideo.com - Catalogue No. 8317/2130)

National Film Board of Canada. (1988). *To a Safer Place: User's Guide: One Woman's Account of Her Life as a Survivor of Childhood Incest* [Videotape]. Montreal, Quebec: Author.

National Film Board of Canada. (1989). *The Crown Prince* [Videotape]. Montreal, Quebec: Author.

Search Institute. (1986). *Human Sexuality: Values and Choices* [Videotape]. Minneapolis, MN: Author.

Psychological Interventions For Surgery Patients

William W. Deardorff

Each year more than 50 million surgeries are performed in the United States (Sobel & Ornstein, 1996), costing the American public billions of dollars in medical expenses and lost wages. Thus one might surmise the enthusiastic adoption of any intervention which was easily applied, safe, side-effect-free, and cost-effective, with the following additional benefits:

- Decreases patient distress before and after surgery.
- Significantly reduces the need for pain medications.
- Results in fewer postoperative complications and fosters a quicker return to health.
- Enhances overall patient satisfaction.
- Empowers patients to take more responsibility for their recovery, thus reducing health care demands.
- Results in potential savings of thousands of dollars per patient surgery.

If such an intervention sounds too good to be true, it's not. Psychological preparation for surgery approaches, in fact, can achieve these remarkable results. Given that these techniques have overwhelming scientific support for their effectiveness and are widely available, why are they only rarely employed in surgical practice? One reason is that surgery has traditionally been viewed in mechanistic terms. In this view, the patient is seen as a passive recipient of a surgical intervention with little influence over the recovery process. Nothing could be further from the truth. Through psychological preparation for surgery, patients can be empowered to significantly impact their healing and recovery.

This contribution reviews enhancing surgical outcome with psychological preparation for surgery. First, the problems associated with surgery are discussed, including growing trends towards shorter hospital stays and outpatient surgery, as well as physical and mental problems associated with surgery. Second, the actual benefits of psychological preparation for surgery are reviewed. Third, specific techniques are outlined, including the actual components of a psychological preparation for surgery program. Fourth, the contribution concludes with a discussion of how these techniques can be added to a psychological practice. For more details about psychological preparation for surgery, please see the book, *Preparing for Surgery: A Mind-Body Approach to Enhance Healing and Recovery* (Deardorff & Reeves, 1997).

THE CHANGING SURGICAL LANDSCAPE

Of the millions of surgeries performed in the United States last year, 20% were in response to an emergency, whereas 80% were considered "elective." Elective surgeries can range from "optional," such as removing a wart or cosmetic surgery, to "necessary," such as tumor removal, coronary artery bypass, hernia repair, hysterectomies, Caesarians, and many spinal surgeries, just to list a few. A psychological preparation for surgery program may be appropriate for any elective surgery done on either an inpatient or outpatient basis. An elective surgery often means there is adequate flexibility in scheduling to allow time for a preparation for surgery program to be completed.

Recent technological innovations in surgical practice, anesthesia, and pain control have made many operations safer than ever before. In the past 25 years, many surgeries have become safer and easier to perform because of advanced surgical instruments that require less invasive procedures, cause minimal tissue destruction, and result in almost no blood loss. In addition, new faster-acting anesthetic agents are much less dangerous and cause far fewer side-effects. Innovations in pain control methods and technology before, during, and following surgery have also dramatically reduced pain and side-effects, thus promoting faster recoveries. Sophisticated pain control techniques can now, in many instances, be effectively and safely delivered and monitored at home following surgery. These remarkable advances have prompted a strong trend toward shorter hospital stays and more outpatient surgeries. In fact, outpatient surgery now accounts for more than half of all surgical procedures performed in the United States (Macho & Cable, 1994). Over 200 kinds of operations now performed on an outpatient basis would have been too dangerous to do without hospitalization even a short time ago.

The managed health care revolution has also propelled the movement toward outpatient surgery in an effort to control costs. As of 1997, nearly three-quarters of all Americans with health insurance were enrolled in some type of health maintenance organization (HMO). Many insurance policies now require that certain operations be performed on a same-day basis. For those surgeries that are done on an inpatient basis, the number of days are "precertified" and kept to a minimum.

As a result of rapidly advancing, safer, less-invasive technology and the growing trend in managed care cost containment practices, the frequency of outpatient surgeries and shorter hospital stays will no doubt continue to increase even more quickly in the years to come. As a result, health care professionals are having less contact with their patients during the entire surgical process. This makes it much more difficult for surgeons to adequately prepare their patients for the procedure as well as monitoring, guiding, and reassuring them during the postoperative phase. This situation creates a fertile ground for complications, including a higher rate of patient dissatisfaction. An article entitled "Losing Patience," published in the *Los Angeles Times* (Levine, 1997) echoes this conclusion. The article noted that "60% of insured Californians are covered by managed care plans, and a 'simmering discontent' has become evident on the part of the public against those plans" (Section E1). It is certainly evident that in order to get the most out of medical care, patients must take more responsibility and play a more active role in their own treatment. A psychological preparation for surgery program is designed to accomplish this goal.

PROBLEMS ASSOCIATED WITH SURGERY

The Doctor-Patient Communication Gap

When patients do not have adequate information about their surgery and how to recover properly, they tend not to fare as well and are prone to more complications. Most epidemiological data indicate that Americans feel there is a significant doctor-patient communication gap, especially when it comes to surgery. A recent survey of consumers by the American Medical Association indicated that only 42% felt that doctors usually explained things well to their patients and only 31% believed that physicians spent enough time with their patients (Ferguson, 1993). This is corroborated by other research that has shown that the average amount of time a general practitioner spends with a patient is 7 minutes, and most doctors interrupt their patients within the first 18 seconds of their explanation of symptoms (Beckman & Frankel, 1984). Considering that the Beckman and Frankel (1984) findings date to the early 1980s before the full impact of managed care, the current situation is likely to be worse as physicians try to keep their production up by increasing patient volume. Given these disconcerting findings, it is not surprising that the vast majority of complaints against HMOs involve the manner in which the medical staff communicates with patients (Ferguson, 1993).

Even if the medical practitioner gives the patient an appropriate amount of time for discussing the surgery, communication problems can still occur. A great body of research demonstrates that most patients will not understand the medical information that is provided to them; nor will they remember it. Inadequate comprehension and retention of information about surgery frequently leads to patient dissatisfaction. This issue will be reviewed in more detail subsequently. These important issues of doctor-patient communication and patient comprehension of information are a primary source of stress, which may result in increased surgical side-effects and poor surgical outcome.

The Stress of Surgery

The stress of an illness or injury and the impending surgery can have a critical impact on both the physical and psychological states of the patient. Surgery and surgical pain are major physical stresses. Chemicals released from the surgically damaged tissue can cause further breakdown of body tissue, increased metabolic rate, increased blood clotting, increased water retention, impaired immune function, and release of stress hormones resulting in the "fight or flight" stress reaction (Benson, 1996). This sequence of events, if left unchecked, can dramatically impede healing and recovery (see Kiecolt-Glaser et al., 1998, for review).

Inadequate pain control is another major physical stress and can be psychologically demoralizing. Research has shown that less than 50% of all surgical patients are provided with adequate pain control following surgery. This alarming fact prompted the government to mandate, through The Agency for Health Care Policy and Research (AHCPR), the establishment of national guidelines for the management of surgical pain (AHCPR, 1992). The guidelines reviewed an abundance of research showing that poorly controlled pain impairs healing and recovery. There are, in fact, many potentially severe and even life-threatening complications that can result from excessive postoperative pain:

- Pain may lead to shallow breathing and cough suppression in an attempt to "splint" or guard the injured area. This results in retained pulmonary secretions ("water in the lungs") that can cause pneumonia.
- Unrelieved pain may delay the return of gastric motility and bowel function following surgery.
- Pain may delay activity such as getting out of bed, moving, and exercising, which are critically important for recovery. Excessive inactivity can increase the risk of inflammation in the veins that may cause dangerous blood clotting.
- Excessive pain can also result in increased requirements for pain medications. These medications, when taken incorrectly, can have side-effects that can negatively impact surgical recovery.

Patients who are provided with adequate pain control become active sooner and show significantly less emotional distress. They heal faster and report much greater satisfaction with the entire surgical experience.

Psychological stress can also affect surgical outcome in a variety of ways (Kiecolt-Glaser et al., 1998). For instance, studies have shown that patients have specific worries about a surgery that are often not addressed or even acknowledged (Johnston, 1988). These include important issues such as whether the operation will be a success, how much pain there will be after the surgery, if the surgeon will make a mistake, and whether the person will survive the procedure. These worries result in significant distress and can impact the surgical process in an adverse manner.

Psychological distress, specifically depression and anxiety, may also affect recovery in many ways. For example, patients who are depressed or anxious may be too unmotivated or fearful to engage in activities that are necessary for a normal recovery. This can cause the same adverse effects as uncontrolled pain, listed previously.

There is now also direct evidence that psychological stress can impair healing. Scientists have known for some time that stress can prevent our immune systems from working at optimal levels thereby making us more vulnerable to infection, but new evidence shows that stress can actually slow the healing time of wounds. For instance, it has been found that people who experience more everyday life stresses had a more difficult recovery from surgery

(B. S. Linn, M. W. Linn, & Klimas, 1988). In another well-controlled study, a group of healthy women who had been caring for a disabled husband or parent for an average of 7 hours per day was compared to a group of women without similar stress. Both groups underwent removal of a small piece of skin from the inner arm below the elbow. The study found that the wounds of the women in the high-stress group took about 9 days longer to heal than the low stress group (Kiecolt-Glaser et al., 1995). There were no other factors that could explain these findings except for the difference in stress levels. If stress can slow the healing of these small wounds, one might speculate that the effect on a major surgery would be even more profound.

BENEFITS OF PSYCHOLOGICAL PREPARATION FOR SURGERY

As discussed previously, there are several factors that clearly have a detrimental effect on surgical healing and recovery. These include recent trends toward shorter hospital stays and outpatient surgical interventions, doctor-patient communication issues, and the physical and psychological stresses of surgery. Unfortunately, these factors that affect surgical outcome and recovery are not adequately addressed during the routine course of events leading up to and following surgery. Psychological preparation for surgery addresses these needs.

Over the past 30 years, more than 200 research studies involving thousands of patients have investigated psychological preparation for surgery. The following specific beneficial effects have been found (see the following reviews: Deardorff & Reeves, 1997; Devine, 1992; Johnston & Vogel, 1993; Prokop et al., 1991):

- Less distress and anxiety both before and after surgery
- Fewer complications related to the surgery and recovery
- Less pain and less need for postoperative pain medication
- Less anesthesia requirements
- Quicker return to health
- Shorter hospitalization period
- Increased patient satisfaction with treatment
- Thousands of dollars in savings per surgery

Johnston and Vogel (1993) reviewed almost 90 scientific studies investigating psychological preparation for surgery. They concluded, "There is now substantial agreement that psychological preparation for surgery is beneficial to patients" (p. 253). In another major review of 191 studies dating from 1963 until the present, Devine (1992) concluded that the positive benefits outlined previously do, in fact, occur with surgical preparation programs. In the following section, specific techniques that are used in a psychological preparation for surgery program will be reviewed. The review will be cursory because most mental health professionals are familiar with these approaches.

SPECIFIC TECHNIQUES OF SURGERY PREPARATION

The specific techniques that are used in a psychological preparation for surgery program include helping the patient to:

- gather accurate information about the surgery and recovery
- get adequate pain control

- learn appropriate cognitive techniques
- learn deep relaxation exercises
- pay attention to spiritual issues
- develop assertiveness skills and control his or her environments

The characteristics of a surgery preparation program are quite flexible depending upon such things as how much time is available before the surgery is to be done, the motivation of the patient, and patient personality variables. Thus, a surgery preparation program may consist of as little as one session with the patient doing most of the exercises in a self-guided fashion, to several sessions or more. As will be discussed later, surgery preparation is amenable to both individual and group formats.

Collecting Information About the Surgery

A long-standing theory in the area of surgery preparation is that the more information a person has about the procedure and recovery, the better he or she will do postoperatively (Johnston, 1988). Information about a surgery can be divided into three specific types: procedural, sensory, and behavioral. Procedural information is factual, objective information about what events will occur and why (Wallace, 1984). Sensory information includes the types of "sensations" a patient is likely to experience throughout the surgery process and recovery. Behavioral information is what the patient will be expected to "do" primarily after the surgery (e.g., "You will be expected to get out of bed and walk the day after surgery in addition to doing breathing/respiratory exercises").

Although the positive benefits of providing information to surgery patients has been established in many studies, these results are tempered by other findings (see Johnston & Vogel, 1993, for review). When individuals are threatened with an aversive event, they show differences in how they manage the information about it. These different personality styles of coping have classified individuals into either "monitors" who are information-seekers or "blunters" who are distractors or information-avoiders (Miller, 1987). This research can be applied to the area of surgery preparation. For those patients who tend to be information-seekers, the more information they are given, the better they seem to do. If they are not given enough information, they will tend to show increased anxiety due to not feeling in control. On the other hand, patients who tend to be "blunters" in the face of the stress may actually do worse if they are given an overwhelming amount of information about their surgery. For blunters, a great deal of information results in more preoperative anxiety which correlates with poorer outcomes. Thus, some level of denial and distraction works best for blunters. For the health care professional, it is important to determine the personality style of the patient to help guide the amount and quality of information that should be provided for optimal results. This determination is done primarily through the clinical interview, although psychological testing can also be helpful (Deardorff & Reeves, 1997).

Research on patients' memory and understanding of medical information is also applicable to this area. As discussed earlier, it has been generally established that patients have a poor understanding of the medical information presented to them and remember little of what they are told (Deardorff, 1986; Ley, 1982; Roter, 1977). Many surgical consent forms are written at the level of scientific journals, beyond the comprehension of most people. Thus, only about 40% of people read the consent forms carefully. In addition, patients only remember about 30% to 50% of simple verbal information they are given about their surgery and only slightly more when it is written. Inadequate comprehension and memory of information about surgery frequently leads to patient dissatisfaction and can compromise treatment (Deardorff & Reeves, 1997).

Pain Control

Almost all surgical procedures cause mild to severe postoperative pain and suffering. Research has shown that postoperative pain is one of the greatest worries of surgical patients. Even so, patients are rarely prepared for the type of pain they will experience after the operation; nor is a systematic pain control approach commonly used. Adequate postoperative pain control is essential to the overall success of the surgery.

It is important to have a pain control plan in place prior to the surgery and to discuss this with the patient. For instance, giving the patient an idea of what to expect relative to postoperative pain, in addition to outlining how the patient is to respond to problems with pain, will greatly decrease complications in this area. It seems that surgeons may have a tendency to "downplay" the postoperative pain issue when discussing it with the patients. This is probably done in an effort to comfort patients and not "put ideas in their heads" about the pain. Unfortunately, this approach often backfires: patients believe something has gone terribly wrong because they were not forewarned about the level of postoperative pain. Agitation, fearfulness, anger, and depression are common responses to postoperative pain that was not expected.

It is beyond the scope of this contribution to review all of the intricacies of appropriate postoperative pain control. Some of the important techniques to consider for adequate pain control include the following (for complete reviews, see AHCPR, 1992; American Pain Society, 1992; Liebeskind, 1991; Melzack & Wall, 1982; Ready & Edwards, 1992):

- It is helpful for the patient to be able to identify the person who will be responsible for his or her postoperative pain management.
- Give the patient accurate expectations about the postoperative pain. This will help alleviate anxiety and worry when the pain occurs and give the patient a greater sense of control.
- Discuss pain medicine options with the patient prior to the surgery. This might include patient-controlled analgesia (PCA), time-contingent scheduling, and options for analgesic medications.
- Inform the patient about pain control options without medications such as cognitive-behavioral methods, relaxation techniques, modalities (e.g., heat and cold, etc.), and transcutaneous nerve stimulation (TNS).
- Help the patient learn how to alert the health care staff about increased pain, including methods to measure it (e.g., rating scales, visual analog scale). This will help the staff "stay ahead of the pain" for more effective management.
- Discuss with the patient how pain control will be managed after discharge from the hospital.

Paying attention to these simple pain control guidelines will result in less patient suffering, reduced complications, and enhancement of overall outcome.

Cognitive Techniques

In his play "Hamlet," Shakespeare wrote, "There is nothing either good or bad, but thinking makes it so." This tenet nicely summarizes the nature of cognitive interventions. These techniques include methods such as distraction, thought stopping, identifying negative automatic thoughts, and developing coping thoughts. Cognitive-behavioral techniques help in surgery preparation in two ways: (a) by directly decreasing the patient's preoperative anxiety and fear and (b) by giving patients the coping skills to help decrease postoperative anxiety and pain (Horne, Vatmanidis, & Careri, 1994).

We all constantly judge and interpret the world around us. These thoughts and judgments, both conscious and unconscious, have been termed "self-talk" because they are like inner dialogues. This inner dialogue or self-talk, which is often out of our awareness, causes emotional and physical reactions. When we are under stress, such as facing a surgery, the self-talk can take on a negative or pessimistic bias. These are called automatic negative thoughts. There are several types or categories of negative automatic thoughts, but the most common ones that occur in preparing for surgery include (see Davis, Eshelman, & McKay, 1995; Deardorff & Reeves, 1997, for a review):

Catastrophizing - imagining the worst possible scenario and then acting as if that will actually happen.

Filtering - focusing only on the negative aspects of a situation to the exclusion of any positive elements or options.

Black and White Thinking - also termed "all-or-nothing" thinking, there is no middle ground nor any shades of gray.

Overgeneralization - an aspect of one situation is applied to all other situations, whether appropriate or not.

Shoulds - Should statements are a key element to negative self-talk. "Should" thinking is operating from a list of inflexible and unrealistic rules about how you (your body) and others "should" act or respond.

Examples of this type of thinking related to surgery include: "What if I never get better?" (catastrophizing); "There is nothing that will help my situation" (filtering); "The surgery either works or it is a failure" (black and white thinking); "With this surgery, I will never have any fun again" (overgeneralization); and "I should never have allowed this to happen" (shoulds).

In preparing for surgery, patients are taught to identify this type of thinking and develop challenging or coping thoughts. This is done through a method called "Stop-Challenge-Reframe" (Deardorff & Reeves, 1997). This involves instructing the patient on how to identify the negative automatic thought when it occurs, challenging the thought through a self-questioning process, and replacing the negative thoughts with coping thoughts. Patients master this technique fairly quickly through the use of a written journal. With a little practice, the negative automatic thoughts begin to diminish and the coping thoughts become more natural. These cognitive exercises can greatly reduce or eliminate anxiety, stress, and dysphoria that often accompany the surgery process.

Relaxation Techniques

The process of going through a surgery is stressful, extending from the time the patient is faced with the decision of whether to have the operation until the recovery is complete. Stress causes deleterious effects on the body including such things as increased blood pressure, increased heart rate, increased muscle tension, rapid and shallow breathing, release of stress hormones, reduced blood flow to certain areas of the body, diminished immune system function, and slowed tissue healing time. Relaxation techniques can effectively block this stress response (Sobel & Ornstein, 1996).

The relaxation response as originally described by Benson (1975) is more than just relaxing. It is a state of deep relaxation in which there are specific physiological changes that are the exact opposite of the stress response. These include a decrease in heart rate, respiration rate, blood pressure, skeletal muscle tension, metabolic rate, and oxygen consumption. Using the relaxation response (RR) throughout the surgery process can help reduce pain, control nausea, enhance immune system function, and improve respiratory function.

There are many methods to achieve the RR, including breathing techniques, progressive muscle relaxation, visualizing a peaceful scene, and meditation, among others. Given the frequent time constraints on a surgery preparation program, a simple deep breathing exercise seems to be the quickest and easiest for patients to master. It involves learning how to breathe diaphragmatically in a slow, paced fashion. Mastering this technique only requires about 10 minutes of practice twice per day. The patient will notice results within 1 or 2 weeks. The deep breathing exercise is generally chosen because it is straightforward, easy to practice, and not very time-consuming as compared with some of the other methods. This increases the probability that patients will actually do it. With a little practice, patients are able to elicit the RR very quickly even in stressful situations.

Once the patient has learned to elicit the RR reliably, cue-controlled relaxation can begin. This is simply the "pairing" of the relaxation response with a specific "cue." The cue can be a muscular signal or a verbal signal such as a word. In the example of using a word, the patient might say "relax" quietly to himself or herself as the RR is practiced at home in a nonthreatening environment. In the case of a muscle cue, we will often have patients touch their forefinger and thumb together while practicing the RR. Once this pairing is practiced for a while, the cue becomes associated with the actual RR and can elicit it in almost any situation. At that point, patients have a powerful tool at their disposal for managing the stresses of going through a surgery. When they are in the stressful situation they simply need to tell themselves to relax or touch their forefinger and thumb together to elicit the RR.

Spiritual Issues

According to a Gallup poll conducted in 1990, 95% of Americans said they believe in God, and 76% said they pray regularly (Gallup, 1990). Even so, there appears to be a doctor-patient spirituality gap and doctors are reluctant to discuss spirituality issues with patients (Wallis, 1996). Many doctors underestimate the importance of religion and prayer to their patients (Larson, 1993), and patients are reluctant to bring these issues up for discussion (Dossey, 1993).

Recent research seems to indicate that belief in a higher power makes a positive contribution to a person's physical health and may help with the surgery process (Larson, 1993; Levin, 1994; Matthews, Larson, & Barry, 1994; Pressman et al., 1990). Spiritual beliefs provide many benefits including giving the person a sense of meaning and purpose, setting health priorities, and giving comfort in the face of illness and crises. All of these can facilitate the surgery process and improve outcomes.

Physicians, surgeons, and other health care professionals can help patients feel comfortable in discussing their spiritual issues related to the surgery process. As an example, Deardorff and Reeves (1997) discuss a patient who had many fears about undergoing a complete hysterectomy (pp. 153-154). She found great comfort in her spiritual practice of Hindu meditation but was reluctant to discuss this with her surgeon. Ultimately, she mustered the courage to talk to her surgeon about her beliefs. The surgeon and a hospital representative made special arrangements for her to have taped recordings of her mantra while in the hospital and to set up a small altar (including a picture of her guru and some flowers) in her room. Her surgery and postoperative recovery went exceptionally well.

This is only one example of how addressing spiritual issues can facilitate the surgery process. Another is how patients will often combine their spiritual beliefs, prayer, and relaxation exercises. Benson found that patients will commonly use prayers as a "mantra" to enhance the relaxation response (1996). He found that this enhanced the RR in many ways including increasing the likelihood that the patient would continue to practice the RR, bringing forth brain waves that are associated with wellness and helping allay feelings of worry and anxiety.

Developing Assertiveness Skills and Controlling One's Environments

The process of surgery and postoperative recovery can bring up many stressful situations in which assertiveness skills will be required for the patient to get good care. As mentioned previously, several interesting findings underscore this point:

> In an extensive survey, only 42 percent of patients felt that their doctor explained things well to them and only 31 percent believed that physicians spent enough time with them.
>
> The average amount of time that a general practitioner spends with a patient is seven minutes. One study found that most doctors interrupt their patients within the first 18 seconds of their explanation of symptoms. (Ferguson, 1993, p. 432)

These findings suggest that patients will have to be assertive with their health care providers to insure that the doctors understand their symptoms and for the patients to get the information they desire. Beyond the preceding findings, other observations indicate that patients also share some of the responsibility for not getting what they need from their health care providers. Kaplan and Greenfield (1989) have determined that the average patient asks fewer than four questions in a 15-minute visit with the doctor. One question frequently asked is, "Will you validate my parking?"

Beyond these issues, being assertive may actually help a patient protect himself or herself during the surgery process (see Griffin, 1996, for a review of this issue). For instance, the chance of getting an infection during a hospital stay is estimated to be between 5% and 10%. Each year, more Americans die from hospital infections than from car accidents and homicides combined. Disturbingly, the Center for Disease Control has found that a great majority of these hospital infections can be prevented. In a review of 37 studies on hand washing, it was found that doctors and nurses typically wash their hands only 40% of the time, even in intensive care units. Being assertive about simple preventative procedures, such as requesting that doctors or nurses wash their hands, could save the patient's life.

Having adequate assertiveness skills can also help patients manage the various environments in which they function. One important way is through adequate time management. Throughout the surgery process, it is important for patients to adequately manage their work, home, hospital, and other situations. Excessive stress in any of these areas has the potential to greatly disrupt the surgery process. Important skills for successfully managing these environments during the surgery process include setting priorities, taking time out for relaxation, delegating responsibilities, and setting appropriate limits. Completing these tasks successfully involves assertiveness behaviors.

THE BUSINESS OF SURGERY PREPARATION

After mental health professionals have become familiar with surgery preparation techniques, they must successfully integrate preparing for surgery into their practice. There are several ways to approach marketing, and given the clinician's particular situation, one or all of them might be pursued. These include offering the program within the surgeon's office, targeting certain types of surgeries, making an arrangement with a local hospital, and contacting insurance companies.

Probably one of the best and most sure ways of gaining access to surgery patients is within the offices of a group surgery practice. Offering the preparation for surgery program either in a group format or individually within the surgeon's office makes it easier for the patient and the physician, as well as increasing the probability that patients will follow through on the recommendation. When approaching surgeons with this proposal, it is important to be as organized and succinct as possible. Focus on making the process easy to implement within another doctor's office and highlight how the program will benefit the surgeon. A few suggestions include: (a) prepare patient pamphlets for the waiting room that describe the program, (b) design referral slips in the form of a prescription pad that the surgeon or assistant can use to make the referral, and (c) make the surgeon a part of the program so that patients see it as being a benefit of the surgery practice.

Adequate space is often an issue in any office. A useful method to address this problem is to use the waiting room of the practice in the evenings to run the preparation for surgery groups. Of course, paying an overhead fee for the use of the space is appropriate. Lastly, the logistics of running the groups should be almost transparent to the surgery practice. The clinician or a designate should handle scheduling, questions about the program, and other program-related issues so that these do not fall upon and overburden the surgery practice. Becoming too much of an administrative "hassle" is the death knell of this type of arrangement.

It can be useful to target a certain surgery population for marketing for at least two reasons. First, providing successful preparation for surgery treatment almost always requires that the clinician have knowledge about the specific procedure (e.g., what the procedure involves, amount of time in the hospital, what the postoperative course is usually like, possible complications, what the psychological issues are likely to be, etc.). Second, some surgeries are highly amenable to advanced scheduling, which allows adequate time for the surgery preparation program. Examples of these include C-sections, most spine surgeries, many heart surgeries, certain organ transplantations, and others.

Another marketing method is to make an arrangement with a local hospital to offer a preparation for surgery program. It can be formulated to the hospital administration as being similar to offering child-birthing classes. Hospitals are always looking for ways to stand out in the public eye. Being able to advertise that they offer a unique program such as preparing for surgery is an excellent item that they can use as part of their marketing to the public as well as doctors.

Insurance companies are another area for potential marketing, although this is bound to be the most frustrating and probably least fruitful. Although you can do a dynamite presentation on how referring patients to a preparation for surgery program can benefit the insurer (e.g., increased patient satisfaction, decreased complications, shorter hospital stays, and overall cost-savings), it can be virtually impossible to get beyond the "red tape" to actually implement the idea.

Depending on a number of factors, practice in this area can often be done outside the constraints of mental health managed care in one of two ways. First, because the program is very amenable to a group format, it can be offered in a structured "class" format rather than as psychological treatment. Patients simply sign up to take the surgery preparation class and pay a fee for the entire class when they register. Under this approach, it would not matter if the clinician were on the managed care panel of any of the class members, because the program is not being offered as treatment. It is important to remember that, if the program is offered as a class, it should be done as such for all members of the group. It would not be prudent to have some members of the class participate on an insurance basis (implying treatment) while others are doing it as a "class."

The class method of running the program is probably the best approach because it really decreases the amount of administrative overhead (e.g., patient and insurance billing, getting preapprovals, etc.) and increases patient motivation to attend each meeting, as it is prepaid. Any patient who required individual treatment beyond the groups (for instance, in the case of medical phobias) could be seen on a different basis at that time. Doing the surgery preparation program as a class follows a model similar to the child-birthing classes or a stress-management class one might take at a local college or hospital.

Second, it is occasionally possible to get approval to provide this treatment under the patient's medical benefits because it directly relates to a surgical intervention. This can be somewhat of a long and arduous process requiring precertification documentation to be supplied about the program, why it should be considered medical treatment, and a referral letter of medical necessity from the surgeon.

Materials

There are several important resources for developing and implementing a preparing for surgery program. *Preparing for Surgery: A Mind-Body Approach to Enhance Healing and Recovery* (Deardorff & Reeves, 1997) is a patient workbook that can be used as the core material for the program. It has structured exercises for the patient to complete and contains an exhaustive list of additional resources. Other books that contain excellent information but are not done in an interactive format include: *A Patient's Guide to Surgery* (Bradley, 1994); *Good Operations, Bad Operations* (Inlander, 1993); *Take This Book to the Hospital With You* (Inlander & Weiner, 1993); *Everyone's Guide to Outpatient Surgery* (Macho & Cable, 1994); *Surgery Electives: What to Know Before the Doctor Operates* (McCabe, 1994); and *The Surgery Book: An Illustrated Guide to 73 of the Most Common Operations* (Youngston, 1993). These latter books were written by surgeons and may tend to frighten patients about the surgery process. They are good professional resources but should be reviewed prior to recommending for patient use. Useful websites for gathering information about surgeries include the following:

http://www.surgeryprep.com
http://www.healthatoz.com
http://www.med-library.com
http://www.cdc.gov
http://www.ampainsoc.org
http://www.health-net.com

CONTRIBUTOR

William W. Deardorff, PhD, ABPP, received his doctorate in clinical psychology from Washington State University, did an internship at the University of Washington Medical School, and then completed a postdoctoral fellowship in behavioral medicine at Kaiser Permanente Medical Center in Los Angeles. Dr. Deardorff is a Fellow of the American Psychological Association, Past-President of the American Academy of Clinical Health Psychology, and assistant clinical professor at the UCLA School of Medicine. He has published extensively in the area of health psychology. Dr. Deardorff can be reached at 120 S. Spalding Drive, Suite 400, Beverly Hills, CA 90212.

RESOURCES

The Agency for Health Care Policy and Research. (1992). *The Practice Guidelines for Acute Pain Management: Operative or Medical Procedures and Trauma.* Silver Springs, MD: Author. (Available for free from The Agency for Health Care Policy and Research [AHCPR] Clearinghouse [800-358-9295], P.O. Box 8547, Silver Springs, MD 20907)

American Pain Society. (1992). *Principles of Analgesic Use in the Treatment of Acute Pain and Cancer Pain* (3rd ed.). Glenview, IL: Author.

Beckman, H. B., & Frankel, R. M. (1984). The effect of physician behavior on the collection of data. *Annals of Internal Medicine, 101,* 692-696.

Benson, H. (1975). *The Relaxation Response.* New York: William Morrow.

Benson, H. (1996). *Timeless Healing: The Power and Biology of Belief.* New York: Scribner.

Bradley, E. L. (1994). *A Patient's Guide to Surgery.* New York: Consumer Reports Books.

Davis, M., Eshelman, E. R., & McKay, M. (1995). *The Relaxation and Stress Reduction Workbook* (4th ed.). Oakland, CA: New Harbinger Publications.

Deardorff, W. W. (1986). Computerized health education: A comparison with traditional formats. *Health Education Quarterly, 13,* 61-73.

Deardorff, W. W., & Reeves, J. L. (1997). *Preparing for Surgery: A Mind-Body Approach to Enhance Healing and Recovery.* Oakland, CA: New Harbinger Publications.

Devine, E. C. (1992). Effects of psychoeducation care of adult surgical patients: A meta-analysis of 191 studies. *Patient Education and Counseling, 19,* 129-142.

Dossey, L. (1993). *Healing Words: The Power of Prayer and the Practice of Medicine.* New York: HarperCollins.

Ferguson, T. (1993). Working with your doctor. In D. Goleman & J. Gurin (Eds.), *Mind-Body Medicine: How to Use Your Mind for Better Health* (pp. 429-450). Yonkers, NY: Consumer Reports Books.

Gallup, G. H., Jr. (1990). *Religion in America.* Princeton, NJ: Princeton Religion Research Center.

Griffin, K. (1996). They should have washed their hands. *Health, November-December,* 82-90.

Horne, D., Vatmanidis, P., & Careri, A. (1994). Preparing patients for invasive medical and surgical procedure I: Adding behavioral and cognitive interventions. *Behavioral Medicine, 20,* 5-26.

Inlander, C. B. (1993). *Good Operations, Bad Operations.* New York: Penguin Books.

Inlander, C. B., & Weiner, E. D. (1993). *Take This Book to the Hospital With You.* Avenel, NJ: Wings Books.

Johnston, M. (1988). Impending surgery. In S. Fisher & J. Reason (Eds.), *Handbook of Life Stress, Cognition and Health* (pp. 79-100). New York: John Wiley and Sons.

Johnston, M., & Vogel, C. (1993). Benefits of psychological preparation for surgery: A meta-analysis. *Annals of Behavioral Medicine, 15*(4), 245-256.

Kaplan, S. H., & Greenfield, S. S. (1989). Assessing the effects of physician-patient interactions on the outcomes of chronic disease. *Medical Care, 27,* 110-127.

Kiecolt-Glaser, J. K., Marucha, P. T., Malarkey, W. B., Mercado, A. M., & Glaser, R. (1995). Slowing of wound healing by psychological stress. *Lancet, 346,* 1194-1196.

Kiecolt-Glaser, J. K., Page, G. G., Marucha, P. T., MacCallum, R. C., & Glaser, R. (1998). Psychological influences on surgical recovery: Perspectives from psychoneuroimmunology. *American Psychologist, 53,* 1209-1218.

Larson, D. B. (1993). *The Faith Factor: An Annotated Bibliography of Systematic Reviews and Clinical Research on Spiritual Subjects* (Vol. 2). Boston, MA: John Templeton Foundation.

Levin, J. S. (1994). Religion and health: Is there an association, is it valid, and is it causal? *Social Science and Medicine, 38,* 1475-1482.

Levine, B. (1997, July 9). Losing patience. *Los Angeles Times,* Section E1.

Ley, P. (1982). Studies of recall in medical settings. *Human Learning, 1,* 223-233.

Liebeskind, J. C. (1991). Pain can kill. *Pain, 44,* 3-4.

Linn, B. S., Linn, M. W., & Klimas, N. G. (1988). Effects of psychological stress on surgical outcome. *Psychosomatic Medicine, 50,* 230-244.

Macho, J., & Cable, G. (1994). *Everyone's Guide to Outpatient Surgery.* Kansas City, MO: Sommerville House Books.

Matthews, D. A., Larson, D. B., & Barry, C. P. (1994). *The Faith Factor: An Annotated Bibliography of Systematic Reviews and Clinical Research on Spiritual Subjects* (Vol. 1). Boston, MA: John Templeton Foundation.

McCabe, J. (1994). *Surgery Electives: What to Know Before the Doctor Operates*. Santa Monica, CA: Carmania Books.

Melzack, R., & Wall, P. D. (1982). *The Challenge of Pain*. New York: Basic Books.

Miller, S. M. (1987). Monitoring and blunting: Validation of a questionnaire to assess styles of information-seeking under threat. *Journal of Personality and Social Psychology, 52*(2), 345-353.

Pressman, P., Lyons, J. S., Larson, D. B., & Strain, J. J. (1990). Religious belief, depression, and ambulation status in elderly women with broken hips. *American Journal of Psychiatry, 147,* 758-760.

Prokop, C. K., Bradley, L. A., Burish, T. G., Anderson, K. O., & Fox, J. E. (1991). Psychological preparation for stressful medical and dental procedures (Chapter 7). In *Health Psychology-Clinical Methods and Research* (pp. 159-196). New York: Macmillan.

Ready, B. L., & Edwards, W. T. (1992). *Management of Acute Pain: A Practical Guide*. Seattle, WA: International Association for the Study of Pain.

Roter, D. L. (1977). Patient participation in the patient-provider interaction: The effects of patient question asking on the quality of interaction, satisfaction and compliance. *Health Education Monographs, 5,* 281-315.

Sobel, D. S., & Ornstein, R. (1996). *The Healthy Mind, Healthy Body Handbook*. Los Altos, CA: Drx.

Wallace, L. M. (1984). Psychological preparation as a method of reducing the stress of surgery. *Journal of Human Stress, 10,* 62-77.

Wallis, C. (1996, June 24). Faith and healing. *Time*, pp. 58-68.

Youngston, R. M. (1993). *The Surgery Book: An Illustrated Guide to 73 of the Most Common Operations*. New York: St. Martin's Press.

Adventure Therapy With Adolescents

Jennifer Davis-Berman and Dene S. Berman

Therapists who work with adolescents understand the limitations of traditional practice settings with this population. Some of these limitations include the confines of a traditional office and the 50-minute hour; the reliance on verbal interchanges between therapist and clients that emphasize cognitive functioning, and the reality of few available levels of care in the current managed care atmosphere (Berman & Davis-Berman, 1995). Adventure therapy is an approach to working with adolescents that overcomes these limitations, contributing to the repertoire of methodologies available to the clinician.

This contribution will present and discuss the use of adventure therapy with adolescents. We will begin by developing a rationale for adventure-based approaches. This will be followed by an explication of the history of the use of adventure as therapy. Different applications of adventure will be presented, followed by a short discussion of the efficacy of these approaches. Finally, we will present and discuss an example of an adventure-based approach to counseling with adolescents.

HISTORICAL PERSPECTIVES ON ADVENTURE THERAPY

The history of the use of the outdoors as a vehicle for growth and change dates back to the early 1900s. At the Manhattan State Hospital, 40 tuberculosis patients were put in tents on the hospital lawn due to lack of space. Interestingly, these patients improved rather dramatically, both physically and psychologically. This same "treatment" was then implemented with the psychiatric patients at the same hospital, again as a space-saving strategy. These patients experienced significant improvements above what would have been expected through traditional treatment. In fact, many of the patients improved enough to justify their discharge (*American Journal of Insanity,* 1906). These initial reports of success generated interest and enthusiasm, but no outcome data other than anecdotal reports accompanied these programs. As America entered the First World War, tenting programs disappeared from the psychiatric literature.

The therapeutic emphasis in outdoor programs resurfaced with Camp Ahmek in 1929 (Dimock & Hendry, 1939). During this early period in the 1900s, there was a strong and important recognition of the natural environment and its ability to stimulate growth and change. There was also an emphasis on activity and the use of adventure in working with people (e.g., Backus, 1947; S. Scheidlinger & L. Scheidlinger, 1947; Zander, 1947). Other early camps included the Michigan Fresh Air Camp (Morse, 1947) and the Salesmanship Club of Dallas, founded by Campbell Loughmiller (Smith, 1958). Loughmiller was a leader in the early therapeutic camp movement. He appreciated and understood the natural environment and its power to facilitate change (Loughmiller, 1965). His ideas have been so influential that they are still referred to today, as is the Salesmanship Club.

One cannot discuss the history of modern outdoor adventure programs without examining the development and implementation of the Outward Bound program. This program was first conceived by Dr. Kurt Hahn, a committed educator. In 1920, Hahn became the Headmaster of the Salem School in Germany. While in this position, Hahn formulated and refined his ideas about education and suggested many innovations. Some of his initial formulations included the inclusion of noncompetitive physical activities in discussions about social cooperation. He also believed that all students should be involved in service to others. Finally, Hahn believed that solitude was essential for learning (James, 1993).

The actual birth of Outward Bound occurred in 1941 in Aberdovey, Wales, by Hahn, who had resettled there. It was there that Hahn applied his notions about the relationship between the physical and the psychological realms to the adjustment and functioning of British merchant seamen (Miner & Boldt, 1981). Later, Kurt Hahn and his dedicated followers worked tirelessly to affect education both within the United States and in the world community. Central components of Hahn's ideas were commitments to service and the pursuit of personal growth and courage through the experience of adventure (Katz & Kolb, 1967).

Although some of the more recent Outward Bound programs are more therapeutic in their focus (James, 1980), the earliest conceptions of Outward Bound lacked reflection and discussion of the experiences gained in the program. Rather, there was a belief that the experience and the environment were healing and therapeutic in and of themselves, and that the mountains speak for themselves (Bacon, 1988). The later formulations of the Outward Bound program involved more debriefing and reflection on the adventure experiences. In fact, some of their programs have become much more therapeutic and include offerings for high-risk groups (e.g., Itin, 1995; James, 1980; Katz & Kolb, 1967; Miner & Boldt, 1981).

Recent years have seen the continued popularity of therapeutic wilderness programs for youth. In an attempt to examine existing wilderness therapy programs more closely, we surveyed 31 programs (Davis-Berman, Berman, & Capone, 1994). The majority of these programs primarily served adolescents, supporting our earlier contention about the popularity of alternatives to traditional programs for adolescents. The activities utilized in these programs ranged from backpacking expeditions to canoeing to ropes courses. There was a wide range of program length, with some occurring over the course of only a few hours, while others were residential in nature, over the course of several months. These long-term programs are usually from 6 to 9 months in length. Participants may live at a base camp, attend school, and participate in both individual and group therapy. Often, wilderness expeditions occur from these base camps (Davis-Berman et al., 1994).

The popularity of wilderness therapy programs is demonstrated in an article by Friese, Hendee, and Kinziger (1998) who were able to identify over 700 programs in the United States that took place in the outdoors and had personal growth, therapy, rehabilitation, education, or leadership/organizational development as their focus. Russell and Hendee (1999) looked at five of the largest expedition-based wilderness therapy programs in the United States. By multiplying the number of clients served in these five programs per year (1,715) by the average number of days in each program (38), they were able to project that there are 65,170 client days of therapy provided by these five programs. These authors projected that industry-wide, there may be as many as 330,000 user days and $60 million in revenue per year generated by one segment of this field, wilderness therapy programs.

DEFINING ADVENTURE THERAPY

Adventure therapy was initially defined in terms of program goals and client characteristics (Gillis et al., 1991). They described programs in terms of whether their primary emphasis was on education and enrichment (personal growth), as an adjunct to therapy, or therapy per se. More recently, Gillis (1995) defined adventure therapy "as an active approach to psychotherapy for people seeking behavioral change . . . that utilizes adventure activities, be they group games and initiatives or wilderness expeditions" (pp. 5-6).

Continued debates in the literature occur regarding what is considered therapy versus what is considered therapeutic. If adventure-based programs take place in outdoor settings, are they automatically considered to be therapy? Are they therapeutic? We have argued (e.g., Davis-Berman & Berman, 1993) that adventure programs, including those in wilderness settings with clinical populations, are not inherently therapy programs. Rather, they may facilitate and accelerate the process of change. The setting and the program type may set the stage for the delivery of therapy itself (Davis-Berman & Berman, 1993, 1994). These issues continue to be hotly debated as the field of adventure therapy continues to try to define itself. In fact, the first international adventure therapy conference was held in 1997, resulting in a publication based on the presentations at that conference (Itin, 1998).

Adventure, when used as a therapy, is an intentional process, containing all the components that one would find in more traditional settings, including assessments, treatment plans, progress notes, and the like (Davis-Berman & Berman, 1994). Adventure therapy is, at heart, a group process (Ringer, in press).

Another critical element that is repeatedly mentioned has to do with the role of reflection on the part of clients. This has not uniformly been so, in that earlier programs, like Outward Bound, minimized reflection and communication as part of the process of growth. Instead, it was espoused that "the mountains speak for themselves" (Davis-Berman & Berman, 1994). More recently, authors have emphasized the importance of reflection. For example, Gass's *Book of Metaphors* (1995) contains a host of activities that can be used with a variety of populations. What makes these activities unique are the narratives that accompany them, suggesting ways of framing the activities so that they can be used as metaphors for growth on the part of the client. Luckner and Nadler (1997), from a narrative therapy perspective, have written about helping clients process their experiences to maximize growth and generalization.

As we previously discussed, adventure therapy programs take many forms and include a variety of settings and techniques. The next section of this contribution briefly discusses some of these variations, including the following adventure therapy program types: games and initiatives, ropes courses, family therapy, adjunctive therapy, psychotherapy, and wilderness therapy.

Games and Initiatives

As one might imagine, there is a very wide range of games and initiatives that are used in some adventure therapy programs. Many of these games and initiatives were developed from the Project Adventure program, a school-related program first begun in the very early 1970s. Project Adventure began with an emphasis on the role and power of experience in the learning process. Thus, rather than lecture about something like communication, games and initiatives were used to help students actually experience communication and its benefits. Project Adventure began as a school-based training program, but rather quickly moved into other spheres of influence. In the early 1980s, this program became a nonprofit corporation and began to train educators and other human service professionals (Schoel, Prouty, & Radcliffe, 1988).

In addition to school and organizational training, Project Adventure staff developed and continue to support a modality referred to as Adventure Based Counseling. Basically, this approach includes adventure, group activity, and community service. This counseling approach has had wide applicability in schools, hospitals, and court-related programs (Schoel et al., 1988).

As defined by Rohnke (1989, p. 59), "A game can be an end in itself [and] can be for personal enjoyment only." Games are often used to introduce group members to each other, stimulate group interactions, or establish a norm for interactions. They can be as elementary and fun as Shoe Bin (Rohnke, 1991), in which group members sit in a circle, blindfolded, and throw their shoes in a pile in the middle. The group is then timed to see how fast they can all locate and put their shoes on. Games are often simple, like throwing balls and saying names, but can also be complex in terms of communication and trust.

Initiatives are tasks that require groups to work together and to cooperate and communicate in solving some kind of problem (Rohnke, 1989). This might involve working as a group to get everyone safely across a pit or getting all participants over a 14-foot-high wall. In Group Juggle (Rohnke, 1989), members of a group in a circle throw and catch a ball. They are asked to establish a sequence. Once started, more balls can be added to the sequence, or clients can be asked to make unique sounds when they catch or throw a ball. Often, games and initiatives are grouped into categories that define their purpose: ice breakers, deinhibitizers, trust and empathy activities, communication activities, decision-making and problem-solving activities, or social responsibility and personal responsibility activities (Schoel et al., 1988).

Games and initiatives tap into a sense of play and fun for participants. Some of them include an element of risk, or at least perceived risk, that adds to the feeling and experience of adventure. In fact, some authors (e.g., Luckner & Nadler, 1997) assert that perceived risk and disequilibrium are necessary antecedents to change.

An example of a very popular activity is the Trust Fall. Rather than talking about trust and how trust is developed, participants actually experience trust through this activity. Basically, the participant stands on a platform or other object that is no more than 5 feet high. Then, the faller, with eyes closed, falls backwards into the interlocked arms of the catchers. This activity, which requires careful setup to assure safety, demands the attention, communication, and, above all, trust between participants (Rohnke, 1989). For many, this activity is often very challenging for participants in that it contains an element of perceived risk.

Often, metaphors are drawn between the activities and real life and are then used to apply lessons learned during the activity to real life. The parallels between the activity and a person's life have been referred to as "isomorphs." Gass (1995) outlined steps in a model for using activities for change that include the selection of activities that have a metaphoric (isomorphic) relationship to the goals and then strengthening this relationship through the verbal and physical setup of the activity and the discussion that follows it.

Games, initiatives, and ropes courses can be processed with the group after the experience ("debriefing"), prior to the experience ("frontloading" or "prebriefing"), or by using some combination of the two. Issues surrounding discussion of activities to maximize change and generalization are discussed in more depth elsewhere (Cain & Joliff, 1998; Itin, 1998; Luckner & Nadler, 1997).

This process can be exemplified by using the activity of Willow in the Wind (Rohnke, 1989, p. 52), where "[t]en to fifteen people stand shoulder to shoulder with one person (the faller) standing rigid and trusting in the center. Remaining rigid, the center person falls slowly in any direction [while those in the circle] redirect the faller's impetus." How a therapist would use this exercise would depend largely on the goals of the activity for this group. In this example, the falling experience may be used as a metaphor for trusting others and letting go of control. This might be discussed as an important aspect of healthy group functioning, and members might be taught to physically insure that the faller is safe. After the activity, elements of safety and trust might be central to a discussion.

Ropes Courses

Ropes courses are often casually referred to as obstacle courses in the skies. Generally ropes courses include both high and low elements that are usually stationary, at a fixed location. Many times, these courses are built in wooded areas, but that is not essential, as they can even be constructed inside.

The first ropes courses in the United States have been credited to Outward Bound in the 1960s and have undergone many changes in the years since. Many of these changes have been in the form of added safety features. Ever since their use, ropes courses have been employed in programs for troubled youth (Rohnke, Tait, & Wall, 1998).

The low ropes elements are constructed close to the ground. Generally, these elements focus more on the group and allow participants to experience group cohesion, cooperation, communication, and trust. The risk in these elements is not so much the physical safety risk as it is the emotional risks of opening up and being vulnerable. Prior to each activity, the leader sets the stage, detailing expectations. An attempt is made to insure that both physical and emotional safety are assured. In this case, emotional safety reflects the need for participants to support each other. Each ropes course can be custom built; thus, the elements and activities vary from course to course. However, some of the more popular elements include: Mohawk Walk, Nitro Crossing, Prouty's Landing, the Spider's Web, and the Wall (see Rohnke et al. [1998] for a detailed explanation of how these activities are set up and run).

All Aboard (Rohnke, 1989; Rohnke et al., 1998) serves as an excellent example of a low ropes course element. Using a sturdy platform 2 feet square and just a few inches off the ground, the goal of the activity is to see how many people as possible can use the platform to keep themselves off the surrounding ground for 10 seconds. This activity requires that the group work together to solve the problem. It also requires communication and cooperation. Finally, this is an activity that requires a great deal of physical contact between the participants in which body size, gender, and appropriate touch can play a role (Rohnke, 1989; Rohnke et al., 1998).

The high ropes elements are generally approached after successfully completing the low elements. These elements tend to be focused more on the individual, rather than on group dynamics. However, others are important, especially those who are on belay (holding the ropes) below. As with the low ropes elements, metaphors are often used in working with clients on the high ropes. For example, facing the fear of heights can be used as a metaphor for facing other fears in life.

For many, the Pamper Pole is the ultimate in the high ropes course experience (see Rohnke et al., 1998, pp. 121-122 for a good discussion of this element in more detail). The goal of this activity is for an individual to climb to the top of a telephone pole, stand on the top of it, and then dive from it to a trapeze that is out of reach. Of course, the person is harnessed, with other safety equipment and considerations to eliminate falls and injury. It is, however, a daunting task to stand on top of a pole that is between 25 and 50 feet tall and dive into the air for a trapeze that seems so far away. The thrill and the fear can be awesome (Rohnke, 1989). It must be reiterated that the use of this activity, which must be conducted under specially constructed and supervised conditions, is therapeutic only to the extent that the challenge is taken willingly by the participant and skillfully put in context and discussed by the therapist.

Family Therapy

The application of adventure techniques and philosophy to family therapy is a fairly recent occurrence. Two of the more prominent books that deal with content on adventure therapy as related to families are *Adventure Therapy* (Gass, 1993) and *Experiential Family Counseling* (Gerstein, 1994). The unit of attention in this approach is the entire family, rather than an identified patient. Obviously, an activity-oriented approach is used to work with families, utilizing many of the games and initiatives discussed previously.

Adventure-based family therapy is different from traditional therapy in its emphasis on both adaptive and maladaptive behaviors of all of the family members. Through the use of activities, interactions and behaviors within the family may be more easily seen by the therapist. The consequences of such behaviors are also more easily seen and experienced, both by the therapist and by the family members themselves. Also, new behaviors may be tried within the context of the activities (Gerstein, 1994).

The goals of adventure and experiential therapy are not really different from the goals of traditional family therapy; it is the mode of practice that is different. The general goals of this approach are open and honest communication, acceptance and understanding of the concerns of other family members, identifying individual and family strengths, becoming more solution focused, increasing the flexibility of family roles, monitoring and modifying discipline in the family, monitoring and adjusting parental roles, and encouraging the family to have fun (Gerstein, 1994). Within this framework, activities are used to serve a number of therapeutic purposes. They can facilitate the gathering of assessment information. Importantly, they can also serve as metaphors for problem areas in the family. This use of metaphor is similar to our previous discussion of the use of metaphor in games and initiatives. Finally, the use of activities can be fun and can lower defenses and resistance to dealing with issues and to making behavior changes (Gerstein, 1994).

An example of an initiative is the Family Obstacle Field. The goals of this initiative are to encourage parents to work as a team and to communicate with their children. Children are also given the opportunity to listen to parents. A final goal involves children seeing parents as authority figures. Obstacles are placed throughout a field that is generally 40 feet long and 10 feet wide. The children are then blindfolded. Parents stand at the end of the field and verbally direct their children around the obstacles. If an obstacle is touched, the child must go back and begin the course again. Many themes for discussion come out of this initiative, such as parental authority, listening skills of children, the need for concrete parental communication, and trust between parents and children (Gerstein, 1994).

Although these therapeutic issues could more than likely be addressed through traditional therapy, the addition of activity and adventure add an element of fun and immediacy to the process.

Adjunctive Therapy

Adventure therapy can be practiced as either the primary therapy approach or as an adjunct to a more traditional therapy program. Gillis and associates (1991) discussed adjunctive therapy as a part of a larger treatment approach. In this type of program, adventure therapy is used in combination with or in addition to other therapy. One of the early examples of adventure therapy as a formal adjunct can be seen in the late 1970s and was affiliated with the Colorado Outward Bound School. Outward Bound has continued to offer these adjunctive programs, working with clients who are sexual abuse survivors, who have experienced physical and emotional trauma, and who are veterans (Itin, 1995).

Adjunctive therapy programs are also often associated with mental health treatment, including inpatient hospital settings. Sometimes this takes the form of ropes courses on the grounds of psychiatric hospitals. A poignant example of the power of adventure therapy as an adjunct comes from a very personal article about this treatment written by a physician who herself was a patient in a hospital. This individual was hospitalized and treated for an ongoing eating disorder and for depression (Eilers, 1997).

In this treatment program, patients are exposed to intensive individual and group therapy, art therapy, and nutritional assistance. The adventure therapy component of this hospital program involved a low and high ropes course. In her personal account, the physician details the impact that the ropes course experiences had on her. In her journal, she reported that "Adventure therapy took me out of the sterile hospital and clinic environment and replaced it with the open outdoors where feelings were accepted, the unexpected happened, and success was not measured by outcome" (Eilers, 1997, p. 61). Being in the outdoor environment seemed to be a strong point of the use of adventure therapy as an adjunct. Eilers (1997) talked of her growth when she said, "I love the outdoors, the beauty of nature. I enjoyed being on the ropes course and seeing the beauty of the sunsets, the sky, the trees. I learned to see and appreciate the beauty of nature and to remember the beauty inside each of us" (p. 64).

It wasn't only a renewed appreciation of the experience of nature that was gained through the adventure therapy experience. Eilers (1997) summarizes the impact of this approach on her when she said: "I learned a lot from each of the methods of therapy; however, in adventure therapy, I came face to face with my personal issues and myself. I saw me. I saw how I functioned. I saw how I did things. It was in adventure therapy that I relived my personal struggles. And I felt the feelings. I felt them intensely. But in adventure therapy I learned new ways of dealing with feelings" (p. 62).

This powerful account helps identify the power of adventure therapy as an adjunct to more traditional approaches. Through the use of activity and action, issues may emerge more quickly and with more immediacy. Additionally, roles and behaviors can be played out through the use of activity. The use of metaphor further encourages self-awareness, consolidates change, and enables clients to make connections between adventure therapy and real life.

Psychotherapy

Adventure therapy can also occur as the primary mode of therapy, taking precedence over other modalities, or even taking place in the absence of other types of therapy. Before we talk about wilderness therapy as an example of a primary adventure therapy program, it is important to mention the act of processing as a precursor to therapy itself.

Briefly stated, one of the primary goals of therapy is change in behavior, attitude, or feelings. In order to effect change, however, some argue that we must move from simply having the experience in adventure therapy to talking about or processing the experiences that we have. Processing is necessary in order to understand, communicate about, and reflect on experience (Luckner & Nadler, 1997). In further discussing processing, Luckner and Nadler (1997) assert that "processing enhances the richness of experience, so it stands out and apart, like the important lines of a page underlined with a yellow high lighter. These unique learnings can be used again and generalized to other settings. When a new experience is processed, integrated, and internalized, individuals are able to grow, and as a result, they have more choices and influence in their lives" (p. 10). Processing the experience is based on a process that involves the individual being placed in a state of equilibrium as a result of being in a novel, yet cooperative, environment. In this setting, the individual is presented with opportunities for problem solving. Hopefully, feelings of accomplishment and success arise from this experience. These successes are enriched by processing the experience, which is finally generalized and transferred to the future (Luckner & Nadler, 1997).

It is important to briefly mention the distinction between adventure therapy and therapeutic adventure. While therapy is an intentional, planned process designed to achieve treatment goals, using techniques that have been demonstrated to be efficacious, therapeutic uses of wilderness may focus on growth and self-awareness, but in a less systematic manner (Berman & Davis-Berman, 1995). Additionally, therapy programs require diagnoses, treatment plans, and certified therapists, while therapeutic programs may not necessarily require this level of credentialing. This distinction is often blurred by programs that would call themselves therapy when, in fact, they are not. The distinction is similarly distorted by those who refer to themselves as therapists or counselors without the credentials to practice as such (Berman & Davis-Berman, 1995; Berman et al., 1997).

A more whimsical example of this obfuscation is provided by Blalock (1977), whose book, *Meet My Psychiatrist*, demonstrates in prose and wonderful photographs just how soothing and healing the wilderness can be. Tongue in cheek, Blalock asks: "Tense? Frustrated? Discouraged? Have a tough decision to make? This may be the time to visit my friendly psychiatrist, Old Doc Log. You'll find him patient, willing to listen. And his price is right" (p. 6). On a more serious and dangerous note are those who believe that the troubled need nothing more than the wilderness to set things right. This point is sadly driven home in the story of Christopher McCandless, who went into the wilderness to soothe his inner turmoil, only to starve to death in the harsh Alaskan winter (Krakauer, 1996). Similarly troubling are the stories in the popular press that chronicle the treatment of youth who have been abused and have even died in programs offering so-called wilderness therapy by staff who have no credentials (Carpenter, 1995; Griffin, 1995).

Wilderness Therapy

Wilderness therapy applies to those activities in which adventure therapy occurs in outdoor settings and is the primary therapeutic modality. Russell and Hendee (1999) succinctly suggested that wilderness therapy involves individual and group therapy provided by professionals who employ formal assessments of client needs and progress. According to Itin (1995), "Wilderness activities can be even more dramatic than other aspects of adventure therapy. Besides the adventure there is also a connection with the natural world [which] can deepen the impact of the programming" (p. 33).

When wilderness therapy is practiced as a primary therapy, a number of aspects of this modality contribute to its significance and effectiveness (Davis-Berman & Berman, 1994). One factor is the ability of the wilderness environment to impose natural consequences on participants. The impact of doing either the right or the wrong thing tends to be felt very readily in this setting. The challenge of an unfamiliar environment also increases the immediacy of therapy in wilderness settings. Positive interactions, cooperation, and good communication skills are necessary for success in the wilderness. Finally, many suggest that the beauty of a pristine wilderness can serve as a catalyst for healing (Davis-Berman et al., 1994). Others write of the ability of the wilderness environment to facilitate pushing out of comfort zones

(Luckner & Nadler, 1997) and of the wilderness as a metaphor for other life experiences (Gass, 1993). Finally, narrative (Luckner & Nadler, 1997) and solution-focused (Gass & Gillis, 1995) approaches have been discussed relative to adventure and wilderness therapy.

We have found that wilderness therapy seems most helpful to adolescents who are depressed, are withdrawn, and have challenges in relating to others; however, others have experienced other clinical results (Ferguson, 1999). This modality also seems effective with adolescents who have trouble controlling their acting-out behaviors (Berman & Anton, 1988; Berman & Davis-Berman, 1989).

Because wilderness therapy programs are therapy, it is essential to develop treatment plan goals for each participant. Ideally, these goals are developed in concert with the participants and their parents if the participants are minors. Additionally, a mental health assessment should be done for each participant prior to the wilderness therapy experience. Of course, this assessment will be incorporated into the treatment plan goals. An attempt should be made to identify strengths, weaknesses, goals, and diagnoses from the *DSM-IV* (American Psychiatric Association, 1994) in a manner consistent with how one approaches conducting therapy in more traditional settings.

Wilderness therapy programs use a wide variety of outdoor activities as their therapeutic modality. Our survey of national programs suggested that backpacking, canoeing, and climbing were commonly used (Davis-Berman et al., 1994). When the wilderness therapy trips actually take place, group therapy becomes an integral part of the experience. In wilderness therapy, the group seems to operate on two levels. First, it becomes a metaphor for life and interpersonal relationships. All conflicts and joys are worked out and processed by and within the group setting. Thus, the group takes on a life of its own and becomes the guiding process of the wilderness therapy program. In addition, traditional therapy issues are dealt with in group therapy. Sometimes the group is topical in nature, for instance, if we focus on loss and grief. With this level of group functioning, the wilderness provides the therapeutic backdrop, and its properties facilitate, encourage, and enrich the more traditional group therapy (Berman & Davis-Berman, 1999a).

Russell and Hendee (1999) summarized information gleaned from five wilderness therapy programs. They described wilderness therapy as a last resort for adolescents who are drug dependent, acting out sexually, in legal trouble, or having intense conflicts with their parents. They describe three phases of wilderness therapy, which also describe the goals of treatment: an initial phase of cleansing in which participants are removed from toxic environments and away from drugs, a phase of personal and social responsibility, and a phase of transition back to the community.

Russell and Hendee (1999) described two basic types of wilderness therapy programs: (a) contained programs that are up to 3 weeks in length, that operate as an expedition, and where clients and staff stay together for the duration of the program; and (b) continuous-flow programs which are up to 8 weeks in length, with clients and staff cycling in and out of the program. They maintain that the former programs used licensed therapists, wilderness guides, and an assistant on each wilderness therapy trip. According to these authors, the latter, continuous programs are staffed by wilderness guides, with therapists visiting the group on a weekly basis. Therapists provide individual and group therapy on this weekly basis.

A recent book by Ferguson (1999) illuminates an insider's view of one of the continuous-flow wilderness therapy programs surveyed by Russell and Hendee (1999). Gary Ferguson is an outdoor writer who signed on as a wilderness guide at a large wilderness therapy program. He tells of the teens who were suicidal, hopelessly depressed, or drug dependent and had not been helped by traditional mental health. To get help for these teens, "escorts" were often hired to take the teens from their beds (a practice now illegal in California) to the wilderness program. Ferguson tells the story, through his own eyes, of the teens and how they grew by being in the wilderness, with caring staff, unlimited metaphors for living, and rituals largely taken from aboriginal people. The book ends with these teens being reunited with families or being placed in other, long-term residential facilities.

Ferguson has an uncanny ability to relate the life stories of the participants and leaders of this program. He also reveals much that goes against the grain of professional care. Examples of this include the fact that staff can be hired after a phone interview, that they are placed in the field after just 6 days of training, or that some staff were former patients in the program. Further concerns are that these caring, but relatively untrained, staff provide the treatment for severely troubled teens, with armchair theorizing about personalities, psychopathology, and the administration of psychoactive prescriptive medications. Therapists came out to the group a few times per week, but the reader is given little information about the training or certification of these therapists, except to learn that all but one of them were untrained in the wilderness. Thus, Ferguson's book (1999) should not be taken as the field manual for wilderness therapy, but it does show the promise of adventure therapy. Nevertheless, testimonials like Ferguson's, while provocative, do little to demonstrate program effectiveness, the topic to which we now turn.

IS ADVENTURE THERAPY EFFECTIVE?

Generally, studies have suggested that adventure therapy programs do promote change, especially in adolescents. These changes tend to be found most often in the form of increasing self-esteem, of building self-concept, and in reducing negative behaviors and general symptoms of distress (Berman & Davis-Berman, 1989; Chenery, 1981; Kaplan, 1974; Krieger, 1973; Shniderman, 1974).

More recent research provides some interesting insight into the effectiveness of adventure therapy programs. Using cooperation as their primary measure, Sachs and Miller (1992) found a significant increase in cooperative behaviors following the completion of a wilderness program. The participants in this program were behaviorally disordered adolescents, whose changes were most dramatic in their school settings. General coping behaviors and self-esteem were used as measures in another recent study. The adventure therapy modality in this program was a transatlantic sailing voyage. Following the completion of this sailing experience, the participants reported significant increases in positive coping behaviors and in self-esteem (Norris & Weinman, 1996).

Another recent adventure therapy program utilized a variety of daily adventure experiences such as games, initiatives, and outdoor experiences. Participants in this program were outpatient mental health clients. Following the completion of the 9-week-long program, clients reported significant increases in self-efficacy, physical self-efficacy, and self-esteem, as compared to a comparison group (Kelley, Coursey, & Selby, 1997). Examining the impact of a wilderness therapy program on families with troubled teens, Bandoroff (1993) found that the functioning of both the families and adolescents significantly improved. Self-esteem also improved among those in the families exposed to the wilderness therapy, as compared to 39 families not included in the program.

The investigation of the efficacy of adventure programs in working with delinquent adolescents has always been a topic of interest in the field. As early as the 1960s, studies suggested that adventure therapy programs facilitated the improvement in a variety of symptoms, and tended to produce lower recidivism rates among those exposed to adventure therapy programs, as opposed to those in more traditional treatment programs (e.g., Kelly & Baer, 1968).

More recent studies have noted mixed and sometimes contradictory results about the effect of adventure programs on recidivism. For example, Castellano and Soderstrom (1992) found a decrease in recidivism in an adventure treatment program as compared to a traditional program. These differences were still apparent at 1 year; however, they had disappeared by the 2-year mark. Another study found no differences in recidivism either at 1 or 2 years between those treated in an outdoor adventure program and those in traditional programs (Elrod & Minor, 1992).

Recently, the evaluation of adventure therapy programs has become more global in scope with the publication of a few meta-analyses. These studies examine a large number of evaluations and attempt to summarize and categorize results in order to make conclusions regarding program efficacy. In this regard, Cason and Gillis (1994) examined 43 studies of adventure-type programs geared toward adolescents. Through this meta-analysis, they concluded that participants in the various adventure programs generally became more internal in their locus of control. Participants in these programs also received better grades, possessed more positive attitudes in general, and had more positive self-concepts after completion of adventure programs. Another meta-analysis concluded that adventure-oriented programs changed in positive directions on the following dimensions: self-concept, leadership, academics, personality, interpersonal relations, and adventure orientation (Hattie et al., 1997).

Finally, Neill and Richards (1999) drew some broad conclusions from their examination of the meta-analyses done on adventure therapy programs. They concluded that adventure programs have a small to medium positive effect on qualities such as self-concept, locus of control, and self-confidence, and that these changes tend to be maintained over time. Generally, these positive, long-lasting changes occur in adults participating in lengthier programs.

Through this sampling of evaluation studies, one can be quite optimistic about the efficacy of adventure therapy programs. However, as the literature has suggested (e.g., Davis-Berman & Berman, 1994), increased attention needs to be paid to the development and implementation of well designed and executed studies. Increased specificity which will allow us to understand the process of adventure therapy will enrich our database. As we have argued elsewhere (Berman & Davis-Berman, 1999b), adventure therapy research is still not at the point where it would be consistent with accepted standards for an empirically validated treatment (Task Force on Promotion and Dissemination of Psychological Procedures, 1995) where there are replicated, controlled studies in which significance is clear, with training manuals and clearly specified clinical populations.

INTEGRATING ADVENTURE THERAPY INTO TRADITIONAL PRACTICE

Integrating adventure therapy into traditional practice settings may be a challenge, but one that is not insurmountable when one considers the potential rewards of gaining new approaches, techniques, and skills. On one level, it may be relatively easy to use adventure programming as an adjunct to traditional therapy. In this regard, the practitioner does not need to be skilled in adventure, just knowledgeable enough to make referrals to these programs and to understand the goals and outcomes of adventure therapy.

How can one begin to use adventure therapy in one's own practice? In that adventure therapy is primarily used with groups, one might begin to use adventure techniques with families and existing groups. In terms of families, it may not be difficult to give families problems to solve in the way of initiatives in order to increase family cohesiveness, cooperation, and trust. The interested reader is referred to Gerstein (1994) for numerous suggestions of activities. For practitioners who work with groups, books by Karl Rohnke (e.g., 1989, 1991) and Jim Cain (Cain & Joliff, 1998) give hundreds of activities in the form of warm-ups and initiatives that are readily translatable into traditional group work. Insight into novel ways of processing these experiences with clients is provided by Luckner and Nadler (1997).

Other aspects of adventure therapy, such as the use of ropes courses and outdoor activities, require specialized training. There is more involved than just learning how to conduct these activities safely. For example, it is possible that a therapist can take courses and become certified as a sea kayak instructor. This does not mean, however, that this will qualify one to use sea kayaking in one's practice. Synthesizing the outdoor and therapy arenas involves either a supervised practice experience (i.e., an adventure therapy practicum) or a partnership between outdoor leaders and therapists, with each having some of the skills of the other professional.

Reimbursement for adventure therapy raises other issues. At least in the United States, mental health care is inextricably involved with third-party reimbursement for services. Receiving reimbursement for adventure therapy programs will largely depend on the qualifications of staff, outcome data, cost-effectiveness, and ability to translate adventure programs into a language that resembles practice settings recognized by insurance companies. It is questionable that wilderness therapy, for instance, will be seen as a practice setting in the same way as are inpatient and outpatient facilities. In addition, there will need to be continued work to amass research data and to educate insurance and managed care companies on the effectiveness of adventure therapy. We must also be prepared to demonstrate the cost-effectiveness of this method and the generalizability and long-term nature of the results.

For those willing to accept the challenge, adventure therapy offers the opportunity to increase one's repertoire of clinical tools, expand into new practice settings, and offer new options to adolescents whose needs too often outstrip the resources available in traditional practice settings.

CONTRIBUTORS

Jennifer Davis-Berman, PhD, is an Associate Professor in the Department of Sociology, Anthropology, and Social Work at the University of Dayton, Dayton, Ohio. She is also Associate Clinical Professor in the Division of Applied Psychology, School of Medicine at Wright State University. Her training is in social work. She is the co-author of *Wilderness Therapy: Foundations, Theory and Research* and numerous articles on adventure therapy. Dr. Davis-Berman can be reached at the Department of Sociology, Anthropology, and Social Work, University of Dayton, Dayton, OH 45469. E-mail: berman@udayton.edu

Dene S. Berman, PhD, is a psychologist whose practice, Lifespan Counseling Associates, includes the Wilderness Therapy Program. He is a Clinical Professor in the School of Professional Psychology and Associate Clinical Professor in the Division of Applied Psychology of the School of Medicine at Wright State University. He is an Instructor for the Wilderness Education Association and the American Canoe Association. He is currently the Chairperson of the Therapeutic Adventure Professional Group of the Association for Experiential Education. Mr. Berman can be reached at 1698 Forestdale Avenue, Dayton, OH 45432. E-mail: dene.berman@wright.edu

RESOURCES

American Journal of Insanity. (1906). p. 63.

American Psychiatric Association. (1994). *Diagnostic and Statistical Manual of Mental Disorders* (4th ed.). Washington, DC: Author.

Backus, R. (1947). Where the new camping tasks begin. *The Nervous Child, 6,* 130-134.

Bacon, S. (1988). *Paradox and Double Binds in Adventure-Based Education* (Eric Document Reproduction Service No. 296832). Greenwich, CT: Outward Bound, USA.

Bandoroff, S. (1993). Wilderness family therapy: An innovative treatment approach for problem youth. *Dissertation Abstracts International, 53*(11-B), 5966.

Berman, D. S., & Anton, M. (1988). A wilderness therapy program as an alternative to adolescent hospitalization. *Residential Treatment for Children and Youth, 5,* 39-52.

Berman, D. S., & Davis-Berman, J. L. (1989). Wilderness therapy: A therapeutic adventure for adolescents. *Journal of Independent Social Work, 3*(3), 65-77.

Berman, D. S., & Davis-Berman, J. L. (1995). Adventure as psychotherapy: A mental health perspective. *Journal of Leisurability, 22,* 21-28.

Berman, D. S., & Davis-Berman, J. L. (1999a). Wilderness therapy for adolescents. In C. Schaeffer (Ed.), *Innovative Techniques for Children and Adolescents* (2nd ed., pp. 161-188). New York: Wiley.

Berman, D. S., & Davis-Berman, J. L. (1999b). Tikkun Olam: A model for healing the world. *Journal of Experiential Education, 22*(1), 24-27.

Berman, D. S., Davis-Berman, J. L., Chamberlain, R., & Dandaneau, C. (1997, November). *Adventure Therapy: What It Takes to Do the Job.* Paper presented at the International Conference of the Association for Experiential Education, Asheville, NC.

Blalock, L. (1977). *Meet My Psychiatrist.* Bloomington, MN: Voyageur Press.

Cain, J., & Joliff, B. (1998). *Teamwork and Teamplay.* Dubuque, IA: Kendall/Hunt.

Carpenter, B. (1995). Taking nature's cure: Do expensive wilderness therapy camps help or hurt troubled teens? *U.S. News and World Report, 118*(25), 54-58

Cason, D., & Gillis, H. (1994). A meta-analysis of outdoor adventure programming with adolescents. *Journal of Experiential Education, 17*(1), 40-47.

Castellano, T., & Soderstrom, I. (1992). Therapeutic wilderness programs and juvenile recidivism: A program evaluation. *Journal of Offender Rehabilitation, 17*(3-4), 19-46.

Chenery, M. (1981). Effects of summer camp on child development and contributions of counselors to those effects. *Journal of Leisure Research, third quarter,* 195-207.

Davis-Berman, J. L., & Berman, D. S. (1993). Therapeutic wilderness programs: Issues of professionalization in an emerging field. *Journal of Contemporary Psychotherapy, 23,* 129-136.

Davis-Berman, J. L., & Berman, D. S. (1994). *Wilderness Therapy: Foundations, Theory and Research.* Dubuque, IA: Kendall/Hunt.

Davis-Berman, J. L., Berman, D. S., & Capone, L. (1994). Therapeutic wilderness programs: A national survey. *Journal of Experiential Education, 17*(2), 49-53.

Dimock, H., & Hendry, C. (1939). *Camping and Character: A Camp Experiment in Character Education.* New York: Association Press.

Eilers, G. (1997). My lessons for living from adventure therapy. *Journal of Experiential Education, 20*(2), 61-65.

Elrod, H., & Minor, K. (1992). Second wave evaluation of a multi-faceted intervention for juvenile court probationers. *International Journal of Offender Therapy & Comparative Criminology, 36*(3), 247-262.

Ferguson, G. (1999). *Shouting at the Sky: Troubled Teens and the Promise of the Wild.* New York: St. Martin's Press.

Friese, G., Hendee, J. C., & Kinziger, M. (1998). The wilderness experience industry in the United States: Characteristics and dynamics. *Journal of Experiential Education, 21,* 40-45.

Gass, M. A. (Ed.). (1993). *Adventure Therapy: Therapeutic Applications of Adventure Programming.* Dubuque, IA: Kendall/Hunt.

Gass, M. A. (Ed.). (1995). *Book of Metaphors* (Vol. II). Dubuque, IA: Kendall/Hunt.

Gass, M. A., & Gillis, H. L. (1995). Focusing on the "solution" rather than the "problems": Empowering client change in adventure experiences. *Journal of Experiential Education, 18,* 63-69.

Gerstein, J. S. (1994). *Experiential Family Counseling: A Practitioner's Guide to Orientation Materials, Warm-Ups, Family Building Initiatives, and Review Exercises.* Dubuque, IA: Kendall/Hunt.

Gillis, H. L. (1995). If I conduct pursuits with clinical populations, am I an adventure therapist? *Journal of Leisurability, 22,* 5-15.

Gillis, H. L., Gass, M. A., Bandoroff, S., Randolph, S., Clapp, C., & Nadler, R. (1991). Family adventure survey: Results and discussion. In C. Birmingham (Ed.), *Proceedings of the 19th Annual Association of Experiential Education Conference* (pp. 29-39). Boulder, CO: Association of Experiential Education.

Griffin, K. (1995). Dangerous discipline. *Health, May/June,* 94-99.

Hattie, J., Marsh, H., Neill, J., & Richards, G. (1997). Adventure education and Outward Bound: Out-of-class experiences that make a lasting difference. *Review of Educational Research, 67*(1), 43-87.

Itin, C. M. (1995). Adventure therapy and the addictive process. *Journal of Leisurability, 22,* 29-37.

Itin, C. M. (Ed.). (1998). *Exploring the Boundaries of Adventure Therapy: International Perspectives.* Boulder, CO: Association of Experiential Education.

James, T. (1980). *Can the Mountains Speak for Themselves?* Unpublished manuscript.

James, T. (1993). *The Only Mountain Worth Climbing: The Search for Roots.* Unpublished manuscript.

Kaplan, R. (1974). Some psychological benefits of an outdoor challenge program. *Environment and Behavior, 6,* 101-115.

Katz, R., & Kolb, D. (1967). *Outward Bound and Education for Personal Growth.* Reston, VA: Outward Bound, USA.

Kelley, M., Coursey, R., & Selby, P. (1997). Therapeutic adventures outdoors: A demonstration of benefits for people with mental illness. *Psychiatric Rehabilitation Journal, 20*(4), 61-73.

Kelly, F. J., & Baer, D. J. (1968). *Outward Bound Schools as an Alternative to Institutionalization for Adolescent Delinquent Boys.* Boston: Fandel Press.

Krakauer, J. (1996). *Into the Wild.* New York: Anchor Books.

Krieger, W. (1973). Study on self-concept change in campers. *Camping Magazine, 45*(4), 16-17.

Loughmiller, C. (1965). *Wilderness Road.* Austin, TX: Hogg Foundation for Mental Health.

Luckner, J. L., & Nadler, R. L. (1997). *Processing the Experience: Strategies to Enhance and Generalize Learning* (2nd ed.). Dubuque, IA: Kendall/Hunt.

Miner, J., & Boldt, J. (1981). *Outward Bound USA: Learning Through Experience in Adventure-Based Education.* New York: William Morrow and Co.

Morse, W. (1947). From the University of Michigan fresh air camp: Some problems of therapeutic camping. *The Nervous Child, 6,* 211-224.

Neill, J. T., & Richards, G. E. (1999). Does outdoor education really work? A summary of recent meta-analyses. *Australian Journal of Outdoor Education, 3*(1), 2-9.

Norris, R., & Weinman, J. (1996). Psychological change following a long sail training voyage. *Personality and Individual Differences, 21*(2), 189-194.

Ringer, T. M. (in press). Groups in adventure therapy: Contributions from psychodynamic approaches. *Insight: The Newsletter of the Therapeutic Adventure Professional Group.* Boulder, CO: Association of Experiential Education.

Rohnke, K. (1989). *Cowtails and Cobras II: A Guide to Games, Initiatives, Ropes Courses and Adventure Curriculum.* Dubuque, IA: Kendall/Hunt.

Rohnke, K. (1991). *Bottomless Baggie.* Dubuque, IA: Kendall/Hunt.

Rohnke, K., Tait, C., & Wall, J. (1998). *The Complete Ropes Course Manual* (2nd ed.). Dubuque, IA: Kendall/Hunt.

Russell, K. C., & Hendee, J. C. (1999). Wilderness therapy as an intervention and treatment for adolescents with behavioral problems. In A. E. Watson, G. Aplet, & J. C. Hendee (Eds.), *World Congress Proceedings on Research Management and Allocation* (Vol. II). Ogden, UT: USDA Forest Service, Rocky Mountain Research Station.

Sachs, J., & Miller, S. (1992). The impact of a wilderness experience on the social interactions and social expectations of behaviorally disordered adolescents. *Behavioral Disorders, 17*(2), 89-98.

Scheidlinger, S., & Scheidlinger, L. (1947). From a camp of a child guidance clinic: The treatment potentialities of the summer camp for children with personality disturbances. *The Nervous Child, 6,* 232-242.

Schoel, J., Prouty, D., & Radcliffe, P. (1988). *Islands of Healing: A Guide to Adventure Based Counseling.* Hamilton, MA: Project Adventure.

Shniderman, C. M. (1974). Impact of therapeutic camping. *Social Work, 19,* 354-357.

Smith, B. (1958). *The Worth of a Boy.* Austin, TX: Hogg Foundation for Mental Health.

Task Force on Promotion and Dissemination of Psychological Procedures. (1995). Training in and dissemination of empirically validated treatments: Report and recommendations. *The Clinical Psychologist, 45,* 3-24.

Zander, A. (1947). The influence of the summer camp on personality development. *The Nervous Child, 6,* 161-165.

Improving Athletic Performance And Motivating Athletes

Bobby L. Stinson, II, Robert D. Friedberg, Richard A. Page, and Michael J. Cusack

Sports and athletic activities appeal to people of all ages and all walks of life. Children as young as 2 and 3 years old are enrolled in activities such as tumbling and swimming. Individuals in their ninth and tenth decade of life continue to exercise and engage in sports. Between those two extremes are the competitive youth, such as Olympic-bound gymnasts and figure skaters; there are high school and college athletes; and, of course, there are professional superstars. At a less competitive level, there are novices who enjoy friendly athletic contests or organized activities through their neighborhoods, local churches, and recreational departments. In fact, you yourself are likely to be an athlete at some level. Most of our friends, family members, colleagues, and associates are athletes to some extent.

When one considers the numerous benefits of participating in sports and athletic activities, it should come as no surprise that individuals of all ages and lifestyles participate. Athletic activities promote physical fitness, including regular exercise and cardiovascular development. Similarly, athletic participation promotes mental health. Participation in athletics can increase one's self-esteem, sense of mastery, and social skills competence, and can assist in basic goal-setting. Yet another way individuals benefit from athletics is simply through the promotion of social activity. For example, individuals involved in athletics often experience camaraderie, develop lasting friendships, and are exposed to team concepts. Athletic participation fosters one's interpersonal development and is conducive to the development of leadership skills. Finally, some individuals are extrinsically rewarded by things such as ribbons, plaques, trophies, and even money. All this and they get to have fun, too!

Unfortunately, however, athletes sometimes drop out of athletics even though they possess numerous traits that have been identified as characteristic of excellent athletes. This is a concern that has gone relatively unaddressed in the literature. Specifically, it is necessary to understand why some athletes are more vulnerable than others to dropping out of athletics. The problem lies in identifying the unique characteristics of athletes who ultimately drop out compared to those athletes who persevere.

This contribution will discuss the relationship between attributional style and athletic performance, including the decision to drop out of athletics. Attributional style is firmly embedded in social psychological and personality theory. Moreover, attributional style has been linked to motivation, persistence, and learned helplessness. These variables are quite likely related to athletic achievement. Finally, attributional style is flexible enough to be measured either directly, through self-report measures, or more unobtrusively, using the Content Analysis of Verbatim Explanations (CAVE; e.g., Rettew & Reivich, 1995; Seligman, 1992) technique (see Clinical Implications, pp. 355-358). Therefore, attributional style not only has support in theory, but it also has practical utility when working with athletes.

Understanding characteristics of athletes that are related to performance and drop-out rates serves several important purposes. For example, clinicians will be able to help athletes to understand how their thoughts affect their behaviors. That is, clinicians will be able to assist athletes in understanding how their attributional style affects their athletic performance and their decision to continue or not to continue in athletics. Subsequently, clinicians could train athletes to use more positive attributions, ultimately resulting in lower attrition rates due to increased self-esteem, higher expectancies for the future, and increased motivation. This contribution will help clinicians become more adept at implementing cognitive-behavioral techniques that result in more functional attributions, which can improve athletic performance and reduce attrition.

Similarly, this information would be useful when clinicians consult with coaches and parents. For instance, clinicians could teach coaches and parents to become more proactive in determining who is most vulnerable to dropping out and then addressing that athlete's attributional style in an attempt to retain that athlete in the athletic program. Additionally, identifying an athlete's attributional style for a coach would be helpful to the coach in deciding who should participate when. Due to their attributional style, some athletes may perform best after a success, whereas they may perform worse after a defeat. In such a case, the coach would be well advised to make substitutions, rotations, and so forth relative to this information.

At the more competitive levels of athletics, clinicians could aid recruiters, saving time, energy, and money. This is particularly important when one considers that the typical division I-A college athletic program spends $286,000 on recruiting and scouting each year, and almost $2.5 million more in grants-in-aid for student-athletes ("Study: Typical I-A Program," 1996). In short, college athletic programs are typically allotting 20% of their expenditures for recruiting and supporting their athletes. Professional organizations such as the National Football League (NFL) already use mental health clinicians as consultants. Many universities in the country employ full-time mental health/sport consultants. Other universities are likely not far behind.

The aim of this contribution is twofold: (a) to provide information that will allow clinicians to help all athletes improve athletic performance and (b) to offer some insight regarding why some athletes decide to drop out while others persevere despite having similar abilities. This information will serve several purposes. Most notably, it will allow clinicians to assist athletes at any level increase their self-esteem, expectations, and overall motivation. Stated another way, clinicians will be able to help athletes by optimizing the latter's athletic performance, decreasing their likelihood of giving up, and increasing their overall quality of life.

ATTRIBUTIONAL STYLE OVERVIEW

Several authors have noted that individuals attempt to make sense of their environment by understanding "why" certain things happen (e.g., Abramson, Seligman, & Teasdale, 1978; Peterson, 1991; Weiner, 1974). In trying to understand why things occur, individuals attribute the outcomes of events to causes. Specifically, the causal explanations (i.e., the reasons why something happened) can be coded into internal-external, stable-unstable, and global-specific categories. Each category has an impact on the individual's future thoughts, feelings, and behaviors (including self-esteem, achievement, and motivation).

Abramson et al. (1978) defined an attribution as *internal* if individuals believe an outcome is the result of a personal attribute of their own. For example, if people assume that others can prevent negative outcomes while they cannot, they will likely blame themselves; that is, they believe the negative outcome must be caused by something within themselves. Conversely, an attribution is defined as *external* if people expect the outcome could not have been altered by anybody (Abramson et al., 1978). That is, external attributions occur when individuals perceive the cause of an event as being external to the individuals involved (e.g., luck, chance, task difficulty). The attribution that is made along the internal-external dimension determines whether or not individuals are likely to suffer an insult to their self-esteem, which can ultimately affect achievement, motivation, and persistence.

In addition to the internal-external dimension, a stability dimension has been proposed (Abramson et al., 1978; Weiner, 1974). *Stable* attributions are long-lived or recurrent (e.g., one's innate potential), while *unstable* attributions are short-lived and nonrecurrent (e.g., luck). The attribution along the stability dimension has an impact on the duration of any self-esteem deficits, which again will ultimately affect one's motivation and persistence as well as one's expectancies for the future.

The final dimension that has been proposed is the globality dimension (Abramson et al., 1978). *Global* attributions affect a wide variety of outcomes, while *specific* attributions refer to specific situations. As such, attributions along the globality dimension have an impact on the pervasiveness of self-esteem deficits, independent of whether they are short-term or long-lived. The previous definitions are summarized in Table 1 (below).

TABLE 1: Attributional Dimensions, Definitions, and Examples

Attributional Dimension	Definition	Example
Internal Attribution	The cause has something to do with you (e.g., effort, ability).	"I'm no good at soccer."
External Attribution	The cause is a result of others, the task, or the environment.	"The refs ripped us off."
Stable Attribution	The cause is constant or long-lasting.	"I'm no good at soccer."
Unstable Attribution	The cause is changing or short-lived.	"The refs ripped us off."
Specific Attribution	Affects one or two areas of your life.	"I'm no good at passing the ball in soccer."
Global Attribution	Affects everything you do.	"I'm not good at anything."

Individuals tend to explain the causes of events in a predictable, habitual way - what has come to be called an "explanatory style" (Peterson, 1991). Some individuals are more optimistic than others. An *optimistic explanatory style* is defined as explaining bad events or negative outcomes with external, unstable, and specific causes. An example would be, "We lost (negative outcome) because our opponents (external) had more practice (unstable) playing under artificial lighting (specific situation)." An individual with an optimistic explanatory style might explain good events or positive outcomes with internal, stable, and global causes. An example of such an attribution follows: "I won (positive event) because I (internal) have the abilities (stable) to be a winner (global)." A *pessimistic explanatory style*, on the other hand, is defined as explaining bad events or negative outcomes with internal, stable, and global causes (e.g., "We're just horrible"). It would be equally pessimistic to describe good events or positive outcomes with external, unstable, and specific causes (e.g., "We only won because of a lucky call at the end of the game").

As Peterson (1991) pointed out, those who are more pessimistic in their explanatory style are more likely to be passive and demoralized and to experience cognitive, emotional, and motivational deficits than are those who are optimistic in their explanatory style. A pessimistic explanatory style has been associated with depression, lowered expectancies, passivity in the face of challenge, and poor achievement. An optimistic explanatory style, on the other hand, has been associated with the opposites, such as higher self-esteem, positive expectancies, perseverance, motivation, and high achievement.

INTERNALITY, STABILITY, AND GLOBALITY IN ATHLETICS

To eliminate confusion, the remainder of this section will be concerned with the repercussions of pessimistic attributions for *failures* (i.e., internal, stable, and global attributions for failures). Nonetheless, it is important to remember that similar findings have been reported for pessimistic attributions for successes (i.e., external, unstable, and specific attributions for successes) (Peterson, 1991). In other words, when discussing *internal* attributions for *failures*, the reader should keep in mind that the same could be said for *external* attributions for *successes*. Similarly, a description of a person who attributes a failure to a stable cause would be similar to the description of a person who attributes a success to an unstable cause. Finally, global attributions for failures have the same results as specific attributions for successes. Stated another way, a person who attributes failures to internal, stable, and global causes will have cognitive, emotional, and behavioral deficits that are similar to someone who attributes successes to external, unstable, and specific causes.

Internal-External Dimension

As noted previously, athletes who make internal attributions for failures have lower self-esteem in comparison to individuals who externalize failures (Abramson et al., 1978; Peterson, 1991). Again, keep in mind that the same could be said of individuals who externalize successes compared to those who internalize successes. In addition, internalizing failures may result in a negative cognitive set as well as feelings of sadness, passivity, incompetence, and worthlessness (Abramson et al., 1978). Individuals who internalize failures have a deficit in self-esteem because they have come to believe that the failure is a result of a personal deficit; they believe that the result is due to a flaw within themselves.

In the case of individuals who attribute failures internally (or successes externally), a vicious cycle may ensue. Those athletes who make internal attributions for failures believe the failure was a result of a personal characteristic or something within themselves. Given that the failure was attributed to a personal characteristic, the athlete feels less confident and experiences lower self-esteem (Abramson et al., 1978). Feeling that way, the athlete puts forth less effort and/or is less motivated in the future. Ultimately, the result may be yet another failure and another internal attribution, as well as further negative self-evaluations and expectations for the future. This self-perpetuating cycle has the potential to hinder achievement at best, and at worst may persuade the athlete to withdraw from athletics altogether.

For the purpose of illustration, consider a basketball player who makes only 3 out of 10 free throws during a game. In an attempt to understand this poor performance, the athlete reconciles, "I just can't shoot free throws. I've never been good at free throws and I never will be." Attributing failure to personal incompetence will lead to greater feelings of inadequacy and hopelessness. Consequently, the athlete comes to believe that there is no use practicing free throws because it is simply something that he or she is incapable of mastering. Due to this negative thinking and a lack of practice, the athlete continues to shoot about 30% from the free-throw line. Over time, these poor performances and continued negative self-evaluations may leave the athlete believing that basketball is not what he or she once thought it was. It may no longer be pleasurable. In other words, this vicious cycle results in basketball losing its reinforcing value for this particular athlete. The consequence may be a lack of interest, further demotivation, and eventually even dropping out.

In fact, as Auvergne (1983) and Seligman et al. (1990) have demonstrated through their studies, high school, college, and professional athletes who internalize failures do perform more poorly in the future than athletes who externalize their failures. Similarly, athletes who externalize successes would be expected to perform more poorly than athletes who internalize their successes (Peterson, 1991).

Stable-Unstable Dimension

It is possible, however, to interrupt a vicious cycle such as the one described above (i.e., negative outcome —▶ internal attribution —▶ poor self-esteem —▶ less motivation —▶ more negative outcomes —▶ more internal attributions, and so on). The interruption of this cycle is likely to depend upon the attribution that is made along the stability dimension. If the athlete's attribution is internal and stable for a failure, the self-fulfilling prophecy described previously is more likely to occur. The reason for this is that the athlete not only has internalized the failure, but also believes that the internal attribution is not likely to go away anytime soon. In other words, it is not only that "I am a horrible free-throw shooter," but more so that "I am a horrible free-throw shooter *and always will be*."

Attributing a poor performance to a deficit in ability is an internal attribution. Therefore, the athlete is susceptible to deficits in self-esteem, which can affect motivation and performance. Additionally, the athlete in this example is inclined to believe that future failures are inevitable because skill level, or one's athletic potential, is not subject to immediate change; that is, it is stable. As such, the athlete is susceptible to *long-lasting* self-esteem deficits, lack of motivation, and a lack of persistence.

On the other hand, if the athlete explains failures with unstable attributions (or is trained by a clinician to make such attributions), he or she will believe that the internal cause for a previous failure will not necessarily apply in future situations. For example, the basketball player earlier could have attributed the poor performance at the free-throw line to a lack of effort. For instance, maybe the athlete was not taking free-throw practice seriously enough or was not spending enough time practicing free throws. Perhaps the individual's attention and concentration were impaired on that night due to a stressful occurrence earlier in the day. These attributions are both internal and therefore may leave the athlete susceptible to deficits in self-esteem (e.g., "I still shot poorly"), which could ultimately lead to less motivation and decreased persistence. However, the fact that effort, attention, and concentration are also unstable provides hope for the future (i.e., increased motivation and persistence). An unstable attribution, in and of itself, implies the potential for change in the future. An unstable attribution that is also internal provides the athlete with the perception of controllability; that is, not only is the result changeable, but the perception is that the athlete has control over that change. Accordingly, athletes are more likely to be motivated and persistent when they realize that outcomes are under their personal control and also quite changeable. Consequently, they can become more optimistic and hopeful.

To summarize this point, the internal-external dimension is very important in terms of the athlete's self-esteem, which can have an impact on motivation and persistence. The duration of the effect on the athlete's self-esteem, motivation, and persistence, however, is dependent upon the stable-unstable dimension. Therefore, the relevance and the impact that the internal-external dimension will have on athletes is essentially dependent upon the stable-unstable dimension. In other words, an internal or external attribution may not be positive or negative per se. Only in the context of the stable-unstable attribution does the attribution along the internal-external dimension become an asset on the one hand, or a liability on the other. For instance, internal-stable attributions for failures leave athletes feeling incompetent with no expectation for change. Internal-unstable attributions for failures, on the other hand, leave athletes feeling a sense of control and hope for change.

Global-Specific Dimension

In addition to the dimensions of internality and stability, it is important to consider the globality dimension. The global-specific dimension will determine whether the cognitive, emotional, and behavioral deficits brought about by the internal-external and stable-unstable dimensions are specific to particular circumstances or more generalized across situations. Someone who makes a global attribution is likely to experience these deficits across different situations (Abramson et al., 1978). In contrast, a person who makes a specific attribution is likely to experience these deficits in rather circumscribed situations. This particular dimension, then, will be important for all athletes. For example, global attributions may result in athletes believing that a poor performance in one contest will be predictive of poor performances in upcoming contests. Once again, this style of thinking results in decreased motivation and hampers performance.

Although the global-specific dimension has implications for all athletes, this dimension may be more relevant depending on the particular athlete and the sport in which the athlete is participating. As alluded to previously, all athletes can experience adverse effects when a global attribution results in expectations for future failures. For some athletes, though, the expectation may go beyond expecting a failure in the next contest. Rather, the effect may be in the next event within a given contest. Alternatively, the generalization may occur from one event in a given contest to multiple events in upcoming contests. For example, a track star who makes a global attribution for a flawed exchange during a 4 x 100-meter relay race may subsequently suffer deficits in other events on the same day (e.g., 4 x 200-meter relay, 100-meter sprint, etc.). A specific attribution, on the other hand, would not necessarily lead to deficits in other events. The implication of a specific attribution is that the cause for the outcome is relevant only to that specific event during that particular competition.

Similarly, multisport athletes who make global attributions for failures in one sport would be more susceptible to subsequently experiencing deficits in another sport. In the same way that an attribution may generalize across events within a given competition, it could generalize across sports. In other words, the generalization that occurs as a result of a global attribution can occur in many forms: from one day to the next in a given sport, from one event within a given sport to the next event, or from one sport to the next sport.

Even athletes who do not play multiple sports or engage in multiple events within a single sport can experience the adverse effects of attributing a negative event to a global cause. For instance, consider the athlete who, either in competition or practice, experiences a failure to which he or she attributes a global cause (i.e., a cause that will be present across numerous different situations). The global attribution leaves the athlete believing and, in fact, expecting further failures. Not only is further failure expected in the same situation, but failures are expected across a broad variety of situations. For example, this athlete may see himself or herself as being less competent in interpersonal relationships. As another example, he or she may experience academic or job difficulties. If similar global attributions are made for negative outcomes or failures in these domains, further failure in his or her life will be expected in general. These expectations for failure may spill back into the domain of athletics, further perpetuating the deficits in this and other domains.

To summarize this section, the three dimensions of internality, stability, and globality are all very important in an attempt to understand cognitive, emotional, and behavioral deficits in athletes. In simple terms, the internality of an attribution essentially determines whether or not self-esteem deficits will be incurred. Moreover, the attribution along the internality dimension will indicate how much control the athlete perceives having over the outcome. The stability dimension will determine the duration of any self-esteem and behavioral deficits. In addition, the stability of the attribution will determine whether perceived control over the outcome or lack thereof is long-lasting or short-lived. Finally, the global-specific dimension will determine whether the consequences of the internality and stability dimensions are circumscribed or more generalized.

GENDER DIFFERENCES

There is an extensive amount of literature supporting a difference in attributional styles between male and female athletes. Generally speaking, males are more likely to show an optimistic pattern of attributing successes to internal factors such as ability and effort, while attributing failures to external and unstable factors, such as luck. Females, on the other hand, tend to show a pessimistic pattern of attributing successes to external and unstable factors such as luck or social support while attributing failures to a lack of ability (e.g., Bird & Williams, 1980; Deaux & Farris, 1977; Nicholls, 1975; Rudisill, 1988).

This gender gap appears to diminish as female athletes gain more experience with competition and success. Furthermore, it appears to be coming more socially acceptable for women to participate in a broad variety of athletic activities. As female athleticism becomes more socially acceptable, female athletes may begin taking more credit for their own successes, which may result in more self-enhancing attributional styles. However, until then, it is worth noting that females may be more likely to exhibit self-defeating attributional styles than males, particularly when they have little experience and fewer past successes.

CULTURAL DIFFERENCES

Peterson (1991) and Peterson, Buchanan, and Seligman (1995) noted that one should consider whether causal attributions may be of particular concern only to residents in Western societies during the late 20th century. In other words, causal attributions may be of relevance only if individuals perceive "self" as distinct from the world, highly endorse individuality, and try to predict and control the events that befall them (Baumeister, 1986; van den Berg, 1983; Weisz, Rothbaum, & Blackburn, 1984).

Research suggests that individuals of different cultures likely do offer causal attributions for behaviors (e.g., Miller, 1984; Si, Rethorst, & Willimczik, 1995). In fact, Peterson (1991) doubts there has ever been a time or place in which individuals did not engage in making sense out of what they see, particularly behaviors by themselves or others. However, it is not clear at the present time if explanations from all cultures can be sensibly described along the dimensions of internality, stability, and globality (Miller, 1984). Even if they can be sensibly described along these dimensions, it is not clear if the same styles across cultures relate to the same outcomes as predicted by the attributional model (Si et al., 1995). Clearly, this is an area in which further research is needed if one expects to generalize findings from the attributional style literature to non-Western cultures. At this time, findings from the attributional style literature should be applied to persons of non-Western cultures only with caution.

CLINICAL IMPLICATIONS

The relationship between attributional style, athletic performance, and dropping out of athletics has compelling implications for a broad range of individuals. This contribution has provided important information that will allow clinicians to help athletes as well as consult with coaches, parents, recruiters, and administrators of athletic programs. How clinicians can assist each of these individuals is discussed more explicitly in this section.

Athletes

Clinicians could be instrumental in educating athletes on how their thoughts affect their behaviors; that is, how their attributional style affects their athletic performance. Even more exciting is that attributional styles are amenable to change. In the same way that cognitive-behavioral therapists help depressed and anxious individuals change their negative thought patterns, athletes can be trained to change their negative attributional styles. A more optimistic style would likely bode well for the athlete. In particular, a specific goal should be for the athlete to attribute successes internally, stably, and globally. On the other hand, the clinician will want to assist the athlete in realizing the instability and specificity of failures while making a balanced attribution along the internality dimension for failures.

As a first step, though, clinicians will need to be adept at assessing an athlete's attributional style. There are several measures that clinicians may find useful in measuring an athlete's attributional style. For example, some authors have reported good results with the Attributional Style Questionnaire (ASQ; Seligman et al., 1990). This instrument measures attributional style in six hypothetical positive and six hypothetical negative affiliation and achievement oriented events along the dimensions of internality, stability, and globality. In addition to analyzing one's responses for each of the three dimensions, it is possible to develop a composite score for positive events, negative events, and an overall composite score. Others have proposed a measure of sport-related attributional style. For example, Hanrahan, Grove, and Hattie (1989) developed the Sport Attributional Style Scale (SASS) which has been reported to demonstrate acceptable psychometric properties and to effectively predict athletic performance (Hale, 1993).

Still others have reported success using a more hands-off approach, such as the Content Analysis of Verbatim Explanations (CAVE) technique (e.g., Rettew & Reivich, 1995; Seligman, 1992). Essentially, this technique uses written or spoken material to derive an attributional style. In particular, events and their causes are extracted and rated along the dimensions of internality, stability, and globality. Once many extractions have been rated and averaged, composite scores can be developed.

In fact, it is conceivable that skilled clinicians could make an informal assessment on their own. However, it is important not to lead athletes by suggesting an explanation for them. For that reason, it is advisable to use open-ended questions whenever possible. For example, one might say to an athlete who had a great performance, "Wow, pretty good night, huh?" On the other hand, one might approach an athlete who had a sub-par performance with, "Tough game, huh?" Often, these comments alone will be enough to solicit a causal explanation.

To increase the validity of a personal assessment and as a way of overcoming impression management effects, the clinician may find it useful to talk with friends and family of the athlete. For example, a clinician might say to the mother, father, sibling, coach, or teammate of an athlete, "I saw in the newspaper that Chris had a big game last week. How did Chris explain that?" A similar question could be posed for an athlete who had a disappointing performance. Finally, one might follow the lead of Seligman (1992) and use athletes' quotes from newspapers to assess their attributional styles.

Pages 359 to 362 provide a worksheet that clinicians might use in their practice to elicit attributional styles. A worksheet such as this one might be used in session with the clinician or it might be explained in session and assigned as homework to the athlete outside of session. Furthermore, the clinician could attend practices and contests, thereby obtaining a sample of the athletes' real-life behaviors. With these samples of actual behaviors, the clinician will better understand the athletes' (and coaches') current attributions and hence where to intervene and what cognitive-behavioral techniques to use. In addition, by attending team functions, the sport consultant will be more adept at using relevant examples in sessions and will conceivably establish better rapport and gain the respect of the coaches and athletes.

Technology may be able to aid in the endeavor of assessing attributional styles in athletes as well. For example, virtual reality simulators could be used to establish a mock athletic event or contest. The athlete's attributional style could then be assessed in the same manner as was discussed earlier. In a similar attempt, computer games or video machines might be utilized.

A caution is in order, though, when assessing another's attributional style. The results are not extremely reliable if we use only one or a few events. In other words, if someone attempts to assess a "style" from a single event or even a few events, he or she is at risk of measuring reality and not a personality characteristic per se (Peterson, 1991). In other words, one runs the risk of observing an attribution that is not characteristic or "typical" of the athlete. However, as the number of events is increased for which attributions are assessed, the reliability of measuring a psychological style is also increased. Consequently, a person's attributional style should be assessed over a series of events rather than basing it on a single attribution. Moreover, every attempt should be made to gather data on both positive and negative events.

After assessing an athlete's attributional style, the second step would be attributional retraining, if necessary. Again, it is worth noting here that an optimistic explanatory style, in particular, will likely lead to greater achievements, more motivation and persistence, and better mental health in general. In particular, athletes should be trained to identify the internal causes for successes (e.g., ability and effort) and the instability of failures. Athletes who are trained in making accurate and functional attributions will take pride and satisfaction in winning. They will learn to accept responsibility for their successes. As a result, athletes will likely have higher self-esteem as well. Athletes will also remain motivated to improve while winning. They will expect future successes and will therefore be motivated to continue putting forth effort. Additionally, they will feel able to change negative outcomes in the future through effort. Finally, athletes with functional attributional styles are more likely to stay focused on the upcoming competition (Leith, 1989).

Pages 363 to 365 provide a worksheet illustrating how clinicians might encourage athletes to make more functional attributions. For example, if the assessment revealed that a particular athlete tends to make stable attributions for failures, then the clinician would want to assist the athlete in realizing how luck and effort can change from one competition to the next. Even task difficulty may be amenable to change (e.g., weather conditions, opponent, etc.). Similarly, if an athlete tended to minimize internal factors for successes, the clinician could be instrumental in helping that athlete realize what role ability and effort played in his or her success. As is true in any cognitive-behavioral treatment, the clinician would need to pay particular attention to negative cognitive distortions and help the athlete identify, evaluate, and replace these distortions with more balanced thinking. To be sure, athletes may need much practice with these exercises before such attributions become "automatic." The athlete may be responsive to an analogy being drawn between such therapeutic exercises and athletic skills. Like athletic skills, these cognitive-behavioral exercises need to be practiced regularly and consistently in order to develop appropriately. Similarly, just as athletes do not wait until the day of a competition to try something new, athletes should not wait until the "heat of the moment" to try these exercises. These exercises should be practiced and reviewed regularly, initially in nonthreatening situations, so that they can be mastered and eventually implemented automatically.

Coaches and Parents

In addition to working with athletes directly, mental health practitioners are serving more and more as consultants to parents and coaches of athletes. Clinicians can play a primary role in helping coaches and parents become aware of their own attributions for successes and failures. Assessment measures and interventions suggested for athletes can be similarly applied to coaches and parents (see previous discussion and worksheets on pages 359-365). Inasmuch that the role of a coach is to teach new skills and fundamentals to his or her athletes, the coach performs an integral role in "teaching" positive attributions. Parents play a similar modeling role in that children often model the behaviors observed in their parents. Specifically, coaches and parents serve as models for appropriate attributions. In other words, athletes may adopt explanations for successes and failures that are consistent with those of the coach or those that they have observed at home. Clinicians may find themselves in the role of providing individual attributional training to coaches. Alternatively, the coaching staff may request or accept an offer for in-service training from a qualified clinician. Again, this modeling of an optimistic explanatory style should result in more functional attributional styles in the athletes, which in turn will result in greater motivation, greater perseverance, and better performance on the part of the athletes.

Clinicians may also serve as consultants in making actual coaching decisions. For example, Seligman et al. (1990) concluded that athletes with optimistic attributional styles will likely do better under pressure than athletes with pessimistic attributional styles. They argue that coaches should consider attributional style when deciding who will participate, particularly when the athlete has suffered a recent defeat or the event is particularly important. Moreover, Seligman (1992) demonstrated that attributional style can predict success beyond an experienced coach's judgment and a handicapper's expertise. Again, then, a consultant could be practically useful to coaches in determining who should participate in particular circumstances. For example, Seligman stated that an athlete who has a pessimistic attributional style should be used primarily after he or she has done well. If the pessimist has experienced a recent failure or shortcoming, and the team is at a crucial juncture, the coach should consider substituting for the athlete with a pessimistic attributional style. A clinician who understands the effects attributions have on athletes and who understands how to assess a person's attributional style could serve as a valuable consultant to coaching staffs.

Recruiters and Administrators

Just as clinicians could serve as consultants to coaches and parents, clinicians could aid recruiters and administrators by saving them time, energy, and money. Obviously, this is only relevant at the higher levels of athletics where administrators utilize recruiting. But, as noted earlier, more and more colleges and many professional organizations are seeking mental health consultants in this regard. In terms of time and energy, recruiters will likely benefit from clinicians who can administer and interpret personality tests that measure attributional style. Although it is not advisable to base the decision to recruit or not to recruit an individual based solely on his or her performance on personality tests, testing can still be beneficial. For example, raw talent being relatively equal, an optimistic athlete will perform better in the long run than a pessimist as measured by personality tests (Scheier, Weintraub, & Carver, 1986; Seligman, 1992). Therefore, it can be concluded that if recruiters are searching for athletes who will be most productive, then recruiters should consider not only the athlete's athletic ability but also his or her attributional style.

Furthermore, measuring attributional style can be helpful beyond assisting in the determination of whom to recruit and whom not to recruit. For example, a recruiter may make the decision that he or she wants to recruit a particular athlete regardless of the athlete's attributional style. Nonetheless, attributional style should not be ignored altogether. Given the fact that the athlete with an optimistic attributional style is likely to perform better over the long run than is the athlete with a pessimistic attributional style, the coaching staff and/or athlete may wish to seek a clinician who can provide attributional retraining. That is, if an athlete is recruited and it is determined that the athlete has a pessimistic attributional style, it is possible to take steps to change that athlete's attributional style to a more optimistic style (see discussion under Athletes [pp. 355-357] and Worksheet for Modifying Attributions in Athletes [pp. 363-365]). Consequently, the athlete will develop a style more conducive to successful athletic performance.

CONCLUSION

Attributional style is a psychological construct that has compelling implications in terms of optimizing athletic performance and decreasing attrition rates in athletes. Embedded in social psychological and personality theory, attributional style has been relatively neglected as an important construct for athletes. However, as outlined in this contribution, attributional style is relevant to the athlete, coaches, parents, recruiters, and administrators. This contribution has provided information that can be used by clinicians to help each of these individuals in improving athletic performance in athletes. Finally, this contribution has offered insight as to why some athletes decide to drop out while others persevere and the role the clinician can play in averting the unfortunate decision to drop out.

Worksheet for Identifying Attributional Styles in Athletes: You Make the Call!*

INSTRUCTIONS: This is where you make the call. You get to determine what type of explanatory style you have. There are three parts to this worksheet. Part I is an example to help you understand how to go about determining your explanatory style. After reading through the example, you get to make the call by imagining or recalling an athletic event and completing your own form in Part II. Finally, in Part III, you will complete the form based on an actual event in which you have just engaged.

PART I: EXAMPLE

As you read through the example be thinking of how you might answer each of the questions, because you will have a chance to do this exercise in just a moment.

A. Think of a recent sporting event that you were a part of, the more recent the better. Maybe you were in practice this evening. Maybe you were practicing some drills by yourself or with a teammate. Maybe you just got home from a competition. Take a few minutes to really picture the scene. Where were you? Who was with you? What was the game situation? What do you remember seeing . . . hearing . . . smelling? What was going through your mind? What happened? Now that you have the image in your head, jot down your responses to the above questions on the lines that follow: *I am thinking of yesterday's basketball game. Actually, I am thinking of the last play in yesterday's game. I was on the left wing. Chris was bringing the ball up the court and I remember Pat was down on the block on my side. There were less than 10 seconds and we trailed by one point. I could tell Chris was going to pass me the ball by the way he glanced at me and then looked away. I knew it was coming to me. I remember hearing Pat call for the ball and I remember hearing the coach yelling to get the ball inside. Chris did pass me the ball. At that point, I don't really remember hearing or smelling anything. I just remember turning toward the basket, jumping (though I do remember seeing Pat open on the block as I jumped to shoot), I released the ball and it went in right at the buzzer!*

B. Then, answer these questions:

1. What was the end result of this situation? *I made the game-winning basket!*
2. Would you consider this a success or a failure? *A success*
3. Explain in some detail the number one reason for this outcome: *Really, it was pretty lucky because to be honest I should have passed the ball to Pat. He's automatic if he gets the ball inside. And quite honestly, I'm a streaky shooter, especially from the left side.*

C. Now look at your explanation in #3 above and answer the following questions:

1. Was the outcome a result of something within you (e.g., ability or effort) or was it contingent upon something outside of you (e.g., luck or task difficulty)? *luck = out*

   a. If the result was due to something within you, circle this "I."
   b. If the result was contingent upon something outside of you, circle this "E."

2. Was the outcome a result of something that was stable (e.g., ability or task difficulty) or something that could change (e.g., effort or luck)? *luck = can change*

   a. If the outcome was the result of something that is stable, circle this "S."
   b. If the outcome was the result of something that could change, circle this "U."

3. Is the explanation appropriate only for this particular event or sport or is it applicable to events in your life in general?
   only for this sport

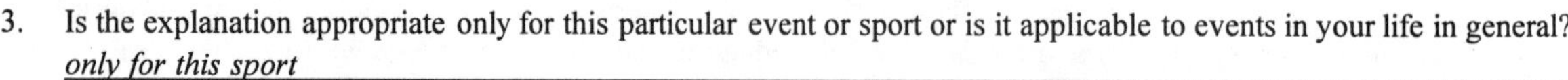

   a. If the explanation is appropriate only for this particular event, circle this "Sp."
   b. If it is applicable to your life in general, circle this "G."

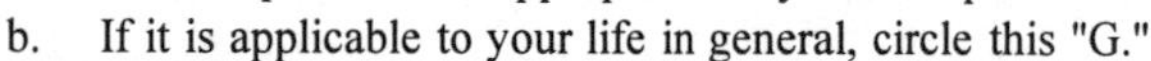

D. Now, complete the following sentence by circling the appropriate items.

"For this success / failure (circle one), my explanation was: I / E (circle one)
S / U (circle one)
G / Sp (circle one)

PART II: IMAGINING OR RECALLING AN EVENT

Now it is your turn to make the call! Read each item below and complete it with as much detail as possible.

A. Think of a recent sporting event that you were a part of, the more recent the better. Maybe you were in practice this evening. Maybe you were practicing some drills by yourself or with a teammate. Maybe you just got home from a competition. Take a few minutes to really picture the scene. Where were you? Who was with you? What was the game situation? What do you remember seeing . . . hearing . . . smelling? What was going through your mind? What happened? Now that you have the image in your head, jot down your responses to the above questions on the lines that follow: ______

B. Then, answer these questions:

1. What was the end result of this situation? ______
2. Would you consider this a success or a failure? ______
3. Explain in some detail the number one reason for this outcome: ______

C. Now look at your explanation in #3 above and answer the following questions:

1. Was the outcome a result of something within you (e.g., ability or effort) or was it contingent upon something outside of you (e.g., luck or task difficulty)? ______

   a. If the result was due to something within you, circle this "I."
   b. If the result was contingent upon something outside of you, circle this "E."

2. Was the outcome a result of something that was stable (e.g., ability or task difficulty) or something that could change (e.g., effort or luck)? ________________

   a. If the outcome was the result of something that is stable, circle this "S."
   b. If the outcome was the result of something that could change, circle this "U."

3. Is the explanation appropriate only for this particular event or sport or is it applicable to events in your life in general?

   ____

   a. If the explanation is appropriate only for this particular event, circle this "Sp."
   b. If it is applicable to your life in general, circle this "G."

D. Now, complete the following sentence by circling the appropriate items.

"For this success / failure (circle one), my explanation was: I / E (circle one)
S / U (circle one)
G / Sp (circle one)

E. If you picked an event that you considered a success last time, this time you will need to pick an event that you consider a failure. Similarly, if you picked an event that you considered a failure last time, this time you will need to pick an event that you consider a success. Take a moment to really picture the scene in your mind. Remember as many details as you possibly can. Think about it for a moment before continuing.

1. Again, explain in some detail the number one reason for this result occurring: ________________

   ____

   ____

   ____

2. Was the outcome a result of something within you (e.g., your ability or effort) or was it contingent upon something outside of you (e.g., luck or task difficulty)? ________________

   a. If the result was due to something within you, circle this "I."
   b. If the result was contingent upon something outside of you, circle this "E."

3. Was the outcome a result of something that was stable (e.g., ability or task difficulty) or something that could change (e.g., effort or luck)? ________________

   a. If the outcome was the result of something that is stable, circle this "S."
   b. If the outcome was the result of something that could change, circle this "U."

4. Is the explanation appropriate only for this particular event or sport or is it applicable to events in your life in general?

   ____

   a. If the explanation is appropriate only for this particular event, circle this "Sp."
   b. If it is applicable to your life in general, circle this "G."

F. Again, complete the following sentence by circling the appropriate items.

"For this success / failure (circle one), my explanation was: I / E (circle one)
S / U (circle one)
G / Sp (circle one)

PART III: DOING AN ACTIVITY

This time, rather than imagine an event, you will actually engage in the event. You can use any event that you want. It will probably be more helpful to do something that is sports related. That way it will be more realistic and more fun, too! For example, you might shoot baskets at a miniature hoop with a nerf ball. As another idea, you might go putt-putting or practice putting on artificial turf in your living room. Have fun with this. It can be anything. The important part is that you will actually be engaging in the event. Remember that it will probably be more meaningful and more fun if it is the actual sport or event, or related to an actual sport or event, in which you participate.

Go Have Fun

You Make The Call!

A. Once you have completed your exercise, answer these questions:

1. What was the end result of this situation? ______
2. Would you consider this a success or a failure? ______
3. Explain in some detail the number one reason for this outcome: ______

______

______

B. Now look at your explanation in #3 above and answer the following questions:

1. Was the outcome a result of something within you (e.g., your ability or effort) or was it contingent upon something outside of you (e.g., luck or task difficulty)? ______

   a. If the result was due to something within you, circle this "I."
   b. If the result was contingent upon something outside of you, circle this "E."

2. Was the outcome a result of something that was stable (e.g., ability or task difficulty) or something that could change (e.g., effort or luck)? ______

   a. If the outcome was the result of something that is stable, circle this "S."
   b. If the outcome was the result of something that could change, circle this "U."

3. Is the explanation appropriate only for this particular event or sport or is it applicable to events in your life in general?

   ______

   a. If the explanation is appropriate only for this particular event, circle this "Sp."
   b. If it is applicable to your life in general, circle this "G."

C. Now, complete the following sentence by circling the appropriate items.

"For this success / failure (circle one), my explanation was: I / E (circle one)
S / U (circle one)
G / Sp (circle one)

Worksheet for Modifying Attributions in Athletes: 100% All the Time*

INSTRUCTIONS: Whenever something happens, our brain tries to understand why it happened. Over time, we develop a "habit" of explaining things in certain ways. That is, we automatically have a thought about why something happened. For example, we may be in the habit of believing that we are always responsible for what happens. Alternatively, we may develop a habit of believing others are always responsible for what happens. If we don't stop to consider them, we will simply assume that our habitual thinking or automatic thoughts are accurate even if they're not. This worksheet will help you identify the possible causes of events, and it will help you break any negative thinking habits you may have. As you begin to change negative thinking habits, you will likely notice improvements in how you feel and perform.

To complete this worksheet, begin by recalling a recent outcome, positive or negative. If you completed the "You Make the Call" worksheet, you may be able to select an outcome from there. Otherwise, you will need to consider a recent event and its outcome. Now, identify as many possible reasons for the outcome as you can. For now, don't worry about how big a role each factor may or may not have played in the final outcome. Simply list as many possible reasons as you can think of for the outcome. Use this worksheet to help you think of all the possible reasons for the outcome.

Now you are to identify as many possible reasons for the outcome as is possible. For now, don't worry about how big a role each factor may or may not have played in the final outcome. Simply list as many possible reasons for the outcome as you can think of. It might help to categorize the reasons under the following headings.

A. **Reasons Associated With the Difficulty of the Task** (It might help to consider the following questions: Was the task too easy? Was the task too difficult? Was this a novel task that you have never participated in before? Was this a task that you could do in your sleep? Was there anything else to do with the difficulty of the task that may have at least partially accounted for the outcome?): ______________________________
____
____
____
____
____
____
____
____

B. Reasons Associated With Luck or Chance (It might help to consider the following questions: Were you especially lucky or unlucky? If there was an opponent, was the opponent especially lucky or unlucky? Did the outcome appear to be a freak occurrence or an act of a higher power? Was there anything else that happened that seemed to be attributable to luck or pure chance?): ______________________________

C. Reasons Associated With Your Effort (It might help to consider the following questions: Did you give your best effort the entire time? Did your teammates, if there were any, give their best efforts the entire time? Were you mentally and physically prepared? Did you practice for this? Was there anything else associated with effort that may have influenced the ultimate outcome?): ______________________________

D. Reasons Associated With Your Ability (It might help to consider the following questions: Do you have the potential to do this? Is there something about you physically or mentally that precludes your doing this? Is there anything else that would indicate your ability might have an impact on the outcome? Be careful, though, not to confuse effort and task difficulty for ability.): ______________________________

E. Any Other Reasons (Are there any other reasons that would not fit under the four categories of task difficulty, luck or chance, effort, and ability?): ______________________________

Now look again at the reasons you have listed. Go back, double check, and think of any other possible reasons for this outcome - be as exhaustive as you can.

Now you will estimate the percentage that each reason played in the ultimate outcome. If we take all the possible reasons and add them together, they should account for 100% of the outcome. Although each reason can hypothetically range from 1%-99%, you may find it easier to round each reason to the nearest 5%. Start with the reason you believe had the least impact on the outcome. Estimate the amount of responsibility (by placing a percentage value on it) that that reason had for the final outcome. Look at the reason that had the next to least impact and estimate its percentage of responsibility. Continue this until you have estimated the responsibility each potential reason had on the ultimate outcome.

1. What percentage fell under Task Difficulty? ______

2. What percentage fell under Luck or Chance? ______

3. What percentage fell under Effort? ______

4. What percentage fell under Ability? ______

5. Was the outcome a result of only Task Difficulty or only Luck or Chance or only Effort or only Ability? ______

6. What percentage can be controlled by you (i.e., what percentage was Effort or Ability)? ______

7. What percentage is susceptible to change in the future (i.e., what percentage was Effort or Luck or Chance or in some circumstances even Task Difficulty)? ______

8. What ultimate conclusion can you derive from this exercise? That is, what do you make of this? ______

CONTRIBUTORS

Bobby L. Stinson, II, PsyD, is a recent graduate of Wright State University School of Professional Psychology. He completed his dissertation in the area of sport psychology and has provided professional and clinical workshops in the area. In addition to sport psychology, his interests include forensic psychology and the application of cognitive therapy. He is currently a Postdoctoral Psychology Resident at Twin Valley Psychiatric System in Columbus, Ohio and works in a group private practice in Springfield, Ohio. Dr. Stinson may be contacted at Twin Valley Psychiatric System, 2200 West Broad Street, Columbus, OH 43223.

Robert D. Friedberg, PhD, is an associate professor and director of the predoctoral internship training program at the Wright State University School of Professional Psychology. His clinical interests include cognitive therapy, childhood depression and anxiety, and training models for cognitive therapy. Dr. Friedberg can be contacted at Wright State University School of Professional Psychology, Ellis Human Development Institute, 9 N. Edwin C. Moses Boulevard, Dayton, OH 45407.

Richard A. Page, PhD, PsyD, is currently an associate professor of psychology at Wright State University. His training is in both social and clinical psychology, and he has taught and published articles in both areas. He maintains a private clinical practice focusing on children's behavioral disorders. Dr. Page may be contacted at the Department of Psychology, Wright State University, Dayton, OH 45435.

Michael J. Cusack, EdD, is currently the Director of Athletics at Wright State University in Dayton, Ohio. His background is in coaching as well as administration. He has written and spoken on a variety of topics, ranging from coaching techniques to the cost of collegiate athletics. Dr. Cusack can be contacted at the Athletic Department, Wright State University, Dayton, OH 45435.

RESOURCES

Cited Resources

Abramson, L. Y., Seligman, M. E. P., & Teasdale, J. (1978). Learned helplessness in humans: Critique and reformulation. *Journal of Abnormal Psychology, 87,* 49-74.

Auvergne, S. (1983). Motivation and causal attribution for high and low achieving athletes. *International Journal of Sport Psychology, 14,* 85-91.

Baumeister, R. F. (1986). *Identity: Cultural Change and the Struggle for Self.* New York: Oxford University Press.

Bird, A. M., & Williams, J. M. (1980). A developmental-attributional analysis of sex-role stereotypes for sport performance. *Developmental Psychology, 16,* 319-332.

Deaux, K., & Farris, E. (1977). Attributing causes for one's own performance: The effects of sex, norms, and outcome. *Journal of Research in Personality, 11,* 59-72.

Hale, B. D. (1993). Explanatory style as a predictor of academic and athletic achievement in college athletes. *Journal of Sport Behavior, 16,* 63-75.

Hanrahan, S. J., Grove, J. R., & Hattie, S. A. (1989). Development of a questionnaire measure of sport-related attributional style. *International Journal of Sport Psychology, 20,* 114-134.

Leith, L. M. (1989). Causal attribution and sport behavior: Implications for practitioners. *Journal of Sport Behavior, 12,* 213-225.

Miller, J. G. (1984). Culture and the development of everyday social explanations. *Journal of Personality and Social Psychology, 46,* 961-978.

Nicholls, J. G. (1975). Causal attributions and other achievement-related cognitions: Effects of task outcomes, attainment value, and sex. *Journal of Abnormal Psychology, 31,* 379-389.

Peterson, C. (1991). The meaning and measurement of explanatory style. *Psychological Inquiry, 2,* 1-10.

Peterson, C., Buchanan, G. M., & Seligman, M. E. P. (1995). Explanatory style: History and evolution of the field. In G. M. Buchanan & M. E. P. Seligman (Eds.), *Explanatory Style* (pp. 1-20). Hillsdale, NJ: Lawrence Erlbaum.

Rettew, D., & Reivich, K. (1995). Sports and explanatory style. In G. M. Buchanan & M. E. P. Seligman (Eds.), *Explanatory Style* (pp. 173-185). Hillsdale, NJ: Lawrence Erlbaum.

Rudisill, M. E. (1988). Sex differences in various cognitive and behavioral parameters in a competitive situation. *International Journal of Sport Psychology, 19,* 296-310.

Scheier, M. F., Weintraub, J. K., & Carver, C. S. (1986). Coping with stress: Divergent strategies of optimists and pessimists. *Journal of Personality and Social Psychology, 51,* 1257-1264.

Seligman, M. E. P. (1992). Sports. In M. E. P. Seligman (Ed.), *Learned Optimism* (pp. 155-166). New York: Pocket.

Seligman, M. E. P., Nolen-Hoeksema, S., Thornton, N., & Thornton, K. M. (1990). Explanatory style as a mechanism of disappointing athletic performance. *Psychological Science, 1,* 143-146.

Si, G., Rethorst, S., & Willimczik, K. (1995). Causal attribution perception in sports achievement: A cross-cultural study on attributional concepts in Germany and China. *Journal of Cross-Cultural Psychology, 26,* 537-553.

Study: Typical I-A program is $1.2 million in the black. (1996, November 18). *The NCAA News, 33,* pp. 1, 10.

van den Berg, J. H. (1983). *The Changing Nature of Man: Introduction to Historical Psychology.* New York: Norton.

Weiner, B. (1974). *Achievement Motivation and Attribution Theory.* Morristown, NJ: General Learning Press.

Weisz, J. R., Rothbaum, F. M., & Blackburn, T. C. (1984). Standing up and standing in: The psychology of control in America and Japan. *American Psychologist, 39,* 955-969.

Additional Resources

Anderson, C. A., Horowitz, L. M., & French, R. D. (1983). Attributional style of lonely and depressed people. *Journal of Personality and Social Psychology, 45,* 127-136.

Anshel, M. H. (1990). Sport psychology: From theory to practice. In M. H. Anshel (Ed.), *Sport Psychology: From Theory to Practice* (pp. 17-48). Scottsdale, AZ: Gorsuch Scarisbrick.

Hendy, H. M., & Boyer, B. J. (1993). Gender differences in attributions for triathlon performance. *Sex Roles, 29,* 527-543.

Hiroto, D. S., & Seligman, M. E. P. (1975). Generality of learned helplessness in man. *Journal of Personality and Social Psychology, 31,* 311-327.

Iso-Ahola, S. E. (1977). Immediate attributional effects of success and failure in the field: Testing some laboratory hypotheses. *European Journal of Social Psychology, 7,* 275-296.

Lirgg, C. C. (1991). Gender differences in self-confidence in physical activity: A meta-analysis of recent studies. *Journal of Sport and Exercise Psychology, 13,* 294-310.

Matteo, S. (1986). The effect of sex and gender-schematic processing on sport participation. *Sex Roles, 15,* 417-432.

Mullen, B., & Riordan, C. A. (1988). Self-serving attributions for performance in naturalistic settings: A meta-analytic review. *Journal of Applied Social Psychology, 18,* 3-32.

Overmier, J. B., & Seligman, M. E. P. (1967). Effects of inescapable shock upon subsequent escape and avoidance learning. *Journal of Comparative and Physiological Psychology, 63,* 28-33.

Robinson, D. W., & Howe, B. L. (1989). Appraisal variable/affect relationships in youth sport: A test of Weiner's attribution model. *Journal of Sport and Exercise Psychology, 11,* 431-443.

Roth, S., & Kubal, L. (1975). Effects of noncontingent reinforcement on tasks of differing importance: Facilitation and learned helplessness. *Journal of Personality and Social Psychology, 32,* 680-691.

Rudisill, M. E., & Singer, R. N. (1989). Influence on causal dimension orientation on expectations, persistence, and performance during perceived failure. *Journal of Human Movement Studies, 15,* 215-228.

Schulman, P. (1995). Explanatory style and achievement in school and work. In G. M. Buchanan & M. E. P. Seligman (Eds.), *Explanatory Style* (pp. 159-171). Hillsdale, NJ: Lawrence Erlbaum.

Seligman, M. E. P., Abramson, L. Y., Semmel, A., & von Baeyer, C. (1979). Depressive attributional style. *Journal of Abnormal Psychology, 88,* 242-247.

Seligman, M. E. P., & Maier, S. F. (1967). Failure to escape traumatic shock. *Journal of Experimental Psychology, 74,* 1-9.

Seligman, M. E. P., & Schulman, P. (1986). Explanatory style as a predictor of productivity and quitting among life insurance sales agents. *Journal of Personality and Social Psychology, 50,* 832-838.

Sweeney, P. D., Anderson, K., & Bailey, S. (1986). Attributional style in depression: A meta-analytic review. *Journal of Personality and Social Psychology, 50,* 974-991.

Vinella, S. (1997, September 14). Budget near $1 million. *Dayton Daily News,* pp. D1, D9.

Wong, A. T. (1979). The contest to become top banana: Chinese students at Canadian universities. *Canadian Ethnic Studies, 11,* 63-69.

Yang, K. S. (1986). Chinese personality and its change. In M. H. Bond (Ed.), *The Psychology of the Chinese People.* Hong Kong: Oxford University Press.

Providing Mental Health Services to the Deaf Community

Robert N. Basil

<Sign> <important> <understand> <full> <first> <THEN> <psychology> <services> <provide> <deaf>. The previous sentence is an example of a "gloss" rendering of an American Sign Language sentence saying "It is important to fully understand American Sign Language before trying to offer psychological services to deaf people." Anthropologists typically define a separate culture or subculture if the group of people use a markedly different language. Certainly American Sign Language (ASL) is quite different from American English. More than any spoken language could be, it uses a different mode of expression, a different grammar, some specialized vocabulary, and a very different way of thinking. To even begin to consider offering the complex and critical mental health services we have been trained to offer, considerable training is required in the variety of nuances involved in sign language, deaf culture, and the deaf perspective on living in both the physical world and in the social world of the Hearing community.

Many hearing people are now gaining more exposure to the deaf world through advertisements, movies, books, and for a time from a TV show, which was unfortunately canceled, called *Deaf World.* In a recent *APA Monitor* article (American Psychological Association [APA] Task Force on Diversity Issues, 1998) entitled "Disability as Diversity: A Guide for Class Discussion," the APA's Task Force on Diversity noted: "Viewing people with disabilities as a specific cultural group within a diverse society is a new development. . . . Yet groups within the Disabled community often share a common language (such as American Sign Language, Braille, terms used to talk about disability or themselves), customs and traditions (such as celebrations of disability consciousness and pride), art (including, poetry, paintings and plays by disabled artists and performers), [and] folklore (such as stories about real or fictional disabled people, from Helen Keller to the mobility-impaired character in 'My Left Foot')" (p. 41). The article goes on to say that although there is an increased willingness to consider disabled populations as minority cultures, there is "thin coverage in the traditional psychological literature of disabled people's psychosocial needs, health concerns, cultural identities and community affiliations" (p. 1). This is especially true for the deaf culture, which makes up roughly 1 % of the U.S. population. Those individuals who identify themselves with the Deaf community frequently prefer to utilize the distinction of "big D Deaf" rather than the small case "d" when deaf is written as "deaf." Throughout this contribution, when this population is indicated, the term "Deaf" will be used.

The Deaf community has much to offer psychology. It is frequently beneficial to a majority group to incorporate the concerns and viewpoints of minority populations, because their different and unexpected views of the world enhance and stimulate the majority's perspectives. The Deaf community has a unique perspective to teach clinicians about many things, including nonverbal or body language communication, visual learning, psychosocial development, language acquisition, communication of empathy, mother/infant communication, cultural impacts of medical advances (e.g. cochlear implants), and family communication and dynamics. Although some areas are considered strengths and others considered weaknesses, all are *different* from the experiences of hearing individuals. Hearing, and the social communication patterns based on hearing, are aspects taken for granted by hearing people. Learning how to "step out" of our world into a different worldview is one of the basic tasks of clinicians as they attempt to understand their clients' behaviors, interactions, and goals.

Few professionals with even beginning training are available for working with deaf individuals, and few interpreters are trained in working in mental health settings. Efforts in both fields of mental health and interpreting are underway to correct this. Two organizations actively involved are the Registered Interpreters for the Deaf (RID) - which is developing a specialized certificate in mental health interpreting, and the mental health committee of the American Deaf and Rehabilitation Association (ADARA). In addition, both APAs, the American Psychological Association and the American Psychiatric Association, have special-interest groups that bring together psychologists and psychiatrists currently working with the Deaf community.

NEED FOR SPECIALIZED TRAINING

Mental health professionals require specialized training to work with deaf clients. No one would consider having a clinician provide services to a Hispanic client who only speaks Spanish - unless the clinician was fluent in Spanish, had received training or supervised experience in the cultural norms of that client's particular Hispanic culture, or at the very least had training in working with a Spanish interpreter. In fact, just having an interpreter present in the sessions does not mean a full understanding has been achieved between the client and the clinician, nor that even adequate service has been provided. To achieve the goal of at least adequate service provision requires that adequate communication and mutual understanding of the concepts exchanged be achieved. Clients must feel they have been understood, while clinicians must feel they have accurately understood the client well enough to appropriately apply their training and experience to the client's situation, at least in an adequately effective manner to achieve the desired treatment goals. Unfortunately, without adequate training, the chances for misattributions and misassumptions are quite high and consequently the chances for effective treatment are quite low.

Implicit cultural norms are present in the design and implementation of psychological research studies. In cross-cultural attempts to "translate" diagnoses, descriptions of psychological processes and phenomena, as well as intervention techniques, it has been evident that although there are commonalities in all cultures (e.g., the facial expression of fear is common worldwide even in congenitally blind subjects), the *meaning* ascribed to various experiences (e.g., the reporting of seeing visions and hearing voices) can vary quite widely among cultures and subcultures. Even when the scientific research is not culturally biased and the relevant scientific knowledge is cross-culturally sound, the *application* of the scientific knowledge can frequently be "colored" or "flavored" by the clinician's cultural background and viewpoint. For example, in working with the deaf, an emergency-room doctor may not realize the error in taking at face value the report of a hearing family member that their deaf relative "looked like they were signing to something that wasn't there" and conclude the deaf individual was hallucinating. In ASL, it is common for the deaf to set up in space a particular person, that is to say, to create a space in front of them which they assign to stand for the person they are discussing who is not present. They may look at this space, gesture to the space, and include the space in their conversation. Visually this is an easy way to refer to "him or her" without having to keep signing their name over and over. It saves time and is understood as a conventional linguistic "grammar" for ASL. If hearing family members and professionals are not knowledgeable about this convention, misattributions can be easily made. It is important to recognize when misattributions are possible and to postpone making attributional conclusions until enough clear evidence is gathered to warrant a diagnosis rather than quickly assigning a diagnosis in order to proceed quickly to treatment.

Interestingly, many cultural aspects of clinicians, even blatantly obvious ones, can be effectively ignored by their clients while other aspects, even seemingly minor ones, may be quite salient. This is true for many different cultures, subcultures, and minority groups, not just with the Deaf community. For example, white clients in therapy with African-American therapists have been observed to make very disparaging remarks about "blacks," "coloreds," and so on, seemingly ignoring the obvious African-American status of their clinician without attributing their remarks to their therapist and without considering whether their therapist would even be offended by their remarks. In contrast, a clinician's "accent," whether in vocal tone and inflection or in signing style and facial expression, can aid or impede the assessment or intervention depending on the cultural expectations of the client. White clients of Appalachian background have left the offices of Indian clinicians refusing to return and complaining, not about the content of the communication, but of the style and accent of the clinician. Similarly, deaf clients can have considerable difficulty lip-reading hearing clinicians who happen to mumble their words or who have full beards. Thus obvious characteristics such as skin color may not have the impediment one would assume, while seemingly insignificant characteristics such as a speaking style in which a person does not move their lips may have a large impact. Many things can interfere with full communication and reduce or even reverse the emotional impact of a clinical intervention. Understanding these various factors and their interactions is critical toward ensuring that what is intended to be communicated is actually received by the client with *the desired emotional impact resulting in the desired treatment goal.*

ETHICAL REQUIREMENTS

APA Ethics

The American Psychological Association Ethical Principles of Psychologists and Code of Conduct (APA, 1992) requires that psychologists offering services to special populations receive training and/or supervision in methods and approaches appropriate to those populations. This is certainly applicable to services provided to the Deaf community. Similar arguments have been made concerning services to Hispanic and African-American communities. Although therapists do not have to be minority members to serve a minority group, they do need to be familiar with the norms, communication styles and idioms, pacing, role expectations, the variety of attitudes toward being a minority member and having "minority status," and the value of empowering minority clients in their efforts to achieve a healthy state of mind with clear behavioral changes needed to sustain their gains.

Ethics regarding the use of psychological assessment instruments with deaf clients are particularly important as most human beings, agencies, organizations, and schools place credence on "hard numbers." Testing and creating a number to represent a measured level of intelligence, a learning disability, a probability of psychosis, or a skill in English or math requires certain assumptions be met. One of the assumptions made by nearly all psychological tests is that the clients are hearing. It has only been in recent years that major efforts have been made to include the deaf population in norming studies. Without a set of "deaf norms," conclusions drawn from tests normed on hearing subjects may be quite inaccurate and widely misrepresent the deaf client's capabilities and characteristics. Frequently, hearing clinicians will hand a deaf client the Minnesota Multiphasic Personality Inventory-2 (MMPI-2; Hathaway & McKinley, 1989). It seems an easy way to assess personality without paying for an interpreter. Most clinicians are unaware that the average reading level for deaf individuals is 4th grade, while the MMPI is written at a 6th-grade level. In addition, several items are inappropriate for deaf clients. For example, "People are talking about me behind my back" is a common occurrence for deaf individuals. Hearing people frequently talk behind a deaf person's back about how the deaf person can't hear.

While working with deaf clients, most therapists unfamiliar with the Deaf population at least recognize some of their limitations. However, with respect to hard-of-hearing clients as opposed to deaf clients, most therapists assume there is no problem in offering services. If the client and therapist generally share a common language, the professional *assumes* the hard-of-hearing person shares a common culture, participates in common activities, and has access to common cultural information. These assumptions may be less accurate than the clinician assumes depending on a variety of factors including the age at which the client began having hearing loss, the amount of loss, the amount of isolation the client has experienced, the hearing losses of other family members, the reaction of others in the family and the social environment to their hearing loss, and the person's own reaction to what the loss *means*. Unlike being born deaf, losing hearing later in life can create a strong sense of loss, particularly if it is the latest in a string of losses. Social isolation is quite common due to misunderstood communications. Hard-of-hearing people become tired trying to lip-read, especially when the conversation moves quickly from one person to another in a group. Unlike ears, which do not rely on muscles to hear, eye muscles can become tired quickly, particularly if required to focus on a very small visual space (i.e., the lips) which shifts position as people move their heads, is covered by mustaches and beards, and may not move much at all by people who mumble their words. Hard-of-hearing individuals may have a sense of isolation that deaf individuals frequently feel, but often without the shared culture, language, and supportive groups available in the Deaf community. This is true even though the Hard-of-Hearing community is made up of roughly 10% of the population, 10 times larger than the Deaf community. Therapists who assume they can "understand" hard-of-hearing individuals may be correct in their assumption regarding the formal language used in communicating, but may be falsely assuming they really "understand" the hard-of-hearing clients' experiences of the world.

Interpreter Ethics

The Registered Interpreters for the Deaf (RID) is the professional organization that governs the ethics that certified interpreters use in their work. Unfortunately, many clinicians who call upon interpreters are not familiar with the rules and requirements governing the work of interpreters and may place interpreters in ethical dilemmas without realizing it. Clinicians have been known to become angry, frustrated, flustered, or embarrassed when an interpreter did not perform in a way that was expected or believed best. The fault, however, is on the clinician for not being trained or supervised in how to work with an interpreter.

Interpreters have ethical limitations on the confidentiality of client information. For example, a clinician cannot ask for history information about clients from the interpreter. The clinician must ask the clients themselves, as is true for hearing clients. Taking advantage of the fact that the interpreter has worked with the client before and likely has relevant information is unfair. The same interpreter is likely to have occasion to interpret for a deaf person in many different situations or settings. The interpreter *must* maintain confidentiality in order for the deaf person to trust them. If an interpreter were to break trust and divulge past information to a therapist, the client would never trust them again. Interpreters are the bridge between the hearing world and the deaf world. Like many "bridges," they can get "burned at both ends," that is to say, by both the professionals they need to work with and by the deaf clients themselves. Some deaf individuals have had little contact with interpreters because they may have been socially isolated by their location or by their families. They too can become angry and frustrated when they confuse the interpreter's role with the clinician's role. They may even believe the clinician's words are actually the interpreter's words and form attachments, associations, and transferences accordingly. Emotional reactions to personality style (e.g., transference and countertransference) may be placed on the interpreter by the clinician as well as by the client. Knowing what service an interpreter can offer and cannot offer (e.g., they do not "babysit" deaf children in the waiting room for clinicians) is critical to the success of the clinician and the interpreter working together with the client as a team.

Most therapists are sufficiently aware of the Deaf community to realize they need an interpreter when trying to offer services to deaf individuals who use sign language, but they may not be aware that trying to write it down may not be sufficient even to give simple information. They also are not generally aware there is a "range" of communication modes in sign language. At one end, American Sign Language is the most different from English, and at the other end Signing Exact English is the closest "manually coded" form of English. In the middle are Signed English, Pidgin (actually a variety of blends of Signed English and ASL), and finger spelling (traditionally called the Rochester method). They also may not be aware they can ask for an "oral interpreter" for deaf or hard-of-hearing individuals who do not use manual communication modes. An oral interpreter mouths the English being spoken by the clinician but without making the sounds. In this situation, interpreters may replace particular words that are difficult to lip-read with words that are easier, although in psychological work this is problematic, as very subtle shifts in meaning may occur.

Although it is frequently tempting for clinicians to use family members as convenient interpreters (including children), even a brief consideration of this practice should alert the clinician to pitfalls inherent in asking one family member "to speak for" another. This is generally not done with hearing families for good clinical reasons. The same reasoning applies to deaf families with hearing members.

Legal Requirements

The passage of the Americans With Disabilities Act (ADA) on July 26 of 1990 strengthened the accessibility of persons with a variety of disabilities and has particularly strengthened the Deaf community's efforts to gain access to services and opportunities that have been difficult and frequently impossible to procure from the hearing culture. Unlike the history with the African-American community in the United States, the Deaf community in the U.S. in general has not been denied access due to active, hostile persecution or prejudicial opposition, but instead, ironically, by patronizing hearing individuals and organizations who felt sorry for deaf individuals and sought to protect them. Also, because 90% of deaf children in the U.S. have hearing parents, the children's parents sought protection and education which, from their natural viewpoint, would bring their children as close to being "hearing" as possible. Unfortunately, the efforts to help them also controlled them.

Deaf people, particularly those who use sign language, make hearing people nervous. Anyone who has spent time in a foreign country knows how uncomfortable it is when you do not understand the communication going on around you. In a foreign country, you have the choice to leave and return to your own country, customs, language, and norms. Deaf individuals in a hearing world are expected to accept the choices made for them by hearing people "for their own good." It is really very hard for hearing people to believe that deaf people are fine, "thank you very much," and can think for themselves and make good choices. The only difference is they cannot hear. Without an appreciation of how much easier it is to communicate in ASL, hearing people naturally respond to deaf people in ways that minimize their own discomfort. Deaf people traditionally have been encouraged to work in printing (which is slightly ironic) or in the post office (because they can read zip codes). Hearing people feel the most comfortable with deaf people in these positions as communication, and frustrations from miscommunication, between workers is minimized. However, the ADA has highlighted deaf individuals' legal right to access services and opportunities the hearing world assumed they could not take advantage of, including education, job training, and modification of work sites. The negative reaction by "abled" populations to the ADA has not altered the fact that the ADA has enabled a variety of diverse populations to challenge the assumptions of American society and allowed a greater chance for the majority population to see the talents and skills the "disabled" groups actually possess.

Unfortunately, there has been a growing backlash by opponents claiming the ADA is "an unfunded mandate" (National Council on Disability, 1995, p. 11). This is not true as "the ADA is, at its core, a civil rights law, grounded in the freedoms guaranteed in the Bill of Rights. As such, the rights and freedoms codified in the ADA should not be subject to a debate on their cost, any more than the rights of women, minorities, or religious groups" (p. 11). With respect to the Deaf community, only 3% of the complaints filed under ADA concerned persons with "hearing impairments." The largest group of disabled persons filing were those with "back impairments" (20%), second were those with "neurological impairments" (12%), and third were those with "emotional/psychiatric impairments" (11%) (p. 41).

There are several areas where the ADA has impacted the accessibility of deaf and hard-of-hearing individuals. Title IV, Telecommunications of the ADA, requires that telephone companies provide telecommunication relay services. These regulations have greatly expanded the Deaf community's access to goods and services, even to ordering a pizza (a high priority in American culture). Title II, Public Services, requires that local, state, and other government agencies are accessible. The responsibility of an agency to provide a sign language interpreter if one is required or requested at the agency's expense, and not the client's expense, is also a major change to providing adequate access to services the Hearing community takes for granted. Title III, Public Accommodations, requires that public accommodations provide "auxiliary aids" (p. 33) but "only if their provision will not result in an undue burden on the business. . . . A public accommodation may choose among various alternatives as long as the result is effective communication" (p. 33).

This may mean writing notes, but it may also mean calling in a certified interpreter who is familiar with the specialized work conducted in a mental health setting. Because psychological and psychiatric work depends so much on accurate communication requiring minimal assumptions in order for correct diagnoses and treatment to be offered, anything that interferes with accurate communication can have dramatic and detrimental effects. The Americans With Disabilities Act requires that reasonable accommodations be made so that adequate services can be provided. The American Psychological Association ethical code (APA, 1992) requires the field to go even beyond that to having psychologists who, in addition to understanding the need to call an interpreter, also understand how to work with an interpreter effectively in service delivery.

DEAF WORLDVIEW

Deaf Community

A great deal has been written about the Deaf community. Readers are referred for a more complete picture to others more qualified as well as to authors who are members of the Deaf community. Several characteristics make the Deaf community unique when compared to other cultures and subcultures. Most people are aware that deaf individuals frequently employ a different language mode (i.e., a visual language vs. an oral language); however, most do not realize the diversity of visual languages (to be discussed) or the diversity of particular individuals in thinking about themselves as "deaf," "big D Deaf," "Hard-of-Hearing," or hearing "with a slight hearing problem." Deafness as a category was dropped from the census (unfortunately for professionals needing these data to apply to funding sources) because, although such persons may have an audiologically defined "severe" or "profound" hearing loss, they may not necessarily call themselves "deaf" or "Deaf" but prefer the label "hard of hearing." Similarly, a person with an audiologically defined "mild" or "moderate" loss may still call themselves "big D Deaf" even though their loss is mild because they may have deaf parents, learned American Sign Language as their first and preferred language, grew up in the Deaf community, and used much of their energy contributing to the advocacy of the Deaf community. This is confusing to hearing persons but is an important identity issue to persons with a hearing loss. The way they think of themselves dramatically affects their attitudes and communication with people in the other groups.

As numbers tend to attract attention (and funding), the Deaf community has a significant disadvantage compared to other minority groups because people who are profoundly deaf and use some form of manual communication comprise roughly only 1% of the U.S. population. This is the same percentage as the number of schizophrenics in the U.S., but the mental health field is certainly more aware of the schizophrenic population than of the Deaf community. Hearing people do not notice deaf individuals because deaf people do not ride in wheelchairs, their skin color is not different, they dress the same, and they frequently act the same (taking nonverbal cues from those around them). It used to be that hearing people would talk for hours on a bus with a deaf person, praising him or her for being "good listeners" but not realize the whole time that the good listener was deaf. Fortunately, sign language is becoming more accepted in public and the Deaf community is learning they can "come out of the closet" and use sign language publicly without so much ridicule as in the past. One notable exception to this is the increased use of "gang signs" by urban gangs which has caused the death of deaf individuals who were mistakenly perceived as members of an opposing gang.

Even when hearing people make efforts to be inclusive of deaf individuals, unless they also learn *how* to relate fairly and equally, hearing people will end up feeling uncomfortable, avoid deaf persons, make decisions that do not include deaf people, and relate in a kind of benign neglect. Hearing people may not realize the impact of their actions, and most would be shocked to think their actions were discriminatory or biased by assumptions. However, deaf people have the same normal intelligence curve as hearing people (with the small exception of a group of mentally retarded deaf children whose disease causes both mental retardation and deafness), yet the unemployment rate for the Deaf community is roughly 50%. The reason for this is not because deaf people do not wish to work nor that they are "disabled" from working. The problem is that hearing people do not know how to communicate *and relate* with deaf people nor how to optimally teach deaf people how to communicate *and relate* back to hearing people.

Most hearing people assume there is only one signed language for deaf people and do not realize there is a whole range of manual communication. At one end of the manual language continuum is American Sign Language (ASL). ASL is a full and complete language. Until the last few decades, hearing professionals have viewed ASL as a "partial" language. By all of the requirements of linguistic analysis, ASL meets the requirements for a language. When not suppressed, it is capable of communicating any concept used in a vocal language. The difficulty has been its suppression. Because hearing people did not understand its grammar and nuances, they assumed that it could not deal with "abstract" thoughts and ideas. The problem was more that hearing people could not conceive of an abstract manual language. Manual languages in hearing cultures had an association with a hunting language or as a language of a "primitive people," as mostly Caucasian people viewed the sign languages used by American Indians. With the more recent support by both the deaf and hearing cultures, ASL is rapidly expanding, broadening its use, and adding more and more terms to its available vocabulary.

At the other end of the continuum of manual languages is Signing Exact English (SEE). There is certainly a question as to whether SEE should be considered an actual language. It is better thought of as a manually encoded form of English because it uses the first letter for many English words, uses English grammar and syntax, was created by hearing people, is used mostly in the schools or universities, and is visually cumbersome and slow. Also, some of the vocabulary is not conceptually fitting (e.g., signing "butter" with "fly" to mean "butterfly"). In this writer's opinion, SEE's best function is as a bridge to learning *written* English.

If one moves across the continuum from SEE, the next manual language is Signed English. There is debate as to whether Signed English can be really considered a separate language. Signed English uses English grammar and syntax, but drops out redundant and conceptually unnecessary articles, endings, and indices used in SEE. Further along the continuum is a mix of Signed English with ASL called Pidgin Signed English. Like any human culture where two languages meet, there usually develops a "pidgin" which borrows elements from both. Pidgin can shift depending on the user and usually does not follow grammatical and marker rules closely. It can be inappropriately used to label persons as having low intelligence. Recently, a new label has arisen for this mix of languages called Conceptually Accurate Signed English (CASE). It was developed to help highlight the need for conceptual accuracy in this freer form of communication.

There is also a form of manual communication that can be drawn on throughout the continuum. This is finger spelling, or what used to be called the "Rochester" method, because it was developed in Rochester, NY. Finger spelling uses the alphabet of the host country (e.g., there is a Greek finger-spelling alphabet for the Greek alphabet) and is used to spell words from the host language. This form of communication allows the inclusion of particularly technical words which have recently developed in English (e.g., autoexec, syscom, etc.).

Most hearing people also assume that deaf people should learn to lip-read because they believe deaf people should be responsible for dealing with the hearing world in English. Lip-reading is really very difficult and not a complete method for communication. Only 20% of the sounds in English are able to be read on the lips. The other 80% occur in the back of the throat and are unreadable. Further, the amount of visual space involved in lip-reading is very small. Simply hold up your thumb and index finger around the space of a person's mouth whom you are looking at. Depending on the distance, the space between your fingers will be either very small or nearly touching. The human capability of attending to such a small space for long periods of time is limited, and if a child or adult has Attention Deficit Disorder it is very limited. A deaf child 5 years old or younger will not attend for very long to a mouth "flapping," but the most important language period is the preschool years. Without adequate access to a language, any child's later learning potential is severely affected. Unfortunately, hearing people still believe deaf people should and must learn to lip-read so they can "function in society." The lip-reading is important, but as an adjunct aid to other communication modes, not as the sole or even primary mode of communication.

Deaf Children of Deaf Parents

Of the deaf children in the US., 90% of them have hearing parents. Said the other way, 10% have at least one deaf parent. This means that only 10% of the Deaf community have had a parent who was in a position *from birth* to pass on their visual language, to teach their culture and values, and to teach their child how to live in the majority hearing world, including how to cope with discrimination in assertive rather than aggressive or passive ways. Deaf children of deaf parents learn their family's language *before* the age when hearing children of *hearing* parents learn their language. This is because the muscles in the vocal cords are quite small and require a longer time for children to learn to manipulate them than the muscles in the arms and hands. Any child who can see is able to learn a manually signed language earlier than a spoken language. All children attend to nonverbal or body language in the first 2 years of life. Learning sign language is simply an extension of this natural process. Watching very young deaf children of deaf parents sign to their friends and family is a delight and wonder at their grasp of language and concepts. They are ahead of their hearing-age peers in their ability to use and understand a language. Unfortunately, this advantage is lost in schools where sign language is not used and the measure of language capability is based on voiced English. Many bright and gifted deaf children are overlooked because of the quest to make them like their hearing-age peers or like their deaf-age peers who have hearing parents emphasizing their oral skills. The percentage difference of 10% versus 90% helps explain why the debate between "oral" and "manual" methods of education has raged for so long. It is extremely difficult for hearing people to "step out" of their reliance on hearing and into the deaf world. They cannot imagine that such an existence could teach them something. They see it as only a loss. The Deaf community sees it as a rich, vibrant community fighting to be understood and given the chance to make contributions and gain the rewards and services granted others.

This does not mean that deaf children should not learn English nor be kept from relating to hearing children and adults. It is unavoidable. The majority culture in the United States is hearing, with English as the majority language. Being only 1% of the population, deaf children cannot avoid hearing people. They are everywhere! The question is better asked, given that deaf children learn in tactile and visual ways, how can they be encouraged to develop language skills initially in their own language and then learn English as a second language? Most of the children in the world are bilingual. Americans have tended to believe their children do not need a bilingual education, but with world internet communications affecting the whole U.S., this assumption is rapidly changing.

Deaf Children of Hearing Parents

With 90% of deaf children having hearing parents, the challenges to raising a child with good language skills, good self-esteem, strong and clear identity, and the ability to contribute to the (now world) community are much greater. What if a doctor were to say to a new American parent, "Here is your new baby, *but* you must raise this child to speak Russian - which means of course you must learn Russian, you must take them to a Russian school which may be hours from your home and have them stay there except for the weekends, you must find some Russian people and make them your friends so your child can play with their children and model from their friend's parents instead of you, and you must attend a Russian Orthodox Church where they can receive the religious message in the Russian language. You may not be Russian, but your child will be." How many parents would actually do this? It is very difficult for hearing parents to learn sign language, enroll their child in the state deaf school, make friends with deaf people whose language grammar is completely different, and find a church with a service that provides sign language (currently usually in Signed English rather than ASL). Some parents persevere, but always wonder if they are making the right choices.

For hearing parents, learning your child is deaf, especially if you did not expect it, creates a strong sense of loss which is not easy to work through. For the deaf adults in the community, watching another family where the deaf child grows up with a hearing parent who finds it hard to imagine a deaf world is also extremely painful. Nearly all of the deaf children will become deaf adults. Hearing parents generally must struggle to understand what this means for their child and for them. Their natural desire to have a child "like me" can, in some very important ways be true, while in other ways will be quite different. Hearing parents may be tempted to access any hope of having their child become hearing. The development of the cochlear implant is *not* the promise of a hearing life. The debate regarding cochlear implants would take a whole chapter, but the reader is referred to *Silent News* (the national deaf newspaper) and *Deaf Life* (the national deaf magazine) for articles on views in the Deaf community. Technology does offer a number of hopes for communication, but all of the devices still require the hearing world to develop a better understanding of the deaf world in order to use them with respect and consideration of deaf individuals.

As hearing parents grapple with the many issues involved in raising a deaf child, the most critical is the choice of an educational environment, including preschool placements. Many hearing parents wish their deaf children to be "mainstreamed" as naturally they wish their children to be close to home and to be culturalized to their particular hearing and ethnic culture. However, as Marta Manfredi noted, "The deaf adolescents attending a school with hearing peers, in order not to succumb, are compelled to use all their energies and resources and to engage in an unequal struggle. . . . They are more aware of the constraints that derive from their impairment, but they are also uncomfortable with it" (Manfredi, 1993, p. 59). Being the minority deaf child in an all-hearing class may give the child the status of "mascot" but will not likely get the child voted class president. Having a self-contained classroom for deaf children with a hearing teacher and adult interpreters will allow the deaf children to have some deaf friends, but on the playground how much of what the hearing children discuss with their friends would be discussed in the same way by telling it through an adult interpreter to a deaf child from a different class? The goal of mainstreaming makes a lot of sense for most of the "disabled" populations. However, with deaf children there is a wide variety of factors to consider and the answers are not always obvious. Helping hearing parents find nurturing *and* empowering choices for their children is critical to the future of the Deaf community.

Hearing Children of Deaf Parents

Hearing children of deaf parents, or Children of Deaf Adults (CODAs) as they are called (as compared to Spouses of Deaf Adults - SODAs), generally have a specific group of experiences which are markedly different from those of other hearing children or from deaf children. Provided their parents use sign language, their first language is a manual language. Because any child can learn a manual language earlier than a vocal language, they develop language skills earlier. Sometimes educators will be concerned about CODAs being behind other hearing children in their English skills when they first start school, but even if CODAs are somewhat behind in the beginning, unless they have a language disability they are able to catch up quite readily. It is simply that English is their second language. However, because 99% of the culture surrounding these children still involves spoken English, these children are not significantly deprived in their exposure to English. How growing up with sign language as their first language affects how they actually think, however, is a question of some debate.

Because a manual language is their first language (generally ASL, but sometimes Signed English), these children learn to associate emotional states, goals, consequences, cues, and desires in terms of a visual language, with all of the rich body language that accompanies it. Any child's first language has the most emotional impact and "colors" how they view the world and conceptualize new situations. Sign language becomes the language of home, mom, dad, personal issues, and private conversations between siblings, whereas English becomes the language of school, hearing friends, TV, music, radio, movies, magazines, and newspapers. Sometimes CODAs will "get away with" using unacceptable or inappropriate language whereupon their hearing friends, or their hearing friends' parents, will naturally wonder "Why don't their parents correct them?" They can't hear them. Children learn very early and very quickly that they can hide language easily. Deaf parents are generally aware of this possibility and most are concerned if their children have violated "hearing norms."

CODAs are frequently caught as "bridges" or "interpreters" between the deaf and hearing worlds. Generally the oldest child will have the role of "family interpreter." They will answer the door; answer the telephone (even if the family has a TTY); read the newspaper; deal with salespeople, shop clerks, income tax people, police, hospital staff, funeral directors, bosses, and insurance salespeople; and so on, all in service of interpreting for their parents what the hearing world requires. So much of the information we take for granted about our own culture comes from overhearing conversations. Deaf people do not overhear a great deal of hearing people's conversations. The "family interpreter" listens in and decides what information gets passed on to the parents and which does not. This gives the family interpreter more power and status in the family than is usual. These "parentified" children (i.e., acting as a third parent) can have emotional difficulties later in life similar to parentified children in alcoholic families.

Deaf and Hearing Siblings

Because it is unusual for all of the children in a family to have exactly the same level of hearing loss at exactly the same age, most families have a mix of "hearing" and "deaf" children. Each family configuration must be considered indepth to provide effective mental health services. The family dynamics can vary considerably depending on a number of important factors. The usual birth-order rights and responsibilities are affected by which of the children are deaf, hard of hearing, or hearing. Which schools - a school with a majority of hearing versus deaf children - or which special classrooms - a self-contained or mainstreamed class - affects the different children in the family. What friends - hearing, hard of hearing, or deaf - are available at school and what friends are available around the home affects the children's play after school. Whether one or both of the parents are hearing, hard of hearing, or deaf affects the likelihood friends will be invited into the home. Whether there are other adults in the family or adults who are "like family" and who "adopt" one or more of the children because of similar hearing status affects the children's identification, sense of actually being a part of the family, and desire to live elsewhere. The parents' experience with different parenting styles for hearing, hard of hearing, or deaf children, and finally the personality types and temperaments, including possible attention, anger control, or learning problems, of the children themselves all have major effects on the problems and successes a child will experience. All of these factors can have a significant impact on the family's ability as a whole to adjust to everyone's communication needs in order to meet the member's emotional needs while standing firm on behavior limits for the children. Given all of these variables and possible conflicts, it is a testimony to the deaf family that is able to resolve them successfully.

There are several issues that arise frequently when there is a mix of hearing, hard-of-hearing, and deaf children in a family. Of course, the major factor is whether the parents are hearing, hard of hearing, or deaf, but of greater concern is the communication mode chosen by the parents for the family to use on a daily basis. The children naturally model the parents, at least initially, and will find some means of communication even if it is limited. Human beings are "wired" to process language information (i.e., body language, gestures, mimes, signs, symbols, icons, lip movements, and, for those with some hearing, sounds, grunts, and words). The *accuracy* of the communication generally improves over time within the family, however, the communication *mode* may vary widely among different groupings of family members. Twins, even two hearing twins, are known to develop their own "language" over the years which is private and based on their mutual experiences.

At various times in a family's development, the role of "interpreter" may shift from the oldest child or daughter to other family members as communication is attempted within the family and with the outside world. This role may be expected by the family and taken for granted, or it may have a higher status with some members of the family but not others. Because language involves the ability and power of information exchange, it can upset the usual power status of family members. A child may be seen to have more power than a parent, and a younger child may be seen to have more power than an older child. The usual American family dynamic of parents sharing equal decision making and information exchange, with the children sharing information among themselves depending on their age, gender, and status as siblings, may be quite different in families with children having mixed hearing capabilities and mixed communication modes. For example, a younger hearing child who has learned American Sign Language or Pidgin better than the hearing father may intentionally or unintentionally misrepresent the older deaf brother's communication to the father. Because the father's signing may be more limited, he may be unable to accurately assess for himself what the older brother is trying to communicate. The father may react inappropriately based on the misinformation and punish the older brother, and the older brother may later, more severely, punish his younger sibling. The potential for triangulation of alliances (i.e., two against one) and coalitions within the family is high. Added to this is the strong influence of each parent's attitude toward deaf children. They may perceive the children as "like me" or "one of us" if the parent is deaf, as "not as good as hearing people" or "broken" if the parent is hearing, as "needing protection" or "my fault" if the parent feels guilt or grief about the hearing loss, and as "unintelligible" or "not like me" if the parent is unable or unwilling to develop an accurate and full communication mode with the child. Siblings who have complete communication access to a parent may "pity," "lord over," "ignore," or "support" a sibling who does not have complete communication with the parent or whose parent has an "attitude problem" toward the deaf child. Children, even without full communication, are usually quick to pick up the body language cues about parental attitudes toward their siblings. Their reaction to those cues depends on their personality temperament and on the parental response to their bid for whatever goal they strive for within the family. These interactions can create coalitions and ostracized individuals within the family.

One might assume these coalitions would follow similar hearing status, that is, hearing children aligning with hearing parents and deaf children aligning with deaf parents. However, it is the desire and willingness to work through problems in communication which tends to form the strongest coalitions. Even in hearing families, coalitions will form along lines of easy communication, as between same gender members in a family that holds strong gender roles. Whether these coalitions are antagonistic to each other greatly depends on the family "cultural atmosphere" created by the adults in the household.

NEED FOR TRAINING EXPERIENCES

Misattributions

The usual processes involved in providing mental health services greatly relies on the accurate perception of the meaning of clients' actions, reactions to the setting, and the clinician. Attributing a reasonable cause for a person's actions is the basis for diagnostic assessment and subsequent treatment. Misdiagnosis of deaf individuals as being mentally retarded, learning disabled, psychotic, manic-depressive, suffering from explosive disorder, or any number of other labels can severely affect the placement, medication, therapy, and follow-up services. Misattributions within psychotherapy can cause misdirection, repeated "going around in circles," lack of rapport, frustration, tension, paranoia, and disgust with the whole process - for both the clinician and the client.

The need for adequate preparation of clinicians prior to treating deaf individuals is obvious. Unfortunately, because the population is small and widely spread out, few agencies and professionals see many deaf individuals in 1 year or even 5 years. Training every mental health professional to a level required for even adequate provision of services is not realistic.

Training every professional about how to work with an interpreter is still less than adequate and probably not realistic. Training every mental health professional to understand that ethically they must refer to other trained professionals is possible and necessary. Changing mental health systems to refer deaf clients to appropriate services is possible and necessary. There is a whole division of the U.S. Department of Justice dedicated to handling lawsuits generated by the Americans With Disabilities Act. The Deaf community has the right of access to equivalent mental health services as compared to the Hearing community. It is the mental health professions' responsibility to train a reasonable portion of their students in methods, approaches, and languages sufficient to serve the Deaf community.

Training Programs

A clinical psychology program has been established at Gallaudet University in Washington, DC. This program graduates PhD psychology students trained to work with the whole range of deaf clients from children to elderly, and the full range of communication modes from lip-reading to American sign language. A few of these graduates are themselves deaf.

Another program offering training is the Mental Health and Deafness Program at the Duke E. Ellis Institute of Human Development at the School of Professional Psychology, Wright State University, Dayton, Ohio. The professional school has hosted for 9 years the Mental Health and Deafness Program, which is a multidisciplinary didactic and experiential program designed to train a variety of mental health students and professionals in working with the Deaf community and to train sign language interpreters in working in mental health settings. The disciplines involved include psychology, psychiatry, mental health counseling, rehabilitation counseling, art therapy, and manual communication.

Other programs in the country include the Center on Deafness at the University of Southern California in San Francisco, California; the psychology residency program at Strong Memorial Hospital in Rochester, New York; and the National Institute for Mental Health and Deafness in Florida. Hopefully the graduates from these various programs will move to other areas of the country to help provide better mental health services to the Deaf community across the United States. Training needs for a particular area may vary considerably. As with other minority populations, certain cities and geographic areas have attracted a high proportion of the Deaf community. However, because the cause of deafness can be from hereditary factors, illness, or injury, deaf individuals exist in all states, counties, cities, and towns at some time or other. Providing access to mental health services is the responsibility of all mental health service providers, and cooperation at all levels will be needed for the Deaf community to truly have equal accessibility.

CONTRIBUTOR

Robert N. Basil, PsyD, is currently a Clinical Faculty member of the School of Professional Psychology at Wright State University in Dayton, Ohio. He has directed the Mental Health and Deafness Program at the Duke E. Ellis Institute of Human Development since 1989. Dr. Basil has a private practice at Health Care Associates, a wholistic health care group, and is a supervisor at Comprehensive Counseling Services, a county mental health center. His training is in clinical psychology with special interests in deafness, giftedness, and attention deficit disorder. Dr. Basil may be contacted at Health Care Associates, 10 Bellemonte Street, Suite C, Middleton, OH 45042. E-mail: rbasil@siscom.net

RESOURCES

American Psychological Association. (1992). Ethical Principles of Psychologists and Code of Conduct. *American Psychologist, 47,* 1597-1611.

American Psychological Association Task Force on Diversity Issues. (1998, February). Disability as diversity: A guide for class discussion. *APA Monitor,* p. 41.

Americans With Disabilities Act of 1990, 42 U.S.C.A. § 12101 *et seq.* (West 1993).

Bonvillian, J. D., & Folven, R. J. (1993). Sign language acquisition: Developmental aspects. In M. Marschark & M. D. Clark (Eds.), *Psychological Perspectives on Deafness* (pp. 229-265). Hillsdale, NJ: Lawrence Erlbaum.

Deaf Life Magazine. Published by MSM Productions Ltd., 1095 Meigs Street, Rochester, NY 14692-3380. E-mail: Deaflife@deaflife.com

Denmark, J. C. (1994). *Deafness and Mental Health*. Bristol, PA: Jessica Kingsley Publishers.

Hathaway, S. R., & McKinley, J. C. (1989). *Minnesota Multiphasic Personality Inventory-2 (MMPI-2)*. Minneapolis, MN: The University of Minnesota Press.

Manfredi, M. M. (1993). The emotional development of deaf children. In M. Marschark & M. D. Clark (Eds.), *Psychological Perspectives on Deafness* (pp. 49-63). Hillsdale, NJ: Lawrence Erlbaum.

Marschark, M. , & Clark, M. D. (Eds.). (1993). *Psychological Perspectives on Deafness*. Hillsdale, NJ: Lawrence Erlbaum.

National Council on Disability. (1995). *The Americans With Disabilities Act: Ensuring Equal Access to the American Dream* (390-329 - 814/20503). Washington, DC: U.S. Government Printing Office.

Paul, P. V., & Jackson, D. W. (1993). *Toward a Psychology of Deafness: Theoretical and Empirical Perspectives*. Boston: Allyn & Bacon.

Silent News. This is a national newspaper for deaf and hard-of-hearing people. It is published monthly by Silent News, Inc., a Non-Profit Corp., 135 Gaither Drive, Suite F, Mount Laurel, NJ 08054-1710. E-mail: silentnews@aol.com

Section V: Selected Topics

This section includes a collection of contributions that address diverse techniques and roles for clinicians in a variety of settings. These contributions represent a sort of potpourri of topics that may not fit neatly into another section of the volume.

Telehealth or telemedicine increasingly underlies health care provision and can be adapted to support nearly any clinical activity. Telecommunication technology also alters sociopolitical contexts and reduces access barriers. In the first contribution of this section, B. Hudnall Stamm offers a model of clinical care across modes of communication including face-to-face and technology-mediated methods suggesting ways telecommunications can be integrated into current models of mental health care.

In the second contribution, Kathryn White introduces readers to the field of alternative medicine. While alternative medicine practices are growing in popularity and patients are turning in large numbers to these options, traditional mental health practitioners have paid little attention to these practices. The contribution presents an overview of four forms of alternative medicine, with an emphasis upon how they are being used to treat psychological disorders.

Dyslexia is the most prevalent type of learning disability, with problems in acquiring reading and language skills the most common symptoms. In the next contribution, George Grosser and Carol Spafford provide some current research-based theoretical underpinnings of dyslexia in such areas as symptomatology, neurophysiological bases, and cognitive-processing deficits and strengths.

Professional and lay primary caregivers to the terminally ill are at heightened risk due to the intensity of the work. Jackson Rainer describes the manifestations of compassion fatigue, which include withdrawal and isolation from others, inappropriate emotionality, loss of pleasure, loss of boundaries with the dying patient, and a sense of being overwhelmed and pressured.

Completing a battery of tests is often a challenge for professionals working with resistant children. In the next contribution, Susan Skinner and Paul Guthrie describe a technique that breaks down a battery of tests into visible steps with ongoing feedback which is effective in completing the needed procedures. Practitioners can replicate and adapt this technique for a variety of children's needs.

In the next contribution, Martin Brodwin and Roy Chen introduce clinicians to the concepts of sexuality and intimacy concerning people who have physical disabilities.

We are all probably tired of hearing about White House affairs. Yet, clinicians frequently work with clients whose relationships are disrupted by sexual affairs. In the last contribution of this section, Emily Brown translates some of the lessons from the President's affair to working with our clients' affairs.

Integrating Telehealth Into Mental Health Care

B. Hudnall Stamm

There are powerful opportunities to expand our current clinical practices by extending through telecommunications the way we transfer information from provider to patient, patient to provider, and provider to provider. Not all extensions will be acceptable, and others will actually be better than traditional face-to-face interactions. The challenge to us now is to examine critically the telehealth options available, imagine new ones, and determine how we can use them to administer the best possible treatment. Because of the rapid changes in and the technological complexities of telehealth it may not ever be possible to "learn" telehealth. Yet, as I have written previously, it is likely that providers will need to know much more about technology than has been the norm (Stamm, 1998). How should one begin to accommodate these knowledge changes? Find what is appealing and focus on that. Ask yourself: *How can it improve my practice? Can I help my patients better if I use it?* For, if it is not a change for the better, why use it? The goal of this contribution is to provide an overview of current telecommunications technology and applications in mental health to help you begin to build a personal-professional vision of telehealth and to see what new professional opportunities wait.

MENTAL HEALTH CARE, TECHNOLOGY, AND SOCIOPOLITICAL CONTEXTS

Telemedicine refers to the use of electronic communications and information technology to provide or support clinical care at a distance (Department of Commerce [DOC], 1997). The broader term, telehealth, encompasses telemedicine and other health care related activities including health education, administration, and training. Nickelson (1998) defines telehealth to include health assessment, diagnosis, intervention, consultation, supervision, and education. Mental health is one of the top specialties using telehealth (DOC, 1997; Grisgby, 1997).

Health care worldwide is becoming more complex and scarcer. Although we think of the patient and provider as being the key elements of the system, the sociopolitical context in which the patient and provider operate is sufficiently powerful that it can overtake and direct the provider-patient relationship (Gaus & DeLeon, 1995; Miller & Farber, 1996). The infrastructure largely determines the type of care that a patient has available or that a provider can offer or even know about. Telehealth expands the patient's and the provider's access to information by diminishing many previously impenetrable isolating boundaries such as economics, climate, geography, or warfare (e.g., Dankins, 1995; Forkner, Reardon, & Carson, 1996; Norton et al., 1997; Preston, F. W. Brown, & Hartley, 1992; Stamm, 1999; Terry, 1999; U.S. Department of Health and Human Services [HHS], 1997).

Because this contribution is about clinical applications, some of the most difficult aspects of health care in general, and telehealth in particular, will be addressed only briefly, if at all. Who pays for the delivery of service is just beginning to be worked out as an increasing number of third-party payment organizations, including Medicare, are including telehealth as reimbursable services. What has not yet been resolved is how licenses and liability will be handled. These are impenetrable problems at this stage of the field's development. In this contribution, few comments are made on the financial, ethical, or legal implications of telehealth (Nickelson, 1998). Similarly, the need for scientific evaluation of telehealth practices is clear but will not be discussed here. This contribution focuses on clinical practices and possibilities by extending current modes of face-to-face communications with the use of telecommunications technology (see Table 1, p. 387).

CLINICAL ACTIVITIES, RELATIONSHIPS, AND MODES OF COMMUNICATIONS

Face-to-Face Relationships

Working with patients as a mental health care provider involves assessment; patient education; crisis intervention; case management; individual, couples, family, and group psychotherapy; and medication support. Providers perform patient-oriented administrative activities such as billing, patient records, and case planning. The latter may include consulting with colleagues, researching the literature, and using other informatics sources to discover the best care alternatives. Mental health care providers participate in routine administrative activities such as departmental meetings. Finally, mental health care providers attend to their own professional development and self-care through individual supervision, peer support, and continuing education (McCarthy, Kulakowski, & Kenfield, 1994; Skorupa & Agresti, 1993; Stamm, 1999). Some activities extend beyond the patient-provider relationship and may include community service, prevention programs, education, and forensic activities.

Thus, clinical interaction can be viewed, by activity or by types of relationships. For example, clinical interventions may involve the provider and the patient in a one-to-one relationship. They may also involve patient-to-peer relationships such as self-help groups. At times, the patient may work alone reading, doing "homework," or experiencing insight. Providers also participate in clinical interventions alone (such as case planning) or with professional peers (as in supervision). Finally, when providers work in the community, the community becomes the "other" in the relationship. The court, too, can become an "other" in the relationship.

Mapping Clinical Activities to Relationships Across Modes of Communications

The first column in Table 1 illustrates how typical face-to-face encounters can be grouped by relationship. For example, in the cell that describes provider and patient, typical activities could include assessment, education, crisis intervention, case management, individual psychotherapy, group psychotherapy, and medication support. Patients and peers might engage in support networks or self-help groups, while providers together might engage in activities such as case conferences or peer support.

Following a primer of technology, the remainder of this contribution will examine common activities of clinical practice, summaries of technology, and how clinical activities can map across various kinds of devices and types of telecommunications technology. Although not exhaustive, the summary illustrates some of the past successes and future possibilities for telehealth in mental health care clinical practice.

A CLINICIAN'S PRIMER OF TELECOMMUNICATIONS TECHNOLOGY

To understand telehealth and telemedicine, it is important to understand the basic technology that fuels it (Crump & Pfeil, 1995). Most providers are not interested in the engineer-

TABLE 1: Possible Technological Adaptations of Clinical Activities

Participants	Mode of Communication						
	Traditional Face-to-Face	**Phone**	**Fax**	**Audio and Video Teleconference**	**Stand-Alone Computer**	**Networked Computer (Intranet, Internet)**	**Virtual Reality**
Patient Alone	• insight	• voice-mail to tx • info. lines • U of VA program	• fax-back info.		• self-help programs	• self-help information • info. searches	• *in vivo* self-exposure trials
Patient and Peer	• support networks • self-help groups	• support networks	• support networks	• support networks • self-help groups		• support networks (e-mail) • self-help group (usenets and listservs)	
Provider and Patient	• assessment • education • crisis intervention • case management • individual psychotherapy • group psychotherapy • medication support	• assessment • education • crisis intervention • case management • individual psychotherapy • medication support	• education • crisis management • case management • medication support (scripts)	• assessment • education • crisis intervention • case management • individual psycho-therapy • group psycho-therapy • medication support	• education • case management • individual psychotherapy • medication support	• education • individual psychotherapy • *in vivo* exposure • medication support	• education • individual psychotherapy • *in vivo* exposure
Provider Alone	• case planning • patient records • billing		• patient records		• case planning • patient records • billing	• on-line searches • archives	
Provider and Provider	• case conferences • individual supervision • group supervision • dept. meetings • peer support • continuing education	• case conferences • individual supervision • group supervision • dept. meetings • peer support	• case conference (send records) • individual supervision	• case conferences • individual supervision • group supervision • dept. meetings • peer support • continuing education	• continuing education	• case conferences • individual supervision • group supervision • dept. meetings • peer support • continuing education	• case conferences • individual supervision • group supervision • continuing education
Provider and Community	• education • community meetings • crisis intervention • prevention programs	• crisis intervention	• education • community meetings • crisis intervention • prevention programs	• education • community meetings • crisis intervention • prevention programs	• education • prevention programs	• education • community meetings • crisis intervention • prevention programs	• education • crisis intervention • prevention programs
Forensic	• education			• education • testifying	• education	• education • research cases	• education • reenactment

ing that makes telehealth possible. But some knowledge of the basic principles allows clinicians to make better judgments about the practicality, desirability, and compatibility of particular technologies and techniques as they apply to clinical care.

The telephone, invented in 1876, is perhaps the oldest application of telecommunications technology to clinical health care (e.g., Benschoter, Wittson, & Ingham, 1965; Field, 1996; Tampas & Soule, 1968). The technology of the telephone - and its related network of cables, transmitters, and satellites - forms the basis of communications technology. Our fears of telehealth may stem from the fact that telecommunications is a complex field with its own technical language that we do not understand. The following section addresses, albeit simplistically, some key concepts and technical terms of telecommunications. The intent is not to teach telecommunications but to provide sufficient information for the reader to form *clinically driven* cognitive maps of how telehealth systems could be used to provide clinical care.

Perhaps the most reassuring thing that can be said is that telecommunication devices are simple in principle. In the simplest form, there is a device at each end connected to a system that transmits information. For example, the telephone is composed of a transmitter (the microphone) and a receiver (the earphone). The microphone converts speech into its electrical form and the earphone translates it back to the sound we recognize as a voice. Passing data from place to place is accomplished (a) in a variety of different ways (mode of transmission), (b) at a variety of speeds (rate of transmission), and (c) in a variety of formats (compression format). These basic principles apply to other devices including fax machines, video teleconferencing units, nodes on a computer network, and even mixed technologies combining several different types of devices.

Mode of Transmission

Copper and Fiber

Sometimes a cable connects two (or more) people point-to-point in a conversation. This cable can be copper or fiber-optic. The first copper TAT-1 transatlantic line, installed in 1958, had a capacity of 36 voice circuits. Currently, a pair of copper wires twisted together (called "twisted pair") can carry 24 telephone signals and is called a T1 line. This line carries an overall equivalent bit rate (a bit is one chunk of information, either a 0 or a 1) of 1.544 million bits per second. Fiber-optic transmission is accomplished by a beam of light passing through a very thin, very pure, glass fiber (invented 1960, general implementation 1970s-1980s). A single strand of glass fiber can carry about 2 gigabits per second (2 billion bits per second) which is about 30,000 telephone signals.

Microwave Transmissions

Sometimes running cable point-to-point is impractical and data is transmitted via very-high-frequency (VHF) radio signals. These signals may be relayed by terrestrial microwave towers which can be located up to about 26 miles apart. These towers must be within "line-of-sight" of each other because the signal cannot travel through solid masses such as buildings or mountains. When it is not possible to use line-of-site microwave transmitters, information may be relayed at super-high-frequency (SHF) via a geosynchronous (same rotation as earth) communications satellite. These satellites orbit at the height they can maintain constant positioning with respect to the earth below, which is about 22,300 miles above earth's surface (circa 1960s). For data, the trip from the origination point to the satellite and on to the destination point is about 12 seconds. Although the 12-second delay is less than ideal, it does allow telephone to remote locations. Sometimes, when communicating to very remote locations, such as the bush in Alaska or Australia, it is necessary to relay the signal twice across the satellite. This results in a "double satellite hop" which creates disturbing 24-second delays. New technologies (e.g., satellites that have switching units on the satellite, circa early 1990s) may reduce the double-hop problem.

Cellular

Cellular telephones (circa early 1980s) use two-way, low-power radio communications. The name cellular was derived from the transmission pattern. Geographical areas are divided into "cells" with a radius of about 8 to 12 miles covered by a radio transmitter with 120 two-way radio channels. The signal is switched from transmitter to transmitter as the mobile user passes over the boundaries of each cell. This technology is the basis for the range of new "wireless" technologies, including the wireless transmission of computer data, images, paging, voice, and e-mail. In the near future, a network of small, relatively inexpensive "low earth orbit" satellites will likely replace and enhance the ground radio transmitters.

Cable

Recent changes in the telecommunications have led to the possibility of using the coaxial cable that delivers cable television as a means of delivery of telephone, fax, or computer data. This is the largest capacity cable coming into most homes or businesses. Coaxial cable is a form of wire that has insulating rings throughout and is well protected from many types of interference. Coaxial cable carries TV transmission, or about 10,000 voice transmissions (660 million bits per second). Cable modems (the device that sits between your computer and the cable) are up to 1,000 times faster than conventional analog modems. One of the major drawbacks of cable modems is that they are one-way. They only receive information; sending must still be done via conventional telephone lines.

Rate of Transmission

Perhaps the most important development in the functional use of telecommunications in the provision of health care has been the changes in the rate of transmission. Only a decade ago, moving data at a rate of 1,200 bits per second was considered fast. Now even the most routine data transfer undertaken by a school child moves 20 or more times that fast. Transmission rate, which is a function of the bandwidth (frequency of the wave), is important because faster rates mean it is possible to move more information. For still-image-based clinical applications such as radiology or dermatology, being able to transfer more information faster means not having to wait as long to see the image being transmitted. For mental health care providers who often use live images, transmission rate may mean the difference between useless information and useful information.

Compression Format

Clearly, it is not possible to move all the information that we want as quickly as we would like. Various forms of data compression exist to address the problems of moving data fast enough to be useful. The key to data compression lies in the fact that much of what exists in any information is repeated information.

The following example, though not technically complete, is a vivid illustration of the theory of compression. Suppose a provider and patient agree to videoteleconference with a specialist at a remote location. Their images are transmitted, similarly to a movie, frame by frame. The device at the remote site receives and displays the picture of the room, which includes the provider, patient, desk, chairs, walls, and so on. Soon the device at the other end has been "trained" to see the room. In future frames, the device can be instructed to transmit only the information *that changes*. Why send a new representation of the desk when the device at the other end already knows what the desk looks like? Unless directed to "update the information," when the computer "refreshes the image" it only adds that information that changes (e.g., the movement of the patient reaching for a tissue). Thus, much less information needs to be transmitted. Some of the newest formulas for data compression can reduce the overall amount of information by ratios of hundreds to one.

CLINICAL APPLICATIONS OF VARIOUS TECHNOLOGIES

Telephony

Telephones figure prominently in a cohesive body of telehealth literature (see Haas, Benedict, & Kobos, 1996, for a complete review). Community hot-lines staffed by volunteer helpers were perhaps the first widely visible use of telephony for clinical care. Grumet (1979) suggests that using the telephone for conducting therapy can be particularly helpful for patients who are anxious and overstimulated by face-to-face office visits. Perhaps more individual telephone-based therapy takes place than is reported in the literature, but few papers report on individual psychotherapy via telephone. Nonetheless, telephones are used in a variety of ways.

A number of papers describe using the telephone to initiate, prompt, or follow up regular face-to-face mental health services. Burgoyne, Acosta, and Yamamoto (1983) report using telephones to prompt keeping first appointments. They postulated that it is the socioeconomic advantages represented by having a telephone that improved attendance, not the prompt itself. This hypothesis is also supported by Shivack and Sullivan (1989), who note improved attendance if patients can be reached directly. Although one study found no improvement (Dooley, Kunik, & Molinari, 1998), several other studies (Carr, 1985; Kourany, Garber, & Tornusciolo, 1990; Warzak, Parrish, & Handen, 1987) found that telephone prompts improved appointment attendance rates. Some treatments use prompts as an adjunctive treatment to face-to-face services. One study found reductions in mild to moderate depression using a telephone-prompted self-help psychotherapy program (Osgood-Hynes et al., 1998). More commonly, the telephone is used to maintain or monitor therapeutic gains during follow-up periods (Cavanaugh, 1990; S. L. Jones, P. K. Jones, & Katz, 1988; McGlynn, 1980; Spevak & Richards, 1980). The telephone is used to bolster adherence to treatment protocols (Schnelle et al., 1979), to support ongoing therapy (Hymer, 1984), or to prompt cognitively compromised individuals (Leirer, Morrow, et al., 1993; Leirer, Tanke, & Morrow, 1993).

Telephones have been used with success to improve auditory comprehension in aphasic adults (Davidoff & Katz, 1985), to reduce anxiety before surgery (Lamarche, Taddeo, & Pepler, 1998), and with smoking cessation (Koffman et al., 1998; Ramelson, Friedman, & Ockene, 1999; Schneider, Schwartz, & Fast, 1995; R. M. Shapiro et al., 1986). Other studies report using telephones for treating phobias: car telephones for *in vivo* treatment for driving phobias (Flynn, Taylor, & Pollard, 1992) and in-house telephones for treatment of panic disorder with agoraphobia (Swinson et al., 1995; Taylor, 1984). Telephones are used for psychological assessment screening (Dorfman et al., 1995; Simon, Revicki, & VonKorff, 1993). One project uses a telephone answering system with multiple options guiding seriously mentally ill people living in the community to medication prompts and a message "bulletin board" (Fox & Blank, 1997). Some therapists use voice mail for centering their dissociative clients between sessions (personal e-mail communications, Indirect-Trauma Discussion List, April, 1997).

Teleconferences may be used for family and group therapy. Several studies among people with physical disabilities who participated in telephone-based group therapy report increased activity and decreased loneliness (Evans, Kleinman, et al., 1984; Evans, Werkhoven, & Fox, 1982; Jaureguy & Evans, 1983) or increased activities accompanied by decreased anxiety (Evans, Fox, et al., 1984). Family therapy also may be enhanced by teleconferencing (DeSalvio, 1988; di Blasio, Fischer, & Prata, 1986; Hines, 1994; Springer, 1991).

Therapeutic contact by telephone has advantages and risks. Haas, Benedict, and Kobos (1996) summarize the work of the American Psychological Association Board of Professional Affairs task force, which documents the pros and cons and ethical dilemmas brought about by using the telephone as an emergency, adjunctive, and primary therapy communication mode. One of the most important conclusions that Haas and colleagues (1996) reach echoes other papers in pointing out the dearth of actual research on the benefits, risks, and outcomes of using the telephone for conducting mental health services.

Facsimile Machines

The Institute of Medicine (IOM) suggests that fax machines - along with e-mail and voice mail - are well suited for some routine clinical communications (Field, 1996). A facsimile (fax) machine is a device that sends an image of the original. Although fax technology has been available for the past century, digital scanning made it practical for common use. Current fax machines usually send images at 14.4 kps using a stand-alone fax or a computer equipped with modem and fax software. Stand-alone machines scan the original by using charge-coupled devices or light-emitting diodes (LEDs) to convert the original into picture elements called pixels, compressing "white" space (blank parts of the page). Computer faxes compress information already encoded digitally and transmit it through the modem to the device at the other end, where it is translated back into an image.

Faxes are a vital part of most patient record systems. As such, measures should be taken to protect the confidentiality of these faxes, such as locating sending and receiving machines in secured areas and treating faxes as confidential records. Under these circumstances, there is less technology-driven potential risk to breach of confidentiality than there is with other data transmissions such as cellular telephone or e-mail. Because of this, fax transmissions are sometimes used to relay identifying information separately from a patient file. For example, a radiological image such as a CT scan from a neuropsychological exam might be transmitted and identified only by a number. The number and patient identification are then faxed separately.

There is not a large amount of information in the literature regarding the use of fax machines for patient care, which may be because faxes are so common no one has felt the need to document fax-based projects. In a study of California licensed psychologists, over three-quarters of the respondents used faxes in their office or home (Rosen & Weil, 1996). There are a few papers that discuss the use of faxes as part of a technology management system (Holt & Crawford, 1992), in support of disaster response (Llewellyn, 1995), or for medication monitoring (Black et al., 1996). There are also reports of using faxes to manage ongoing chronic conditions such as AIDS (Huba, V. B. Brown, & Melchior, 1995) or asthma (Watson & Young, 1995). Other papers discuss clinical supervision (Cole et al., 1994; Rustin, 1998; Stamm, 1999).

Audio and Video Teleconferencing

Over and above family therapy via audio teleconference (ATC) mentioned previously, many projects and consultations take place via ATC. Standard telephones often come equipped with teleconferencing functions. However, even with the frequent use of ATC, video teleconferencing (VTC) is the most identifiable application of telehealth to mental health. In many ways, VTC has been synonymous with "telepsychiatry" or "tele-mental-health." While ATC passes one set of data (voice), generally, VTC passes two sets of data simultaneously. One set contains the image (picture) and the other set contains the sound (voice). In VTC, the bandwidth and compression algorithms determine the quality of the data that passes from one location to the other. Because of bandwidth limitations, some video teleconferencing is what is called half-speed video, 15 frames per second instead of full speed of 30 frames per second. If there is interference on the lines (i.e., the lines are "dirty"), the rate of transmission slows. Better compression algorithms mean better transmissions but may also involve higher equipment costs. Units that do only VTC, that is "dedicated" VTC, generally do a better job at compressing (and uncompressing) data than video cameras added to desktop computers, although the quality is rapidly improving. They may also cost 100 times as much as desktop units. It is critically important that the necessary quality of transmission drive the application purchasing choices. Cheaper may not be better if the quality is not sufficient for the task at hand (see Cukor, O'Laughlen, & Bauer, 1995, for a review). One important thing to consider is whether or not the system is proprietary or "open platform," meaning that it can "talk" to other brands, which is highly preferable.

Although there is some concern that diagnosis via VTC is inadequate (Montani et al., 1996) or economically unfeasible, most recent papers on diagnosis and assessment by VTC suggest that results compare favorably to face-to-face encounters, especially for schizophrenia (Ball et al., 1993, 1995; Salzman et al., 1996; Zarate et al., 1997). One paper also reports favorable results with Obsessive-Compulsive Disorder (Bauer et al., 1995). Kavanaugh and Wellowlees (1995) report positive reactions to the use of VTC in Australia; patients were more involved in decision making, and they perceived the VTC to be less threatening than face-to-face encounters. Similar positive results were observed in an inner-city pilot study (McLaren et al., 1996), rural children (Ermer, 1999), and a project on a remote island in the

Pacific (Delaplain et al., 1993). In one study on the use of VTC in an acute psychiatric service, most of the 105 clinical interactions were successful, with only a few refusals by patients (e.g., a paranoid schizophrenic who had delusions of being controlled by TVs, a bulimic woman who worried about how she looked on camera) (McLaren et al., 1995). Refusals by staff were generally based on concern that the patient might feel the VTC was dismissive when giving bad news (e.g., telling patients they had to leave the ward, or consulting with an HIV-positive patient). Patients and providers were satisfied with the technical quality of the transmissions. Some difficulties arose due to patients and providers accidentally moving out of camera range, and providers did express concern about their fatigue after 30 to 40 minutes in a session. In fact, human factors such as these are of major concern in using VTC comfortably (Cukor & Bauer, 1994).

Stand-Alone Computers

As previously mentioned, faxes and VTC can be done with desktop computers. It is unlikely, though, that anyone would own a computer solely for these purposes. In one survey, nearly three-fourths (72%) of California psychologists reported using a computer in their practice (Rosen & Weil, 1996). The most common application was word processing (69%), followed by record keeping (52%). About one-third (31%) of the psychologists used computers for scoring psychological tests, although most computer scoring was done by mailing tests to a centralized scoring facility. Few used computers to administer psychological tests (11%) or to provide direct client assistance (6%). Like individuals, hospitals are more likely to use computers for correspondence and financial record keeping (95%). Davis (1994) projected the changes in applications of technology in hospitals over the next decade. Little change was expected in financial applications, while increases of 15% to 20% were expected in patient care areas. This may be because the use of financial applications is already at ceiling (95%) and patient care applications baselines are considerably lower: 20% to 50% (Davis, 1994).

Informatics

One growing area of use of computers is in storing and accessing clinical and research information. The increase of information available on CD-ROM or DVD disks (compact disks for computers) offers previously unparalleled access to information. These disks are comparatively inexpensive and can store massive amounts of information in a small space, thereby reducing production and storage costs in comparison to reference books and paper files. Additionally, locating information on stored disks is generally faster. The increased ease of use of computer operating systems, coupled with increasing amounts of material available on disk, makes the stand-alone computer an underused resource for patient and provider education.

Assessment

There is a vast literature on using computers for psychological assessment. Readers are referred to Butcher (1994), Wetzler and Marlowe (1994), or Kobak and colleagues (1996) for more thorough reviews. With some limitations, most papers report good interrater reliability between computers and clinicians. Many of the major assessment instruments have been computerized, including the Composite International Diagnostic Interview (Wittchen, 1993), the Structured Clinical Interview for Diagnosis (SCID; Raffoul & Lyles, 1993; Williams et al., 1992), the Center for Epidemiological Studies Depression Scale (CES-D; Munoz, Gonzalez, & Starkweather, 1995), and the Diagnostic Interview Schedule (DIS; Bucholz et al., 1996). Assessment using speech recognition has also been tested with favorable results compared to human clinicians, even with multiple languages (Gonzales, Spiteri, & Knowlton, 1995; Munoz et al., 1995) and across languages in a geriatric population (Saz et al., 1996). In addition to the aforementioned CES-D, other tests for depression have been computerized (Kobak, Reynolds, & Greist, 1994; Mezaros et al., 1995). Some patients who completed a computerized form of the Hamilton Rating Scale for Depression reported differences between the human clinicians and the computers. They were less embarrassed to give data to the computers but felt that the clinicians were more likely to understand them (Kobak et al., 1994).

Psychotherapy

Interestingly, the literature on psychotherapy and computers is even larger than that of computer-aided assessment. Computers have been used for cognitive behavioral therapies (CBT). For example, CBT therapy administered by computer did equally as well as face-to-face group therapy among test-anxious college students when compared on GPA and reduction of anxiety symptoms (Buglione, DeVito, & Mulloy, 1990). One case history using computer-delivered CBT suggests staff interaction regarding the use of the computer program is critical for effective psychotherapy (Stuart & LaRue, 1996). Finkel (1990) posits that although computers are not likely to be good at interpreting messages for insight therapy, they do offer potential benefits for psychological symptom reduction, even among the elderly who are traditionally considered to be negatively oriented to computers. There are several review papers that cover psychotherapy and stand-alone computers (Bloom, 1992; Ford, 1993; Plutchik & Karasu, 1991; Wetzler & Marlowe, 1994).

One of the potential problems in using computers to sort, store, retrieve, and analyze information is that the speed and level of complexity at which they operate may outstrip our ability to articulate or understand our questions. This puts us at risk for obtaining information that we perceive as meaningful to turn out to be not meaningful at all (Sommer et al., 1994; Stamm, 1999). On the positive side, computers may enhance our ability to document, improve, and justify our work in the face of pressure from health care reform.

Networked Computers

Perhaps being "on-line" is the most talked-about use of technology of the past few years. On-line resources, for professionals and laity alike, have exploded with the development of easy user interfaces such as web browsers and commercial services. Once the purview of hard-core "computer geeks," networked computers are now frequented by perhaps 30 million or more people worldwide. Consider these facts: In 1993 there were only 130 web sites in the world, in June 1995 there were about 23,500, and in the next 12 months, more than 200,000 *new* web sites came on-line (O'Malley & Rosenzweig, 1997). By 1999, no one seemed to be able to count the number of web sites. As early as 1996, two different studies (Rosen & Weil, 1996; Rudolph, 1996) reported figures showing that about one-quarter of mental health care providers had at least sampled the Internet. Furthermore, Rudolph (1996) notes that about 50% of the respondents have e-mail and Internet access available, with about 25% using it regularly.

Types of Networks

Local Area Networks (LANs) and Wide Area Networks (WANs) connect computers with one another. There are myriad ways individual computers are connected to networks. The most common are digital links (usually an "ethernet" card) on smaller networks which act as gateways to larger networks or via a modem that connects the user by telephone lines. Modems are devices that translate between digital computers and analog telephone lines. Once connected, a host of activities are possible, including document sharing, image transfers, e-mail, listservs, database searches, synchronous communications (when parties are on-line at the same time, for example, chat sessions), Internet audio/video telephone, and store-and-forward applications.

A network may have tens of thousands of computers on it or as few as two computers (a host and a node). LANs are common in offices; they may serve only to share one printer between machines or may have elaborate networks for patient records, and so forth. Controlled access *intranets* are designed to be secure from access by nonapproved users. For example, the U.S. Department of Veterans Affairs (VA) maintains an intranet for patient records, which connects LANs to the VA WAN. This system connects VA facilities around the United States (Dayhoff & Maloney, 1992; Dayhoff, Kuzmak, & Kirin, 1994). A sister system operates in the Indian Health Service (Curtis, 1994). These are but two of many different systems designed to link patient records, ranging from large, well-funded projects (Gustafson et al., 1992; McDaniel, 1994; Forslund & Kilman, 1996) to small, BWCW (because we can't wait) systems which operate on nearly no funding at all (Terry, 1999).

The Internet

Certainly the most celebrated WAN is not a private, secured *intranet* network, but the anarchic, open, free-for-all, "Internet." The range of activities on-line is so great that no paper could do justice to the Internet. Sterling (1993) offers a history of the Internet, and O'Malley and Rosenzweig (1997) offer a history of the development of the World Wide Web (WWW), which is a graphical interface on the Internet. Perhaps the most thorough literature on mental health and the Internet are Haung and Alessi (1996) and Grohol (1999). Other papers discuss applications to clinical training and supervision (Lim, 1996; Stamm 1999).

Databases and Discussion Groups

Many resources exist on-line for professionals and laypersons alike. It is possible to categorize activities roughly into two groups: databases and human exchanges. Databases for professionals are of particular interest to readers of this contribution. One such database is the Telemedicine Information Exchange (TIE) (http://tie.telemed.org), which maintains a searchable database of professional telehealth and telemedicine papers, meetings, and programs. Increasingly, full texts of journals can be found on-line at databases such as Medline (www.nlm.nih.gov). The cornerstone of human exchange is discussion lists. InterPsych (IP) (http://www.InterPsych.org) is the oldest professional, on-line mental health organization. Established in February of 1994 by Ian Pitchford, IP maintains over 40 different discussion forums serving over 10,000 subscribers in more than 40 countries worldwide.

Unlike IP, which is focused primarily toward professionals, some resources cater to professionals and laypersons alike. For example, CyberTowers (CT) (www.cybertowers.com) is a large web site (over 2,000 pages) which combines fee-for-service with free service. Lay, self-help networks can be an important part of a treatment plan. In a survey of members of an Obsessive Compulsive Disorders (OCD) self-help group, 90% of the participants reported finding the list "somewhat helpful" to "definitely helpful" in living with OCD (Stein, 1997). Both on-line (Isenberg, n.d.) and print (Ferguson, 1996) overviews of the on-line self-help environment exist. Baldwin (1997) predicts continued good support for patients and providers alike. In addition to these resources, there are a number of culturally driven on-line organizations. The Waseskun Network (WN) (www.waseskun.net) is an example of a culturally driven project that serves laity and professionals. WN is a Canadian First Nation's site specializing in supporting mental health care for First Nation's people.

On-Line Psychological Assessment and Psychotherapy

Another form of on-line human exchange - more controversial than databases or support networks - is psychological assessment and psychotherapy. You can take personality tests on-line (for free or for fee) and receive computer-generated feedback that no human has ever touched during the testing cycle (see www.queendom.com). Some tests are similar to those obtained through self-help programs or vocational counseling services, and others are linked to profit ventures. For example, there is a test of "burnout" that offers a link to a job placement service if the score is above a cutoff point for job burnout.

Therapy via e-mail is one of the most controversial applications. Although it may be a good alternative if no better one exists (C. Johnson, 1996), there are risks and ethical concerns (Lloyd, 1996; Schlosser, 1996; D. E. Shapiro & Schulman, 1996, Stricker, 1996). Maheu, Callan, and Nagy (in press) review the Ethical Principles of Psychologists and conclude that it is not ethical for a psychologist to practice traditional psychotherapy on-line. When it can work, it is more likely to be used as an adjunctive intervention than a primary means of contact (Stamm, 1998).

Store-and-Forward

One of the best and least controversial uses of the Internet for the support of mental health services is "store-and-forward." Consultations and supervision, with appropriate attention to protection of patient information, can take place between private parties via e-mail. A host of different types of data (multimedia) can be sent including text, records, photographs, videotape, and test results. This removes the need for both parties to be present at the same time; the message is stored-and-forwarded to be opened at the convenience of the recipient. Data can be sent on secured intranets or, with accommodation for protection of privacy, over a nonsecured Internet. Beyond direct patient care, store-and-forward technology can be a good way of supporting an isolated or less skilled caregiver in the community without disrupting the community (see Stamm, 1999). It may also be used for licensure supervision at some time in the future.

Virtual Reality (VR)

No application of technology better exemplifies employing multiple media than Virtual Reality (VR). VR is actually a form of multimedia computer presentation, which may or may not be stand-alone. VR is very striking. To create the "virtual reality," computer-generated three-dimensional images are projected on a screen that is placed in proximity to the user. Images are projected biocularly and connected to units that track head movements to replicate ordinary vision. The head-tracking units, along with other electronic sensors and cameras, are attached to the user and feed information about the user's movement back to the computer, which then incorporates the user's movements into the projected image. Ordinary auditory devices create sound. Depending on the speed of the computer and the quality of the graphics simulation (which is directly related to costs), the image can be small and not very complex or quite compelling and disorienting. Many people experience similar feelings to motion sickness in VR, although this usually decreases with practice.

VR is not limited to stand-alone applications. Systems exist that project the virtual reality - sound and image - via phone lines. Although the possibilities seem limitless, there is likely a greater potential risk for harm with VR than with some other forms of computer-aided psychotherapy because VR can "trick" the central nervous system into interpreting as present things that are not (Zyss, 1994). Most VR applications are not all that glamorous or risky. For example, trainers can practice on "virtual patients" created by projections of computer replicated humans on screens (N. M. Thalmann & D. Thalmann, 1994; Wittson & Dutton, 1956). Or, this type of scenario could be adapted to provide ongoing feedback to a therapy trainee during a session with the supervisor watching through a one-way mirror or a video link. Another use of VR is the creation of *in vivo* scenes for treatment of various phobias. North and colleagues (M. M. North, S. M. North, & Coble, 1997) report treating fear of flying with VR. Rothbaum and colleagues report positive results in both case studies (Rothbaum et al., 1996) and in small sample psychotherapy studies with wait-list controls (Rothbaum et al., 1995). Camara (1994) provides more information about possible mental health care uses of VR.

SUMMARY AND CONCLUSIONS

In summary, telehealth can be potentially useful for initial evaluation, emergency care, preadmission and discharge planning, medication management, evaluation and diagnosis, management of chronically ill patients, consultations with and supervision of primary care providers, and educational and administrative activities. It can support people in pursuit of mental health self-care (Ferguson, 1997) and can provide rich opportunities for training and supervision (Bhatara, Fuller, & Fogas, 1995; Fairbanks & Viens, 1995; Heidenreiter, 1995; McLaren et al., 1995; Stamm, 1999). Telehealth can be adapted to support nearly any activity that can be done by traditional face-to-face methods.

There are legal and ethical issues to be resolved, and there is a disturbing lack of data on the effectiveness of various techniques. Even with these limitations, there is a world of opportunity for creative and satisfying extensions of our traditional practice. Given the potential benefits in removing barriers to treatment and training, telehealth is worthy of our consideration. We may find that it is not a "thing" at all but that it is just one of the collection of tools with which we seek to provide our patients and trainees the best possible care.

CONTRIBUTOR

B. Hudnall Stamm, PhD, is currently a Research Associate Professor and Assistant Director of the Institute of Rural Health Studies at Idaho State University. Having received undergraduate and masters degrees from Appalachian State University and his doctorate from University of Wyoming, the author has held appointments at the VA National Center for PTSD, Dartmouth Medical School, and University of Alaska. Working primarily with rural underserved peoples, Dr. Stamm focuses on traumatic stress where telehealth figures prominently. He is President Emeritus of InterPsych and a member of American Psychological Association committees. The editor of three other books, Dr. Stamm is currently working on *Behavioral Healthcare in Rural and Frontier Areas* with APA Books. Dr. Stamm can be contacted at www.isu.edu/~bhstamm

RESOURCES

Baldwin, D. (1997). Peering into the Internet's future (part II). *Traumatic Stress Points, 2*(11), 7-8.

Ball, C. J., McLaren, P. M., Summerfield, A. B., Lipsedge, M. S., & Watson, J. P. (1995). A comparison of communication modes in adult psychiatry. *Journal of Telemedicine and Telecare, 1*, 22-26.

Ball, C. J., Scott, N., McLaren, P. M., & Watson, J. P. (1993). Preliminary evaluation of a low-cost videoconferencing (LCVC) system for remote cognitive testing of adult psychiatric patients. *British Journal of Clinical Psychology, 32*, 303-307.

Bauer, L., Cuker, P., Jenike, M., Leahy, L., O'Laughlen, J., & Coyle, J. T. (1995). Pilot studies of telemedicine for patients with obsessive-compulsive disorder. *American Journal of Psychiatry, 152*(9), 1383-1385.

Benschoter, R. A., Wittson, C. L., & Ingham, C. G. (1965). Teaching and consultation by television. *Mental Hospital, 16*(3), 99-100.

Bhatara, V. S., Fuller, W. C., & Fogas, B. S. (1995). An educational perspective of reservation mental health service deficit: The South Dakota experience. *American Indian & Alaska Native Mental Health Research, 6*(3), 56-68.

Black, L. L., Greenidge, L. L., Ehmann, T., Ganesan, S., & Honer, W. G. (1996). A centralized system for monitoring clozapine use in British Columbia. *Psychiatric Services, 47*(1), 81-83.

Bloom, B. L. (1992). Computer-assisted psychological intervention: A review and commentary. *Clinical Psychology Review, 12*(2), 169-197.

Brown, F. W. (1995). A survey of telepsychiatry in the USA. *Journal of Telemedicine and Telecare, 1*(1), 19-21.

Bucholz, K. K., Marion, S. L., Shayka, J. J., Marcus, S.C., et al. (1996). A short computer interview for obtaining psychiatric diagnoses. *Psychiatric Services, 47*(3), 293-297.

Buglione, S. A., DeVito, A. J., & Mulloy, J. M. (1990). Traditional group therapy and computer-administered treatment for test anxiety. *Anxiety Research, 3*(1), 33-39.

Burgoyne, R. W., Acosta, F. X., & Yamamoto, J. (1983). Telephone prompting to increase attendance at a psychiatric outpatient clinic. *American Journal of Psychiatry, 140*(3), 345-347.

Butcher, J. N. (1994). Psychological assessment by computer: Potential gains and problems to avoid. *Psychiatric Annals, 24*(1), 20-24.

Camara, E. (1994). Virtual reality: Applications in medicine and psychiatry. *Hawaii Medical Journal, 52*(12), 332-333.

Carr, V. C. (1985). Telephone prompting to reduce missed CMHC appointments. *Hospital and Community Psychiatry, 36*(11), 1217-1218.

Cavanaugh, R. M. (1990). Utilizing the telephone appointment for adolescent follow-up. *Clinical Pediatrics, 29*(6), 302-304.

Cole, D. R., Johnson, M. S., Heaton, C. J., & Petti, M. (1994). Fax/Modem board communications decrease preceptor communication costs. *Family Medicine, 26*(7), 418-420.

Crump, W. J., & Pfeil, T. (1995). A telemedicine primer: An introduction to the technology and an overview of the literature. *Archives of Family Medicine, 4*(9), 796-803.

Cukor, P., & Bauer, L. (1994). Human factors issues in telemedicine: A practical guide with particular attention to psychiatry. *Telemedicine Today, 2*(2), 9-18.

Cukor, P., O'Laughlen, J., & Bauer, L. (1995). Gazing in the crystal ball: Trends in video conferencing R & D. *Telemedicine Today, 3*(3), 9-18.

Curtis, A. C. (1994). The patient care component: Patient-centered horizontal integration in a vertical world. *Proceedings of the Symposium on Computer Applications in Medical Care*, pp. 580-584.

Dankins, D. H. (1995). Plugging into success: Clinical applications from around the globe. *Telemedicine and Telehealth Networks, 12*, 19-21.

Davidoff, M., & Katz, R. (1985). Automated telephone therapy for improving auditory comprehension in aphasic adults. *Cognitive Rehabilitation, 3*(2), 26-28.

Davis, M. W. (1994). *Computerizing Healthcare Information: Developing Electronic Patient Systems.* Chicago: Probus Press.

Dayhoff, R. E., Kuzmak, P. M., & Kirin, G. (1994). Integrated clinical workstations for image and text data capture, display, and teleconsultation. *Proceedings of the Symposium on Computer Applications in Medical Care*, pp. 1060-1064.

Dayhoff, R. E., & Maloney, D. L. (1992). Exchange of veterans affairs medical data using national and local networks. *Annals of New York Academy of Science, 670,* 50-66.

Delaplain, C. B., Lindborg, C. E., Norton, S. A., & Hastings, J. E. (1993). Tripler pioneers telemedicine across the Pacific. *Hawaii Medical Journal, 52*(12), 338-339.

Department of Commerce. (1997). *Telemedicine Report to Congress* (DOC Publication). Washington, DC: Author [On-line]. Available: www.ntia.doc.gov

DeSalvio, F. J. (1988). Family telephone therapy in university counseling and psychological service centers: A family systems approach. *Journal of American College Health, 37*(2), 71-76.

di Blasio, P., Fischer, J., & Prata, G. (1986). The telephone chart: A cornerstone of the first interview with the family. *Journal of Strategic and Systemic Therapies, 5*(1-2), 31-43.

Dooley, R., Kunik, M. E., & Molinari, V. (1998). Reminder call on appointment compliance in geropsychiatric outpatients. *Clinical Gerontologist, 19*(2), 82-88.

Dorfman, R. A., Lubben, J. E., Mayer-Oakes, A., Atchison, K., et al. (1995). Screening for depression among a well elderly population. *Social Work, 40*(3), 295-304.

Ermer, D. J. (1999). Experience with a rural telepsychiatry clinic for children and adolescents. *Psychiatric Services, 50*(2), 260-261.

Evans, R. L., Fox, H. R., Pritzl, D. O., & Halar, E. M. (1984). Group treatment of physically disabled adults by telephone. *Social Work in Health Care, 9*(3), 77-84.

Evans, R. L., Kleinman, L., Halar, E. M., & Herzer, K. (1984). Predicting change in life satisfaction as a function of group counseling. *Psychological Reports, 55*(1), 199-204.

Evans, R. L., Werkhoven, W., & Fox, H. R. (1982). Treatment of social isolation and loneliness in a sample of visually impaired elderly persons. *Psychological Reports, 51*(1), 103-108.

Fairbanks, J., & Viens, D. (1995). Distance education for nurse practitioners: A partial solution. *Journal of American Academy of Nurse Practitioners, 7*(10), 499-503.

Ferguson, T. (1996). *Health Online.* New York: Addison-Wesley.

Ferguson, T. (1997, May). *A Guided Tour of Self-Help Cyberspace.* Presented at 1996 Partnerships for Networked Consumer Health Information Conference, Rancho Mirage, CA [On-line]. Available: http://odphp.osophs.dhhs.gov/confrnce/partnr96/ferg.htm

Field, M. J. (Ed.). (1996). *Telemedicine: A Guide to Assessing Telecommunications in Health Care.* Washington, DC: National Academy Press.

Finkel, S. I. (1990). Psychotherapy, technology and aging. *International Journal of Technology and Aging, 3*(1), 57-61.

Flynn, T. M., Taylor, P., & Pollard, C. A. (1992). Use of mobile telephones in the behavioral treatment of driving phobias. *Journal of Behavior Therapy and Experimental Psychiatry, 23*(4), 299-302.

Ford, B. D. (1993). Ethical and professional issues in computer-assisted therapy. *Computers in Human Behavior, 9*(4), 387-400.

Forkner, M. E., Reardon, T., & Carson, G. D. (1996). Experimenting with feasibility of telemedicine in Alaska: Successes and lessons learned. *Telemedicine Journal, 2*(3), 233-240.

Forslund, D., & Kilman, D. (1996). The virtual patient record: A key to distributed healthcare and telemedicine [On-line]. Available: http://www.acl.lanl.gov/TeleMed/Papers/virtual.html

Fox, G., & Blank, M. (1997, April). *Informal Systems and Social Support.* Paper presented at Research to Practice: A Conference on Rural Mental Health Research, Oxford, MS.

Gaus, C. R., & DeLeon, P. H. (1995). Thinking beyond the limitations of mental health care. *Professional Psychology: Research and Practice, 26*(4), 339-340.

Gonzales, G. M., Spiteri, C. B., & Knowlton, J. (1995). An exploratory study using computerized speech recognition for screen depressive symptoms. *Computers in Human Behavior, 11*(1), 85-93.

Grisgby, B. (1997). *ATSP Report on U.S. Telemedicine Activity.* Portland, OR: Association of Telemedicine Service Providers [On-line]. Available: http://www.atsp.org

Grohol, J. M. (1999). *The Insider's Guide to Mental Health Resources Online.* New York: Guilford.

Grumet, G. W. (1979). Telephone therapy: A review and case report. *American Journal of Orthopsychiatry, 49*(4), 574-584.

Gustafson, D. H., Bosworth, K., Hawkins, R. P., Boberg, E. W., & Bricker, E. (1992). CHESS: A computer-based system for providing information referrals, decision support and social support to people facing medical and other health-related crises. *Proceedings of the Symposium on Computer Applications in Medical Care,* pp. 161-165.

Haas, L. J., Benedict, J. G., & Kobos, J. C. (1996). Psychotherapy by telephone: Risks and benefits for psychologists and consumers. *Professional Psychology: Research and Practice, 27*(2), 154-160.

Haung, M. P., & Alessi, N. E. (1996). The Internet and the future of psychiatry. *American Journal of Psychiatry, 53*(7), 861-869.

Heidenreiter, T. J. (1995). Using videoteleconferencing for continuing education and staff development programs. *Journal of Continuing Education in Nursing, 26*(3), 135-138.

Hines, M. H. (1994). Using the telephone in family therapy. *Journal of Marital and Family Therapy, 20*(2), 175-184.

Holt, N., & Crawford, M. A. (1992). Medical Information Service via telephone: The pioneer of physician consultation services. *Annals of the New York Academy of Science, 670,* 155-162.

Huba, G. J., Brown, V. B., & Melchior, L. A. (1995). Fax-in forms as a technology for evaluating community projects: An example of HIV risk reduction. *Educational and Psychological Measurement, 55*(1), 75-83.

Hymer, S. M. (1984). The telephone session and the telephone between sessions. *Psychotherapy in Private Practice, 2*(3), 51-65.

Isenberg, D. H. (n.d.). Health care consumers: Cruising the information highway. *Self-Help and Psychology* [On-line]. Available: http://www.shpm.com/articles/health/hlthinfo.html

Jaureguy, B. M., & Evans, R. L. (1983). Short term group counseling of visually impaired people by telephone. *Journal of Visual Impairment and Blindness, 77*(4), 150-152.

Johnson, C. (1996). Psychiatrist says counseling via e-mail may be yet another medical use for Internet. *Canadian Medical Association Journal, 155*(11), 1606-1607.

Jones, S. L., Jones, P. K., & Katz, J. (1988). Health Belief Model intervention to increase compliance with emergency department patients. *Medical Care, 26*(12), 1172-1184.

Kavanaugh, S. J., & Wellowlees, P. M. (1995). Telemedicine - Clinical applications in mental health. *Australian Family Physician, 24*(7), 1242-1247.

Kobak, K. A., Greist, J. H., Jefferson, J. W., & Katzelnick, D. J. (1996). Computer-administered clinical rating scales: A review. *Psychopharmacology, 127*(4), 291-301.

Kobak, K. A., Reynolds, W. M., & Greist, J. H. (1994). Computerized and clinician assessment of depression and anxiety: Respondent evaluation and satisfaction. *Journal of Personality Assessment, 63*(1), 173-180.

Koffman, D. M., Lee, J. W., Hopp, J. W., & Emont, S. L. (1998). The impact of including incentives and competition in a workplace smoking cessation program on quit rates. *American Journal of Health Promotion, 13*(2), 105-111.

Kourany, R. F., Garber, J., & Tornusciolo, G. (1990). Improving first appointment attendance rates in child psychiatry outpatient clinics. *Journal of the American Academy of Child and Adolescent Psychiatry, 29*(4), 657-660.

Lamarche, D., Taddeo, R., & Pepler, C. (1998). The preparation of patients for cardiac surgery. *Clinical Nursing Research, 7*(4), 390-405.

Leirer, V. O., Morrow, D. G., Tanke, E. D., & Pariante, G. M. (1993). Elders' nonadherence: Its assessment and medication reminding by voice mail. *Gerontologist, 31*(4), 514-520.

Leirer, V. O., Tanke, E. D., & Morrow, D. G. (1993). Commercial cognitive/memory systems: A case study. *Applied Cognitive Psychology, 7*(7), 675-689.

Lim, R. F. (1996). The Internet: Approaches for mental health clinicians in clinical settings, training and research. *Psychiatric Services, 47*(6), 597-599.

Llewellyn, C. H. (1995). The role of telemedicine in disaster medicine. *Journal of Medical Systems, 19*(1), 29-34.

Lloyd, M. (1996). Have you had a long-distance therapeutic relationship? You will. *Ethics and Behavior, 6*(2), 169-172.

Maheu, M., Callan, J. E., & Nagy, T. F. (in press). Call to action: Ethical and legal issues for online psychological services. In S. F. Buckey (Ed.), *Comprehensive Textbook of Ethics and Law in the Practice of Psychology.* New York: Plenum.

McCarthy, P., Kulakowski, D., & Kenfield, J. A. (1994). Clinical supervision practices of licensed psychologists. *Professional Psychology: Research and Practice, 25*(2), 177-181.

McDaniel, J. G. (1994). Simulation studies of a wide area health care network. *Proceedings of the Symposium on Computer Applications in Medical Care,* pp. 438-444.

McGlynn, F. D. (1980). Successful treatment of anorexia nervosa with self-monitoring and long distance praise. *Journal of Behavior Therapy and Experimental Psychiatry, 11*(4), 283-286.

McLaren, P. M., Ball, C. J., Summerfield, A. B., Lipsedge, M., & Watson, J. P. (1992). Preliminary evaluation of a low cost videoconferencing system for teaching in clinical psychiatry. *Medical Teacher, 1*(14), 43-57.

McLaren, P. M., Ball, C. J., Summerfield, A. B., Watson, J. P., & Lipsedge, M. (1995). An evaluation of the use of interactive television in an acute psychiatric service. *Journal of Telemedicine and Telecare, 1,* 79-85.

McLaren, P. M., Blunden, J., Lipsedge, M. L., & Summerfield, A. B. (1996). Telepsychiatry in an inner-city community psychiatric service. *Journal of Telemedicine and Telecare, 2,* 57-59.

Mezaros, A., Englesmann, F., Meterissian, G., & Kusalic, M. (1995). Computerized assessment of depression and suicidal ideation. *Journal of Nervous and Mental Disease, 183*(7), 487-488.

Miller, B., & Farber, L. (1996). Delivery of mental health services in the changing health care system. *Professional Psychology: Research and Practice, 27*(5), 527-529.

Montani, C., Billaud, N., Couturier, P., Fluchaire, I., Lemarie, R., Malterre, C., Lauvernay, N., Piquard, J. F., Frossard, M., & Franco, A. (1996). "Telepsychometry": A remote psychometry consultation in clinical gerontology: Preliminary study. *Telemedicine Journal, 2*(2), 145-150.

Munoz, R. F., Gonzalez, G. M., & Starkweather, J. (1995). Automated screening for depression: Toward culturally and linguistically appropriate uses of computerized speech recognition. *Hispanic Journal of Behavioral Sciences, 17*(2), 194-208.

Nickelson, D. W. (1998). Telehealth and the evolving health care system: Strategic opportunities for professional psychology. *Professional Psychology: Research and Practice, 29*(6), 527-535.

North, M. M., North, S. M., & Coble, J. R. (1997). Virtual reality therapy for fear of flying. *American Journal of Psychiatry, 154*(1), 130.

Norton, S. A., Burdick, A. E., Phillips, C. M., & Berman, B. (1997). Teledermatology and underserved populations. *Archives of Dermatology, 133,* 197-200.

O'Malley, M., & Rosenzweig, R. (1997). Brave new world or blind alley? American history on the World Wide Web. *Journal of American History, 84*(1), 132-155.

Osgood-Hynes, D. J., Greist, J. H., Marks, I. M., Bauer, L., Heneman, S. W., Wenzel, K. W., Manzo, P. A., Parkin, J. R., Spierings, C. J., Dottl, S. L., & Vitse, H. M. (1998). Self-administered psychotherapy for depression using a telephone-accessed computer system plus booklets: An open U.S.-U.K. study. *Journal of Clinical Psychiatry, 59*(7), 358-365.

Plutchik, R., & Karasu, T. B. (1991). Computers in psychotherapy: An overview. *Computers in Human Behavior, 7*(1-2), 33-44.

Preston, J., Brown, F. W., & Hartley, M. (1992). Using telemedicine to improve health care in distant areas. *Hospital and Community Psychiatry, 43*(1), 25-32.

Raffoul, P. R., & Lyles, E. (1993). (Mini-SCID): Structured clinical interview for DSM-III-R. *Computers in Human Services, 10*(1), 65-69.

Ramelson, H. Z., Friedman, R. H., & Ockene, J. K. (1999). An automated telephone-based smoking cessation education and counseling system. *Patient Education & Counseling, 36*(2), 131-144.

Rosen, L. D., & Weil, M. M. (1996). Psychologists and technology: A look at the future. *Professional Psychology: Research and Practice, 27*(6), 635-638.

Rothbaum, B. O., Hodges, L., Hodges, L. F., Kooper, R., Opdyke, D., Williford, J. S., & North, M. (1995). Effectiveness of computer-generated virtual reality graded exposure in the treatment of acrophobia. *American Journal of Psychiatry, 152*(4), 626-628.

Rothbaum, B. O., Hodges, L., Watson, B. A., Kessler, C. D., & Opdyke, D. (1996). Virtual reality exposure therapy in the treatment of fear of flying: A case report. *Behavior Research and Therapy, 34*(5-6), 477-481.

Rudolph, J. M. (1996). *Compassion Fatigue, Mental Health Care Providers, and Mental Health Care Policy.* Unpublished master's thesis, University of Alaska, Anchorage.

Rustin, M. (1998). Observation, understanding and interpretation: The story of a supervision. *Journal of Child Psychotherapy, 24*(3), 433-448.

Salzman, C., Orvin, D., Hanson, A., & Kallinowski, A. (1996). Patient evaluation through live video transmission [Letter to the editor]. *American Journal of Psychiatry, 153*(7), 968.

Saz, P., Dia, J .L., de la Camara, C., Carreras, S., et al. (1996). Reliability and validity of the Spanish version of the GMS - AGECAT package for the assessment of dementia and cognitive disturbances. *International Journal of Geriatric Psychiatry, 11*(8), 721-728.

Schlosser, B. (1996). Transmitter v. hedonia. *Ethics and Behavior, 6*(2), 169, 172-174.

Schneider, S. J., Schwartz, M. D., & Fast, J. (1995). Computerized, telephone-based health promotion: I. Smoking cessation program. *Computers in Human Behavior, 11*(1), 135-148.

Schnelle, J. F., Gendrich, J., McNees, M. P., Hanna, J., & Thomas, M. M. (1979). Evaluation of outpatient client progress: Time-series telephone interview data. *Journal of Community Psychology, 7*(2), 111-117.

Shapiro, D. E., & Schulman, C. E. (1996). Ethic and legal issues in e-mail therapy. *Ethics and Behavior, 6*(2), 107-124.

Shapiro, R. M., Ossip-Klein, D. J., Gerrity, E. T., & Stiggins, J. (1986). Perceived helpfulness of messages on a community-based telephone support service for ex-smokers. *International Journal of the Addictions, 20*(11-12), 1837-1847.

Shivack, I. M., & Sullivan, C. W. (1989). Use of telephone prompts at an inner-city outpatient clinic. *Hospital and Community Psychiatry, 40*(8), 851-853.

Simon, G. E., Revicki, D., & VonKorff, M. (1993). Telephone assessment of depression severity. *Journal of Psychiatric Research, 27*(3), 247-252.

Skorupa, J., & Agresti, A. A. (1993). Ethical beliefs about burnout and continued professional practice. *Professional Psychology: Research and Practice, 24*(3), 281-285.

Sommer, J. F., Williams, M. B., Stamm, B. H., & Harris, C. J. (1994). The development of ethical principles for post-traumatic research, practice, training, and publication. In M. B. Williams & J. F. Sommers (Eds.), *Handbook of Post-traumatic Therapy* (pp. 520-539). Westport, CT: Greenwood Press.

Spevak, P. A., & Richards, C. S. (1980). Enhancing the durability of treatment effects: Maintenance strategies in the treatment of nail-biting. *Cognitive Therapy and Research, 4*(2), 251-258.

Springer, A. K. (1991). Telephone family therapy: An untapped resource. *Family Therapy, 18*(2), 123-128.

Stamm, B. H. (1998). Clinical applications of telehealth in mental health care. *Professional Psychology: Research and Practice, 29*(6), 536-542.

Stamm, B. H. (1999). Creating virtual community: Telehealth and self care updated. In B. H. Stamm (Ed.), *Secondary Traumatic Stress: Self-Care Issues for Clinicians, Researchers and Educators* (2nd ed., pp. 179-207). Lutherville, MD: Sidran Press.

Stein, D. J. (1997). Psychiatry on the Internet: Survey of an OCD mailing list. *Psychiatric Bulletin, 21,* 95-98.

Sterling, B. (1993, February). A brief history of the Internet. *The Magazine of Fantasy and Science Fiction.* Cornwall, CT: Fantasy and Science Fiction [On-line]. Available: http://www.eff.org/pub/Publications/Bruce_Sterling/FSF_columns/fsf.05Feb1993

Stricker, G. (1996). Psychotherapy in cyberspace. *Ethics and Behavior, 6*(2), 169, 175-177.

Stuart, S., & LaRue, S. (1996). Computerized cognitive therapy: The interface between man and machine. *Journal of Cognitive Psychotherapy, 10*(3), 181-191.

Swinson, R. P., Fergus, K. D., Cox, B. J., & Wickwire, K. (1995). Efficacy of telephone-administered behavioral therapy for panic disorder with agoraphobia. *Behavior Research and Therapy, 33*(4), 465-469.

Tampas, J. P., & Soule, A. B. (1968). Experiences with two-way television in a teaching hospital complex. *Journal of the American Medical Association, 204*(13), 83-85.

Taylor, I. (1984). Self-exposure instructions by telephone with a severe agoraphobic: A case study. *Behavioral Psychotherapy, 12*(1), 68-72.

Terry, M. J. (1999). Kelengakutelleghpat: An Arctic community-based approach to trauma. In B. H. Stamm (Ed.), *Secondary Traumatic Stress: Self-Care Issues for Clinicians, Researchers and Educators* (2nd ed., pp. 149-178). Lutherville, MD: Sidran Press.

Thalmann, N. M., & Thalmann, D. (1994). Towards virtual humans in medicine: A Prospective view. *Computerized Medical Imaging and Graphics, 18*(2), 97-106.

U.S. Department of Health and Human Services [HHS]. (1997). *Exploratory Evaluation of Rural Applications of Telemedicine* (HHS Publication). Washington, DC: Author [On-line]. Available: ftp://158.72.84.9/ftp/finalabt.pdf

Warzak, W. J., Parrish, J. M., & Handen, B. L. (1987). Effects of telephone intake procedures on initial appointment keeping in a child behavior management clinic. *Journal of Compliance in Health Care, 2*(2), 143-154.

Waseskun Network. (1997). *The Waseskun Network.* Waseskun, Canada: Author [On-line]. Available: www.waseskun.net

Watson, E., & Young, L. (1995). Re-engineering care delivery to improve the health outcome of asthmatics in Campbelltown, New South Wales. *Medinfo, 8*(1), 545.

Wetzler, S., & Marlowe, D. B. (1994). Clinical psychology by computer? The state of the "art." *European Journal of Psychological Assessment, 10*(1), 55-61.

Williams, J. B., Gibbon, M., First, M. B., Spitzer, R. L., Davies, M., Borus, J., Howes, M. J., Kane, J., Pope, H. G., Rounsaville, B., et al. (1992). The Structured Clinical Interview for DSM-III-R (SCID) II. Multisite test-retest reliability. *Archives of General Psychiatry 49*(8), 630-636.

Wittchen, H. (1993). Computer scoring of CIDI diagnoses. *International Journal of Methods in Psychiatric Research, 3*(2), 101-107.

Wittson, C. L., & Dutton, R. (1956). A new tool in psychiatric education. *Mental Hospital, 7,* 11-14.

Zarate, C. A., Weinstock, L., Cukor, P., Morabito, C., Leahy, L., Burns, C., & Bauer, L. (1997). Applicability of telemedicine for assessing patients with schizophrenia: Acceptance and reliability. *Journal of Clinical Psychiatry, 58*(1), 22-25.

Zyss, T. (1994). The techniques of virtual reality: A new tool in research of the production of symptoms in psychiatry. *Psychiatria Polska, 28*(3), 355-363.

Alternative Medicine's Contribution to Mental Health Treatment

Kathryn P. White

A 6-year-old boy with an Attention-Deficit/Hyperactivity Disorder is ricocheting off the walls of a medical clinic waiting room, while his mother cuddles her newborn daughter. But the mother refuses to put her son on Ritalin, because she considers the side effects to be as harmful as the disorder. Instead, she has chosen an alternative approach: acupuncture. According to the *Journal of the American Medical Association*, this mother is typical of 42% of Americans who seek alternatives to orthodox medicine and prescription drugs (Eisenberg et al., 1998). The journal reported that in 1997, Americans spent an estimated $21.2 billion on alternative treatments for depression, anxiety, back pain, headaches, and other conditions, with more than two-thirds of this amount coming directly out of pocket (i.e., not paid for by third-party payors). These statistics suggest that many psychotherapy patients, if they show similar utilization rates to the general public, may be receiving care from alternative practitioners for psychological and medical conditions.

It is not only the American public that is becoming enamored with Oriental medicine and other holistic medical approaches. Many venerable Western medical schools and hospitals are discovering the "new" treatments from the East that are thousands of years old. UCLA Medical Center boasts an East-West Medical Center. The University of Miami Medical School has opened its own acupuncture training program within the medical school. Hennepin County, MN, Faculty Associates has been offering since 1993 a 2-year training program for physicians in "integrative medicine," the term coined to denote practices integrating orthodox and alternative medicine. In 1997, the University of Arizona Medical School enrolled its first physicians in a 2-year fellowship in integrative medicine. The University of California, San Francisco, Medical School recently established four endowed chairs to direct the new UCSF Center for Integrative Medicine. A survey of U.S. medical schools showed that more than half (66) of the 124 medical schools accredited by the American Association of Medical Colleges (AAMC) are providing one or more courses in alternative and complementary medicine (Bhattacharya, 1998). New schools in integrative medicine also are springing up. In Washington, DC, the Capitol University of Integrative Medicine offers 2-year programs for physicians, chiropractors, osteopaths, and naturopaths leading to a Doctor of Integrative Medicine degree or a Doctor of Physiotherapy degree, and in Los Angeles, the new American University of Complementary Medicine offers certificate and advanced degree programs in several forms of complementary and alternative medicine for health professionals and others.

Acupuncture in particular has received two unprecedented endorsements by the medical establishment. On November 6, 1997, a National Institutes of Health (NIH) Consensus Development Conference, after reviewing research evidence demonstrating acupuncture's efficacy, ruled that this ancient procedure provides an effective treatment for certain disorders, and on March 29, 1996, the Federal Drug Administration (FDA) removed the "investigational status" designation of acupuncture needles and declared acupuncture an effective medical procedure. NIH established an Office of Alternative Medicine (OAM) to fund research on unconventional medical practices in 1993; this office was upgraded to center status in 1998 and is now called the National Center for Complementary and Alternative Medicine (NCCAM).

Patients and professionals are turning to unconventional medicine because of their frustration at contemporary Western medicine's typical piecemeal, symptomatic approach to treatment, giving one set of pills for one disorder and another set of pills for another disorder. Western practitioners separate psyche and soma, with psychologists typically neglecting the body and most medical doctors disregarding the mind. Many alternative medical practices, by contrast, seek to understand and treat a person's body-mind-spirit from an integrated perspective. They presume relationships between inflexibilities in one's personality - such as fixed ideas or stubbornness - and inflexibilities in one's body - such as chronic back pain or arthritis. Similarly, therapies affecting the body are recognized as having the capacity to influence the mind, and vice versa. The paradigms in alternative medicine focus upon the whole person, not the disease, and address energetic imbalances in a person's body-mind. These approaches present great opportunities for collaboration between therapists of the mind and therapists of the body (Seem, 1987) and offer exciting possibilities for paradoxically accelerating and deepening the level of change in patients.

Despite this major sociological trend of Americans exploring unconventional medicine, the field of psychology has paid little attention to these practices. A recent computer search of *PsychInfo* showed few articles on alternative medicine in mainstream psychology journals. This contribution is designed to introduce psychologists and other mental health professionals to the field of alternative medicine. After defining terms, I will present an overview of four forms of alternative medicine, with an emphasis upon how they are being used to treat psychological disorders. I also will describe roles mental health professionals can play in interaction with these emerging fields in the United States.

DEFINITION OF TERMS

Several terms have been used to refer to alternative medicine, including "alternative," "unconventional," "complementary," "holistic," "natural," "energy," and "integrative" medicine. The term "alternative medicine" emphasizes practices that can be used as alternatives to orthodox medicine, such as chiropractic, Yoga, herbology, and homeopathy. Weil (1993) offered the following definition: "Alternative medicine is a vast collection of theories and practices, some very ancient, some very recent, some sensible and worthy of study, others not so sensible" (p. 9). W. Jonas (1996), Director of NIH's former Office of Alternative Medicine, defined alternative medicine differently: "What constitutes alternative medicine right now is a definition by exclusion. If you can't get it in a hospital, if it's not reimbursed, if there isn't much research support for it, if your doctor doesn't know about it, or pooh-poohs it, then we'll call it alternative medicine" (p. 12). W. Jonas's definition excludes as alternative practices acupuncture, chiropractic, herbology, homeopathy, and naturopathy because practitioners of these disciplines are licensed in some states, serve as members of some hospital staffs, are increasingly being covered by third-party payers, and can point to a growing body of research demonstrating the efficacy of their practices in treating physical and psychological disorders. The term "unconventional medicine" is used as a synonym for "alternative medicine." Many physicians prefer the term "complementary medicine," which emphasizes the use of these practices as "complements" to conventional medicine. Eisenberg et al.'s (1993) study indicates that most Americans do use alternative practices in conjunction with conventional medicine. Their data showed that 83% of American patients using alternative medicine reported they had seen their physician for the same problem, although only 72% had told their physicians about their use of alternative care. Eisenberg et al. found that about 1 in 5 Americans utilized unconventional practices alone, while Austin (1998) found that only 4.4% of his respondents stated they relied primarily on alternative forms of health care.

Weil pointed out that the term "traditional" medicine more appropriately is applied to such alternative practices as acupuncture, herbalism, and Ayurvedic medicine, which have existed for several millennia, than it is to modern-day, conventional medical practices. He suggested use of the term "orthodox medicine" to refer to contemporary, conventional medicine. "Holistic medicine" connotes practices - be they alternative or orthodox - that consider the whole person - body, mind, and spirit - and that encourage patient responsibility for health. "Natural medicine" refers to the use of natural remedies to enhance the body's innate healing mechanisms. Weil (1993) wrote, "Healing is a natural process, common to all life. Wounds heal by themselves in people just as in animals and plants" (p. 8). "Energy" medicine is a phrase used to refer to those alternative practices that conceive healing to occur through changes in the life force, vital force, *Prana* (Ayurvedic term), or *Qi* (Chinese medical term). The concept of life force as the healer will be explored more fully later. "Integrative medicine," as explained previously, is the latest term, referring to efforts to integrate conventional and alternative medicine. Recently, I coined the term "integrative medical psychology" to describe coordinated treatments blending alternative medicine and Western mental health practices. In this contribution, I will discuss four medical systems that can be used as alternatives or complements or that can be integrated with conventional medicine and psychology.

CLASSICAL AND TRADITIONAL CHINESE MEDICINE

Classical and Traditional Chinese Medicine refer to a comprehensive system of medicine practiced over the last 3,000 years that is currently used by about one-quarter of the world's population (World Health Organization [WHO], 1991). Based upon a worldview that diverges significantly from Western orthodox medicine, Chinese medicine looks for energetic imbalances in an individual's entire body, mind, and spirit, and seeks to treat underlying causes of imbalance that create disease. Chinese medicine conceptualizes health and disease as resulting from either a balanced or an imbalanced flow of *Qi*, the life energy that is responsible for the creation and sustenance of life in humans, plants, and animals. According to Chinese medicine, *Qi* flows in a series of energy pathways, meridians, or channels that cover the entire interior and exterior of the human body. In all, there are six types of meridians, each with 6 to 16 individual channels, and each of the individual channels is composed of from 6 to 67 individual acupuncture points. Although the idea of energy pathways may be foreign to most Westerners, French researchers (De Vernejoul, 1985) who injected radioactive isotopes into acupuncture and nonacupuncture points in humans and followed the movements of the isotopes with a gamma imaging camera have presented evidence that supports the existence of meridians. The radioisotopes injected into acupuncture points traversed 30 centimeters along the meridians in 4 to 6 minutes, whereas the radioisotopes injected into non-acupuncture points did not behave similarly.

In Classical Chinese Medicine, the meridians represent not only energetic physiology, but also psychology. A whole theory of psychological development is written in the energy pathways to those who know how to decipher it. Psychologically, five of the six different types of meridians represent our ways of posturing ourselves in the world and relating to others in our external environment as seen through our musculature (Sinew channels); our conscious or subconscious attempts to hold or suppress conflicting emotions and thoughts as well as physical toxins (Luo-connecting channels); the psychological tasks of postnatal life including surviving, interacting with others, creating meaning in our lives, and differentiating ourselves (the Regular meridians); chronic rigidities in the way we think and approach the world, manifesting as personality disorders or chronic degenerative diseases such as cancer, arthritis, and lupus (the Divergent meridians); and the development of our sense of self, our constitution, and our genetics (the Extraordinary meridians) (Yuen, 1995). (The sixth type of meridian, the Lutaneous Zones, have little meaning for psychology and are almost never used for medical treatments either.)

Classical and Traditional Chinese Medicine contend that disease occurs with blockages or other disruptions in the flow of *Qi*, which in time create physical or psychological pathology. The flow of energy in the meridians also reflects the psychological issues and interests we have prioritized in our lives (Yuen, 1997). According to Classical Chinese Medicine, blockages develop when we become habituated and rigid in life, failing to make appropriate changes in response to shifting life circumstances. Healing involves reestablishing the natural flow of energy through the injured body parts or the whole body; the reattuned life energy, in turn, repairs the anatomical damage or injuries (Yogananda, 1986). Chinese medicine uses acupuncture, acupressure, massage, herbal medicine, nutritional programs, lifestyle counseling, a chiropracticlike technique known as *Tui Na*, meditation, and energetic practices such as *Tai Qi* and *Qi Gong* to right the flow of energy and thereby reestablish health. Acupuncture involves the practice of inserting hair-thin needles into various acupuncture points on the surface of the body, to stimulate the flow of *Qi* in one or more of the various meridians that flow on the surface, just under the surface, or deep into the interior of the body. Acupressure attempts to achieve a similar effect by using the practitioners' fingers on various acupuncture points rather than needles. Chinese herbs are seen as having energetic properties that determine the meridians they enter and influence; they are not simply used on the basis of their clinical functions. Foods also are conceptualized as having various energetic properties, thereby affecting the flow of *Qi*. Chinese medicine additionally recognizes the influence a person's thoughts and emotions can have on the flow of *Qi*. Suppressed anger, for example, is said to constrict *Qi* in the lower abdominal and genital regions, with the potential of causing hernias, fibroids, endometriosis, or intestinal or urinary dysfunctions, while anger that is expressed directs *Qi* upward, potentially causing hypertension and migraine headaches (Yuen, 1995). In Chinese medicine, *Qi* is seen as the dynamic, all-important, unseen intermediary between the mind and the body, with the three parameters not fully separate from one another. Chinese medicine also describes various types of *Qi*, including *Qi* that represents a person's relationship with the exterior world (*Wei Qi*), *Qi* that symbolizes a person's relationship with his or her internal world (*Ying Qi*), and *Qi* that reflects a person's deepest sense of self (*Yuan Qi*) (Yuen, 1995). Each organ of the body also is seen as having its own individual *Qi*, with the proper working of the organ depending upon the harmonious flow of the organ's *Qi*.

The concept of *Qi* gives Chinese medicine an edge over Western orthodox medicine in the area of disease prevention, proponents claim. Chinese medical diagnostic techniques are reported to enable practitioners to detect subtle energetic imbalances in the mind and body before these imbalances spawn physical pathology. Chinese medical treatments can then be used to correct these energetic imbalances before they crystallize into physical diseases. For example, based upon a comprehensive examination of a patient's pulse, one doctor of Chinese medicine told a man that his *Heart Qi* was weak and that he needed to take herbal medicine that would strengthen his *Heart Qi* to prevent problems. The man dismissed the advice, because he had just seen his cardiologist who had told the patient that his examination and EKG revealed no problems. In this particular case, the man suffered a heart attack within 2 weeks of seeing the Chinese medical doctor. Had he undergone Chinese medical procedures to strengthen his *Heart Qi*, the Chinese medical doctor believed, the patient may have averted the heart attack.

Acupuncture in America and Elsewhere

New York Times correspondent James Reston, who received acupuncture while recuperating from a surgery in China in the early 1970s, is largely responsible for introducing Americans to acupuncture in the 20th century. But records in Washington and Idaho indicate that acupuncture was practiced in America by traveling Chinese physicians in the 1800s. Because of Reston's and other journalists' focus on acupuncture, it is this modality rather than the complete system from which it originates and the system's many other modalities that caught the interest and fascination of Americans. In the United States, 39 states plus the District of Columbia license or regulate the practice of acupuncture and/or Oriental medicine. To become eligible for licensure in most states, practitioners must complete a 3-year acupuncture or 4-year Oriental medical degree program, leading to the award of master's degree, with some programs requiring approximately the same number of units as do PhD or PsyD programs in psychology. (In contrast to professional acupuncturists, most MDs who practice acupuncture have completed 200-300 hours of training, much of which has been done through home study.) The field of acupuncture and Oriental medicine features two prominent national professional organizations, an accreditation commission recognized by the U.S. Department of Education, a council of accredited colleges, and a national commission that develops licensing examinations in acupuncture and Chinese herbology. In some states (e.g., California, Florida, and New Mexico), licensed acupuncturists are considered primary health care providers.

Acupuncture and Oriental medicine feature a wide variety of traditions, with many diverse techniques and theoretical approaches. Most professional acupuncturists in America practice a style of acupuncture known as Traditional Chinese Medicine (TCM), which is composed of the various theories and techniques taught in postrevolution Communist China. Although spiritual and psychological dimensions of the medicine were deemphasized in the Cultural Revolution due to political factors, TCM still effectively treats many psychological and physical conditions. Classical Chinese Medicine (CCM) is the name given to pre-Cultural Revolution Chinese medicine, which is primarily being taught via oral traditions in China and America by practitioners trained in apprenticeships. Its proponents contend that CCM provides more in-depth understandings of physical and psychological development and more comprehensive and integrated mind-body treatments than does TCM. More than 1,000 years ago, Chinese medicine also was transmitted to countries that are now known as Vietnam, Japan, and Korea; each of these cultures has introduced inter- and intracultural diversity. In the 20th century, practitioners in France, England, and America also have developed new schools of acupuncture, such as the Five Elements tradition and auriculotherapy (i.e., ear acupuncture). Some (e.g., Seem, 1987) have talked about creating a distinctly American school of acupuncture as well. Thus, the field of traditional East Asian medicine, in which acupuncture is rooted, is composed of diverse traditions and practices, each with its distinctive approaches to the treatment of psychological problems.

Chinese Medicine and the Treatment of Psychological Disorders

Chinese medicine is being used in America to treat the full gamut of psychological disorders, including adjustment, stress, affective, anxiety, addiction, pain, psychosomatic, psychotic, and even personality disorders. East Asian medical diagnosis of psychological disorders diverges significantly from *Diagnostic and Statistical Manual of Mental Disorders* (*DSM-IV*; American Psychiatric Association, 1994) diagnoses, which means that patients need a separate full evaluation and assessment by a Chinese medical practitioner in addition to any Western medical diagnosis. For example, a patient with a *DSM-IV* diagnosis of Generalized Anxiety Disorder may present as any one of 12 different diagnostic syndromes in TCM, each with its own signs and symptoms. Other Oriental diagnoses would be given by those practicing Korean Constitutional medicine, Japanese Meridian Therapy, CCM, Five Elements acupuncture, auriculotherapy, and so forth. East Asian medical diagnosis considers not only psychological symptomatology, but also details of sleep patterns, appetite, sense of vitality, color of the tongue body and coating, various qualities of the radial pulse, responses to palpation of acupuncture points and meridians, and seemingly unrelated details about a person's menstrual cycles, urination, defecation, food preferences, and a host of other phenomena.

Although Western research in acupuncture and East Asian medicine has been riddled with problems due to differences in paradigmatic assumptions, diagnostic entities, and the general individualized approach to treatment of Chinese medicine, a variety of studies have supported acupuncture's usefulness in treating depression (Hitt, Allen, & Schnyer, 1995; Luo, Jia, & Zhan, 1985; Yang et al., 1994); anxiety (Guizhen et al., 1998; Lanza, 1986); pain (e.g., Birch & Hammerschlag, 1996); drug and alcohol abuse and dependence (e.g., Brewington, Smith, & Lipton, 1994); and sequelae of stroke (Hu et al., 1993; K. Johansson et al., 1993; Naeser et al., 1992; Sallstrom et al., 1996; Zhang et al., 1987). Research has demonstrated acupuncture's influence on various neurotransmitters, such as ACTH (adrenocortico-tropic hormone) and cortisol levels (Wen et al., 1978a, 1978b), serotonin and norepinephrine (Han & Terenius, 1982; Sytinsky & Galebskaya, 1979), and 5-HT (Lewith & Kenyon, 1984). Controlled clinical trials with Chinese herbs in areas relevant to psychology have not been published in U.S. journals to date.

AYURVEDIC MEDICINE

Ayurvedic medicine is the comprehensive medical system indigenous to India which originated at least 5,000 years ago and which is being promoted in the United States by Western orthodox physician Deepak Chopra, Indian-trained Ayurvedic physicians Vasant Lad and Robert Svoboda, and acupuncturist and Doctor of Oriental medicine David Frawley. Ayurveda is not simply a medical system, but a "complete philosophy of life" (Joshi, 1997, p. 15). With "Ayur" meaning "life" and "veda" meaning "science," Ayurveda literally is translated as the "science of life." Ayurvedic medicine, built on the foundation of Hinduism and Yoga, construes health as involving a balanced, coordinated relationship among the soul (*atma*), mind (*manas*), senses (*indriyas)*, life force (*Prana*), and body (*sharira*), while disease is said to develop when these aspects of life become disconnected and inharmonious (Joshi, 1997). Records indicate that Ayurvedic physicians were skilled surgeons and practiced plastic surgery on the face and other parts of the body and fitted amputees with artificial limbs as early as 2000 B.C. (Feuerstein, Kak, & Frawley, 1995), but Ayurveda as it is practiced in America and India today generally uses natural remedies. Traditionally, psychiatry and psychology comprised one of the eight branches of Ayurvedic medicine (Ranade, 1993).

In contrast to the numerous 5- to 8-year medical school programs in Ayurvedic medicine in India, only one university offers master's and doctoral degree programs in Ayurveda in America. Most of the training in Ayurveda consists of correspondence or in-residence certificate programs. Ayurvedic practitioners are licensed in the state of Massachusetts. Many persons purporting to practice Ayurveda are physicians or nonphysicians who have had little formal training in Ayurvedic medicine.

The Gunas and the Doshas

According to Ayurveda, the mind is composed of three fundamental qualities, or *gunas*: *sattva, rajas,* and *tamas*. *Sattva*, which manifests as a clear intelligence and an enlightened state of mind, predominates over the others in psychological health. *Rajas* indicates the activating or energetic principle that underlies either *sattva* or *tamas*, and *tamas* refers to destructive and lethargic states of mind (Yogananda, 1983). These three qualities of the mind are related to the three metabolic body-mind types in Ayurveda - *Vata*, *Pitta*, and *Kapha* - which determine a person's constitutional type. The *doshas* that define the general health picture of an individual are of central importance in treating a person with psychological or physical disorders. Determining a person's constitution requires careful discrimination and really should be done by an experienced Ayurvedic diagnostician. The true *doshic* nature sometimes is hidden by imbalances resulting from years of unhealthy behavioral and eating patterns. Once determined, the constitution is a major factor in almost all clinical decisions. Most people are a mixture of *doshic* characteristics, with one usually predominating over another. A rare few are *tridoshic*, manifesting equal proportions of all three *doshas*. A person's *doshic* body type usually matches his or her mind type, but occasionally a person's body and mind types diverge, often in a way that suggests they counterbalance each other (Frawley, 1996). For example, a flighty *Vata* mentality may be balanced with a solid and stable *Kapha* body in one individual. Each of the types thrives with specific treatments, diets, psychotherapeutic strategies, exercise plans, and lifestyles.

Vata types tend to be slender persons with small eyes, dry, cool, and rough skin and hair, and variable appetites, sleep patterns, and energy levels. Psychologically, they tend to be moody, enthusiastic, and impulsive and are the Ayurvedic type most prone to psychological problems (Ranade, 1993). *Vata* psychological disorders include extreme reactivity, anxiety, fear, insomnia, agitation, and in the extreme, bipolar or schizophrenic disorders with delusions and hallucinations. In psychotherapy, they tend to be overly enthusiastic in the beginning but become quickly frustrated and want to quit. They seek quick fixes and magical healing. Ayurveda recommends that therapists approach them "like a flower" (Frawley, 1996, p. 159), cordially and calmly. Therapists should help them develop daily regimens to stabilize, calm, and protect them, as they are exquisitely sensitive to upsets. Besides psychotherapy,

Ayurvedic practitioners may recommend a *Vata*-calming diet, sedative herbs, therapeutic enemas, nasal cleaning, quiet walks in peaceful, natural surroundings, gentle exercise, the development of emotional support from family and friends, mental concentration and memory-strengthening exercises, and the use of *mantras*, which are Sanskrit seed words said to be imbued with healing powers (Frawley, 1996).

Pitta types tend to have moderate body frames and weight, soft, oily, and red skin and hair, and piercing eyes, with good to excessive appetites. Psychologically, they are intelligent, articulate, passionate, and critical, with fiery tempers (Ranade, 1993). When psychologically unhealthy, *Pittas* tend to be self-centered and antisocial, projecting blame onto other people and engaging in aggressive and possibly violent behavior. If they become psychotic, they tend to have paranoid delusions or delusions of grandeur. In psychotherapy, *Pittas* often can be recognized by their tendency to become angry if therapy doesn't proceed the way they want, dictate to their therapists, and question the latter's qualifications. Ayurveda recommends that psychotherapists approach *Pitta* types tactfully and diplomatically, appealing to their intelligence and logic, and helping them come to their own truths and insights. Once they see the need to change, they are the best of the three types in implementing changes. Other Ayurvedic medical techniques for treating *Pitta* imbalances include a *Pitta*-calming diet, antipyretic herbs, therapeutic purgation, blood-cleansing, moderate exercise, and instructions to walk at night and gaze at the sky, cultivate kindness and courtesy with others, learn to listen to other persons' points of view, and practice anti-*Pitta* mantras (Frawley, 1996).

Kapha persons usually have large, thick builds, a tendency to be overweight, thick, oily skin and hair, and large, round eyes with thick eyelashes. Their metabolism and energy level tend to be lethargic and slow (Ranade, 1993). *Kaphas* usually are the least likely of the three metabolic types to have psychological problems. When imbalanced, *Kaphas* tend to be passive, dependent, low in motivation, depressed, sorrowful, and clinging. *Kapha* persons typically must be confronted and sometimes even shaken up to change. They remodel themselves slowly even when they know it is necessary, as they typically are stuck in the inertia of deeply ingrained patterns. Ayurveda recommends that psychotherapists confront *Kapha* types, not comfort them. Once they begin the path to change, they usually continue on their own. Other Ayurvedic techniques for treating *Kapha* imbalances include an anti-*Kapha* diet, expectorant and decongestive herbs, therapeutic emesis (which is used to treat depression, grief, and attachment), nasal cleansing, vigorous hiking or walking, strong aerobic exercises, and instructions to cultivate detachment and release greed and attachment and to practice anti-*Kapha mantras* (Frawley, 1996).

The *doshas* also exist in different proportions within every cell of the body. *Vata* energizes the body, overseeing respiration and circulation; *Pitta* metabolizes food, water, and air and controls enzymatic activity; and *Kapha* provides the structure of bones, muscles, and fat and protects and nourishes the body. When the *doshas* are well-calibrated for one's constitution, a person enjoys radiant health. When this balance falters owing to psychological and physical stress, a person becomes prone to disease, unless he or she takes preventive dietary, lifestyle, or other measures that reestablish harmony among the *doshas* (Svoboda, 1992). Ayurveda also emphasizes the role of *ama* or toxicity in psychological and physical disease formation. *Ama* builds up in the gastrointestinal tract when undigested food remains in the body and eventually is carried into various body tissues. *Ama* is distinct from the normal waste products that are excreted as urine, feces, and sweat (Svoboda, 1992).

Ayurvedic Treatments and Research

Some of the natural healing strategies of Ayurveda are diet, exercise regimens, meditation and spiritual practices, counseling, herbal treatments, massages, limited sunbaths, breathing exercises, five special cleansing and detoxification procedures called *Panchakarma,* and rejuvenation techniques, called *Rasayana,* used after cleansing regimens. *Panchakarma* consists of five purification methods used to reverse disease mechanisms by transporting toxic waste products from the tissues back to the digestive tract and expelling them from the body. What is distinct about *Panchakarma* is its recognition of a person's *doshic* make-up in the healing process.

Panchakarma techniques include (a) the inhalation of medicated substances (*Nasya*), which eliminates toxic congestion in the perinasal sinuses seen in *Kapha* conditions; (b) therapeutic vomiting (*Vamana*), which removes toxic congestion in the stomach, also seen in *Kapha* disorders; (c) the use of strong natural, herbal purgatives (*Virechana*) to induce bowel movements to cleanse the intestines and remove excess *Pitta*; (d) colonics (*Basti*) with medicated liquids to remove excess *Vata*; and (e) therapeutic blood-letting (*Raktamokshana*) to remove excess *Pitta*. Each of these procedures requires proper preparation and proper aftercare, and they typically are performed in certain seasons and times of day (Joshi, 1997).

Ayurvedic research is in its infancy in America, especially in areas relevant to psychology. NIH's former Office of Alternative Medicine (OAM), however, funded four studies. Simon (1993) at Sharp Healthcare in San Diego, CA, compared the benefits of subjects practicing an Ayurvedic (consisting of a *dosha*-specific diet, Hatha Yoga exercises, and meditation) versus a Western (composed of a low-fat, low-salt diet, an aerobic exercise routine, and a relaxation technique) healthy lifestyle program for 1 year. For the 88 subjects who completed the program, the subjects in the Ayurvedic group demonstrated significantly greater improvement than the Western healthy lifestyle group in their overall health status as measured by indices such as blood pressure, weight, serum cholesterol, high-density lipoprotein (HDL), low-density lipoprotein (LDL), and number of visits to health care providers, although both treatment groups did better than control subjects. Shannahoff-Khalsa (1997) compared the benefits of a meditation technique known as Kundalini Yoga to a combined regimen of relaxation therapy and mindfulness meditation in the treatment of 25 patients with obsessive-compulsive disorders. After a 3-month treatment, the subjects randomly assigned to the Kundalini Yoga therapy group showed significant improvement in obsessive-compulsive symptomatology, whereas the subjects randomly assigned to the combined relaxation and mindfulness meditation therapy group did not. Another study found that weekly practice of Hatha Yoga was as effective as group therapy in enhancing outcomes in methadone maintenance programs (Shaffer, LaSalvia, & Stein, 1997), while a fourth study demonstrated the superiority of an Ayurvedic herb over L-DOPA in the treatment of Parkinsonian disease in rats (Manyam, 1994).

NATUROPATHY

Naturopathy is a system of medicine formalized in the past two centuries that treats diseases by stimulating a person's innate healing capacities and using natural remedies and techniques. Some of Nature's resources employed include fresh air, pure water, bright sunlight, natural diet, proper and timely sleep, water therapies, homeopathic remedies, and natural herbs. Rather than focusing upon a single modality, naturopathy comprises a variety of techniques. Although the term naturopathy was not used until the 19th century, its practice and philosophy are rooted in ancient Ayurvedic, Chinese, Native American, and Greek medical traditions.

Health, according to naturopathy, involves a harmonious balance among physical, mental, social, and spiritual aspects of a person's life. As one early 20th-century naturopath wrote, "A healthy person feels well, delights in work, easily bears troubles, is able to sleep soundly, possesses natural appetites, and has a positive outlook on life" (Kulkarni, 1930/1997, p. 5). Psychological and physical diseases occur primarily through a process of autointoxication caused by eating unnatural, toxic foods, breathing polluted air, breathing rapidly and shallowly, spending no time in sunlight, exercising irregularly or not at all, overworking, feeling troubled and burdened, and living in inharmonious environments. In health, a person rids himself or herself of waste materials through natural means, such as through the urine, feces, sweat, and acute illnesses. Naturopaths view acute disorders as a person's body and mind's way of attempting to cleanse itself and release toxins and rarely would interfere with these natural mechanisms by using antiinflammatory herbs or other procedures that suppress the natural healing response. Naturopaths consider disease itself "a curative process" which a person employs when other natural methods of elimination have failed (Boyle & Saine, 1988).

Naturopaths seek to treat the underlying cause of conditions, which can stimulate a temporary exacerbation of symptoms called a "healing crisis," which is thought to help move the patient toward health. Other tenets of naturopathy include treating the whole person, using illness as an opportunity to educate and empower patients, and focusing upon prevention.

Naturopaths are licensed or regulated in 13 states and the District of Columbia. In some states (e.g., Washington and Oregon), they have parity as primary care physicians with orthodox medical doctors. Naturopaths typically attend a 4-year medical school program, which requires premedical course work for entry. The first 2 years focus upon training in anatomy, physiology, pathology, and other clinical sciences, while the last 2 years comprise clinical training in natural healing methods. The education culminates in the award of a Doctor of Naturopathy (ND) or Doctor of Naturopathic Medicine (NMD).

Naturopathic Treatments

Naturopathic treatment techniques include the use of sunlight and water therapies. Sunbaths in moderation are recognized as curative for destroying microbes and revitalizing the body and mind. Hydrotherapy or water therapies involve the "application of water in any form, either externally or internally, in the treatment of disease and the maintenance of health" (Boyle & Saine, 1998, p. 19). Typically, hydrotherapeutic treatments make use of water, ice, or steam to heal disorders or restore health and include such practices as steam baths, saunas, sitz baths, full body immersion, colonic irrigation, and the application of hot and/or cold compresses. Hydrotherapy is designed to regulate the quantity and quality of blood flowing through specific areas of the body, increasing circulation in some cases and decreasing it in others. Naturopaths contend that by improving blood flow through the organs of elimination - which include the skin, liver, kidneys, and intestines - hydrotherapy helps the person to rid himself or herself of waste products and toxins. Actually, hydrotherapy is a misnomer, because these water treatments really involve the treatment of disease through applications of hot or cold. "In hydrotherapeutics, water is the medium and heat (or cold) is the message. . . . Neither water nor heat nor cold heals; only the body heals; but hot and cold via water can enhance the capacity of the body to heal" (Boyle & Saine, 1988, p. 24). For certain depressions construed to be caused by congestion in the head region, naturopaths may use hydrotherapeutic applications of hot water to the face over the maxillary artery to draw blood away from the middle meningeal artery, which branches deep into the brain.

Naturopaths contend that good air and proper breathing also are important in living and healing. Accordingly, they suggest we spend part of each day in fresh air. Deep and natural breathing is said to purify blood, strengthen the heart, facilitate circulation, vitalize the whole body, bolster immunity, and improve one's mental powers and clearsightedness (Kulkarni, 1930/1997). Naturopaths in this country also perform or recommend psychotherapy for patients, contending that a healthy mind is necessary to have a healthy body.

A major focus in naturopathic medicine is proper eating habits and balanced diets, elements that naturopaths contend most medical doctors and mental health practitioners overlook. Studies have shown that deficiencies of vitamin B_1 or thiamin can cause depression, anxiety, confusion, and neurological deficits, all part of the syndrome of beriberi. In advanced stages, a niacin deficiency can give rise to delusions and other psychotic symptoms. As Hoffer (1973) pointed out, "If all the vitamin B_3 were removed from our food, everyone would become psychotic within 1 year" (p. 203). Nobel prize-winning chemist Linus Pauling, who introduced the term "orthomolecular psychiatry," spent years reviewing studies demonstrating that vitamin deficiencies can result in depression, schizophrenia, and mental retardation (Miller, 1996).

Other naturopathic techniques include the use of Yogic postures, massage and physical manipulations, homeopathy, and nontoxic Western herbal therapies. Naturopaths employ a wide variety of individual herbs for treatment of disease, including psychological disorders. One of the best-known Western herbs to treat depression, for example, is the highly publicized herb Hypericum perforatum, or St. John's Wort. More than 26 double-blind, controlled studies have demonstrated that this herb is as effective as standard antidepressants in alleviating symptoms of depression but with fewer side effects (Murray, 1995). In 1997, NIH's former OAM released a request for proposals for a million-dollar, multisite, coordinated clinical trial of St. John's Wort. Duke University Medical School is now coordinating this study. Another herb shown to have antidepressive as well as antianxiety effects is Kava Kava (Murray, 1995).

HOMEOPATHY

Homeopathy is a complete system of medicine developed in 18th-century Germany by physician Samuel Hahnemann in which massively diluted solutions of herbs and other substances are given to patients to stimulate their "vital force" to effect healing. Homeopathy's name is derived from the Greek words *homoisos*, meaning "similar," and *pathos*, meaning "suffering," referring to a basic tenet in homeopathy that substances that cause certain symptoms in healthy individuals will cure those same symptoms in ill persons (Ullman, 1991). For example, the remedy *Arsenicum Album*, which is made from arsenic, typically ameliorates ill patients who manifest the symptoms that healthy persons do when they take an extremely low dose of arsenic. A high dose of arsenic, of course, will kill a person. But homeopathic microdoses of *Arsenicum Album* often are used to treat highly insecure patients who suffer from an overwhelming sense of anxiety and fear for their well-being and material security. The homeopathic principle that "like cures like" occasionally is employed in orthodox medicine when a stimulant like *Ritalin* is used to treat hyperactivity or small doses of bacteria in vaccinations are used to induce immunity.

Homeopathy has been identified by WHO as a traditional medicine that should be promulgated around the world. Estimates of its usage range up to 500 million persons worldwide (Bannerman, Burton, & Chieh, 1983). In the United States, however, homeopathy has suffered a checkered history. In the early 1900s, 1 in 3 American physicians was a homeopath. The American Medical Association (AMA) gained ascendancy in the early part of this century by organizing to bar homeopaths from medical practice, effectively running homeopaths out of the country until the 1970s, when Americans began looking at this natural form of medicine once again (Cook, 1989). Homeopathic remedies are recognized by the FDA as drugs and they are listed in the official compendium *Homeopathic Pharmacopoeia of the United States*. At present, three states license homeopaths, although several other states give physicians, acupuncturists, chiropractors, or naturopaths the right to practice homeopathy under their respective licenses. One university in the United States grants a Master of Arts degree in homeopathy, but certificate programs abound in growing numbers. In other countries, such as the United Kingdom or India, homeopaths complete a 5-year medical school program and enjoy the rights and privileges of physician status.

Hahnemann defined health as a state in which "the spirit-like vital force (or *dynamis*), animating the material human organism, reigns in supreme sovereignty. It maintains the sensations and activities of all parts of the living organism in a harmony that obliges wonderment. The reasoning spirit who inhabits the organism can thus freely use this healthy living instrument to reach the lofty goals of human existence" (1982, p. 15). In ill health, the vital force becomes "untuned," which sparks the symptoms known as disease. Because Hahnemann viewed disease as an energetic disorder of the life force, he believed that energy locked into the form of "potentized" homeopathic remedies could best right the disturbed vital force. For this reason, he developed energetic medicines, made from material substances that have been diluted to the point at which no trace of the original molecules are left, in most cases. With each step in the dilution process, the homeopathic solution is vigorously shaken 100 times against a hard-back book, a process Hahnemann termed "succussion." The step-by-step process of diluting and succussing a remedy is called "potentization," which is thought to make a remedy strong and effective. In fact, generally the more a remedy is potentized, the more powerful and longlasting is its effect (Ullman, 1991). Cook (1989) contended that one must look to quantum physics to understand the mechanisms of action of homeopathic remedies. One study employing nuclear magnetic resonance (NMR) imaging found that 23 different remedies each showed singular readings, whereas placebo substances did not (Smith &

Boericke, 1968). In America, a review of 135 articles in the toxicology literature showed that very small, but potentized dilutions appeared to be able to protect organisms from damage by environmental toxins (L. K. Jonas et al., 1994).

Homeopathy and the Mind

Homeopaths select remedies through an individualized and comprehensive process that integrates information about a person's mental state, physical condition, sleep habits, dreams, eating habits, likes and dislikes, medical and psychological history, and other seemingly irrelevant details. Hahnemann himself was quite psychologically minded, having worked as the medical director of an insane asylum. He considered the mental state of the patient to be the most essential determinant in choosing a correct homeopathic medicine for disorders with physical or psychological presentations. Some modern-day homepaths such as Rajan Sankaran contend that all diseases, even those with purely physical symptomatology, involve cognitive distortions or delusions, which result in a person adopting "false postures" (Sankaran, 1994, p. 28) that are inappropriate to situations. These homeopaths suggest that people look for circumstances that confirm their false perceptions; when they cannot find outside of themselves situations that support their misperceptions, they develop physical pathology. Physical pathology thus is seen as "an indirect way of actualizing" (Sankaran, 1994, p. 28) a person's cognitive distortions or delusions. In this form of classical homeopathy, each homeopathic remedy is conceptualized as treating a particular psychological posture as well as various physical tendencies and symptoms. Sankaran also has developed a psychotherapeutic-like technique called "homeopsychotherapy," in which practitioners make patients aware of their cognitive distortions or delusions. Having observed sessions of "homeopsychotherapy" by Sankaran in his Bombay office, I can attest that his interventions are quite similar to those of many American clinical psychologists. Sankaran (1991) wrote, "Once a patient appreciates his own delusion, this begins to work on him like a homeopathic remedy" (p. 249).

Because of the highly individualized approach to the selection of remedies and medical politics, research in homeopathy has been slow to develop in the United States, and no double-blind studies have been published in the area of psychological disorders. Controlled clinical trials have demonstrated homeopathy's effectiveness in treating childhood diarrhea (Jacobs, Jimenez, & Gloy, 1994), rheumatoid arthritis (R. G. Gibson et al., 1980), and fibromyalgia (Fisher et al., 1989). One multicase study of 10 women and 2 men who received homeopathic treatment for depression or social phobia showed that on the basis of the Clinical Global Improvement (CGI) Scale, 58% of the 12 patients responded positively to homeopathic treatment. Interestingly, half of these patients had not received benefit from standard psychiatric medication (J. R. T. Davidson et al., 1997).

ROLES FOR MENTAL HEALTH PRACTITIONERS

Alternative medicine is a new frontier worthy of exploration for mental health practitioners looking for ways to expand their range of professional activities and expertise. The study of alternative medicine can offer practitioners new paradigms for understanding the interaction of body and mind, natural alternatives to medication for some patients who need more than talk therapies, and increased opportunities for practice, education, and research. Increasing numbers of hospitals and outpatient clinics are incorporating alternative and complementary practices into their services, many of which need mental health consultants. Mental health specialists also can consider developing referral relationships with a variety of complementary medical providers or joining alternative medical group practices. As with the establishment of any new referral source, it is important for mental health providers to become familiar with alternative practices and interview and develop confidence in possible complementary medical practitioners to whom they may wish to refer patients. Before making referrals, practitioners may wish to explore their patients' expectations about alternative treatments and help them make informed choices. With the high utilization rates of alternative medicine, mental health practitioners should ask all patients whether they are using any form of alternative care (Eisenberg, 1997).

In the field of education, mental health specialists may wish to apply for faculty appointments in Oriental, naturopathic, homeopathic, and Ayurvedic colleges, teaching and training alternative medical students about psychological issues and practice. Given the widespread usage of complementary medicine in America, graduate programs in psychology and social work should incorporate training about alternative medicine into their curricula. Research opportunities abound for mental health practitioners in the field of alternative care. As most complementary medical providers are not rigorously trained in research methods and statistics, psychologists and other providers can lead the efforts to critically examine these practices, which are being used to treat the mind as well as the body.

Some mental health practitioners are integrating theories and techniques from alternative medicine into their practices, developing holistic conceptualizations of their patients, and more fully appreciating the interaction of body and mind. Breathing exercises, lifestyle counseling, consideration of diet and exercise, instruction in meditation, and other techniques easily can be incorporated into a mental health practice. Other providers are choosing to undergo formal education in a field of complementary medicine. I personally know at least 12 mental health practitioners who hold advanced degrees in alternative medicine.

Whether our interest is casual or serious, patients' usage demands that we at least familiarize ourselves with models of complementary medicine. A list of organizations offering additional resources and referrals can be found on page 413.

Information Resources for Education and State Licensure

Acupuncture

The American Association of Oriental Medicine
433 Front Street
Catasauqua, PA 18032
(610) 266-1433
www.aaom.org

National Acupuncture and Oriental Medical Alliance
14637 Starr Road SE
Olalla, WA 98359
(253) 851-6896
www.acuall.org

National Certification Commission for
Acupuncture and Oriental Medicine
11 Canal Center Plaza, Suite 300
Alexandria, VA 22314
(703) 548-9004
www.nccaom.org

Ayurvedic Medicine

American Institute of Vedic Studies
PO Box 8357
Santa Fe, NM 87504-8357
505-983-9385
www.vedanet.com

American University of Complementary Medicine
11543 Olympic Boulevard
West Los Angeles, CA 90064
(310) 914-4116
www.aucm.org

Ayurvedic Institute
11311 Menaul, NE
Albuquerque, NM 87112
(505) 291-9698
www.ayurveda.com

California College of Ayurveda
1117-A East Main Street
Grass Valley, CA 95945
(503) 274-9100
www.ayurvedacollege.com

International Ayurvedic Institute
111 N. Elm Street, Suite 103-105
Worcester, MA 01609
(508) 755-3744

Homeopathy

American University of Complementary Medicine
11543 Olympic Boulevard
West Los Angeles, CA 90064
(310) 914-4116
www.aucm.org

Homeopathic Educational Services
2124 Kittredge Street
Berkeley, CA 94704
(510) 649-0294
www.homeopathic.com

National Center for Homeopathy
801 North Fairfax Street, Suite 306
Alexandria, VA 22314
(703) 548-7790
www.homeopathic.org

Massage Therapy

American Oriental Bodywork Therapy
Association National Headquarters
Glendale Executive Campus, Suite 510
1000 White Horse Road
Voorhees, NJ 08043
(609) 782-1616
AOBTA@prodigy.net

National Certification Board for Therapeutic
Massage and Body Work
8201 Greensboro Drive, Suite 300
McLean, VA 22102
(800) 296-0664
www.ncbtmb.com

Naturopathy

American Association of Naturopathic Physicians
601 Valley Street, Suite 105
Seattle, WA 98109
(206) 328-8510
www.infinte.org/NaturopathicPhysician

CONTRIBUTOR

Kathryn P. White, PhD, LAc, is a licensed psychologist, licensed acupuncturist, board-certified herbologist, and doctor of homeopathic medicine who serves as Assistant Clinical Professor of Medical Psychology at UCLA Medical School, Professor at the California School of Professional Psychology, Los Angeles, and President of the American University of Complementary Medicine. She also has served as Academic Dean at two nationally accredited Oriental medical schools, Samra University of Oriental Medicine in Los Angeles and Emperor's College of Traditional Oriental Medicine in Santa Monica, CA. Dr. White practices clinical psychology and complementary medicine in Pacific Palisades, California.

Dr. White earned a PhD in clinical psychology from the University of North Carolina at Chapel Hill, interned at Harvard Medical School, and completed a NIMH Postdoctoral Fellowship in Clinical Psychology at UCLA Neuropsychiatric Institute and Hospital. In terms of alternative medical education, she earned a Master of Traditional Oriental Medicine degree from Emperor's College of Traditional Chinese Medicine and interned at Shanghai People's Hospital Number Six and Shanghai Mental Health Center. Dr. White also completed a Doctor of Homeopathic Medicine degree at Hahnemann College of Homeopathy in the United Kingdom, and interned in homeopathic clinics in Bombay, India. She has taken course work in Ayurvedic medicine.

Dr. White has presented at national and international conferences on psychology and complementary and alternative medicine, authored articles on the subject, and currently is working on a book. Dr. White may be contacted at California School of Professional Psychology, Los Angeles, 1100 South Fremont Avenue, Alhambra, CA 91803. E-mail: kwhite@mail.cspp.edu

RESOURCES

Cited Resources

American Psychiatric Association. (1994). *Diagnostic and Statistical Manual of Mental Disorders* (4th ed.). Washington, DC: Author.

Austin, J. A. (1998). Why patients use alternative medicine. *Journal of the American Medical Association, 279*(19), 1548-1553.

Bannerman, R. H., Burton, I., & Chieh, W. (Eds.). (1983). *Traditional Medicine and Health Care Coverage*. Geneva, Switzerland: World Health Organization.

Bhattacharya, B. (1998). M.D. programs in the United States with complementary and alternative medicine education: An ongoing list. *The Journal of Alternative and Complementary Medicine, 4*(3), 325-335.

Birch, S., & Hammerschlag, R. (1996). *Acupuncture Efficacy: A Compendium of Controlled Clinical Studies.* Terrytown, NY: National Academy of Acupuncture and Oriental Medicine.

Boyle, W., & Saine, A. (1988). *Lectures in Naturopathic Hydrotherapy.* Sandy, OR: Eclectic Medical Publications.

Brewington, V., Smith, M., & Lipton, D. (1994). Acupuncture as a detoxification treatment: An analysis of controlled research. *Journal of Substance Abuse Treatment, 11*(4), 289-307.

Cook, T. (1989). *Homeopathic Medicine Today: A Study.* New Canaan, CT: Keats Publishing.

Davidson, J. R. T., Morrison, R. M., Shore, J., Davidson, R. T., & Bedayn, G. (1997). Homeopathic treatment of depression and anxiety. *Alternative Therapies, 3*(1), 46-49.

De Vernejoul, P. (1985). Study of acupuncture meridians using radioactive tracers. *Bulletin de L'Academie Nationale de Medicine,* pp. 1071-1075.

Eisenberg, D. M. (1997). Advising patients who seek alternative medical therapies. *Annals of Internal Medicine, 127*(1), 61-69.

Eisenberg, D. M., Davis, R. B., Ettner, S. L., Appel, S., Wilkey, S., Van Rompay, M., & Kessler, R. C. (1998). Trends in alternative medicine use in the United States, 1990-1997. *Journal of the American Medical Association, 280*(18), 1569-1575.

Eisenberg, D. M., Kessler, R. C., Foster, C., Norlock, F. E., Calkins, D. R., & Delbanco, T. L. (1993). Unconventional medicine in the United States. *The New England Journal of Medicine, 328*(1), 246-252.

Feuerstein, G., Kak, S., & Frawley, D. (1995). *In Search of the Cradle of Civilization: New Light on Ancient India.* Wheaton, IL: Quest Books.

Fisher, P., Greenwood, A., Huskisson, E. C., Turner, P., & Belon, P. (1989). Effect of homeopathic treatment on fibrositis (primary fibromyalgia). *British Medical Journal, 299,* 365-366.

Frawley, D. (1996). *Ayurveda and the Mind: The Healing of Consciousness.* Twin Lakes, WI: Lotus Press.

Gibson, R. G., Gibson, S. L. M., MacNeill, A. C. D., & Watson, B. W. (1980). Homeopathic therapy in rheumatoid arthritis: Evaluation by double-blind clinical therapeutic trial. *British Journal of Clinical Pharmacology, 9,* 453-459.

Guizhen, L., Yunjun, Z., Linxiang, G., & Aizhen, L. (1998). Comparative study of acupuncture combined with behavioral desensitization for treatment of anxiety neuroses. *American Journal of Acupuncture, 26*(2/3), 117-120.

Hahnemann, S. (1982). *The Organon of Medicine* (6th ed.). New York: William Radde.

Han, J., & Terenius, L. (1982). Neurochemical basis of acupuncture analgesia. *American Review of Pharmacological Toxicology, 22,* 199-220.

Hitt, S. K., Allen, J. J. B., & Schnyer, R. N. (1995). Acupuncture as a treatment for major depression in women. *Proceedings of the Third Symposium of the Society for Acupuncture Research, 3,* 135-149.

Hoffer, A. (1973). Mechanisms of action of nicotinic acid and nicotinamide in the treatment of schizophrenia. In D. Hawkins & L. Pauling (Eds.), *Orthomolecular Psychiatry: Treatment of Schizophrenia* (pp. 202-262). San Francisco: W. H. Freeman.

Hu, H. H., Chung, C., Liu, T. J., Chen, R. C., Chen, C. H., Chou, P., Huang, W. S., Lin, J. C. T., & Tsuei, J. J. (1993). A randomized controlled trial on the treatment for acute partial ischemic stroke with acupuncture. *Neuroepidemiology, 12,* 103-113.

Jacobs, J., Jimenez, L. M., & Gloy, S. S. (1994). Treatment of acute childhood diarrhea with homeopathic medicine: A randomized clinical trial in Nicaragua. *Pediatrics, 93,* 719-725.

Johansson, K., Lindgren, I., Widner, H., Wiklund, I., & Johansson, B. B. (1993). Can sensory stimulation improve the functional outcome in stroke patients? *Neurology, 43,* 2189-2192.

Jonas, L. K., Melchart, D., Warku, F., Wagner, H., & Eitel, F. (1994). Critical review and meta-analysis of serial agitated dilutions in experimental toxicology. *Human Experimental Toxicology, 13,* 481-492.

Jonas, W. (1996). Issues of concern for the Office of Alternative Medicine. *Bridges [ISSSEEM Magazine], 7*(1), 12-14.

Joshi, S. V. (1997). *Ayurveda and Panchakarma: The Science of Healing and Rejuvenation.* Twin Lakes, WI: Lotus Press.

Kulkarni, V. M. (1997). *Naturopathy: Art of Drugless Healing.* New Delhi: Sri Satguru Publications. (Original work published in 1930)

Lanza, U. (1986). The contribution of acupuncture to clinical psychotherapy by means of biofeedback training. *International Journal of Acupuncture & Electro-Therapeutics Research, 11*(1), 53-57.

Lewith, G., & Kenyon, J. (1984). Physiological and psychological explanations for mechanism of acupuncture as a treatment for chronic pain. *Social Science Medicine, 19,* 1367-1378.

Luo, H., Jia, Y., & Zhan, L. (1985). Electro-acupuncture v. amitriptyline in the treatment of depressive states. *Journal of Traditional Chinese Medicine, 5,* 3-8.

Manyam, B. (1994). Method of evaluating Ayurvedic drug in Parkinsonism. *National Institutes of Health, Office of Alternative Medicine On-Line Research Reports* [On-line]. Available: altmed.od.nih.gov

Miller, M. (1996). Diet and psychological health. *Alternative Therapies, 2*(5), 40-48.

Murray, M. T. (1995). *The Healing Power of Herbs.* Rocklin, CA: Prima Publishing.

Naeser, M. A., Alexander, M. P., Stiassny-Eder, D., Galler, V., Hobbs, J., & Bachman, D. (1992). Real versus shum acupuncture in the treatment of paralysis in acute stroke patients: A CT scan lesion study. *Journal of Neurological Rehabilitation, 6,* 163-173.

Ranade, S. (1993). *Natural Healing Through Ayurveda.* Salt Lake City, UT: Passage Press.

Sallstrom, S., Kjendahl, A., Osten, P. E., Stanghelle, J. H., & Borchgrrevink, C. F. (1996). Acupuncture in the treatment of stroke patients in the subacute stage: A randomized, controlled study. *Complementary Therapies in Medicine, 4,* 193-197.

Sankaran, R. (1991). *The Spirit of Homeopathy*. Bombay, India: Homoeopathic Medical Publishers.

Sankaran, R. (1994). *The Substance of Homeopathy.* Bombay, India: Homoeopathic Medical Publishers.

Seem, M. (1987). *Bodymind Energetics: Towards a Dynamic Model of Health.* Rochester, VT: Thorsons Publishers.

Shaffer, H. J., LaSalvia, T. A., & Stein, J. P. (1997). Comparing hatha yoga with dynamic group psychotherapy for enhancing methadone maintenance treatment: A randomized clinical trial. *Alternative Therapies, 3*(4), 57-66.

Shannahoff-Khalsa, D. (1997). Yoga therapy for Obsessive-Compulsive Disorder. *National Institutes of Health, Office of Alternative Medicine On-Line Research Reports* [On-line]. Available: altmed.od.nih.gov

Simon, D. B. (1993). Ayurvedic Medicine Demonstration Project. *National Institutes of Health, Office of Alternative Medicine On-Line Research Reports* [On-line]. Available: altmed.od.nih.gov.

Smith, R. B., & Boericke, G. W. (1968, November/December). Changes caused by succussion on N.M.R. patterns and bioassay of Bradykinin Triacetate (BKTA) succussions and dilution. *Journal of the American Institute of Homeopathy, 61,* 197-212.

Svoboda, R. E. (1992). *Ayurveda: Life, Health, and Longevity.* New York: Penguin Books.

Sytinksy, I., & Galebskaya, L. (1979). Physiologico-biochemical bases of drug dependence treatment by acupuncture. *Addictive Behavior, 4,* 97-120.

Ullman, D. (1991). *Discovering Homeopathy: Medicine for the 21st Century.* Berkeley, CA: North Atlantic Books.

Weil, A. (1993). Introduction: Why a book on natural medicine? In A. E. Guinnes (Ed.), *Family Guide to Natural Medicine* (pp. 8-15). New York: The Reader's Digest Association, Inc.

Wen, H., Ng, Y., Ho, W., Wong, H., Mehal, Z., Ng, Y., & Ma, L. (1978a). Acupuncture in narcotic withdrawal: A preliminary report on biochemical changes in the blood and urine of heroin addicts. *Bulletin of Narcotics, 30,* 31-39.

Wen, H., Ng, Y., Ho, W., Wong, H., Mehal, Z., Ng, Y., & Ma, L. (1978b). Reduction of adrenocorticotropic hormone (ACTH) and cortisol in drug addicts treated by acupuncture and electrical stimulation (AES). *Comparative Medicine East & West, 6,* 61-66.

World Health Organization (WHO). (1991). *A Proposed Standard International Acupuncture Nomenclature: Report of a World Health Organization Scientific Group.* Geneva, Switzerland: Author.

Yang, X., Liu, X., Luo, H., & Jia, Y. (1994). Clinical observation of needling extrachannel points in treating mental depression. *Journal of Traditional Chinese Medicine, 14,* 14-18.

Yogananda, P. (1983). *Autobiography of a Yogi.* Los Angeles: Self-Realization Fellowship.

Yogananda, P. (1986). *The Divine Romance.* Los Angeles: Self-Realization Fellowship.

Yuen, J. (1995, May). *Chronic Degenerative Disorders.* A Continuing Education Course presented at Emperor's College of Traditional Oriental Medicine, Santa Monica, CA.

Yuen, J. (1997, October). *Primary Meridian Energetics Part II.* A Continuing Education Course presented under the auspices of Kathryn P. White, PhD, in Los Angeles, CA.

Zhang, W., Li, S., Chen, G., Zhang, O., & Wang, Y. (1987). Acupuncture treatment of apoplectic hemiplegia. *Journal of Traditional Chinese Medicine, 7,* 157-160.

Additional Resources

Benfield, H., & Korngold, E. (1995). Chinese traditional medicine: An introductory overview. *Alternative Therapies, 1*(1), 44-52.

Bullock, M., Culliton, P., & Olander, R. (1989). Controlled trial of acupuncture for severe recidivist alcoholism. *Lancet,* 1435-1439.

Bullock, M., Umen, A., Culliton, P., & Olander R. (1987). Acupuncture treatment of alcoholic recidivism: A pilot study. *Alcoholism: Clinical and Experimental Research, 11,* 292-295.

Clement-Jones, V., McLoughlin, L., Lowry, P., Besser, G., Res, L., & Wen, H. (1979). Acupuncture in heroin addicts: Changes in met-enkephalin and beta endorphin in blood and cerebrospinal fluid. *Lancet,* pp. 380-382.

Clevel, F., Benhamou, S., Company-Huertas, A., & Flamant, R. (1985). Helping people to stop smoking: Randomized comparison of groups being treated with acupuncture and nicotine gum with control group. *British Medical Journal, 291,* 1538-1539.

Elder, N. C., Gllcrist, A., & Minz, R. (1997). Use of alternative health care by family practice patients. *Archives of Family Medicine, 6*(2), 181-184.

Furnham, A., & Forey, J. (1994). The attitudes, behaviors and beliefs of patients of conventional vs complementary (alternative) medicine. *Journal of Clinical Psychology, 50*(3), 455-469.

Furnham, A., & Kirkcaldy, B. (1996). The health beliefs and behaviors of orthodox and complementary medicine clients. *British Journal of Clinical Psychology, 35,* 49-61.

Kiser, R., Khatami, M., Gatchel, R., Huang, X., Bhatia, K., & Altshuler, K. (1983). Acupuncture relief of chronic pain syndrome correlates with increased plasma metenkephalin concentrations. *Lancet, 2,* 1394-1396.

Lipton, D. S., Brewington, V., & Smith, M. (1994). Acupuncture for crack-cocaine detoxification: Experimental evaluation of efficacy. *Journal of Substance Abuse Treatment, 11,* 205-215.

Margolin, A., Avants, S. K., Chang, P., & Kosten, T. R. (1993). Acupuncture for the treatment of cocaine dependence in methadone-maintained patients. *American Journal of Addiction, 2,* 194-201.

Oleson, T. (1996). *Auriculotherapy Manual* (2nd ed.). Los Angeles: Health Care Alternatives.

Pert, A., Dionne, R., Ng, L., Bragin, E., Moody, T., & Pert, C. (1981). Alterations in rate central nervous system endorphins following transauricular electro acupuncture. *Brain Research, 224,* 83-93.

Pomeranz, B. (1978). Do endorphins mediate acupuncture analgesia? In E. Costa & M. Trabucchi (Eds.), *Advances in Biochemical Pharmacology* (Vol. 18, pp. 351-359). New York: Raven Press.

Pomeranz, B. (1982). Acupuncture and the endorphins. *Ethos, 10,* 385-393.

Pomeranz, B., & Chiu, D. (1976). Naloxone blockage of acupuncture analgesia: Endorphin implicated. *Life Sciences, 19,* 1757-1762.

Reilly, D., Taylor, M. A., Beattie, N. C. M., Campbell, J. H., McSharry, C., Aitchison, T. C., Carter, R., & Stevenson, R. D. (1994). Is evidence for homeopathy reproducible? *Lancet, 344,* 1601-1606.

Sjohund, B., & Eriksson, M. (1976). Electroacupuncture and endogenous morphine. *Lancet, 2,* 1085.

Sjohund, B., & Eriksson, M. (1979). Endorphins and analgesia by peripheral nerve conditioning stimulation. In J. Bonica, J. Liebeskind, & G. Albe-Fessard (Eds.), *Advances in Pain Research and Therapy* (Vol. 3, pp. 587-592). New York: Raven Press.

Wen, H. (1975). Role of acupuncture in narcotic withdrawal. *Medical Progress, 2,* 15-16.

Dyslexia: Overview And Treatment*

George S. Grosser and Carol S. Spafford

"The books looked like gemstones with their red, green, black, and blue covers. They lay in orderly stacks on the white metal shelves . . . each book a treasure. . . . College Grammar . . . Calculus . . . Fluid Mechanics . . . Anthology of English Literature . . . inevitably there were paragraphs of words to read. . . . [When] I read, 'the man tr a v ve l ed, traveled a great a great dis dis tan ce to see the won to see the won derfu wonderful cas castle by the D D Dan [Danube] River. . . . The man had plannnned this trip to Gerrrmany for many years.' . . . tears of frustration, embarrassment . . . flowed down my cheeks. . . . A young child or adult with a learning disability will need to have others give them *a lot of help in learning*. . . . Being read to and listening to books on tape opened up a vast world of knowledge for me."

(J. Nuttall, personal communication regarding continued word recognition problems associated with his dyslexia condition during PhD Studies, April 1999).

Dyslexia is the most prevalent type of learning disability. Its meaning can be partially abstracted from the word itself: *"dys"* and *"lexia,"* or an *"inability"* to [adequately] process *"words."* Dejerine (1892), W. P. Morgan (1896), and Bastian (1898) are considered some of the first clinicians to identify the dyslexia condition which was referred to by W. P. Morgan as "word blindness." It wasn't long before multisensory approaches were introduced to alleviate the word recognition difficulties of dyslexics (Fernald, 1943; Gillingham & Stillman, 1970; Orton, 1937; Slingerland, 1976).

Word identification and fluency are central to the problems of dyslexics, who struggle to acquire reading and language skills commensurate with their age and developmental levels. In many cases, reading and language difficulties can lead to other, more widespread problems such as social misperceptiveness, less than satisfactory social interactions, school failure, and a poor self-image. However, many individuals with dyslexia have special gifts and talents that allow them to excel and succeed in many life and career situations. Understanding the nature of the syndrome, in addition to using relevant diagnostic and remedial procedures, can positively contribute to the support systems/strategies required for dyslexics to develop compensatory and strategic school and life adjustments to be academically and socially successful.

The influence of famous dyslexics who have made significant contributions to society (e.g., Ann Bancroft [arctic explorer], Baruj Benacerraf [Nobel prize winner], Agatha Christie, a son of George and Barbara Bush, Prince Charles, Cher, Bill and Camille Cosby's son [Ennis], Leonardo da Vinci, Walt Disney, Dwight D. Eisenhower, Whoopi Goldberg, Robert and John F. Kennedy, Greg Louganis, Mozart, Edgar Allen Poe, Steven Spielberg, etc.) has destigmatized this sometimes debilitating condition. Dyslexia is a lifelong condition of which

*This contribution is dedicated to our families, the Grossers, Spaffords, and Sullivans, and to the memory of our dear friends, Dr. Robert Bohlke, Dr. James Brennan, Francesca DiVenuto, Pat Hunter, Pat Jones, David Lees, Paul Mason, Carrie Sarkozi, Gilbert Schimmel, William Schwartz, Margie Sullivan, Tim Sunstrom, and Dr. Ken Winetrout.

the negative symptoms can only be alleviated or diminished. This contribution will attempt to present some current research-based theoretical underpinnings of the learning disabilities field (which includes dyslexia) in such areas as definition and correlating symptomatology, neurophysiological bases and anomalies, and cognitive processing deficits/strengths. Our intent is to present and discuss research-driven and proven educational, social, assessment, and remedial practices that clinicians can adopt and recommend to teachers, professionals, parents, and students.

DEFINITION AND PREVALENCE

Learning Disabilities Defined

Although some practitioners recognized that there were children with average to above average intelligence whose reading impairment could not be explained (e.g., Hinshelwood, 1917), the learning disabilities "condition" was not given formal recognition until the 1960s. In fact, S. A. Kirk (1963) coined the term *learning disability.* He described children with learning disabilities as "a group of children who have disorders in development, in language, speech, reading, and associated communication skills for social interaction" (cited in S. A. Kirk & W. D. Kirk, 1976, pp. 255-256). Dyslexia, a reading disability, is the most common learning disability. Learning disabilities do involve one or more of the psychological processes required for understanding, or for using, either spoken or written language; the individual may suffer deficits in one or more of the areas of listening, speaking, thinking, spelling, reading, writing, or mathematics (Grosser & Spafford, 1995).

Learning disabilities can be diagnosed after individual and collective test results/evaluations show a pattern of unexpected and discrepant academic and/or social deficiencies in a specific area (e.g., written language disability or dyslexia/reading disorder) and when specific diagnostic criteria (e.g., *Diagnostic and Statistical Manual of Mental Disorders* [*DSM-IV*]; American Psychiatric Association, 1994) are identified. However, in some cases, when so-called "average" test results (i.e., on each individual measure given) are combined, depressed academic achievement can also be evidenced. This might include problems in the areas of reading, mathematics, and written expression that together interfere with academic achievement even though tests of each component skill *do not* show substantially lower performance than expected given the individual's chronological age, measured intelligence, and age-appropriate education. In other words, a student could be classified as learning disabled (LD) even though test results in individual areas show adequate performance. According to the *DSM-IV* (APA, 1994), this condition is a type of learning disability and is labeled a "Learning Disorder Not Otherwise Specified" (p. 53). According to Spafford, Pesce, and Grosser (1998), *dyslexia* is a specific type of learning disability involving a severe impairment in reading ability that affects and disrupts a person's language development and functioning.

Dyslexia Terminology

Frequently the term "dyslexia" is interchanged with such diagnostic classifications as "reading disability," "reading problem," and "reading disorder." The *DSM-IV* (APA, 1994) uses the "reading disorder" terminology to denote the general condition of dyslexia. Critchley (1970) offered a fundamental definition of dyslexia that was embraced by the World Federation of Neurology and this definition can be considered the foundation for most definitions used today. Critchley referred to dyslexia as a disorder of constitutional origin that is characterized by difficulties in learning to read even when adequate intelligence is apparent and conventional instruction and sociocultural opportunities are afforded to the learner.

"Dyslexia" Also Known as a "Reading Disorder"

Dyslexia or reading disorder is seen when "reading achievement . . . falls substantially below that expected given the individual's chronological age, measured intelligence, and age-appropriate education. . . . The disturbance in reading significantly interferes with academic achievement or with activities of daily living that require reading skills. . . . If a sensory deficit is present, the reading difficulties are in excess of those usually associated with it" (*DSM-IV*; APA, 1994, p. 48). Although several researchers have established that students with dyslexia or reading disabilities exhibit variability in reading performance, more often than not these individuals display a decoding deficit characterized by inefficient phonological processing (Adams, 1990; I. Y. Liberman, Shankweiler, & A. M. Liberman, 1989; Morris et al., 1998; Murphy & Pollatsek, 1994; Stanovich, 1988; Vellutino, 1991). Deficits in the speed of processing words (Hultquist, 1997; Wolf & Obregon, 1992) are also evident.

Prevalence of Dyslexia

"It is estimated that at least 2.625% to 5% (and perhaps even more) of the entire population suffer from dyslexia, which is the most prevalent type of learning disability" (Spafford et al., 1998, p. 84). Lerner (1989) estimates that 80% of those diagnosed with learning disabilities are reading disabled. Additionally, "from 60% to 80% of individuals classified as, 'Reading Disorder' (Dyslexia) are males. . . . The disorder has been found to occur at more equal rates in males and females when careful diagnostic ascertainment and stringent criteria are used rather than traditional school-based referral and diagnostic procedures" (*DSM-IV;* APA, 1994, p. 49). Shaywitz et al. (1990) have corroborated this observation regarding gender and agree that equal numbers of males and females are affected. For practical purposes, checklists and observation guides have been created by several practitioners to help teachers, parents, and clinicians identify the "warning signs" of dyslexia. It is necessary, however, to keep in mind that no two individuals with dyslexia display identical symptoms (or every symptom listed), and display the symptoms to varying extents.

SALIENT CHARACTERISTICS

Correlating Behaviors of Dyslexia

There are several correlating behaviors of dyslexia that alert practitioners to the possibility of the presence of dyslexia. The degree of severity ranges from mild to severe, with autism seen by some as a severe instance. When dyslexia is identified early, treatments/programs can be individually designed to alleviate many of the primary presenting problems of dyslexia (see Table 1 below).

TABLE 1: Early Warning Signs of Dyslexia

- Familial pattern
- A discrepancy in apparent natural abilities or intelligence and the rate or development in acquiring reading, writing, and spelling skills/strategies/concepts
- Age-appropriate reading, writing, and spelling tasks seem tedious and overwhelming
- Phonemic awareness (i.e., the awareness that words can be broken down into smaller units of sound) and the basic phonic ability of matching sounds to printed letters are problem areas
- Hyperactivity, inattention, and low frustration tolerance
- Delays in language and speech development
- Poor or less than satisfactory peer relations
- Distractibility
- Poor self-image and low self-esteem
- Mood swings and some cases of depression
- Difficulties in time and space concepts
- Directional confusions (i.e., left/right)
- Disorganization in planning, following directions, and problem solving
- Difficulties in copying
- Slowness in completing tasks
- "The Clumsy Child Syndrome"

Co-Morbidity of Dyslexia With Other Primary/Secondary Disorders

Adults (and children) with Learning Disorders (learning disabilities) may also exhibit Conduct Disorder (CD), Oppositional Defiant Disorder (ODD), Attention-Deficit/Hyperactivity Disorder (ADHD), Major Depressive Disorder (MDD), or Dysthymic Disorder. Learning Disorders are often found to be associated with such medical conditions as lead poisoning, fetal alcohol syndrome (FAS), or fragile (frag) X syndrome (APA, 1994). The biogenic implications involved in dyslexia, and other possible coexisting conditions, have led many researchers to use a medical model and to investigate neurobiogenic causes/factors. Current research focuses on three causal theories: (a) language-deficiency processing, (b) visual and/or auditory processing deficits, and (c) temporal processing dysfunctioning within the visual and/or auditory systems. Although there is a lack of consensus in the field regarding a definitive causal link, a range of studies (e.g., Byrne et al., 1997; Hallgren, 1950; Scarborough, 1989) does show a familial/genetic connection.

NEUROBIOGENIC FACTORS/IMPLICATIONS

The Role of Genetics

Pennington et al. (1991) and others have found that dyslexia tends to run in families, implying a genetic link. Grigorenko et al. (1997) indicated that a gene for dyslexia may occur on chromosome 15 and that another gene for reading disability may be found on chromosome 6. The gene on chromosome 6 was related to two common symptoms of dyslexia: (a) a lack of phonological awareness and (b) poor reading of single words. The gene on chromosome 15 was related to symptom (b).

Cortical Anomalies

Several case studies conducted during the past 15 years have pointed to cortical abnormalities in some cases of dyslexia (e.g., Galaburda et al., 1985; Hynd et al., 1990). ERP evidence with dyslexics (*e*vent-*r*elated *p*otentials: modified electroencephalogram [EEG] brainwave patterns in which peaks and valleys in positive and negative electrical voltage are recorded during reading/language activities) points to aberrant brain patterns during the processing of phonological tasks (e.g., McPherson et al., 1998). PET scan (positron emission tomography: a modified computerized axial tomography [CAT] scan that is used to identify areas of high and low activity in the brain) studies (e.g., Wood et al., 1991) have yielded similar results. Although many researchers concede that learning disabilities are developmentally related to cortical anomalies and central nervous system dysfunctioning (e.g., Hammill, 1990), more extensive research needs to be undertaken before definitive conclusions can be drawn regarding the nature and causes of the dysfunction and cortical anomalies.

Language-Deficiency Processing Theories

The most sophisticated part of the brain, the cerebral cortex, has been the object of intense research efforts to locate the neurological basis of reading and dyslexia. Several authors (Catts, 1999; Shaywitz, 1998; Vellutino, 1987) have attributed all dyslexia to language-related areas of the brain. The cortex is subdivided into a left and right hemisphere, separated at the body's midline by a deep grove called the longitudinal fissure. Each hemisphere's external surface consists of four sectors: the frontal lobe, the parietal lobe, the occipital lobe, and the temporal lobe.

The Planum Temporale

At the back of the temporal lobe in the left hemisphere is Wernicke's area, the brain's organ for the understanding of spoken language. Some researchers have implicated a part of Wernicke's area, the planum temporale, in dyslexia and other learning disabilities (e.g., Duane, 1989; Galaburda & Kemper, 1978). In proficient readers, the left hemisphere's planum temporale is larger than the planum temporale on the right side, but, in some dyslexics' brains, the size of the planum temporale on the right is equal to or greater than the left planum temporale. Carlson (1995) posits that dyslexia might occur when the development of the left hemisphere is suppressed to the point where normal development does not occur. Humphreys, Kaufmann, and Galaburda (1990) trace this phenomenon to the developing fetus who receives antibodies that attack cells that comprise the capillaries and small arteries in the cerebral cortex during a "critical" stage in prenatal development. It is assumed that the mother possesses a genetic predisposition to dyslexia.

Hynd and his associates (Hynd, Marshall, & Gonzalez, 1991; Hynd et al., 1990) and A. E. Morgan and Hynd (1998) have discovered that the dyslexia-brain relationship (e.g., the planum temporale issue) is a complicated one. One complication is that some dyslexics have the standard planum temporale asymmetry (planum temporale in the left hemisphere greater than the planum temporale in the right hemisphere) while some proficient readers have equal-sized left and right plana (A. E. Morgan & Hynd, 1998; Rumsey et al., 1997). Ridder et al. (1997) and Williams (1999) hypothesize that different types of dyslexia account for different kinds of cerebral abnormalities such as the one described. For example, Williams (1999) proposes right hemispheric malfunctioning in the brains of dyseidetic (visual) dyslexics who have a tendency to view printed or written words as just another type of visual stimulation. Regardless, the relationship between non-leftward plana asymmetry and corresponding deficits in phonological processing and language, with dyslexia, cannot, in and of itself, account for all instances of dyslexia (A. E. Morgan & Hynd, 1998).

Visual and/or Auditory Processing Deficits - Theories and Implications

The Role of Vision/Visual Perceptual Theories

Most of the research on the neurophysiological bases of dyslexia has focused on language-related areas of the brain. The present authors (Grosser & Spafford, 1989, 1990, 1998; Spafford & Grosser, 1991) along with others (e.g., Geiger & Lettvin, 1987; Livingstone, 1993; Lovegrove, Martin, & Slaghuis, 1986; Pavlides, 1985; Ridder et al., 1997) describe disruptive neuroanatomical aberrations/behavioral manifestations in the visual nervous system. The visuospatial and visuomotor functions attributed to reading can be traced to Brodmann area 8 and the premotor cortex (Brodmann area 6) in the frontal lobe of the brain (Cheng et al., 1995). The processing of individual visual stimuli (i.e., the printed word) into more complex wholes seems to be carried out with different functions assumed by the left hemisphere and the right cerebral cortex. The left cortex integrates stimuli over time, as in language, deductive logic, and mathematical reasoning, whereas the right hemisphere deals with complex spatial gestalts.

Specifically, Grosser and Spafford (1998) and Spafford et al. (1995) found that individuals who demonstrated a dysphonetic type of dyslexia showed poorer contrast sensitivity, that is, the ability to detect sine-wave gratings of both high (thick black-and-white lines) and low (thin black-and-white lines) spatial frequencies on a wall chart when either clear or colored lenses were used. Carroll, Mullaney, and Eustace (1994) explain related findings by proposing that the visual deficit observed in some individuals with dyslexia begins "at the retinal rod photoreceptor level, involves the magnocellular pathway, and extends to the visual cortex" (p. 140).

Grosser and Spafford's preliminary research suggests that visual screening with gratings charts might be useful in a comprehensive diagnostic assessment, although some research (e.g., Demb et al., 1998) proposes that motion discrimination tasks might be more sensitive psychophysical predictors of dyslexia than contrast sensitivity tasks. Grosser and Spafford's gratings findings were similar to those of Lovegrove et al. (1986). The lower-level processing of visual information has been referred to as "parvo" or "magno," for which several researchers have discussed two distinct visual processing systems: the "magnocellular or transient visual system" (responsible for detection of visual motion and of gross details) and the "parvocellular or sustained visual system" (responsible for the resolution of fine details as in a page of print and color vision). The gratings results may be a result of deficits in dyslexics in the visual "magno" pathway, whereas the "parvo" visual system appears to be intact (Raymond & Sorensen, 1998). However, Ridder et al. (1997) and others infer that the apparent magnocellular deficiency affects only some individuals with dyslexia - the dysphonetic dyslexics.

Theories of Auditory Processing Deficits

There appear to be some auditory processing deficits exhibited by individuals with dyslexia, for example, in dichotic listening research. A dichotic listening task is a type of auditory evaluation in which the sound message sent to the left earphone is different from the message arriving at the right earphone; the individual is typically asked what he or she hears in either ear or in both. Individuals with dyslexia or reading disabilities find it difficult to change their response patterns when asked to attend to a different earphone. Proficient readers do not experience this auditory analysis difficulty (Asbjornsen & Bryden, 1998). Additionally, Schulte-Korne et al. (1998) found that some children with dyslexia demonstrate specific auditory speech processing deficits at an early age, and as such, these deficits can be used as indicators of developmental dyslexia.

Theories Related to Temporal Processing Deficits

In more recent times, deficits in temporal and spatial processing have been cited as the major impairment to reading/language acquisition in students who are dyslexic (e.g., Eden et al., 1995). Temporal and spatial processing refers to both auditory and visual components. In order to process the printed page, the individual must decode visual symbols that are spatially arranged in a temporal sequence, from one fixation to the next fixation, which is known as the span of perception.

Stein and Walsh (1997) postulate that the language, motor, and visual temporal processing systems are implicated in the problems of dyslexics. The end result is that individuals with dyslexia may not be able to process incoming sensory information efficiently. Because of the academic and social manifestations of the dyslexia problem, the evaluation and recommendations sections will focus on the educational domain.

THE EVALUATION PROCESS

Diagnosticians seeking to determine a dyslexia diagnosis need to conduct a comprehensive assessment that begins with the educational and familial history. "The child's developmental status, or his/her relative abilities as compared to his/her age group peers, is determined through the use of both formal and informal measures. A record review and parent interview is used to investigate pre-natal, medical, and familial factors that may relate to the child's developmental status [and learning problems]" (Garbett, 1993, p. 17). Table 2 (below) lists the features of a thorough dyslexia evaluation that need to be reviewed before a definitive diagnosis can be made.

TABLE 2: Comprehensive Diagnostic Assessment of Dyslexia

1. Conduct an *educational and family history.*
2. *Rule out medical problems* such as eye and ear problems.
3. Administer an IQ measure to determine *intellectual capacity* for learning and verbal short-term memory capacity.
4. Administer and/or examine formal and informal *reading and language evaluation* results to assess word recognition, comprehension, spelling, and writing proficiency.
5. Administer and/or evaluate achievement measures in a number of areas so as to determine *academic strengths and weaknesses.*
6. Determine *discrepancy differences between* quantified achievement results and IQ scores with significant differences (i.e., discrepancy differences) indicated from state or federal criteria.
7. Observe and record *positive and negative social/behavioral symptoms/actions.*
8. Conduct a *motor skills assessment* (if relevant).
9. Arrange student, teacher, and family *interviews.*

In many instances, an evaluative academic deficit model is presented without corresponding strengths noted. However, some research (e.g., Padget, 1998) cites a number of strengths shown by individuals with dyslexia. For example, many individuals with dyslexia have been observed to utilize (a) context support during word recognition, (b) adequate handwriting and word processing abilities, (c) good to excellent expressive vocabulary when spelling skills are in the average range, (d) appropriate math knowledge when computing and reasoning through math problems, and (e) good to excellent ideas/concept formation/proficiency in specific academic areas, the arts, and sports. Academic strengths need to be identified and are considered critical initial areas to focus on because individuals with dyslexia need to have motivation and a purpose for reading/learning.

Experiencing endless reading difficulties can make language processing tedious and cumbersome. Most school systems have extensive and mandated testing requirements, and these test results, along with other more informal performance-based assessment measures, can be used to pinpoint academic strengths. Both academic strengths and weaknesses need to be aligned to student performance relative to curriculum standards, and documentation of student performance needs to be linked with those standards (Farrar, 1999).

The use of diagnostic-reflective portfolios in the diagnostic process is currently stressed with students who are dyslexic; this can be an effective tool when developing reflective narratives of student performance relative to the curriculum. In essence, the teacher, over time, collects diagnostic information, work samples, and goals for learning that best portray a student's academic progress and literacy development. The student is actively involved in the selection, organization, and collection of materials for his or her portfolio. This diagnostic portfolio process encourages teachers and students to work together to assess acquired literacy skills and the strategies the student uses to achieve comprehension of the printed page (Courtney & Abodeeb, 1999).

Canney et al. (1999) highlight special considerations for the limited English proficient (LEP) student. These include anecdotal observations with recorded weekly observations of effective methods and conditions for the student's learning. This running record could be included in the diagnostic portfolio. According to Canney et al. (1999), a "profile should emerge of each student's skills, interests, and needs that you can use to plan instruction" (p. 543). Canney and his colleagues stress the use of multiple evaluative measures with LEP students when assessing and evaluating literacy interests, attitudes, self-perceptions of reading ability, and overall progress. Specific areas of strength and weakness will emerge with an intense study of the phonological processing abilities of the student required if dyslexia is suspected. Stanley and Spafford's (1998b) portfolio measures that address cultural factors and personalized assessment measures so as to provide special sensitivity to all ethnic minority students are outlined in Table 3 (below).

TABLE 3: Cultural Portfolio Considerations/Inclusions
Adapted from the Work of Stanley and Spafford (1998b)

1. Cross-cultural learning.
2. Personal collections of artifacts that express cultural identities/family ties/community resources.
3. International exchanges.
4. Interactive dialoguing.
5. Daily communications about learning (e.g., daily math communications).
6. Cooperative constructivism where learning episodes are mutually discovered.
7. Autobiographical information/subject histories/personal experiences/personal anecdotes/attitudes/interests/goals/likes/dislikes/fears/difficulties/needs about a subject(s) and learning.
8. Self-evaluations of learning growth and development so as to encourage independent, confident, reflective, and competent learners.

There is a consensus in the field that most individuals with dyslexia display a phonologic deficit that significantly impairs reading/language acquisition (Bradley & Bryant, 1983; Schulte-Korne et al., 1998; Stanovich et al., 1997). According to Shaywitz (1998), an examination of language deficits must focus initially on word identification abilities as many individuals with dyslexia perform at higher achievement levels on comprehension evaluations than on measures that involve decoding isolated words. Decoding the printed page is considered the most important lower-level processing requirement in the achievement of comprehension or deriving meaning from the printed page (Perfetti, 1985). Pages 427 to 430 identify some commonly used evaluative measures (early intervention) in the schools that can be used to detect phonological awareness/decoding problems with corresponding recommendations for teachers and parents.

ADDITIONAL PROGRAM/ TREATMENT RECOMMENDATIONS

Remediating dyslexia can involve "fine-tuning" the match between assessment and treatment based on the type of dyslexia observed (Lyon, 1985). There is currently a lack of consensus in the field regarding a unitary subtype scheme with classification systems specifying one to several dyslexia types. The present authors, Grosser and Spafford, propose three basic subtypes of dyslexia that are similar to those presented by Boder (1973) and A. V. Manzo and U. C. Manzo (1993), with recommendations for remediation based upon a current review of the literature. The three subtypes are (a) *visual dysphonetic type* (individuals display a poor or unsatisfactory understanding of phoneme-grapheme correspondences and poor phonological awareness knowledge), (b) *dyseidetic type* (individuals show poor or unsatisfactory ability to recognize sight words with some intact phonological processing abilities), and (c) *dysphonetic-dyseidetic type* (individuals exhibit poor or unsatisfactory phonological processing/sight word knowledge). Identification is based on specific word recognition deficiencies observed for each type. This subtyping conceptualization can be used to more specifically plan additional remedial strategies as seen on pages 431 to 432.

ACADEMIC

Pages 433 to 434 summarize several key instructional practices in the field to include those emanated from a report sponsored by the National Academy of Sciences and U.S. Department of Education (Snow, Burns & Griffin, 1998). This comprehensive project emphasized developing clear guidelines for educators and professionals to use with children who are at-risk for reading problems and reading disabilities, keeping in mind that "there is little evidence that children . . . with identifiable learning disabilities need radically different sorts of supports than children at low risk, although they may need more intensive support. . . . Excellent instruction is the best intervention for children who demonstrate problems learning to read" (p. 3). As in all good teaching programs, culturally appropriate materials (Au, 1980) are interwoven across disciplines. Finally, research has proven that the most basic statement, "We learn best to read by reading," is critically fundamental to individuals who are dyslexic or reading disabled, as they often have fewer opportunities to read (e.g., informational text) than proficient readers (Allington, 1984).

Academic evaluations and interventions finally need to consider individual learning styles (J. M. Hebert, 1997), keeping in mind that all children can learn and be stimulated in their environment with linguistic, logical-mathematical, spatial, musical, kinesthetic, interpersonal, and intrapersonal encounters (Gardner, 1991). Gardner (1991) points to a bias in our educational system toward linguistic and logical-mathematical learning episodes while stressing the need for determining a child's preferred intellectual style. As an example, Levasseur (1997) studied the cognitive learning styles of Passamaquoddy American Indians and found that the presentation of content in the traditional textual, sequential manner undermined the Passamaquoddy children's learning preference for hands-on, activity-based learning that involved visuo-spatial processing and simultaneous reasoning skills. Levasseur further indicates that "a teacher's most effective teaching style may not correspond to the student's most effective learning style" (p. 3). As such, the teacher must take individual cognitive learning styles into consideration (Swanson, 1993) and adapt instructional/assessment practices to the cognitive learning strengths of the students. Social and behavioral implications result from the many academic/social failures that occur from the repeated inability of many students with learning challenges and disabilities (i.e., dyslexia) to succeed in traditional school programs.

SOCIAL IMPLICATIONS

Although dyslexia is considered a reading disability, repeated academic failures and apparent reading/language deficits can diminish feelings of positive self-worth and self-esteem. Kavale and Forness (1996) estimate that up to 75% of all students with dyslexia and other learning disabilities experience social skills deficits. Many studies have reported that individuals with dyslexia and other learning disabilities are "rejected more by peers" and receive more negative peer and adult feedback (Conners, 1997).

Dyslexics who experience social problems are often at-risk for social rejection and neglect (Vaughn & Haager, 1994) leading to feelings of depression and isolation. More severe instances of depression arise when individuals with dyslexia "are inundated with failure experiences that produce, for example, the phenomenon of learned helplessness" (Leary, 1992, p. v).

The current authors believe that neurophysiological evidence from studies with dyslexics negates, to a large degree, causal attributions of depression and other social problems to family dysfunctioning, school failures, and/or personality disturbances (Spafford & Grosser, 1993). Rather than focus on blame or negative consequences, it is recommended that appropriate clinical/professional/community/family groups collectively brainstorm to create social action plans that result in more positive and productive social/life outcomes for the individual with dyslexia. The recommendations outlined on page 435 emerged after specific characteristics/behavioral manifestations of the social problems of dyslexics were identified through a comprehensive research study (i.e., over 100 studies) (Spafford & Grosser, 1993). Many researchers have concluded that social-academic strategies need to be explicitly taught and modeled, as students with dyslexia often lack what proficient learners use to be successful in school (e.g., Deshler & Schumaker, 1993; Gersten, 1998).

Clinicians must create and capitalize upon social environments where students with dyslexia can self-manage and positively interact with others. Parent involvement is a critical variable to optimal social understandings/growth and effective teaching/learning. Parents should be involved in every aspect of the student's educational career. Progress reports, journals, and newsletters need to communicate as much information as possible (and in the language of the home) so parents feel more connected to the school (Koenig & Spafford, 1999). Parents can facilitate problem solving, help develop respect and trust in the educational process, and initiate the acquisition of insightful understandings that help to create successful learning experiences (Matlock, 1999).

SUMMARY

We have attempted to present an overview of the condition of dyslexia for those professionals and clinicians not immersed in the learning disabilities field. Dyslexia, a reading disability, is the most frequently occurring learning disability (up to 5% of the entire population) and is considered cross-cultural, persists across a lifetime, and tends to run in families. There is a consensus in the field regarding the primary presenting problem of the dyslexic, namely, a phonological processing dysfunction. This is considered a significant impairment in language processing as the individual does not excel at age and/or developmental expectations. As a result, reading comprehension is mildly to severely impaired. On the basis of the findings and recommendations abstracted from numerous studies, conclusions may be drawn regarding correlating symptoms of dyslexia, possible causal factors, evaluation issues, and academic/social considerations. In addition to strategic educational planning, there needs to be a focus on developing and reinforcing many of the positive characteristics seen in some of the more famous and visible dyslexics (e.g., Steven Spielberg). These include but are not limited to an enhanced self-esteem, resiliency, stick-to-it-iveness, empathy, a reflective cognitive learning style, and creative thinking. Clearly the role of the clinician is to provide guidance and support systems for teachers, counselors, and families of dyslexics that will be particularly useful in creating optimal social/learning environments that are inclusive, challenging, and enriching.

Diagnosing and Remediating Dyslexia: Additional Factors and Recommendations

Identifying Phonological Awareness Factors

Academic Symptom or Related Factor	Example(s) and/or Definition	Supporting Research	Some Remedial Suggestions
Lack of phonological awareness*	the sound structure of words, includes • alphabetic knowledge • phonemic awareness • rhyme awareness • awareness of onset and rhyme	Frith (1985) Bradley and Bryant (1983)	teaching the alphabetic principle directing exposure to print to enhance the acquisition of patterns, rhythm, and sounds of language
Doesn't fully understand the alphabetic principle (written letters and words represent sounds of spoken words)	giving the names and sounds of alphabet letters	Adams (1990) Johnston (1998)	practice in saying and writing the alphabet teaching the sounds of letters both in isolation and in the context of words
Phonemic awareness (awareness that words consist of sound segments)	breaking words down into consonants and vowels using multisensory approaches	Badian (1997) Wagner and Torgesen (1987) Oakland et al. (1998)	phonemic identification and segmentation games at the level of the phoneme
Lack of rhyme awareness	"cat" rhymes with "sat," "bat," and "hat"	Bradley and Bryant (1983)	orally show rhyming patterns by reading from text, singing songs, and so on categorizing sounds identifying or tapping syllables heard
Lack of awareness of onset and rhyme in word recognition	onset: initial phoneme rhyme: rest of word	Goswami and Bryant (1990)	segmenting words orally in onset and rhyme positions

*best predictor of reading achievement at this level

Additional Phonological Awareness Factors to Consider in a Dyslexia Diagnosis:

Factor:

- Students tend to minimize the value of phonemic awareness training.

Additional Recommendations:

- Have children self-select rhymes, poetry, songs, raps, stories, and so on for homework so phonemic awareness skills can be reinforced and valued by parents (Hayden, Anderson, & Gunderson, 1997); nursery rhymes, word games, and word play provide valuable opportunities for children to learn about and understand the segmental structure of words (Lerner, 1997).

- Present motivating phonological awareness programs (e.g., *The Lindamood Phoneme Sequencing Program for Reading, Spelling, and Speech* [LiPS; 3rd ed.] by C. H. Lindamood & P. C. Lindamood, 1998) and games that key in on phonemic word parts in relation to whole words.

Factors:

- Continued lack of ability/proficiency to blend, delete, segment, and count phonemes (A. M. Liberman, 1998).
- Impaired nonword decoding (nonword decoding = e.g., /l/ - /a/ - /k/ = lak; decoding = recognizing the printed word) (Rack, Snowling, & Olson, 1992).

Additional Recommendations:

- Incorporate direct teaching of word recognition strategies in lesson presentations: (a) teach to use phonological awareness knowledge, (b) analogize to known words, and (c) use sentence context (Ehri, 1991).
- According to Blachman (1997): (a) review sound-symbol associations, (b) formally instruct in phonemic analysis and blending by manipulating letters in small pocket charts, (c) review regular words and high frequency irregular words to develop fluency, (d) read stories from phonetically controlled readers/basal readers/trade books, and (e) dictate and write regular words and sentences. Burns (1999) emphasizes the necessity to develop programs that target the phonological deficits commonly at the root of the language problems experienced by dyslexics. Burns provides evidence to support computerized training exercises that reinforce language-processing skills. Specifically, Burns cites the work of Drs. Tallal, Miller, Jenkins, and Merzenich who devised computerized training programs that emphasize decoding exercises and cognitive tasks (word exercises, for example). They tried to choose programs that are research based and clinically tested (Tallal et al., 1997). Tallal and associates recommend a sixth remedial step for dysphonetic dyslexics, namely, the use of a computerized program that prolongs a consonant sound. This allows the student to recognize consonant phonemes that begin syllables, a skill they would otherwise lack (see Merzenich et al., 1996).

Factor:

- Impaired sight word recognition (Ehri, 1997).

Additional Recommendations:

- Provide many opportunities for repeated exposure to print; reading connected text allows students to view relevant language usage in functional and meaningful ways (K. S. Goodman, 1986; K. S. Goodman & Y. M. Goodman, 1979).
- Key in on word recognition deficits and reinforce areas of strength by scheduling 15 minutes of daily 1:1 individualized instruction (C. R. Hebert, 1998); individual literacy needs can only be met with high expectations (and learning goals) set for the teacher/student (Rizzo, 1999); and devise informal curriculum-based assessment measures that monitor subsets of individual learning goals and change (word recognition) teaching methods if goals are not being met (L. S. Fuchs, D. Fuchs, & Hamlett, 1989).
- Continue to have students make connections between letters in spellings of words and sound pronunciations (Chall, 1967) as weaknesses in phonological processing impede the acquisition of sight words (Lyon & Moats, 1997).

Factor:

- Deficient phonological naming speed (McBride-Chang & F. R. Morris, 1996) (e.g., use the RAN or *R*apid *A*utomatized *N*aming of colors, objects, numbers, and letters with letters most predictive (RAN; Denckla & Rudel, 1974).

Additional Recommendations:

- Facilitate daily assisted and repeated readings of connected text so as to facilitate speed/accuracy in word recognition; slightly increase the difficulty level.
- Encourage independent and leisure reading at home; use much and varied practice in reading to acquire fluency and accuracy.

Factor:

- Deficient sentence memory (Badian, 1997; Torgesen, 1988) (ask child to repeat increasingly longer sentences and compare to what proficient readers can do at that level).

Additional Recommendations:

- Present many expressive language tasks that involve sentence completion, sentence repetition.
- For older students, teach mnemonic techniques that have been found to be effective with LD populations (Scruggs & Mastropieri, 1991).
- Provide many opportunities to make reading-writing connections as reading knowledge is more fully developed with purposeful writing (Templeton, 1991).

Factor:

- Deficiencies in spelling at all levels (Carlisle, 1987; Treiman, 1998); spelling is highly correlated with phonemic awareness skills (Reopel, 1997).

Additional Recommendation:

- Include formal spelling instruction within the curriculum and games that involve analyzing initial and final letter clusters.

Factors:

- Studies continue to report that students of color do not succeed at the same levels as their white counterparts on literacy measures of achievement placing them at "greater risk" for learning difficulties and learning disabilities. Students of color are disproportionately placed in special education programs before other alternative educational strategies are used.
- The most important aspects of school change are relationships, relationships, relationships. *Cultural changes* are considered paramount in school efforts that are focused on helping students of color overcome (learning obstacles and) the negative effects of the past, promote self and group appreciation, and find personal adequacy and meaning in life (Comer, 1997).
- School success is largely the result of relationships, climate, child development, and *then learning* (Comer, 1997). Relationship building begins with the development of positive personal identities.

Additional Recommendations:

- Developing positive personal identities in all children will empower them to transcend diversity problems/issues. Personal identity formation allows one to answer the questions, "Who am I?" "Who can I be?" "Who am I ethnically and/or racially?" (Tatum, 1999). Tatum (1999) stresses an open and respectful dialogue that acknowledges the identity struggles of people of color.
- View different learning styles, as often shown in populations who differ from the "mainstream," as learning strengths as opposed to learning deficiencies.
- Specifically consider the perspective of racial and minority students because there are cultural and cognitive differences in learning styles which necessitate alternative pedagogical practices (Dei et al., 1997).
- All students need to understand how literacy *connects us to others* (Burke, 1999). Burke (1999) cites the work of Clifton Taulbert who helps children to reflect upon how rich, complex, and satisfying life can be because of one's literary experiences. Burke challenges all community members to be "risk takers" in helping all children reach their maximum potentials in reading and writing.
- The skills, talents, and experiences that all students bring to their education need to be considered as valid starting points for future schooling. "Equity . . . includes equal educational opportunities . . . and the real possibility of equality of outcomes for a broader range of students" (Nieto, 1996, p. 10).
- Chira (1999) has provided specific equity education suggestions that are far-reaching and adaptive to inclusive classrooms. Initially, students develop a working "map" of their own equity education goals and objectives and teaching methods and materials needed to meet them. They continue to research and present team equity projects and complete individual equity portfolios that allow them to put their conceptual and procedural knowledge into practice. Dialogue journals are maintained which include reflective responses to class issues and dialogues with journal partners. Additionally, students can create eq-

uity autobiographies, participate in a mock school meeting, develop their own lesson plans and critiques, plan in-class teaching demonstrations, present a team presentation project on an equity issue, collaboratively select weekly cultural art pieces, and initiate an outside school observation that centers on an equity issue.

- Share positive relevant research findings (i.e., there is research that demonstrates well that children from low-income families are frequently exposed to rich and elaborate narratives from family members thus enriching communicative effectiveness) that can help enrich literacy initiatives.
- Since the "home is still the most significant determinant of educational outcomes" (Stotsky, 1999, p. 277), literacy outreach strategies need to be initiated that involve all family members.
- Families need to be encouraged to nurture confidence and self-esteem, interaction skills, thinking and articulating one's thoughts, defending arguments, pulling apart and solving problems, and embracing cultural literacy (Comer, 1997).
- The "[familial] cultures, languages, and experiences (of students from all backgrounds) need to be acknowledged, valued, and used as important sources of their education" (Nieto, 1996, p. xix).
- Finally, "It is very important that we build relationships and communicate our knowledge and ideas to our leaders through letters, phone calls, and personal visits" (Wall, 1999, p. 18). Wall emphasizes the importance of sharing important educational perspectives with our leaders who can impact change at all levels.

Issues to Check for Assessment; Basic Remediation on Diagnosed Subtypes

1. Does the primary problem appear to be phonetic (i.e., Grosser & Spafford's *Visual-Dysphonetic* Type)?

   Yes, if a. auditory analysis ability is impaired (i.e., segmenting and blending aurally presented words)
   and b. nonwords or pseudowords cannot be decoded phonetically
   and c. spelling errors have no relation to phonics principles
   and d. irregularly spelled words do not provide additional problems
   and e. comprehension is impaired

2.

   No, if a. auditory analysis ability is adequate (i.e., can segment and blend aurally presented words)
   and b. nonwords or pseudowords can be decoded phonetically
   and c. spelling errors do have a relation to phonics principles
   and d. irregularly spelled words are misspelled due to the misapplication of phonic principles
   and e. reading accuracy is improved when large-type font is used

   Number 2 is an example of the Dyseidetic (dys = difficulty with; eidolon = an image) type of dyslexia (visual processing problems as opposed to phonological processing problems); comprehension is also impaired in this type of dyslexia.

3. If patterns in both #1 and #2 appear to be equally present, with a concomitant comprehension (severe) deficit, this type of dyslexia is referred to as a "Mixed" or "Dysphonetic-Dyseidetic" Type.

The *recommendations* below are made assuming program efforts are inclusive except in the case of students with severe disabilities who may require some 1:1 and small group instruction outside of the regular classroom setting; curriculum content requirements/school standards should be the same - only curriculum adaptations/additional support are required.

A. If *Visual-Dysphonetic Type,*

- training in speedier processing of consonants may be in order.
- phonetic training programs are needed (e.g., direct teaching of sound separations, phonemic matching, finding sound/word differences, etc.)
- both visual and auditory modalities (i.e., paired oral reading)
- writing process programs with access to word processors/spell checks/poor spellers' dictionaries (peer/teacher editing)
- explicit spelling instruction with a strong phonics base

B. If the *Dyseidetic Type,*

- training in coordinating all of the senses is in order so that in the recognition of letters, phonological processing can be as fast as lexical processing
- multisensory instruction such as in the "Orton-Gillingham" and "Slingerland" programs (work on phonemic segmentation, sound blending, and so on)
- writing process programs with access to word processors/spell checks/poor spellers' dictionary (peer/teacher editing)
- explicit spelling instruction with a focus on irregular English spellings; incorporate phonics
- use of larger-type fonts to provide more success in reading

C. If *Mixed Dysphonetic-Dyseidetic Type,*

- both sets of treatments discussed in A and B.
- books on tape/access to tutors/individuals who can transcribe dictated materials
- access to tutors or individuals who can prepare/review content (orally) for quizzes/tests
- the student has a relatively severe disability and will require some 1:1 instruction on a daily basis

A Summary of Key Literacy Recommendations

Current Research Findings Abstracted and Summarized From the Work of Snow et al. (1998):

- A systematic approach to phonics and word identification is required for students with reading disabilities.
- The 1997 reauthorization of Pub. L. No. 94-142 addressed such issues as effectively integrating special education and regular classroom instruction (e.g., inclusion); maintaining high expectations for students with learning disabilities; and reducing the numbers of students requiring specialized service delivery and utilizing research-based/proven methods and teachers who are professionally prepared to teach students with disabilities.
- Programs that offer services to students with reading disabilities and disadvantaged students need to focus on educational program planning that incorporates challenging state standards as opposed to restructuring efforts that "water down" curriculum efforts.
- Greater learning gains are made by children whose teachers engaged in professional development efforts that tapped into current/appropriate strategic planning for students with disabilities.
- Class size does make a difference; the smaller, the better.
- In reference to early intervention programs, it has been found that: (a) writing is an important feature, (b) intervention efforts need to occur on a daily basis all year, (c) increased instructional time must occur in reading/writing areas, (d) literacy planning must emphasize word study strategies needed for decoding, and (e) assessments need to monitor the outcomes/responses of the child to interventions given.
- The use of thematically based curriculum and teaching is particularly effective for students with disabilities.
- Many and varied opportunities for reading exposure are necessary.
- Be wary of interventions for students with reading disabilities that have no confirmed or validated research findings such as the nutritional therapies, cerebellar-vestibular stimulation, optometric visual training alone, neurophysiological retraining, and so on.
- Regarding bilingual students, initial reading instruction in the child's language (spoken in the home) creates a positive incentive to literacy attainment for both English and the language spoken in the home.
- Parents need support/guidance in working with children who have dyslexia.

Additional Research Recommendations:

- "There is no single method or single combination of methods that can successfully teach all children to read. Therefore, teachers must have a strong knowledge of multiple methods for teaching reading and a strong knowledge of the children in their care so they can create the appropriate balance of methods needed for the children they teach" (*Using Multiple Methods of Beginning Reading Instruction: A Position Statement of the International Reading Association* - Contact IRA via the web site www.reading.org). "Decisions about grouping, instruction, and assessment practices need to be made collaboratively by generalists and specialists with the students' best interests in mind" (Turpie et al., 1998-1999, p. 10).
- Graves (1999) points out that "the children study you from the moment you enter the classroom in the morning until you leave in the afternoon. . . . They are interested in what you want. They want to feel what you feel passionate about - a book, a current event. They wonder how you learn and what you do when things don't work" (p. 118). "Our students need to see us as readers, writers, and life-long learners" (Lowe, 1999, p. 15) who "have a passion for learning" (Tuttle, 1999, p. 19).
- Model attentive listening. If teachers show they are good listeners, students are more likely to listen attentively (Mezzetti, 1999). The development of effective "attentive listening" will facilitate Read-Aloud activities, motivating effective learning times that help develop better readers (Freeman, 1995; Landry, 1999). "Research has shown that literacy activities (i.e., Read-Alouds) that help the reader-learner establish a reading purpose, while at the same time invite them to interact with the text, are most effective. This is especially true for the student with dyslexia as more cognitive attention and resources must be expended than by proficient readers to achieve and sustain satisfactory reading behaviors" (Spafford & Grosser, 1996, p. 120). Freeman (1995) offers several Read-Aloud learning extensions that can help motivate all reluctant learners as she delves into such areas as story telling, creative drama, Reader's Theater, book talks, and creative writing. Simpson (1999) recommends reading aloud to children every day regardless of grade level.
- Focused reading/writing activities should occur 90 minutes per day to include guided reading activities. Guided Reading is one literacy method that allows teachers to work with "small groups who have similar reading processes. The teacher selects and introduces new books and supports children reading the whole text to themselves, making teacher points during and after reading" (Fountas & Pinnell, 1996, p. 22)

- Lipson and Wixson (1997) emphasize the interrelatedness of reading/writing remediation and the fact that instructional programs need to provide daily writing opportunities to "plan, draft, edit, revise, and/or publish written work" (p. 135). Calkins (1991) and Graves (1994) explain that effective writing programs need to (a) provide frequent, predictable, and productive opportunities for varied writing activities; (b) create supportive, challenging, and purposive activities where real audiences can interchange ideas and provide feedback; and (c) teach the basic writing conventions where students have easy access to materials and support/feedback.
- Reading achievement will improve if greater emphases are placed on guided and supported reading by the teacher than on games and workbook activities (e.g., Zigmond, Vallecorsa, & Leinhardt, 1980).
- Teachers need to design authentic assessment tasks that measure ambitious learning outcomes. Close examination of student learning can be most effective using multiple sources of evidence such as scoring rubrics, work samples in portfolios, and qualitative records of student development in literacy (Sykes, 1999) and mathematics subject areas (Stanley & Spafford, 1998a)

Social/Behavioral Correlates of Dyslexia and Positive Environmental Actions

Areas of Impaired Social Adjustment* in Students With Dyslexia and Other Learning Disabilities:

Characteristic	Results in
• more negative peer interactions	• more peer rejection
• lower social standing in the eyes of significant adults	• more teacher rejection
• misinterpretations of facial expressions, body language, voice inflections/tone	• more social rejection/ignoring/neglect
• diminished self-concept	• increased feelings of rejection
• lowered self-esteem	• a more negative attitude toward oneself
• subject or school avoidance because of repeated failures	• episodes of anxiety; severe cases = school phobia
• few to several episodes of depression	• fewer coping skills
• learned helplessness and diminished self-efficacy	• an external locus of control (i.e., one doesn't control one's own destiny - others do)
• unawareness of developmentally appropriate social conventions	• socially inappropriate behavior

*Not all individuals with dyslexia have social skills deficits. Those who experience social-behavioral difficulties do so on a continuum from mild to severe with severe instances requiring counseling services. Many individuals with LD display positive self-concepts with corresponding positive feelings of self-efficacy (Meltzer et al., 1998; Winne, Woodlands, & Wong, 1982).

Some Recommended Environmental Actions to Alleviate Some of the Social Problems Experienced by Students With Dyslexia and Other Learning Disabilities:

- Ensure remedial/counseling support for students in academic/social difficulties (capitalizing on individual strengths) so as to allow them to experience school successes.
- Reduce unnecessary ambiguity in the classroom by setting up procedures for such "administrivia" as leaving the classroom, sharpening pencils, and so on (Kline, 1999) as disruptive behaviors could interrupt classroom instruction/social acceptance.
- Teach social coping strategies (i.e., teach ways to participate constructively in various aspects of social activities; creative problem solving).
- Teach academic stress management behaviors (Knapp & VandeCreek, 1994) such as how to reduce test anxiety, how to overcome anxiety or fears about specific academic subjects/school (e.g., math anxiety; school phobia), time management, study skills strategies, and the importance of having a sense of humor.
- Teach specific ways to cope and manage stress within "inclusive classroom" settings (i.e., being on time, respecting and being interested in what other students have to say, following directions, completing assignments).
- Teach positive assertive actions and behaviors that foster independence and an internal locus of control.
- Teach "other" students in the classroom how to "attend to" and "respond to" students who need help (e.g., explaining directions, finding one's place in reading, etc.) when the teacher is unable to assist; peer tutoring can be very effective (Hall, 1997).
- Encourage families of children with dyslexia to reinforce and support their personal growth and independence.
- Increase the level of communication between students with dyslexia and their families by giving them "tips" and "communication strategies" (i.e., set aside 15 minutes per day - at the same time if possible - for special time with that child so that the child can "expect" a special family conference time).
- Suggest to parents that they try to have more conversations with their child.
- Encourage parental involvement with outside institutions and activities such as religion (if appropriate), recreation, team sports, the arts, and politics. If these are extended to students with dyslexia, the cohesiveness of the family unit can be increased.
- Allow students to participate in decision-making processes that impact their social well-being.
- Try to understand the needs of students with dyslexia before beginning efforts at teaching social skills to those children.
- Provide consistent positive reinforcement every time an improved behavior is exhibited; this will yield more positive social adjustments.

CONTRIBUTORS

George S. Grosser, PhD, is currently an Associate Professor of Psychology at American International College in Springfield, MA. He received his PhD in Experimental and Physiological Psychology from Boston University in 1957. Dr. Grosser has been engaged in several graduate-level and doctoral teaching and research studies in the field of learning disabilities which have addressed such areas as cognitive functioning, cultural considerations, social factors, assessment practices, and neurophysiological implications. Dr. Grosser is the author or co-author of 5 books and 25 journal articles. He is a member of the New York Academy of Sciences, the American Psychological Society, and the Division of Learning Disabilities, the Council for Exceptional Children. Previous to his education/research career, Dr. Grosser was a full-time psychological scientist. Dr. Grosser may be reached at American International College, 1000 State Street, Springfield, MA 01109-3189. E-mail: grossr@javanet.com

Carol S. Spafford, EdD, is an author and educator who has extensive public school and college teaching experiences. She received her EdD from American International College in 1987. Dr. Spafford has participated in several doctoral and private research endeavors in the field of learning disabilities and has authored four books and more than a dozen publications in this area. She is an active member in a number of professional organizations, including the American Psychological Association, the Massachusetts Reading Association, and the Division of Learning Disabilities, the Council for Exceptional Children. Dr. Spafford can be contacted at 734 Bliss Road, Longmeadow, MA 01106. E-mail: css.prof@aol.com

RESOURCES

Adams, M. G. (1990). *Beginning to Read.* Cambridge, MA: MIT Press.

Allington, R. L. (1984). Context coverage and contextual reading in reading groups. *Journal of Reading Behavior, 16,* 85-96.

American Psychiatric Association. (1994). *Diagnostic and Statistical Manual of Mental Disorders* (4th ed.). Washington, DC: Author.

Asbjornsen, A. E., & Bryden, M. P. (1998). Auditory attentional shifts in reading-disabled students: Quantification of attentional effectiveness by the Attentional Shift Index. *Neuropsychologia, 36*(2), 143-148.

Au, K. (1980). Participation structures in a reading lesson with Hawaiian children. *Anthropology and Education Quarterly, 11,* 91-115.

Badian, N. A. (1997). Dyslexia and the double deficit hypothesis. *Annals of Dyslexia, 47,* 69-87.

Bastian, H. C. (1898). *A Treatise on Aphasia and Other Speech Defects.* London: H. K. Lewis.

Blachman, B. A. (1997). Early intervention and phonological awareness: A cautionary tale. In B. Blachman (Ed.), *Foundations of Reading Acquisition and Dyslexia* (pp. 409-430). Mahwah, NJ: Lawrence Erlbaum.

Boder, E. (1973). Developmental dyslexia: A diagnostic approach based on three atypical reading-spelling patterns. *Developmental Medicine and Child Neurology, 15,* 663-687.

Bradley, L., & Bryant, P. E. (1983). Categorizing sounds and learning to read - A causal connection. *Nature, 301,* 419-421.

Burke, G. (1999). The habits that bind. *MRA Connection, 5*(2), 4.

Burns, M. S. (1999, March). *Scientific Disciplines Unite to Identify Causes and Improve Outcomes for Children With Language and Reading Problems.* Paper presented at the American International College in Springfield, MA.

Byrne, B., Fielding-Barnsley, R., Ashley, L., & Larsen, K. (1997). Assessing the child's and the environment's contribution to reading acquisition: What we know and what we don't know. In B. Blachman (Ed.), *Foundations of Reading Acquisition and Dyslexia* (pp. 265-285). Mahwah, NJ: Lawrence Erlbaum.

Calkins, L. M. (1991). *Living Between the Lines.* Portsmouth, NH: Heinemann.

Canney, G. F., Kennedy, T. J., Schroeder, M., & Miles, S. (1999). Instructional strategies for K-12 limited English proficiency (LEP) students in the regular classroom. *The Reading Teacher, 52*(5), 540-544.

Carlisle, J. (1987). The use of morphological knowledge in spelling derived forms by learning disabled and normal students. *Annals of Dyslexia, 27,* 90-108.

Carlson, N. R. (1995). *Foundations of Physiological Psychology.* Needham Heights, MA: Allyn & Bacon.

Carroll, T. A., Mullaney, P., & Eustace, P. (1994). Dark adaptation in disabled readers screened for scotopic sensitivity syndrome. *Perceptual and Motor Skills, 78,* 131-141.

Catts, H. W. (1999, February). *Language Basis of Reading Disabilities: Implications for Early Identification and Remediation.* Paper presented at the American International College, Springfield, MA.

Chall, J. S. (1967). *Learning to Read: The Great Debate.* New York: McGraw-Hill.

Cheng, K., Fujita, H., Kanno, I., Miura, S., & Tanaka, K. (1995). Human cortical regions activated by wide-field visual motion: An H_2(15) O PET study. *Journal of Neurophysiology, 74*(1), 413-427.

Chira, D. (1999). *Teaching and Reaching Every Child: Equity Education Theory and Practice.* Unpublished master's thesis, American International College, Springfield, MA.

Comer, J. P. (1997). *Waiting for a Miracle: Why Schools Can't Solve Our Problems - How We Can.* New York: Penguin Group.

Conners, B. D. (1997). *Personality and Cognitive Factors Found in Students With Learning Disabilities Identified With Social Skills Difficulties.* Unpublished doctoral dissertation, American International College, Springfield, MA.

Courtney, A. M., & Abodeeb, T. L. (1999). Diagnostic-reflective portfolios. *The Reading Teacher, 52*(7), 708-714.

Critchley, M. (1970). *The Dyslexic Child.* London: Heinemann.

Dei, G. J. S., Mazzuca, J., McIsaac, E., & Zine, J. (1997). *Reconstructing "Drop-Out": A Critical Ethnography of the Dynamics of Black Students' Disengagement From School.* Toronto, Canada: University of Toronto Press.

Dejerine, J. (1892). Contribution a l'etude anatomopathologique et clinique des differents varietes de cecite verbale. *Comptes Rendus des Seances de la Societe de Biologie, 4,* 61-90.

Demb, J. B., Boynton, G. M., Best, M., & Heeger, D. J. (1998). Psychophysical evidence for a magnocellular pathway deficit in dyslexia. *Vision Research, 38,* 1555-1559.

Denckla, M. B., & Rudel, R. (1974). Rapid "automatized" naming of pictured objects, colors, letters and numbers by normal children. *Cortex, 10,* 186-202.

Deshler, D. D., & Schumaker, J. B. (1993). Strategy mastery by at-risk students: Not a simple matter. *Elementary School Journal, 94,* 153-167.

Duane, D. (1989). Neurobiological correlates of learning disorders. *Journal of the American Academy of Child and Adolescent Psychiatry, 28,* 314-318.

Eden, G. F., Stein, J. F., Wood, H. M., & Wood, F. B. (1995). Temporal and spatial processing in reading disabled and normal children. *Cortex, 31,* 451-468.

Ehri, L. C. (1991). Development of the ability to read words. In R. Barr, M. L. Kamil, P. Mosenthal, & P. D. Pearson (Eds.), *Handbook of Reading Research* (2nd ed., pp. 383-417). New York: Longman.

Ehri, L. C. (1997). Sight word learning in normal readers and dyslexics. In B. Blachman (Ed.), *Foundations of Reading Acquisition and Dyslexia* (pp. 163-189). Mahwah, NJ: Lawrence Erlbaum.

Farrar, R. D. (1999, March 25). *Teaching for Concepts in Content Area Reading.* Paper presented at the 30th annual conference of the Massachusetts Reading Association, Sturbridge, MA.

Fernald, G. (1943). *Remedial Techniques in Basic School Subjects.* New York: McGraw-Hill.

Fountas, I. C., & Pinnell, G. S. (1996). *Guided Reading: A Good First Teaching for All Children.* Portsmouth, NH: Heinemann.

Freeman, J. (1995). *More Books Kids Will Sit Still For.* New Providence, NJ: Bowker.

Frith, U. (1985). Beneath the surface of developmental dyslexia. In K. Patterson, J. Marshall, & M. Coltheart (Eds.), *Surface Dyslexia* (pp. 301-330). London: Lawrence Erlbaum.

Fuchs, L. S., Fuchs, D., & Hamlett, C. L. (1989). Computer and curriculum-based measurement. *School Psychology Review, 18,* 112-125.

Galaburda, A. M., & Kemper, T. L. (1978). Cytoarchitectonic abnormalities in developmental dyslexia: A case study. *Annals of Neurology, 6,* 94-100.

Galaburda, A. M., Sherman, G. F., Rosen, G. D., Aboitiz, F., & Geschwind, N. (1985). Developmental dyslexia: Four consecutive patients with cortical anomalies. *Annals of Neurology, 18,* 222-233.

Garbett, R. (1993). *Can the Early Screening Inventory (ESI) Be Utilized to Predict Later Reading Ability?* Unpublished doctoral dissertation, American International College, Springfield, MA.

Gardner, H. (1991). *The Unschooled Mind: How Children Think and How Schools Should Teach.* New York: Basic Books.

Geiger, G., & Lettvin, J. Y. (1987). Peripheral vision in persons with dyslexia. *New England Journal of Medicine, 316,* 1238-1243.

Gersten, R. (1998). Recent advances in instructional research for students with learning disabilities: An overview. *Learning Disabilities Research & Practice, 13*(3), 162-170.

Gillingham, A., & Stillman, B. (1970). *Remedial Training for Children With Specific Difficulty in Reading, Spelling, and Penmanship.* Cambridge, MA: Educators Publishing Service.

Goodman, K. S. (1986). *What's Whole in Whole Language: A Parent-Teacher Guide.* Portsmouth, NH: Heinemann.

Goodman, K. S., & Goodman, Y. M. (1979). Learning to read is natural. In L. B. Resnick & P. A. Weaver (Eds.), *Theory and Practice of Early Reading* (Vol. 1, pp. 137-154). Hillsdale, NJ: Lawrence Erlbaum.

Goswami, U., & Bryant, P. E. (1990). *Phonological Skills and Learning to Read.* Hove, UK: Erlbaum.

Graves, D. H. (1994). *A Fresh Look at Writing.* Portsmouth, NH: Heinemann.

Graves, D. H. (1999). *Bring Life Into Learning: Create a Lasting Literacy.* Portsmouth, NH: Heinemann.

Grigorenko, E. L., Wood, F. B., Meyer, M. S., Hart, L. A., Speed, W. C., Shuster, A., & Pauls, D. L. (1997). Susceptibility loci for distinct components of developmental dyslexia on chromosomes 6 and 15. *American Journal of Human Genetics, 60,* 27-39.

Grosser, G. S., & Spafford, C. S. (1989). Perceptual evidence for an anomalous distribution of rods and cones in the retinas of dyslexics: A new hypothesis. *Perceptual and Motor Skills, 68,* 683-698.

Grosser, G. S., & Spafford, C. S. (1990). Light sensitivity in peripheral retinal fields of dyslexic and proficient readers. *Perceptual and Motor Skills, 71,* 467-477.

Grosser, G. S., & Spafford, C. S. (1995). *Physiological Psychology Dictionary.* New York: McGraw-Hill.

Grosser, G. S., & Spafford, C. S. (1998). *Contrast Sensitivity Responses of Dyslexics and Proficient Readers to Luminance Gratings of Various Spatial Frequencies.* Paper presented at the American International College, Springfield, MA.

Hall, E. C. (1997). *Inclusion is Here to Stay.* Unpublished master's thesis, American International College, Springfield, MA.

Hallgren, B. (1950). Specific dyslexia ("congenital word - blindness"): A clinical and genetic study. *Acta Psychiatrica et Neurologica Scandinavica, 65*(Suppl.), 1-287.

Hammill, D. D. (1990). On defining learning disabilities: An emerging consensus. *Journal of Learning Disabilities, 23,* 78-84.

Hayden, R., Anderson, J., & Gunderson, L. (Eds.). (1997). Literacy learning from a multicultural perspective. *The Reading Teacher, 50*(6), 514-516.

Hebert, C. R. (1998, September). *Guided Reading and Shared Writing for Struggling Students.* Paper presented at the Pioneer Valley Reading Council workshop, Mont Marie Center, Holyoke, MA.

Hebert, J. M. (1997). *The Usefulness of the Wisconsin Card Sorting Test and the Rey-Osterrieth Complex Figure Test in Assessing the Learning Styles of the Student With or Without Attention-Deficit Hyperactivity Disorder.* Unpublished doctoral dissertation, American International College, Springfield, MA.

Hinshelwood, J. (1917). *Congenital Word Blindness.* London: Lewis.

Hultquist, A. M. (1997). Orthographic processing abilities of adolescents with dyslexia. *Annals of Dyslexia, 47,* 89-114.

Humphreys, P., Kaufmann, W. E., & Galaburda, A. M. (1990). Developmental dyslexia in women: Neuropathological findings in three patients. *Annals of Neurology, 28,* 727-738.

Hynd, G. W., Marshall, M., & Gonzalez, J. (1991). Learning disabilities and presumed central nervous system dysfunction. *Learning Disability Quarterly, 14,* 283-296.

Hynd, G. W., Semrud-Clikeman, M., Lorys, A. R., Novey, E. S., & Eliopulos, D. (1990). Brain morphology in developmental dyslexia and attention deficit disorder/hyperactivity. *Archives of Neurology, 47,* 919-926.

Johnston, R. S. (1998). The role of letter learning in developing phonemic awareness skills in preschool children: Implications for explanations of reading disorders. In C. Hulme & R. M. Joshi (Eds.), *Reading and Spelling: Development and Disorders* (pp. 287-301). Mahwah, NJ: Lawrence Erlbaum.

Kavale, K. A., & Forness, S. R. (1996). Social skills deficits and learning disabilities: A meta-analysis. *Journal of Learning Disabilities, 29*(3), 226-237.

Kirk, S. A., & Kirk, W. D. (1976). *Psycholinguistic Learning Disabilities: Diagnosis and Remediation.* Chicago: University of Illinois Press.

Kline, J. E. (1999). President's message. *MRA Primer, 28*(1), 2.

Knapp, S., & VandeCreek, L. (1994). *Anxiety Disorders: A Scientific Approach for Selecting the Most Effective Treatment.* Sarasota, FL: Professional Resource Press.

Koenig, A., & Spafford, C. (1999). *Dyslexia: The Myths and Realities.* Unpublished manuscript.

Landry, D. I. (1999). Ten ways to help your children read better. *MRA Primer, 28*(1), 13.

Leary, C. (1992). *A Study of the Reynolds Adolescent Depression Scale as It Relates to Learning Disabled Adolescents.* Unpublished doctoral dissertation, American International College, Springfield, MA.

Lerner, J. W. (1989). Educational interventions in learning disabilities. *Journal of the American Academy of Child and Adolescent Psychiatry, 28,* 326-331.

Lerner, J. W. (1997). *Learning Disabilities: Theories, Diagnosis, and Teaching Strategies.* Boston, MA: Houghton Mifflin.

Levasseur, R. M. (1997). *Cognitive Learning Style Profiles With Passamaquoddy Native American Indians.* Unpublished doctoral dissertation, American International College, Springfield, MA.

Liberman, A. M. (1998). Why is speech so much easier than reading? In C. Hulme & R. M. Joshi (Eds.), *Reading and Spelling: Development and Disorders* (pp. 5-17). Mahwah, NJ: Lawrence Erlbaum.

Liberman, I. Y., Shankweiler, D. P., & Liberman, A. M. (1989). The alphabetic principle and learning to read. In D. P. Shankweiler & I. Y. Liberman (Eds.), *Phonology and Reading Disability: Solving the Reading Puzzle* (IARLD Monograph Series, pp. 1-33). Ann Arbor: University of Michigan Press.

Lindamood, C. H., & Lindamood, P. C. (1998). *The Lindamood Phoneme Sequencing Program for Reading, Spelling, and Speech* (LiPS) (3rd ed.). Austin, TX: PRO-Ed.

Lipson, M. Y., & Wixson, K. K. (1997). *Assessment & Instruction of Reading and Writing Disability: An Interactive Approach.* New York: Longman.

Livingstone, M. (1993). Parallel processing in the visual system and the brain: Is one subsystem selectively affected in dyslexia? In A. M. Galaburda (Ed.), *Dyslexia and Development* (pp. 237-256). Cambridge, MA: Harvard University Press.

Lovegrove, W., Martin, F., & Slaghuis, W. (1986). A theoretical and experimental case for a visual deficit in specific reading disability. *Cognitive Neuropsychology, 3,* 225-267.

Lowe, D. L. (1999). Advice to educators in 1999 from past MRA presidents. *MRA Primer, 28*(1), 15.

Lyon, G. R. (1985). Identification and remediation of learning disability subtypes: Preliminary findings. *Learning Disability Focus, 1,* 21-35.

Lyon, G. R., & Moats, L. C. (1997). Critical conceptual and methodological considerations in reading intervention research. *Journal of Learning Disabilities, 30*(6), 578-588.

Manzo, A. V., & Manzo, U. C. (1993). *Literacy Disorders: Holistic Diagnosis and Remediation.* New York: Harcourt Brace Jovanovich.

Matlock, S. A. (1999). *Metamorphosis: Reflections of a First Year Teacher.* Unpublished manuscript.

McBride-Chang, C., & Morris, F. R. (1996). Structural invariance in the associations of naming speed, phonological awareness, and verbal reasoning in good and poor readers: A test of the double deficit hypothesis. *Reading and Writing: An Interdisciplinary Journal, 8,* 323-339.

McPherson, W. B., Ackerman, P. T., Holcomb, P. J., & Dykman, R. A. (1998). Event-related brain potentials elicited during phonological processing differentiate subgroups of reading disabled adolescents. *Brain and Language, 62,* 163-185.

Meltzer, L., Roditi, B., Houser, R. F., & Perlman, M. (1998). Perceptions of academic strategies and competence in students with learning disabilities. *Journal of Learning Disabilities, 31*(5), 437-451.

Merzenich, M. M., Jenkins, W. M., Johnston, P., Schreiner, C., Miller, S. L., & Tallal, P. (1996). Temporal processing deficits of language-learning impaired children ameliorated by training. *Science, 271,* 77-81.

Mezzetti, K. (1999). *Substitute Teachers' Survival Guide.* Unpublished master's thesis, American International College, Springfield, MA.

Morgan, A. E., & Hynd, G. W. (1998). Dyslexia, neurolinguistic ability, and anatomical variation of the planum temporale. *Neuropsychology Review, 8*(2), 79-93.

Morgan, W. P. (1896). A case of congenital word-blindness. *British Medical Journal, 2,* 1378-1379.

Morris, R. D., Shaywitz, S. E., Shankweiler, D. P., Stuebing, K. K., Fletcher, J. M., Lyon, G. R., Francis, D. J., & Shaywitz, B. A. (1998). Subtypes of reading disability: Variability around a phonological core. *Journal of Educational Psychology, 90*(3), 347-373.

Murphy, L., & Pollatsek, A. (1994). Developmental dyslexia: Heterogeneity without discrete subgroups. *Annals of Dyslexia, 44,* 120-146.

Nieto, S. (1996). *Affirming Diversity: The Sociopolitical Context of Multicultural Education.* New York: Longman Publishers.

Oakland, T., Black, J. L., Stanford, G., Nussbaum, N. L., & Balise, R. R. (1998). An evaluation of the dyslexia training program: A multisensory method for promoting reading in students with reading disabilities. *Journal of Learning Disabilities, 31,* 140-147.

Orton, S. (1937). *Reading, Writing and Speech Problems in Children.* New York: Norton.

Padget, S. Y. (1998). Lessons from research on dyslexia: Implications for a classification system for learning disabilities. *Learning Disabilities Quarterly, 21,* 167-178.

Pavlides, G. T. (1985). Eye movement differences between dyslexics, normal, and retarded readers while sequentially fixating digits. *American Journal of Optometry and Physiological Optics, 62,* 820-832.

Pennington, B. F., Gilger, J. W., Pauls, D., Smith, S. A., Smith, S. D., & DeFries, J. C. (1991). Evidence for major gene transmission of developmental dyslexia. *Journal of the American Medical Association, 266,* 1527-1534.

Perfetti, C. A. (1985). *Reading Ability.* New York: Oxford University Press.

Rack, J. P., Snowling, M. J., & Olson, R. K. (1992). The nonword reading deficit in developmental dyslexia: A review. *Reading Research Quarterly, 27,* 29-53.

Raymond, E., & Sorensen, R. E. (1998). Visual motor perception in children with dyslexia: Normal detection but abnormal integration. *Visual Cognition, 5*(3), 389-404.

Reopel, R. (1997). *A Validation Study of the Relationship of the WISC-III and PIAT-R Spelling Test With a Sample of Normally Achieving Fourth and Fifth Grade Elementary School Children.* Unpublished doctoral dissertation, American International College, Springfield, MA.

Ridder, W. H., III, Borsting, E., Cooper, M., McNeal, B., & Huang, E. (1997). Not all dyslexics are created equal. *Optometry and Vision Science, 74,* 99-104.

Rizzo, C. (1999). Advice to educators from past MRA presidents. *MRA Primer, 28*(1), 19.

Rumsey, J. M., Donohue, B. C., Brady, D. R., Nace, K., Giedd, J. N., & Andreason, P. (1997). A magnetic resonance imaging study of planum temporale asymmetry in men with developmental dyslexia. *Annals of Neurology, 54,* 1481-1489.

Scarborough, H. S. (1989). Prediction of reading disability from familial and individual differences. *Journal of Educational Psychology, 81,* 101-108.

Schulte-Korne, G., Deimel, W., Bartling, J., & Remschmidt, H. (1998). Auditory processing and dyslexia: Evidence for a specific speech processing deficit. *NeuroReport, 9,* 337-340.

Scruggs, T., & Mastropieri, M. (1991). *Teaching Students Ways to Remember: Strategies for Learning Mnemonically.* Cambridge, MA: Brookline Books.

Shaywitz, S. E. (1998). Dyslexia. *The New England Journal of Medicine, 338*(5), 307-312.

Shaywitz, S. E., Shaywitz, B. A., Fletcher, J. M. & Escobar, M. D. (1990). Prevalence of reading disability in boys and girls: Results of the Connecticut Longitudinal Study. *Journal of the American Medical Association, 264,* 998-1002.

Simpson, M. J. (1999). Read, read, and write, write, write then *read* and write some more. *MRA Primer, 28*(1), 17.

Slingerland, B. (1976). *A Multisensory Program for Language Arts for Specific Language Disability Children: A Guide for Primary Teachers.* Cambridge, MA: Educators Publishing Service.

Snow, C. E., Burns, M. S., & Griffin, P. (Eds.). (1998). *Current Research Preventing Reading Difficulties in Young Children: National Research Council.* Washington, DC: National Academy Press.

Spafford, C. S., & Grosser, G. S. (1991). Retinal differences in light sensitivity between dyslexic and proficient reading children: New prospects for optometric input in diagnosing dyslexia. *Journal of the American Optometric Association, 62,* 610-615.

Spafford, C. S., & Grosser, G. S. (1993). The social misperception syndrome in children with learning disabilities: Social causes versus neurological variables. *Journal of Learning Disabilities, 26*(3), 178-189, 198.

Spafford, C. S., & Grosser, G. S. (1996). *Dyslexia: Research and Resource Guide.* Needham Heights, MA: Allyn & Bacon.

Spafford, C. S., Grosser, G. S., Donatelle, J. R., Squillace, S. R., & Dana, J. P. (1995). The use of chromatic lenses during visual search and contrast sensitivity among proficient and disabled readers. *Journal of Learning Disabilities, 28,* 240-252.

Spafford, C. S., Pesce, A. J. I., & Grosser, G. S. (1998). *The Cyclopedic Education Dictionary.* New York: Delmar.

Stanley, C. A., & Spafford, C. S. (1998a, August 4). *Authentic Math Assessment Applications for Diverse Student Populations.* Packet presented at the National Council of Teachers of Mathematics (NCTM) Conference, Washington, DC.

Stanley, C. A., & Spafford, C. S. (1998b). MARCS and MAPP: Professional portfolio inclusions. In C. S. Spafford, A. J. I. Pesce, & G. S. Grosser (1998), *The Cyclopedic Education Dictionary* (pp. 363-368). New York: Delmar.

Stanovich, K. E. (1988). Explaining the differences between dyslexic and the garden-variety poor reader: The phonological core variable difference model. *Journal of Learning Disabilities, 21,* 590-604.

Stanovich, K. E., Siegel, L. S., Gottardo, A., Chiappe, P., & Sidhu, R. (1997). Subtypes of developmental dyslexia: Differences in phonological and orthographic coding. In B. Blachman (Ed.), *Foundations of Reading Acquisition and Dyslexia* (pp. 115-141). Mahwah, NJ: Lawrence Erlbaum.

Stein, J., & Walsh, V. (1997). To see but not to read: The magnocellular theory of dyslexia. *Trends in Neuroscience, 20,* 147-152.

Stotsky, S. (1999). *Losing Our Language: How Multicultural Classroom Instruction Is Undermining Our Children's Ability to Read, Write, and Reason.* New York: Free Press.

Swanson, H. L. (1993). Learning disabilities from the perspective of cognitive psychology. In G. R. Lyon, D. Gray, J. Kavanagh, & N. Krasnegor (Eds.), *Better Understanding Learning Disabilities* (pp. 199-228). Baltimore: Paul Brookes.

Sykes, G. (1999). Teacher and student learning: Strengthening their connection. In L. Darling-Hammond & G. Sykes (Eds.), *Teaching As the Learning Profession: Handbook of Policy nd Practice* (pp. 151-179). San Francisco: Jossey-Bass.

Tallal, P., Miller, S. L., Jenkins, W. M., & Merzenich, M. M. (1997). The role of temporal processing in developmental language-based learning disorders: Research and clinical implications. In B. Blachman (Ed.), *Foundations of Reading Acquisition and Dyslexia* (pp. 49-66). Mahwah, NJ: Lawrence Erlbaum.

Tatum, B. D. (1999). *"Why Are All the Black Kids Sitting Together in the Cafeteria?"* New York: Basic Books.

Templeton, S. (1991). Teaching and learning the English spelling system: Reconceptualizing method and purpose. *The Elementary School Journal, 92,* 185-201.

Torgesen, J. K. (1988). Studies of children with learning disabilities who perform poorly on memory span tasks. *Journal of Learning Disabilities, 10,* 605-612.

Treiman, R. (1998). Beginning to spell in English. In C. Hulme & R. M. Joshi (Eds.), *Reading and Spelling: Development and Disorders* (pp. 371-393). Mahwah, NJ: Lawrence Erlbaum.

Turpie, J. T., McCormack, R. L., Sorokoff-Segall, C. B., Aucoin, M. G., & Lumnah, S. (1998-1999). *Teaching Literacy in an Elementary Inclusive Setting: Does One Size Fit All?* A Studies and Research Committee Publication of the Massachusetts Reading Association, Massachusetts.

Tuttle, J. L. (1999). Advice to educators in 1999 from past MRA presidents. *MRA Primer, 28*(1), 19.

Vaughn, S., & Haager, D. (1994). The measurement of assessment of social skills. In G. R. Lyon (Ed.), *Frames of Reference for the Assessment of Learning Disabilities: New Views of Measurement Issues* (pp. 555-570). Baltimore: Paul Brooks.

Vellutino, F. R. (1987). Dyslexia. *Scientific American, 256*(3), 4-41.

Vellutino, F. R. (1991). Introduction to three studies on reading acquisition: Convergent findings on theoretical foundations of code-oriented versus whole language approaches to reading instruction. *Journal of Educational Psychology, 83,* 437-443.

Wagner, R. K., & Torgesen, J. K. (1987). The nature of phonological processing and its causal role in the acquisition of reading skills. *Psychological Bulletin, 101,* 192-212.

Wall, E. L. (1999). Advice to educators in 1999 from past MRA presidents. *MRA Primer, 28*(1), 18.

Williams, K. (1999). *Differential Diagnosis of Dyslexia Subtypes.* Unpublished doctoral dissertation, American International College, Springfield, MA.

Winne, P. J., Woodlands, M. J., & Wong, B. Y. L. (1982). Comparability of self-concept among learning disabled, normal, and gifted students. *Journal of Learning Disabilities, 15,* 470-475.

Wolf, M., & Obregon, M. (1992). Early naming deficits, developmental dyslexia, and a specific deficit hypothesis. *Brain and Language, 42,* 219-247.

Wood, F., Flowers, L., Buchsbaum, M., & Tallal, P. (1991). Investigation of abnormal left temporal functioning in dyslexia through rCBF, auditory evoked potentials, and positron emission tomography. *Reading and Writing: An Interdisciplinary Journal, 3,* 379-393.

Zigmond, N., Vallecorsa, A., & Leinhardt, G. (1980). Reading instruction for students with learning disabilities. *Topics in Language Disorders, 1,* 89-98.

Compassion Fatigue: When Caregiving Begins to Hurt

Jackson P. Rainer

The daughter* of a dying mother told this story to her friend: "I'm so ashamed," she said, "Mother has been sick for months now. She continues to go downhill, but will not die, though we all know what's coming - later rather than sooner, it seems to me. Even though I love her dearly and am grateful for all she has meant to me, I'm tired and sick to say that I can't stand to take care of her any more. But what can I do? I swallow hard and go back in, because of the obligation I hold and the guilt I feel. Some days I feel like I'm the terminal one and that keeping on doing what I am doing is going to kill me first."

There is a cost to caring for the terminally ill. Persons who are facing the inevitability of death communicate a different perspective from those who will continue to live ordinary lives. Beliefs, attitudes, and behaviors taken for granted in predictable, routine, and ordinary days are called into question for the patient whose lively rhythms have been disrupted by the trauma of illness. Caregivers enter into the world of the dying patient as emissaries of healing from the prevailing culture, which may or may not be an accurate representation of the worldview of the patient. Discordance may be created between the lived experience of the caregiver and the dying experience of the terminally ill patient. For the caregiver, the insidious nature of distress that arises from the dissonance found in extending care to a loved one in great distress can be disruptive to the compassionate delivery of the work at hand. The body of literature describes this phenomenon occurring when the caregiver "has taken over the pathology of the client" (English, 1976, p. 191). This seems to manifest as the caregiver progressively struggles with the demands related to the interaction and activities associated with the sick or traumatized individual. If the patient's needs are perceived by the caregiver to be beyond his or her personal and professional resources, then the probability of distress increases. Caregivers say, "I've lost myself" or "I can't go on." This type of burnout has been originally described in the literature as "secondary victimization" and is now known as "compassion fatigue" (Figley, 1983).

The diagnosis of Posttraumatic Stress Disorder (PTSD) is readily accepted and understood in the mental health community. There is a wide body of research found in the literature describing the treatment of traumatized individuals. The *Diagnostic and Statistical Manual of Mental Disorders - 4th Edition (DSM-IV*; American Psychiatric Association, 1994) describes PTSD as developing "characteristic symptoms following exposure to an extreme traumatic stressor involving direct personal experience of an event that involves actual or threatened death or serious injury, or other threat to one's physical integrity; or witnessing an event that involves death, injury, or a threat to the physical integrity of another person; or learning about unexpected or violent death, serious harm, or threat of death or injury experienced by a family member or other close associate" (p. 424).

It is now known that caregivers can experience distress, with similar PTSD-like symptoms, in parallel to the traumatized patient (Colligan & Murphy, 1979). Indeed, the psychological constellation defining the attributes of sympathy and compassion requires relational proximity between two individuals - one in pain and distress, the other able to empathize

*Names and characteristics in all case examples have been changed to protect privacy.

with the plight of his or her companion. Some caregivers are able to maintain a sense of autonomy and integrity in the presence of caregiving for the terminally ill; others lose their boundaries and are swept up by darker demands of the life-and-death proceedings. It is important to know how these supporters and providers of care, whether professionals or family members, become upset or traumatized as a result of exposure to the patient and his or her dying. By understanding the process, caregivers might be inoculated against the "infection" of compassion fatigue, or at least be sensitized to the potential for distress. Ultimately, understanding and increasing caregiver adaptive strategies can enhance the quality of care for the dying patient.

BURNOUT AND SECONDARY STRESS

The story was told that one sister looked to another sister as they cared for their elderly, dying mother. The eldest sister sat by her mother's bed, wiped tears from her eyes, and rasped as she talked with a sore throat caused by the flu, not grief. The other tripped over her mother's bedside commode and cursed the appliance. Both looked at each other and started laughing. The sisters sighed in concert with each other, saying, "Now, who's the patient?"

In his book *Healing and the Mind* (1993), Bill Moyers defines caregivers as "people who are willing to listen to ill persons and to respond to their individual experiences. Caring has nothing to do with categories; it shows the person that her life is valued because it recognizes what makes her experience particular. . . . Care is inseparable from understanding, and like understanding, it must by symmetrical. Listening to another, we hear ourselves. Caring for another, we either care for ourselves as well, or we end in burnout and frustration" (p. 22).

Burnout has been defined as a collection of symptoms associated with emotional exhaustion, or as a depletion of energy experienced when people feel overwhelmed by others' problems (Freudenberger, 1986). Alternately, burnout is described as "a syndrome of emotional exhaustion, depersonalization, and reduced personal accomplishment . . . as a result of the chronic emotional strain of working extensively with other human beings, particularly when they are troubled" (Maslach, 1982, p. 3). It is described as a process, rather than an event, that begins gradually and becomes progressively worse. In a comprehensive review of the empirical research on the condition, five clusters of symptoms have been identified in the syndrome: physical distress (fatigue, depletion, disruption of sleep), emotional pain (irritability, anxiety, depression, increase of guilt, helplessness), behavioral concerns (defensiveness, cynicism, substance abuse, aggression), work-related problems (absenteeism, theft, accident-proneness, declining performance), and interpersonal strain (withdrawal from others, dehumanized contact) (Kahill, 1988). A definition originating from the hospice environment presents burnout as a coping mechanism used by staff members to distance themselves from the patient emotionally, thus enabling them to continue working in the field (Masterson-Allen et al., 1985).

In contrast to the traditional definitions of burnout, researchers believe that secondary stress, that is, compassion fatigue, can emerge suddenly and with little warning (Figley, 1988). In addition to rapid onset of symptoms, there is an increased sense of helplessness and confusion, a sense of isolation from the support of others, and an increased sense of disconnection from the caregiving tasks. The dictionary defines compassion as "a feeling of deep sympathy and sorrow for another who is stricken by suffering or misfortune, accompanied by a strong desire to alleviate the pain or remove its cause" (*Websters Encyclopedic Unabridged Dictionary of the English Language,* 1989, p. 299). To experience compassion fatigue, the caregiver becomes depleted in caring activities and feels diminished or distressed in reaction to generally defined compassionate actions offered on behalf of the dying patient.

Compassion fatigue emerges as a natural by-product of the process of caring for another, or multiple others, in emotionally charged, intense, ongoing caregiving circumstances. When an individual is dying, caregivers enter into the patient's experience through the doorway of empathy. As the patient's life energies wane, empathic caregivers must find fluid and varying emotional and spiritual connections to the patient. It is taught to budding young psychotherapists, and practiced as a fundamental "truth," that the bridge between therapist and client is empathy. It does not require a strong leap of faith to appreciate that empathic caregivers would then touch their own death as they enter the patient's world. In a further extrapolation, the potential for compassion fatigue is amplified when caregivers have unresolved trauma in their life about death and dying. Entering into the dying experience of another is likely to provoke the power of past experiences on current functioning.

A man had cared for his wife during her cancer experience for 14 months before he began to experience compassion fatigue, and spent another 2 months before he guiltily disclosed these feelings to his therapist. "I don't know whether I'm coming or going," he said. "There is a ball of contradiction in my gut. I love my wife and am terrified of her dying, and am numb to the bone with caring for her. I've gotten her the best care that is available in this part of the country, and still feel helpless. I'm not going anywhere, but I would love to run away." The gentleman began to struggle with the arousals and anxieties of attachment/detachment, fight/flight, rescue, and acceptance/denial, and had progressively difficult days in caring for himself as he cared for his wife in this hyperaroused state. At one point he cried, saying, "I've lost my way . . . I'm losing her, I'm losing myself. I can't see the forest for the trees. I can't even see the tree because my nose is slammed against the bark."

MANIFESTATIONS OF COMPASSION FATIGUE

When caregivers begin to lose themselves to the demands brought on by the stress of the illness and impending death of the patient, the body of research suggests that a predictable constellation or pattern of symptoms emerge, requiring careful consideration in order to heal and effectively reenter the patient's world.

The experience of another's dying process creates ambiguity in terms of belief and subjective meaning (Lazarus & Folkman, 1984). Called appraisals, these cognitive processes involving attribution of meaning to experiences include the components of sensory perceptions, past learning, and the composite view of oneself, including role functioning and the sense of mastery. The appraisals of meaning become progressively easy to dissociate and split from consciousness when constructs of alternate realities of life and death are held in close emotional proximity, particularly those that challenge an individual's fundamental or routinized, habitual beliefs about life.

The reliving and avoidance of traumatic experiences constitute the core of PTSD (Horowitz, 1976). For caregivers, a similar pattern emerges. Secondary appraisal of meaning to the dying experience psychically constricts the individual as fatigue deepens and the perception of dangerousness in thought and cognition intrude. One young man, caring for his father, literally yelled at a family friend who inquired about his health, saying, "Don't ask me how I am! I don't have time to wind my watch, much less think of how I am. Maybe someday I'll have the luxury of making sense out of all of this. Right now, I'm scared and can't do anything but move on." What had been asked in a fairly innocuous way was perceived as a threatening challenge to the gentleman's capacity to care for his loved one and, perhaps, how he cared for and soothed himself in an anxiety-producing circumstance.

This may be the most fundamental disruption for caregivers who experience a disruption of frame of reference, including an individual sense of identity and spirituality. The young fellow questioned who he was as man, son, and human. When caregivers actively question themselves and feel progressively jaded, confused, or depleted, then compassion fatigue should be considered. A second aspect of this frame of reference is the disruption of worldview, including understandings of causality, life philosophy, and moral principles. One woman cried as she sat with her dying child, "Life's not fair, it's cruel . . . I'll never be able to trust anyone or anything again! And, you know what? I don't care! I just don't care." Her belief in a just world where people who live good lives can influence good outcomes was shaken to her core - another characteristic of compassion fatigue. The mother's loss of hope and idealism of connection with others as well as the larger body of the community and universe, and her devaluing of her own experience, characterize the constellation of diminished spirituality. The larger sense of meaning and connection is crucial for psychological well-being in general and critical for anyone facing loss, grief, and bereavement. Its inhibition is a marker of compassion fatigue.

Self-capacities are the inner and intrapersonal abilities that allow the individual to maintain a continuous, relatively positive sense of self, and are seen as critical for self-soothing and affect tolerance (Pearlman & Saakvitne, 1995). The emotional self is potentially disrupted in the presence of anxiety and depression, affective states that have been noted as common stress responses. Anticipatory grief is also associated with depression and physical illness (Raphael, 1984). One researcher (Schmale, 1972) describes the "given-in/given-up" syndrome, characterized by caregiver helplessness and hopelessness in the presence of the dying patient. There are multiple reports that emphasize the strength of family and community support as antidotes to an individual's loss of capacity to adapt to trauma (Figley, 1986, 1989; Mileti, Drabek, & Haas, 1975). Emotional care, comfort, love and affection, encouragement, advice, companionship, and tangible aid have been identified as characteristics of support that increase an individual's capacities to cope through adaptive responses to a stress event/process. Given the present discussion, it is possible to hypothesize that family members and other helpers might become vulnerable to their own distress *through* their empathy and might develop a secondary stress disorder. Signs that these capacities may be disrupted include overextending oneself, overindulging or compulsively consuming to manage or avoid affect, frequent or intense self-criticism or self-loathing, hypersensitivity to emotional material (that formerly would have evoked no response), and a sense of isolation in the world and disconnection from loving others, both interpersonally and in one's inner world. One man attending to his dying wife described his experience: "I've been with her through this whole cancer thing. My choice . . . wouldn't be anywhere else. In the last few days, though, I see her dead so clearly in my mind's eye and I feel betrayed. I really didn't know what 'till death do us part' meant. It's almost more than I can swallow." When asked about his support system, he said, "Who can I tell about such an awful feeling? There are days that I just hate myself. No, I don't talk to anybody else about this. I've just started eating. I've gained 20 pounds, eating comfort foods. I guess that's a pretty good metaphor, huh? My favorite carbohydrates help me swallow those feelings that are so hard to digest."

Certain basic psychological needs - safety, trust, esteem, control, and intimacy - that motivate behavior are particularly susceptible to change through traumatic experiences (McCann, Sakheim, & Abrahamson, 1988). When, as a result of trauma, an individual begins to believe that these basic needs cannot and will not be met, for example, "I am never safe" or "I'm not worthy of being alive," these beliefs shape relationships, identity, and access to hope or despair.

A paradigm addressing this concern has been proposed by Valent (1995), who suggests that a rescuing-care-altruism survival loop is commonly evoked in caregivers as they provide for their terminally ill charges. Social beliefs and attitudes shape the content in which values are formed. Contemporary views on death and dying are focused on an attitudinal shift that acknowledges the reality of death along two dimensions: first motivated to protect the dying person and, later, to spare him or her from suffering. One researcher suggested that this is a misplaced concern and created an artificial environment in which the dying were expected "to behave in ways that do not offend the living" (Aries, 1974, pp. 86-87). He further stated: "An acceptable death is a death which can be accepted or tolerated by survivors" (Aries, 1974, p. 89). Caregivers generally enter into the care of those with terminal illnesses sufficiently ready to meet the demands of the illness, calling forth their ideals, enthusiasm, altruism, and their own personal health. When caregivers sense a need to rescue, protect, or provide in order to enable others to survive, a one-way investment of energy is evoked, because the patient is unable to return the energy in a complementary fashion. The adaptive value of this strategy is associated with feelings of care, empathy, devotion, and responsibility that caregivers will attribute to themselves in order to provide the needed ministrations for the patient. The danger is created when the crisis becomes the focal point, and sometimes the only basis, of the relationship. When the responsibility is too great, and the caregivers cannot cope with the realities of the impending death of the patient, there is potential for the building of a sense of resentment toward the needy, a sense of depletion of strained personal resources, and consequently neglect and even rejection of unwanted burdens. Altruism turns to self-concern. Caregivers and their patients' alternate realities may become abrasive. A self-centered view of the world that disregards the reality experienced by others creates tension between individuals, and caregivers, who will survive the death of the patient, are likely to need replenishment and rejuvenation from the irritating experience.

One man described the paradigm in this way: "When my friend was diagnosed with AIDS, I was ready to do anything I could to help him live. We weathered the first couple of infections - particularly when he bounced back - quite well. Lots of family and friends were around to help. Let me tell you, though, I was in a completely different place when it became apparent that he wanted to start talking about dying and being dead. I couldn't reconcile it, and would try to quiet him down from what I thought was talk that would 'jinx' him. I finally just had to back off from him for awhile. I wanted to talk with him about his life, not about his death. Others had to do that. Even after he died, I still wanted to remember events about his life, not the misery of his death." The surviving friend had a difficult time acknowledging and holding the coexistence of different constructions of reality and the contradictions of life and death that exist in the interpretations of experience. In order to survive with an internally consistent and valid belief system, the young man distanced from his disillusionment by withdrawing from the pain of his friend's death.

Another gentleman reported "taking on the health care system" when his daughter became ill and was subsequently diagnosed with a terminal disease. "I became the Lone Ranger," he said. "I was the one fighting the bad guys - the system - who couldn't do anything to save her. I believed that I single-handedly was working for her good." Although this is an engaging image in its bravado and machismo, the story of the Lone Ranger was that he fought in a hostile world. He was not a part of a community, but acted alone. In this example, when several of the "Lone Ranger's" friends helped him to refocus and channel his efforts in a constructive fight to engage care, he found many more affiliative points for relating to the system providing his daughter's end-of-life care. The "you-and-me-against-the-world" mentality set up a stereotypical response that no one could effectively care for his daughter. This influence diluted care and drained the caregiver of his psychological energies.

The paradigm shift described previously required this fellow to accept a major loss, that is, death of a loved one, and to grieve it. His lack of willingness to do so only postponed the process. Grief cannot be prohibited. The psychosocial adaptation to acceptance is to yield to the mourning, which ultimately turns into hope for a new future (Valent, 1995). In the presence of maladaptive compassion fatigue, individuals feel progressively overwhelmed and helpless, leading to withdrawal into depression, and finally giving in to despair. When individuals give in to despair and its manifestations, they may fully and vulnerably be exposed to the full continuum of psychic elements. They will ultimately succumb to these elements, which is seen as a common element of the experience of distress and trauma. It is important to notice shifts in these beliefs; they may represent accurate representations of the world. It would be unwise to feel safe in dangerous situations, for example. However, such a shift in belief may represent compassion fatigue: a newly developed inability to feel safe even in situations where there is a reasonably low likelihood of danger.

Caring for a chronically or terminally ill individual requires coming together with the patient and becoming trusted partners in the process of meeting the demands of the disease. Such a collaboration creates mutual essentials. For caregivers, reciprocity of energy may not be immediate; such caring for another must be seen as altruistic. Reciprocal altruism, a termed coined by Tivers (1971), establishes a social glue characterized by giving and taking and mutual obligation. It is seen in the social constructs of cooperation and generosity.

Such reciprocal altruism is a natural phenomenon and is observed in the biological paradigm (Tivers, 1971). Colloquially, it is manifest by "you scratch my back and I'll scratch yours." Adaptive cooperating is associated with the emotions of trust, mutuality, reciprocity, sharing, and love. Its outcome is creativity and synthesis. A maladaptive breeding ground emerges out of patients' inability to energetically return the gifts of their caregiver. An interesting phenomenon unfolds. Paradoxical gratitude is observed: There is initial identification and appeasement of the patient by the caregiver. As one caregiver said, "I was taking care of her - doing whatever she needed - believing that she would get better." Shortly after, feelings of betrayal, exploitation, and theft emerged. The caregiver continued: "I couldn't believe she didn't get better. She was on a slippery slope, downhill all the way. I was horrified that the disease could steal her life, right in front of our eyes." Caregivers feel stagnant and begin to sense a disintegration in the relationship, rather than an ongoing sense of creativity and synthesis. As caregivers continue to give without a larger sense of the greater good, they begin to feel alienation and decay. One woman saw a counselor in this regard. Her precipitating complaint was, "I'm falling apart. My husband has been sick for nearly 3 years. He looked at me a couple of months ago and said, 'You're wearing yourself out. You aren't the one on chemotherapy, I am. You don't have to take my sickness on. . . . You've got enough to take care of me.' You would think I'd have gotten tired before now, but this is a new and terrible feeling. He needs me the most as we speak, and I'm no good. I'm as far removed from this as I can be. Doesn't that sound selfish? That's how I feel. I feel like I've betrayed him and our marriage because I can't care more." The woman could not articulate her distress at the lack of reciprocal altruism from her husband. Unconsciously, she had manifested an expectation of generosity and gratitude for otherwise thankless tasks. When it was not forthcoming as she needed to rebalance, she found herself in the presence of disappointment and a feeling of exploitation.

CARING FOR THE CAREGIVER

Compassion fatigue is defined as a negative transformation of inner experience resulting from empathic engagement with a patient's distress. Exposure to the graphic nature and realities of life-threatening disease leaves caregivers too vulnerable to their own personal distress to continue mustering the resilience needed for work with the terminally ill. By definition, the effects of compassion fatigue on an individual include significant disruption in one's sense of meaning, connection, identity, and worldview, as well as a diminishment of one's affect tolerance, psychological needs, beliefs about self and others, interpersonal relationships, and sensory imagery (Pearlman & Saakvitne, 1995).

Professional and lay caregivers who work with the terminally ill report an interesting phenomenon as they successfully emerge from the experience of compassion fatigue. They report profound and marked changes in core aspects and psychological foundations of themselves. These alterations include shifts in individual identity and worldview, and in the ability to manage strong feelings and to maintain a positive sense of self and connection with others. They further report a shift in spirituality or sense of universal meaning, expectation, and awareness, as well as in basic needs for and schemata about safety, esteem, trust, dependency, control, and intimacy. Some will also report a heightened vulnerability to intrusive imagery and other posttraumatic stress symptomatology as they struggle to integrate the death of the patient and the profound personal changes such a loss brings, but find a greater tolerance for such PTSD-type symptoms.

A hospice nurse told the story of caring for her dying mother. "Well," she said, "I had been working with dying patients for a decade, and let me tell you, it didn't prepare me at all for my mother's death. Seeing her physically deteriorate was like watching her live in reverse. I had always seen her as the biggest and strongest adult in the world. Then she got sick and grew weaker and more childlike in her need for care every day. And I became the parent - the protector, the nurturer, the conductor, and the traffic director for all of the tasks provided on her behalf. She's been dead now for nearly 2 years, and it's taken me just about that long to join the world again. I was afraid I'd live the rest of my life a bitter old woman. I've learned how close we all are to death. . . . I never knew that before. Our world is full of contingencies and we are just one step away from trouble. Know what else I've learned? I've needed a lot more help than I ever wanted to believe. Tennessee Williams wrote about the lesson in *A Streetcar Named Desire.* As Blanche DuBois said, 'I've become dependent on the kindness of strangers.' That's been the hardest lesson of all - to learn that help is available to me. I'll never forget it, now that I've learned it. And I'm better for it. What a way to learn." The shifts described by this woman reflect the specific characteristics described and give clear examples of learning that occurred in context of the caregiving, and of the lessons applied in a differential fashion following the death of her mother.

She learned that traumatic events can happen to any one of us or our loved ones at any time. She also learned it is almost intolerable to accept the fact that our lives can be permanently changed in a moment. The concomitant sudden experience of losing control or being pushed beyond one's perceived ability to cope makes change an undeniable, terrifying possibility for all of us. Working with her mother, the daughter's professional denial which was needed as a hospice nurse, eroded. She gained an inescapable reminder of her own personal vulnerability to traumatic loss as she participated in the death of her mother.

The experience of compassion fatigue is different from "soul sadness," described as more of a universal response from working long-term with dying patients (Chessick, 1978). This response develops as a result of caring for clients who struggle with despair and is experienced with a sense of global perspective. It is not taken in as personal diminishment. Soul sadness is also to be differentiated from the fatigue that can result from working in a field that requires the maintenance of empathic attunement, selflessness, and the capacity to form and hold connections with a range of individuals with varying diagnoses. Compassion fatigue can accurately be characterized by a disillusionment with the nature of caring that diminishes the capacity to enter into or stay connected to the system and world of the dying person. The individual experiencing compassion fatigue feels demoralized in a way that approaches cynicism. Such an affective hardening breeds criticism and harsh judgment for others' caregiving activities. Caregivers become progressively alienated from friends, colleagues, and family. They become poorer "team players" in the efforts made on behalf of the patient, and may be unavailable to others in their support system, yet may unconsciously pull for extra support and bolstering from the larger environment. Caregivers may not know where to turn for help, and often are too reluctant to acknowledge the need for help until their distress becomes so great that physical or emotional impairment become evident.

There are interventions that can serve to ameliorate the impact of compassion fatigue once the condition has been recognized. Initially, caregivers can benefit from identifying disrupted schemas. Such disruption becomes evident in the presence of particularly distressing imagery, generally centering around themes related to five salient need areas: safety, trust, esteem, intimacy, and control (Pearlman & Saakvitne, 1995). If caregivers know their own needs and can articulate the distress associated with those needs, it becomes possible to tease out the theme or "moral of the story" that has become distressing or troublesome. Armed with this self-knowledge, the imagery becomes less intrusive and the caregivers begin to use the distress as a red flag indicator for examination, in conscious awareness, of the personal life lessons held in context of the relationship with the dying patient.

One middle-aged woman described the experience following her mother's death. She said, "Daddy died nearly 10 years ago. It wasn't till mother was critically ill some years later that I realized that I had put so much of my grief about him on the shelf as I tended to her. As she came closer to dying, his death came back to me. It took me some time to understand that I didn't feel safe grieving his loss while she was still alive. For the decade after his death, I never dreamed or really could recall much about my dad's life. Coming home from her funeral, though, I had an image - almost hallucinatory - that he peacefully came to me and told me I could rest with their memories. Once I got that 'sign,' I began to feel safer and more trusting that I could get back to the real world." Placing the distress in context, she connected the memory to her own salient themes of safety and trust and was able to use these memories to consciously attribute meaning to the process of caring and grieving for her parents.

To combat the effects of compassion fatigue, it is necessary and essential to have a fulfilling personal life outside the boundary of caregiving activities. Though the breadth of activities may be limited in favor of the demands required by the disease, a sense of balance is needed in order to maintain perspective. The explicit acknowledgment of oneself as deserving of care and of one's needs as valid and important is essential. One cancer patient recognized the signs of compassion fatigue in her companion. She lovingly told him, "I'm the one who is sick. It isn't going to help me if you get sick and tired of taking care of me. Take care of me by taking care of yourself." Her companion found a mutual friend who was willing to spend an evening, once a week at dinner, in an effort to maintain his sense of mastery and balance.

Caregivers report that compassion fatigue places psychological blinders on the identification of personal healing activities. There are many important ways to engage in restorative self-care at a personal level. There are no specific prescribed activities, just the acknowledgment that in the presence of distress, loss of choice of lively activity deepens pain and the sense of helplessness. Therefore, choice becomes necessary for renewal and vitality. It is not unusual that caregivers will be asked to create a concrete list of healing activities, distribute it to their support systems, and gain commitment and encouragement for self-care on a regular, routine basis. Such replenishment means participating in other activities, in addition to the caregiving, that are challenging and different.

The support system can help absorb the secondary trauma associated with the loss by diffusing its effects among many people and by demonstrating that the survivor's feelings are understood, while still enabling the caregiver to maintain the valued role as a healing presence to the dying patient. The caregiver's role as a healing presence to the dying person is, in some ways, similar to the role of a parent caring for a child. When the metaphorical parent is primary caregiver to the client, the support system fills a complementary role as encouraging the care. In contemporary terms, such a process has been described as "it takes a village." Donald Winnecott (1964) identified three different ways in which the support system's complement to caregivers is valuable: helping caregivers feel well cared for and providing a sense of social security and hope for the future; supporting the authority of caregivers while allowing for individual variances that do not destroy anyone in the system; and enriching the life of the one receiving care through the personal qualities, ideals, knowledge, and liveliness of the other.

Additionally, the spiritual damage, that is, the loss of meaning, connection, and hope that can signal compassion fatigue, becomes profoundly destructive to facilitating the patient's care and to the caregiver's sense of self-efficacy. Attending to spiritual health is critical for survival and growth. Developing or reconnecting with the spiritual self is unique to the individual and entails finding ways to restore faith in something larger than oneself, either through the engagement with the best of all that is human, with nature, or with God. Consciously expanding personal frames of reference through risk taking, finding loving connections, and exploring joy in ordinary moments address the fundamental disruption in meaning created by compassion fatigue. The cynicism caused by overgeneralized negative expectancies can be neutralized by the pursuit of the spiritual. One man told of his understanding of this concept. He said, "I got to the point that my 'well' was dry. I had to drive 20 back-road miles through the country to the hospital where my wife was receiving care. One morning as I was grousing about the misery of the entire circumstance of her sickness, I noticed what a pretty drive it was. I decided that I could dust off my old 35-mm camera and take pictures of the beauty of the mountains and valley on the drive to the hospital. The richness of the natural environment helped me to balance the starkness of the clinical surroundings of the hospital. My wife enjoyed the pictures, too. It gave me a creative outlet and a new way to engage with her. It was almost like I took her out for a drive with me every time I stopped to take a picture. I started feeling more resourceful, like my well was being refilled."

PREVENTION OF COMPASSION FATIGUE

There is no simple and straightforward explanation for the evolution of psychological distress in caregivers as has been described. There *is* a conspiracy of silence around compassion fatigue, because most primary caregivers to the terminally ill are high-functioning individuals and can conceal their suffering from themselves and others until it reaches severe proportions (Schieber, 1983). Reports vary about the nature of caregiving for the terminally ill, though all writers and researchers agree that to effectively provide care, one must be vulnerable to the dying process and to the personal and unique integrity of the patient. This vulnerability places caregivers at risk for stress-related problems. Certain aspects of the care of the chronically and terminally ill, such as feelings of failure resulting from the patient's death, only enhance the likelihood of distress.

There is a school of thought that suggests that distortions in the goals and process of caregiving place an individual at higher risk for compassion fatigue. One unhealthy path is for caregivers' self-worth to be completely tied to productivity of the caring process and living up to "great potential," defining such productivity-potential as mastery. One family member described her nurse/sister's caring for a dying father, saying, "She's the best nurse I've ever known. And now with Daddy, she can do anything. I believe she could save him." Impracticable expectations and ideals are a fundamental element in the appearance of compassion fatigue. If death is not regarded as an acceptable outcome (and it rarely is in the medical/health care community), then the caregivers' skewed sense of efficacy, defined by attributes such as achievement and competition (i.e., beating the disease), is lost to the humanity found in caring for the terminally ill. This process can be amplified when caregivers enter into the patient's system with a sense of narcissistic entitlement. Caregivers easily become the watchdog for health and life, and find themselves unable to tolerate "unacceptable" behaviors from others because of the primacy of the hard work and the inflation of the importance of the mission to be accomplished (Martin & Julian, 1987). A hospice team was quite concerned with the depleted spouse who refused to leave his wife's bedside. His mantra was, "No one can take care of her like I do," even as his personal hygiene and mental status deteriorated. Another caring spouse was reprimanded by the dying patient when she entered his room asking, "How are *we* today?" The patient responded, "I'm dying and feel awful. I hope you don't feel the same way I do or then *we* are both in big trouble."

The bulk of the popular and professional literature suggests that prevention of compassion fatigue is best managed through reduction of internal stressors. Cultivation of an internal locus of control is recommended as fundamental (Riordan & Saltzer, 1992). For professional caregivers, this requires an ongoing assumption of responsibility for choosing work in an intense, emotionally charged environment. Mentoring and supervision help to ensure congruent expectations with the work at hand. For the family member of a dying loved one, an internal locus of control is encouraged through a steady, gentle reevaluation of reason for involvement in the caregiving process, while concurrently evaluating ways to maintain individuality in the context of the caring relationship. One caregiver reported, "I get up every morning and ask myself if I am strong enough today to take care of my sister and wise enough to learn the lessons in her life and death. If I can answer yes to those two questions, I know it'll be a good day. If the answer is no, then I have to take that very seriously." Grief counseling and intermittent psychotherapy are useful sources of guidance and support (Rando, 1986). Support groups offer safe places for catharsis, a critical element in facilitating the grieving process. Groups also become a place to share information that fosters better understanding of the dying process (Thacker, 1984).

A frequently cited preventive measure to compassion fatigue revolves around the development of a self-care/wellness program, particularly when caregivers are involved in caring for a chronically ill individual. Those holistic programs that incorporate stress-reducing practices in the four aspects of daily life - physical, psychological, intellectual, and spiritual - are most favored (Glogow, 1986; Rando, 1986). Researchers agree that caregivers must make a dedicated effort to incorporating such a self-care program into the daily routine of meeting the demands of the disease. Physical exercise continues to be seen as the best stress reducer (Leighton & Koye, 1984). The development of a heightened sense of body awareness is also viewed as an adaptive mechanism that helps caregivers attend to the numbing manifestation of compassion fatigue (Coffey-Lewis, 1982). One progressive hospital offers primary caregivers of the terminally ill day passes to the campus fitness center. At the patient's intake, the staff social worker orients and encourages caregivers' use of the facilities.

Cognitively and spiritually, journaling, meditation, and prayer are all encouraged as self-soothing and focusing mechanisms for caregivers (Borysenko, 1987; Rando, 1986). Laughter is also seen as a great stress reducer, and developing and maintaining a sense of humor is seen as helpful (Larson, 1986). Others suggest specific cognitive exercises to prevent or ameliorate the sense of "stuckness" that characterizes compassion fatigue. Approaching stress in the caregiving relationship from a problem-solving approach is a powerful orientation. By identifying those concerns, points of distress, and difficulty, caregivers mobilize choice, which enhances functioning and self-esteem. Discovering silence is one of the most favorable and accessible strategies (Wakefield, 1998). Cognitively, it is thought that taking a break from inner and outer noise can facilitate a feeling of clarity, leading to a heightened awareness of individual need. As noted earlier, compassion fatigue is numbing. Most individuals take their senses for granted. When caregivers begin to feel less attentive to the environment, cognitively increasing attention to the sensual day can help reconnect to the world of ideas, metaphors, and creativity. Looking in detail at the environment and recalling sensory memory can encourage this sense of balance. One man told this story: "I was taking my wife's flowers home one afternoon and really smelled the carnations, like it was the first time I had ever smelled them. If pink had a scent, I decided that's what pink would smell like. I felt a small, but real, sense of rejuvenation, and decided that I would literally 'stop and smell the flowers' from that point forward. It's a little thing, but with the enormity of my wife's illness, I'll take whatever I can get."

There is a large body of literature that suggests a spiritual belief system provides nourishment and nurturance in the presence of death and loss, either through traditional religious practice or a private belief system (Glogow, 1986; Munley, 1983). Adopting as playful an attitude, whenever possible, supports caregiving as a spiritually light and lively activity, even amidst the serious nature of death. For those not oriented to an organized faith system, listening to nighttime dreams and journaling can become a rich source of encouragement (Wakefield, 1998). Dreams provide unconscious messages and bring images and themes oriented to growth and replenishment.

When the high cost and personal impact of caregiving for the dying is not balanced by appropriate coping mechanisms and personal resources, consequences develop. One researcher suggests a novel observation with regard to prevention. The distortion of emotional perspective has been discussed earlier in this contribution as a manifestation of compassion fatigue. Small concerns become obstacles, and caregivers muster an exaggerated sense of their own importance or of the significance of certain incidents and events. This loss of perspective can involve seeing problems become too big to influence or change. It can also involve a minimization or denial of personal feelings. Along with a distorted perspective, caregivers may experience a heightened sense of emotionality surrounding events and circumstances, referred to as the "drama" of caregiving (Lattanzi-Licht, 1995). This "drama" response includes significant personalization, where caregivers begin to envision themselves progressively at the center of all critical events related to the patient and family. One family member angrily told his parent's attending physician, "We are living her death. . . . It's not just *her* that's dying." These extrensic activities associated with drama deplete the sense of balance that is more effectively guided through innerdirectedness and maintenance of support systems (Jaffee & Scott, 1984). Some caregivers find heightened personal and systemic power in caregiving activities. It is not unusual for caregivers who might feel diminished in other areas of their lives to become more invested and caught in the "script," the "play," or the "role" that manifests as extrensic activities to "managing" the disease. Suggestions of inappropriate treatments, doubts about the value of others' attempts to care, and the caregiver who becomes the absolute expert are signs of entrance into drama. Some caregivers become jealous of the interaction and depth the dying person achieves with others. One mother had an extreme degree of difficulty acknowledging that she no longer had exclusive rights to give and receive love and care to her young adult daughter, dying of a blood-related cancer. She did not hesitate to make it known that although others might enter the system for a while, she expected them to comply and perform according to her directions regarding the daughter's care. Her anguish and woundedness in the progressive loss of her daughter was transformed into a consuming mixture of rage and hope which behaviorally sounded like demands, harassment, and self-proclaimed expertise when she referred to herself as "Dr. Mom." (Until a loving friend stepped in, the mother stridently attempted to require all of her daughter's health care professionals to refer to her only in this way, "Dr. Mom.") Maintenance of the quietness, of the "person-ality," and of the unique and private mustering of care for the patient encourages a proactive orientation away from drama and toward an intrinsically rewarding relational stance.

Social support is frequently mentioned as a means of relieving dysfunctional effects that result from difficult life events. The concept is defined as resources (actual or perceived) available from one or more others to assist an individual in the management of stress experiences and to increase the experience of well-being (McIntosh, 1991). Two dimensions consistently identified are the *source* and *type* of support. With regard to compassion fatigue, social support can be operationalized in terms of its structure and function.

It is worthy to note that a social network has not been useful in prediction of health or illness (House & Kahn, 1985). Social networks and social support are conceptually confused with each other in terms of relevance, type, and dimension. Definitions will aid in clarifying how social support is functionally manifest.

Numbers of people defines a social network. The existence of persons caregivers may use as confidants is a component of social support. There is some evidence that suggests an optimum number of persons in whom caregivers might confide. Assuming a reciprocity of relationship, too few persons may result in a restricted resource, increasing the potential for isolation, while too many may add additional burden to the system, potentially emerging through the experience of "drama" as previously discussed (Cohen & Willis, 1985). Amount of support is defined in terms of how much supportive resource is available. The focus for determination of "how much" is held in the nature of the instrumental or emotional assistance offered to the individual for handling stressful situations. The perception of support adequacy varies from person to person and is defined as the amount of support available compared to the amount needed or desired. Following his wife's funeral, a man looked at the enormity of food brought to his home and sighed, "It would have been good to have some of these fine dishes these last few months while I was eating cheese and crackers." The adequacy of his support system was incongruent with his needs.

In models of stress prevention, social support is hypothesized as having main and moderating effects (House, 1981). Main effects operate by changing the amount of stress the individual perceives in a situation, which directly affects well-being. Moderating effects change the relationship between the perception of a stressful event and the degree of the strain experienced. One caregiver reported having several friends who "would do anything I asked them to do. One even cleaned my house and washed my clothes for me while I was so far in over my head trying to take care of my dying wife." This is an example of a main effect of the social support system. The fellow continued in his conversation: "I have an old friend that I've known since high school - so you know I mean old. He just showed up to sit with me on those days my wife had surgery. We never really talked about her illness, and soon as we heard my wife was done with whatever the procedural things had been prescribed, he would leave and go on about his day. His sitting with me 'lightened the load' so much. I could've sat by myself, but I sure was glad to have his company." This is an example of a moderating effect of the social support system.

SUMMARY

Clinical experience reveals that death, dying, life, and loss place their own emotional burdens on the caregiver. In our contemporary society, great emphasis is placed on work as a gauge for worth. One grandmother described her granddaughter's caregiving for her as she died as "a thankless task." Certainly, caregiving for a dying individual is an intense, emotionally draining experience. When compassionate individuals put the needs of the dying patient exclusively at the forefront of their own lively self-care, the ability to respond to self and, therefore, to others, is at risk. The greatest risk is found in loss of meaning for the caring activities, and loss of meaning of the process of life and death. As Carl Jung said, "To give deep meaning to one's life makes it possible to endure many things, anything, maybe. . . . The absence of such deep meaning, makes existential fulfillment out of reach and in a certain way, is the equivalent of sickness" (1983, p. 231).

Compassion fatigue emerges as a potential for all caregivers of the terminally ill and requires the individual to seek self-renewal through the activities described in this contribution. Martin Buber (1964) describes this resilience that can be discovered in the presence of such distress in a story: News was brought to the rabbi that his friend had fallen ill. The rabbi cared, nursed, and comforted his dying friend. On the sabbath he said his name over and over and prayed for his recovery. Then he put on new shoes made of the finest leather, laced them up, and danced. Another friend who was present said, "Power flowed forth from his dancing. Every step was a powerful mystery. An unfamiliar light suffused the house, and everyone watching saw the heavenly hosts join in his dance" (p. 90).

CONTRIBUTOR

Jackson P. Rainer, PhD, is an Associate Professor of Psychology at Gardner-Webb University in Boiling Springs, North Carolina, and a practicing psychotherapist with Woodridge Psychological Associates in Rutherfordton, North Carolina. Dr. Rainer is Chair of the Publication Board for the Division of Psychotherapy of the American Psychological Association. He is on the editorial boards of the journals *In Session, Psychotherapy,* and *Healthcare Financial Management.* He is a nationally known expert on issues related to death, dying, grief, and bereavement as a teacher and consultant with the American Academy of Bereavement, Tucson, Arizona. Dr. Rainer can be contacted at Gardner-Webb University, Department of Psychology, Box 7251, Boiling Springs, NC 28017.

RESOURCES

American Psychiatric Association. (1994). *Diagnostic and Statistical Manual of Mental Disorders* (4th ed.). Washington, DC: Author.

Aries, P. (1974). *Western Attitudes Toward Death.* Baltimore: Johns Hopkins University Press.

Borysenko, J. (1987). *Minding the Body, Mending the Mind.* Menlo Park, CA: Addison-Wesley.

Buber, M. (1964). *Tales of the Hasidim: The Later Masters.* New York: Schocken Books.

Chessick, R. (1978). The sad soul of the psychiatrist. *Bulletin of the Menninger Clinic, 42,* 1-9.

Coffey-Lewis, L. (1982). *Be Restored to Health.* New York: Ballentine Books.

Cohen, S., & Willis, T. (1985). Stress, social support, and the buffering hypothesis. *Psychological Bulletin, 98,* 310-357.

Colligan, M., & Murphy, L. (1979). Mass psychogenic illness in organizations: An overview. *Journal of Occupational Psychology, 52,* 77-90.

English, O. S. (1976). The emotional stress of psychotherapeutic practice. *Journal of the American Academy of Psychoanalysis, 4,* 191-201.

Figley, C. R. (1983). Catastrophe: An overview of family reactions. In C. R. Figley & H. I. McCubbin (Eds.), *Stress and the Family: Vol. 2. Coping With Catastrophe* (pp. 3-20). New York: Brunner/Mazel.

Figley, C. R. (1986). Traumatic stress: The role of the family and social support system. In C. R. Figley (Ed.), *Trauma and Its Wake: Vol. 2. Traumatic Stress Theory, Research, and Intervention* (pp. 120-151). New York: Brunner/Mazel.

Figley, C. R. (1988). Toward a field of traumatic stress. *Journal of Traumatic Stress, 1*(1), 3-16.

Figley, C. R. (1989). *Treating Stress in Families.* New York: Brunner/Mazel.

Figley, C. R. (1993, February). Compassion stress and the family therapist. *Family Therapy News,* pp. 1-8.

Freudenberger, H. (1986). The issues of staff burnout in therapeutic communities. *Journal of Psychoactive Drugs, 18*(2), 247-251.

Glogow, E. (1986). Research note: Burnout and loss of control. *Public Personnel Management, 15,* 79-83.

Horowitz, M. (1976). *Stress Response Syndromes.* New York: Jason Aronson.

House, J. (1981). *Work, Stress, and Social Support.* Reading, MA: Addison-Wesley.

House, J., & Kahn, R. (1985). Measures and concepts of social support. In S. Cohen & S. Syme (Eds.), *Social Support and Health* (pp. 81-121). Orlando, FL: Academic Press.

Jaffee, D., & Scott, C. (1984). *Self-Renewal.* New York: Fireside.

Jung, C. (1983). *L'Homme et ses Symboles.* Paris: Robert Laffont.

Kahill, S. (1988). Interventions for burnout in the helping professions: A review of the empirical evidence. *Canadian Journal of Counseling Review, 22*(3), 310-342.

Larson, D. (1986). Developing effective hospice staff support groups: A pilot test. *Hospice Journal, 2*(2), 41-55.

Lattanzi-Licht, M. (1995). Professional stress: Creating a context for caring. In C. Figley (Ed.), *Compassion Fatigue: Coping With Secondary Traumatic Stress in Those Who Treat the Traumatized* (pp. 486-525). New York: Brunner/Mazel.

Lazarus, R., & Folkman, S. (1984). *Stress, Appraisal, and Coping.* New York: Springer.

Leighton, S., & Koye, A. (1984). Prevention and self care for professional burnout. *Family and Community Health, 6*(4), 44-56.

Martin, C., & Julian, R. (1987). Causes of stress and burnout in physicians caring for the chronically and terminally ill. *The Hospice Journal, 3*(2), 121-146.

Maslach, C. (1982). *Burnout - The Costs of Caring.* Englewood Cliffs, NJ: Prentice-Hall.

Masterson-Allen, S., Mor, V., Laliberte, L., & Monteiro, L. (1985). Staff burnout in a hospice setting. *The Hospice Journal, 1*(3), 1-15.

McCann, I., Sakheim, D., & Abrahamson, D. (1988). Trauma and victimization: A model of psychological adaptation. *Counseling Psychologist, 16*(4), 531-594.

McIntosh, T. (1991). Identification and investigation of properties of social support. *Journal of Organizational Behavior, 12,* 201-217.

Mileti, D., Drabek, T., & Haas, J. (1975). *Human Systems in Extreme Environments.* Boulder: University of Colorado, Institute of Behavioral Science.

Moyers, B. (1993). *Healing and the Mind.* New York: Doubleday.

Munley, A. (1983). *The Hospice Alternative.* New York: Basic Books.

Pearlman, L., & Saakvitne, K. (1995). Treating therapists with vicarious traumatization and secondary traumatic stress disorders. In C. Figley (Ed.), *Compassion Fatigue: Coping With Secondary Traumatic Stress in Those Who Treat the Traumatized* (pp. 380-421). New York: Brunner/Mazel.

Rando, T. (1986). *Loss and Anticipatory Grief.* Lexington, KY: Lexington Books.

Raphael, B. (1984). *The Anatomy of Bereavement.* London: Hutchinson Publishers.

Riordan, R., & Saltzer, S. (1992). Burnout prevention among health care providers working with the terminally ill: A literature review. *Omega, 25*(1), 17-24.

Schieber, S. (1983). Emotional problems in physicians: Nature and extent of problems. In S. C. Schieber & B. B. Doyle (Eds.), *The Impaired Physician* (pp. 3-10). New York: Plenum.

Schmale, A. (1972). Giving up as a final common pathway to changes in health. *Advances in Psychosomatic Medicine, 8,* 20-40.

Thacker, J. (1984). Using psychodrama to reduce burnout or role fatigue in the helping professions. *Journal of Group Psychotherapy, Psychodrama, and Sociometry, 37*(1), 14-26.

Tivers, R. (1971). The evolution of reciprocal altruism. *Quarterly Review in Biology, 46,* 35-57.

Valent, P. (1995). Survival strategies: A framework for understanding secondary traumatic stress and coping in helpers. In C. R. Figley (Ed.), *Compassion Fatigue: Coping With Secondary Traumatic Stress in Those Who Treat the Traumatized* (pp. 245-261). New York: Brunner/Mazel.

Wakefield, D. (1998, April 15). Creativity doesn't belong solely to artists. *Bottom Line,* p. 9.

Webster's Encyclopedic Unabridged Dictionary of the English Language. (1989). New York: Gramercy Press.

Winnecott, D. (1964). *The Child, the Family, and the Outside World.* Reading, MA: Addison-Wesley.

A Simple Technique to Aid in the Assessment of Resistant Children

Susan K. Skinner and Paul C. Guthrie

Completing a battery of tests is often a challenge for professionals working with resistant children. A technique that breaks down a battery of tests into visible steps with ongoing feedback is effective in completing needed procedures. This technique has been found to be effective with children identified as having Attention-Deficit/Hyperactivity and Oppositional Defiant Disorders, with very young children who have no intrinsic interest in test procedures or in examiner authority, and with children who have severe communication limitations. Practitioners can replicate and adapt this technique for a variety of children's needs.

INTRODUCTION

The difficulties involved in the psychological assessment of resistant children are well known to child psychologists. Children with Attention-Deficit/Hyperactivity Disorder (ADHD) and/or Oppositional Defiant Disorder are among those frequently referred for testing. Also frequently referred are children with communication difficulties and young children with varied special needs. Sattler (1992) listed "inability to focus, sustain, and organize attention, and to inhibit impulsive responding" (p. 625) in his discussion of the assessment of ADHD children. The presence of oppositionality only adds to these difficulties. Communication disabilities interfere with a clinician's ability to reason with, bargain with, or reassure a child in testing, and very young children often have no interest in attending to the usually structured tasks required by test protocols. The conundrum for clinicians, however, is that those children who are most difficult to test are those who are most likely to require assessment services. Assessment of intellectual functioning, academic skills, personality characteristics, and adaptive living skills are only a few of the areas that may need to be assessed in order to make decisions regarding differential diagnosis, treatment, and placement. This multitude of questions frequently results in the need to administer a time-consuming battery of tests, which can present a distinct challenge in maintaining the attention and motivation of resistant children.

The frequent necessity of performing multiple tests on this population has resulted in the development by the authors of a number of strategies designed to maximize motivation, participation, and persistence in the assessment task. Typically, these approaches include breaking the battery into time-limited substeps and providing frequent reinforcement throughout and upon completion of the battery. In addition, every clinician who evaluates these children has probably developed techniques of his or her own to facilitate the process with greater or lesser success. These techniques are notably absent in the testing literature, however, as a computer search yielded no information on this topic. Literature with regard to behavioral and emotional characteristics and treatment methods abounds, yet no information addressing methods for engaging such children in necessarily structured assessments was identified.

The following is a technique that has proven to be helpful in maintaining the interest and participation level of oppositional defiant children on numerous occasions. Its development was preceded by numerous evaluation sessions with findings being "unable to test." These outcomes were unsatisfactory to parents, other services involved with the children, and the authors. The technique will be described first, with two examples of its use to follow.

TESTING PROCEDURE

The first step in this technique is to break down the test battery into its component parts. On a piece of paper, usually titled "JOBS," tasks are enumerated for the child to see. In this way, the child has a visual representation of the task at hand. Upon completion of each task, the child places a check mark next to the appropriate number. He or she receives generous praise for completion of each task and a reminder of the reinforcement to be received at the completion of the battery. The child thus receives reinforcement, tangible evidence of progress (and evidence that the battery is not, in fact, interminable), and a reminder of reinforcement yet to come. For a battery of tests, representing each test with a number is helpful. For a single test comprised of subtests, enumerating each subtest is usually effective. The number lists, with no task descriptions are used because written language is typically of no more interest to these children than spoken language. Our experience is that children who are otherwise difficult to keep on task usually respond well to this technique, and the testing process is made substantially less onerous for all involved. The use of this technique and specific case examples in clinical settings will be described next.

CASE EXAMPLES*

Example A

The client in this case is a 6-year-old boy who had previously been diagnosed as having a bilateral, moderately severe, sensorineural hearing loss. He had been fitted with hearing aids, to which he was reported to have trouble adjusting. He had been evaluated as functioning within the Well Below Average range of intelligence in both verbal and nonverbal areas and evidenced disruptive classroom behaviors, inattention, and aggression. He was referred by his public school to rule out the possibility of a serious emotional disturbance.

The check mark system was used in this evaluation in an effort to minimize the client's distractibility and impulsivity. First, the child was informed that there were six activities that needed to be completed. The numbers one through six were then placed in a column on a piece of paper. He was told that he would be allowed to check off each task when it was complete, and then when all the tasks were done, he would earn a sticker. The sticker used was the child-oriented kind commonly available in grocery stores and discount stores. This client, like the others with whom this technique has been used, seemed to enjoy and respond well to this approach. Although distractibility and impulsivity were clearly not eliminated, the client was motivated to give his best effort. The check-off sheet used with this child can be seen in Figure 1 (p. 457).

The examiner made the first check mark, and the remainder were made by the child. It is interesting to note the deterioration in the client's check marks, which reflect his gradual loss of control over the course of the testing session.

Example B

The second example is an 11-year-old girl who had been diagnosed with Attention-Deficit/Hyperactivity Disorder, Combined Type, and Oppositional Defiant Disorder. This child was being evaluated for specialized school services. All previous attempts to administer standardized tests had required multiple sessions, with brief sessions being held over several days. The youngster was both unable and unwilling to remain seated and attend to instructions. She also showed no desire to earn praise from the examiner. In this case, use of the

*Identifying characteristics in all case examples have been changed to protect confidentiality.

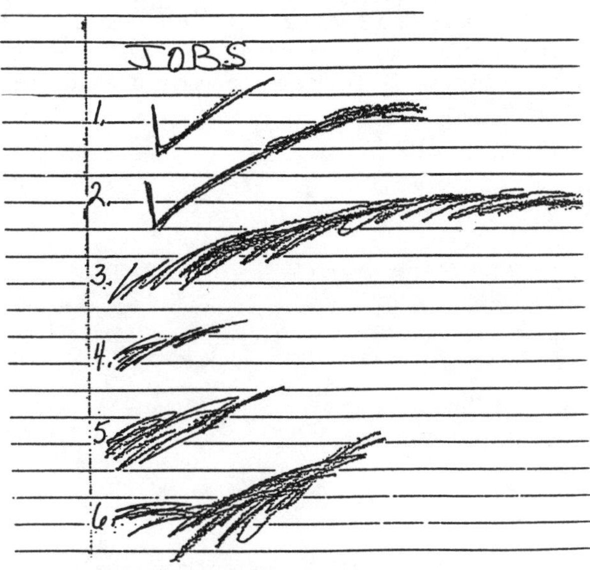

Figure 1. Checklist Technique Used With 6-Year-Old Child.

checklist enabled testing to be completed in one 2-hour session. The child was still restless and needed frequent reminders to attend, but she remained sufficiently cooperative to complete the battery in a much more timely manner than was typically the case. In addition, she was observed to be sufficiently involved with test tasks for the examiner to be able to accept the test results as valid estimates of her abilities.

The check mark system may also be useful in testing preschoolers, who are often unimpressed with the need for formal assessment. Check marks in different colors, paired with enthusiastic applause, have been observed to increase the motivation and cooperation of children as young as 3 or 4 in the administration of developmental tests. Interestingly, young deaf children respond as well to the checklist/applause combination as young hearing children.

SUMMARY

This technique is offered as a suggestion for improving the assessment of resistant children. The specifics of its use will, of course, depend on the specific assessment tasks to be used and the characteristics of the child. Children with emotional disturbances, autism, mental retardation, and deafness also represent potential target populations for whom use of this technique would aid in the assessment process.

CONTRIBUTORS

Susan K. Skinner, PhD, is currently Program Director of the Deaf Outreach Center, Arkansas Rehabilitation Services, in Little Rock, Arkansas. She also maintains a part-time private practice. Dr. Skinner has published research in the area of assessment of children who are deaf and has presented numerous workshops on assessment of individuals with hearing disabilities. Dr. Skinner may be contacted at Deaf Outreach Center, 4601 West Markham Street, Little Rock, AR 72205.

Paul C. Guthrie, PhD, is currently an Associate Professor of Psychology at Midwestern State University in Wichita Falls, Texas. He also maintains a private practice and is a consultant to the Helen Farabee Mental Health Retardation Center and the Wichita Falls State Hospital. Dr. Guthrie has published research in the area of personality assessment and is currently involved in collaborative research on the changing nature of psychology curricula. Dr. Guthrie can be contacted at Midwestern State University, Department of Psychology, Wichita Falls, TX 76308.

RESOURCE

Sattler, J. M. (1992). *Assessment of Children* (3rd ed.). San Diego: Author.

Marital and Sexuality Issues In Clients With Disabilities

Martin G. Brodwin and Roy K. Chen

The purpose of this contribution is to introduce clinicians to the concepts of sexuality and intimacy concerning people who have physical disabilities. This contribution is limited to a discussion of individuals who have physical disabilities, although many of the concepts and discussion also relate to persons with other kinds of disabilities. The professional literature seldom discusses the subjects of sexuality, intimacy, and marriage as related to people with disabilities. The limited information that is published is found primarily within rehabilitation and disability resources and not usually in psychology-specific journals and books.

Historically, as early as the 1910s, several federally funded vocational training and placement programs were developed to cope with both the surging numbers of injured veterans returning from World War I and disabled workers suffering from industry-related accidents and illnesses during the peak of the second industrial revolution. Despite passage of rehabilitation-oriented acts, such as the Smith-Hughes Act of 1917 and the Soldier Rehabilitation Act of 1918, the social climate in which people with disabilities lived was far from accepting (Danek et al., 1996; Jenkins, Patterson, & Szymanski, 1998). People with disabilities faced patterns of oppressive treatment similar to that faced by ethnic minority groups.

Since enactment of the Americans With Disabilities Act (ADA) in 1990, persons with disabilities have become more visible in all aspects of American society; clinicians are seeing these individuals in their offices with increasing frequency. Familiarity with disability-related issues will help professionals more effectively treat clients who have disabilities and chronic, debilitating illnesses. The ADA prohibits discrimination against persons with disabilities in virtually every aspect of society, including employment, housing, transportation, telecommunications, and accessibility to public facilities (restaurants, all retail establishments, hotels, libraries, museums, and schools, to name a few). Throughout history, persons with disabilities have been segregated physically and isolated socially from mainstream society; the ADA is a legislative attempt to at least partially remedy this situation. This legislation is a turning point in public policy away from the federal government as caretaker for persons with disabilities toward empowerment, including the assurance of individual rights and full participation in mainstream society. We have seen a more positive and enlightened attitude toward people with disabilities since passage and enactment of the ADA. As stated by Dart and West (1995), the ADA has often been described as the emancipation proclamation for persons who have disabilities, comparable in significance to the Civil Rights Act of 1964 for cultural minorities in this country.

MISCONCEPTIONS AND ASSUMPTIONS REGARDING DISABILITY

Intrapersonal and interpersonal misconceptions that may impede the emotional and social development of persons with disabilities include the following (Vargo, 1987, 1989):

1. My disability is a punishment.
2. All of my difficulties are caused by my disability.
3. Asking for help is a sign of personal weakness.
4. It is impossible for a person with a disability to be happy.
5. I am of less value as a person because I am not able-bodied.
6. No one can possibly understand how I feel.
7. I cannot continue to live like this.
8. I cannot do things the way I used to, so why do anything at all.
9. I could never succeed in anything.
10. Life cannot possibly be fulfilling for me.

Research has shown that it is the limitations in social-role performance, not the extent of a disability, that lowers life satisfaction among people with disabilities (Atkinson & Hackett, 1998; Nosek, Fuhrer, & Potter, 1995).

Fine and Asch (1988) outlined this set of incorrect and misleading assumptions about disability made by others and by people with disabilities:

1. Disability is a biological condition that is synonymous with the person and therefore the cause of others' behaviors and attitudes.
2. Problems encountered by the person with a disability are a result of the disability.
3. People with disabilities are "victims."
4. The disability of the person is central to his or her self-definition, social comparison, and reference group.
5. Disability is synonymous with needing help and social support.

Based on current research, there is a trend toward more positive attitudes toward people with disabilities. Notwithstanding, "the acceptance and integration of people with disabilities continues to be limited by the negative attitudes, misconceptions, and prejudicial stereotypes of health professionals, employers, coworkers, educators, peers, and neighbors" (Antonak & Livneh, 1995, p. 3). Hahn (1988) suggested that rather than looking at a disability as a tragic fate, people with disabilities could view their disabilities as opportunities to effect changes in the meaning of their lives. He noted that very few people in history have taken advantage of such an opportunity for life satisfaction.

SOCIETAL ATTITUDES TOWARD DISABILITY

From the beginning of time, Western civilization has defined its standard of beauty and health by the image of an impeccable and physically fit body. The obsession with a tall, slim, and beautiful appearance is exemplified by adoration of mythical characters such as Apollo and Venus. Unfortunately, the inner beauty of people with physical disabilities is often overshadowed by a less attractive outer appearance. Research has shown that attitudes toward individuals with disabilities are typically negative and often block accessibility to opportunities available to physically nondisabled people (Gething, LaCour, & Wheeler, 1994; Yuker, 1995). Both mainstream white culture and minority cultures perceive persons with disabilities as weak, unattractive, and undesirable. Among Americans, the social stigma attached to disability partially depends on whether or not the disabled individual is perceived as being responsible for his or her own state of limitation (Chubon, 1994; Fine & Asch, 1988). For example, people tend to be more tolerant of mental retardation and less sympathetic toward drug abuse or alcohol-caused disabilities. Thus, an individual who has a physical disability will tend to be viewed more positively if that person is perceived as not having caused or contributed to the disability.

Studies have demonstrated that women with disabilities are more likely to be stigmatized than their male counterparts (Danek, 1992; Lloyd, 1992). An Australian university study asked 80 undergraduate students their opinions about social issues related to sexuality and disability (Chandani, McKenna, & Maas, 1989). These researchers discovered significant nonacceptance of the sexuality of women with disabilities as compared to nondisabled women. Solomon (1993) found that women with disabilities were devalued and marginalized in American culture, often being ostracized, neglected, and harassed. A woman of minority ethnicity with a disability endures threefold discrimination. She is devalued by the stereotypes associated with her gender, minority status, and negative attitudes toward her disability. "Denial of a woman's sexuality is denial of her very humanness, and may negatively affect her view of herself as well as her place in the world" (M. G. Brodwin, Parker, & DeLaGarza, 1996, p. 172). Atkinson and Hackett (1998) found that persons with disabilities have lower incomes and face higher rates of unemployment and underemployment than do persons without disabilities. This is true to an even greater extent for persons with disabilities belonging to minority cultures, and for women. In a sense, a person with a disability from a minority background faces "double" discrimination, where a minority woman with a disability, as discussed previously, may encounter "triple" discrimination (M. G. Brodwin, Hong, & Soriano, 1992).

Livneh (1991) suggested that the sight of a person with a mobility limitation or a physical abnormality rekindles anxiety and fear associated with death. Disability reminds us how fragile human life is, and that it can be taken away or altered by unforeseen illnesses or accidents. Being unable to move at will or control undesirable movements leads to devaluation from society. To nondisabled people, the possibility of loss of body function due to accidents and chronic, debilitating illnesses invokes great anxiety and fear. Through the defense mechanism of denial, some people may unconsciously choose to be hostile toward individuals with disabilities as a means to hide their insecurity and to confirm their belief in personal superiority.

Yuker (1992, 1995) stated that attitudes are, in great measure, a function of the variables of contact, information, and role characteristics, as well as the attitudinal norms of the environment. Positive attitudes from people with disabilities usually result in warm feelings and positive interactions and behaviors from others, while negative attitudes usually result in bias and discrimination. Negative societal attitudes result in the creation of barriers that impede persons with disabilities from full participation in that society. Past interaction with persons with disabilities affects one's attitudes. Interaction that has been personal, rewarding, and characterized by cooperation and intimacy tends to provide positive information and to result in positive attitudes. People with close friends or associates who have disabilities typically have positive attitudes.

In a study published in 1989, Vargo reviewed research on attitudes of the general public toward persons with disabilities. This review found that the more industrialized a culture is, the more accepting it is of people with disabilities. On the other hand, the more agrarian the culture, the less tolerant it is of people with disabilities. This researcher also found that, in cultures where women are assigned low status, women with disabilities face far more serious obstacles than women without disabilities or men with disabilities.

REACTIONS TO DISABILITY BY PEOPLE WITH DISABILITIES

Due to the stigmatizing effects of disability in society, many people with disabilities tend to develop negative feelings about their own disabilities. When a physical disability is acquired, there is considerable resistance to the sudden change of body image which may damage and debase one's self-esteem (Schilder, 1964). Rubin and Roessler (1995) noted that denial of the alteration of body image is a common defense mechanism used by people with disabilities to fend off the devaluation imposed on them. Other defensive reactions include overdependency, withdrawal, aggression, and secondary gain through manipulation. Robinault (1978) noticed a similar pattern of reaction to the sudden onset of a disability; many individuals claimed they would rather die than be dependent on others for their basic needs. Although a person with a disability can find the courage and energy to cope with physical or mental limitations most of the time, there are times the individual has difficulty coping. Even a great and wise man such as Franklin Delano Roosevelt went to great lengths to shield his disability from the American public. Of the hundreds of official pictures taken while he was already in office as the 32nd president, only a few showed him using a wheelchair. It is not known why President Roosevelt hid his disability; possible reasons that have been postulated include concerns about national security, feelings of personal maladjustment, or living in an unsympathetic social climate that devalues people who have disabilities.

Although some remain bitter and fail to acquire the necessary coping skills to accommodate their disability, not all people with disabilities react negatively. Goffman (1963) noted that stigmatized individuals may avoid interaction with other people because they are uncertain as to nondisabled individuals' acceptance or rejection of people who have disabilities. He also stated that disabled people vacillate between hostile and bravado attitudes toward the world as a reaction to the differing attitudes and behaviors of able-bodied groups. Weinberg (1984) found that it takes time for people with disabilities to come to terms with their physical conditions. Despite having to learn to use wheelchairs, become knowledgeable about assistive equipment, or have personal attendants to compensate for their impairments, persons with disabilities felt adjusting to societal attitudes was the most difficult. Vash (1981, 1994), in discussions of the psychology of disability and psychospiritual aspects of rehabilitation, noted that some individuals embrace their disabilities for various reasons such as God's intervention or fate. Depending on the locus of control by which a person with a disability operates, some will forever be depressed, blaming the world and the people around them for their perceived suffering. Others will internalize the ideal of becoming a "complete" person by taking responsibility for ensuring better outcomes for their own lives.

If persons with disabilities have positive attitudes toward their disabilities (self-acceptance, disability acknowledgment, and disclosure), this often has a positive effect on the attitudes and actions of others toward them. Further, persons with disabilities who have good social skills are positively evaluated by others. When others perceive interaction with persons with disabilities as personal, rewarding, and characterized by cooperation, intimacy, and equal status, positive attitudes and behaviors are the result. Research (Yuker, 1992, 1995) has shown that attitudes are largely a function of the variables of contact, information, role characteristics, and the attitudinal norms of the environment.

DISABILITY AND SEXUALITY

As previously noted, there is a lack of information on the subject of disability and sexuality. Persons with disabilities have generally been perceived as nonsexual beings, incapable of achieving and maintaining intimate relationships with other people. Adjustment and adaptation to a physical disability recently acquired is a gradual process. To the extent that a person learns to value new sexual capabilities and establishes positive levels of communication, the individual will begin to attain a satisfying and more fulfilling sexual adjustment (Ducharme, 1993, 1995).

Perhaps the most important single variable in adjustment is communicating one's sexual needs and desires. Psychological considerations and physical functioning are equally important. "Usually, people will indicate their readiness by asking questions regarding attractiveness, dating, relationships, and intimacy" (Ducharme, 1995, p. 670). Clinicians need an awareness of this as they counsel persons with disabilities. Restrictions on the expression of sexuality originate from cultural biases, social ignorance, and unfounded fears regarding persons with disabilities.

Physical disability can affect individual sexuality in other ways. As related by Chubon (1994), the mere presence of a physical disability sometimes has a "desexing" effect on individuals. The portrayal of sex in the media is that of a human quality that borders on perfection, reserved for the young and beautiful. Persons viewed as unattractive and weak are often considered lacking in sexuality. Because people with physical disabilities have less than this perfect body image, frequently they are considered nonsexual beings and rejected as potential mates.

A physical disability may affect the ability to function sexually. One needs an awareness and knowledge of compensatory or alternative techniques. Without a good understanding, the individual may come to erroneous conclusions regarding interpersonal relationships, marriage, and parenthood, and these may be adversely affected. Positive family support may affect adjustment; the best measure of adjustment may be self-esteem and the ability to maintain satisfying relationships (Chubon, 1994; Kelley & Lambert, 1992).

Boyle (1998) provided some common sense guidelines for rehabilitation professionals addressing sexuality issues and concerns with clients who have disabilities. These guidelines apply to all mental health clinicians who work with disability issues.

1. Counselors need to sincerely believe that sexuality is a valid and important rehabilitation issue.
2. Professionals should have come to terms with their own sexuality.
3. Counselors must learn to accept and appreciate sexual lifestyles very different from their own.
4. Counselors need to be sensitive, but direct, about issues of sexuality.
5. A sense of humor about sexuality can serve both professional and client well.
6. Counselors should not expect their counseling efforts in the area of sexuality to be a "quick-fix" for rehabilitation clients.

DATING AND MARRIAGE

In medieval times, love was not seen as a reason for marriage (Murstein, 1976). The freedom of women to choose a marriage partner was curtailed, largely due to their illiteracy and financial dependency. Before the early 1900s, the sole function of dating was to select a suitable marriage partner. Adolescents started to date as soon as they entered puberty, between the ages of 12 and 16. Dating today is more for enjoyment and provides an informal social environment for young people to explore the dynamics of interpersonal relationships (Cobb, 1995).

Marriage is both an emotional and a legal bond between two persons. It serves as a shelter for a person, especially during times of emotional stress. According to Horenstein (1974), there are three bases for marriage: sexual gratification, companionship, and reproduction. For a marriage to last, he believed that at least two of these components must be present. In the conventional institution of marriage, the union of a man and a woman is seen as the plateau of commitment to a relationship. Yet, there are other reasons people get married. Steward (1964) stated that the most important reason for wanting a marriage is the desire for companionship with a person of the opposite sex. People also marry to gain financial support, to escape from an unhappy home, and as a safeguard against loneliness.

Heterosexual relationships are not the sole form of interpersonal attraction. As more and more famous celebrities reveal their sexual orientation, gay and lesbian relationships have gained wider acceptance. Despite the gradual subsidence of homophobia over the last few decades, disabled individuals with a same-gender sexual orientation are intimidated from expressing their true sexuality. Wohlander and Petal (1985) estimated that there are about 3 million people with disabilities whose sexual orientation is same-gender, many of whom find they need to hide their sexual preferences. Yet, keeping one's true sexual identity secret can result in heightened emotional tension and anxiety.

INTERPERSONAL ATTRACTION AND INTIMACY

Attraction and intimacy are central factors in all interpersonal relationships. Because of societal attitudes toward persons with disabilities, these factors become even more central in relationships where one of the partners has a physical disability. E. Walster and G. Walster (1976) defined interpersonal attraction as "an individual's tendency or predisposition to evaluate another person or symbol of that person in a positive way" (p. 280). Berscheid and E. Walster (1978) discussed three interesting features that reflect how much one person is attracted to another. First, individuals tend to avoid eye contact with somebody with whom they are not comfortable, but will look people they like directly in the eye, longer and more often. Secondly, body posture and distance can serve as a gauge to show the desire for closeness to another person. People have a tendency to lean toward and stand closer to individuals they like and lean away from individuals they dislike. Individuals are more likely to do favors for those in whom they take an interest and to react less warmly toward those for whom they do not genuinely care.

Masters, Johnson, and Kolodny (1995) identified several of the components of interpersonal intimacy, including caring, trust, commitment, sharing, honesty, empathy, and tenderness. Intimacy is not a discrete event and takes time to develop (Burling, Tarvydas, & Maki, 1994). The willingness to self-disclose feelings to one's partner is vital to the growth of an intimate and trusting relationship. Cohesion develops when two individuals in a relationship discover their similar feelings and are willing to share their "ups and downs" (G. Corey & M. S. Corey, 1997). Intimacy does not, however, mean that two people involved in the relationship must share the same interests and always agree with each other.

People tend to change over time, and their values have to adjust to new norms and social trends. It is unrealistic to expect that emotional passion for the other person will not fade as time and outside influences affect the relationship. External factors such as illness, work, and family all exert strong pressure on the two partners' internal worlds. The degree of willingness to resolve problems depends on each partner's commitment. Moreover, without continued empathy and understanding, both partners may fail to continue relating to each other and gradually drift apart.

PARTNER SELECTION THEORIES

Social psychologists have conducted much empirical research on mate selection preference. With very few exceptions, men look more for superficial attributes when it comes to choosing a partner for intimate involvement. Studies have demonstrated that males are strongly drawn to physically attractive women (Bernstein et al., 1983; Huston, 1973). Sprecher, Sullivan, and Hatfield (1994) found that men gave more weight than women to factors such as physical attractiveness and youth, across all age groups and races. Keller and Young (1996) determined that similar physical traits are usually the first criteria people use to choose compatible partners. The selection process becomes more complicated when factors such as social and economic status are taken into consideration. Partner selection theory plays a significant role when one of the individuals in the relationship has a disability. This is due, in part, to the importance of physical attractiveness when seeking intimate relationships, especially for men in this country. Someone with good social attributes is more likely to end up with a potential partner of comparable qualities.

DISABILITY AND MARRIAGE

Isolation and loneliness are two stressful aspects of life that are accentuated when a person has a disability. When it comes to marriage, the disabled population has as much a right as any other group to be autonomous in making marital choices. When two persons decide to live together and share their lives, whether through marriage or cohabitation without marriage, the underlying need is the sense of belonging to a mate, a major function of marriage (DeLoach & Greer, 1981; Lim-Kee, 1994).

Researchers have conducted studies to dispel the myth that people with disabilities have no interest in having relationships with the opposite sex. Cromer et al. (1990) administered the Offer Self-Image Questionnaire for Adolescents (Cromer et al., 1990) to a group of 58 teenagers with chronic disabilities to assess their knowledge, attitudes, and behavior related to sexuality and marriage. The results showed that an overwhelming 88% of the respondents expressed a desire to marry. Additionally, individuals with less severe disabilities seemed to have more knowledge about sexuality than their counterparts who had more limited body functions.

Although the general public is more accepting of persons with disabilities as colleagues or casual friends, people are hesitant to perceive individuals with disabilities as potential dating or marriage partners (DeLoach, 1994; Kelly, 1996). Myths, prejudice, and misunderstandings of disabling conditions continue to make people shy away from intimate relationships with persons who have disabilities. Kroll and Klein (1995) believed that the most difficult challenge in a relationship in which one partner has a disability and the other does not is the constant negative experiences the couple encounter in society. Discouragement becomes a common deterrent to development of a potential relationship. This is particularly true at the beginning stages of a relationship, when its development is under scrutiny by people around the couple.

REASONS PERSONS WITH DISABILITIES OFTEN REMAIN SINGLE

Intermarriage between persons with disabilities and nondisabled people is rare; even when it does occur, the able-bodied marriage partner usually is assumed to have a "lesser" value (i.e., earning less, being less educated, or perceived as less attractive). A nondisabled person who forms a relationship with a person with a disability may be incorrectly interpreted by society as psychologically maladjusted. A fear of ostracism also discourages interaction between these two groups. However, to say that all rejections of disabled individuals by people without disabilities are due to a lack of physical attraction does not present the entire picture. A high level of anxiety, strong need for social approval, poor self-concept, and ethnocentrism are some factors that lead to nonacceptance of persons with disabilities (Lim-Kee, 1994; Livneh, 1982, 1991; Smith-Hanen, 1976).

Self-Concept

Evans and Conine (1985) indicated that chronic illness and disabling conditions inevitably delay the normal sexual development of youngsters, resulting in an impaired sense of self. Confusion over sexual feelings caused by delayed psychosocial development often leads to low self-esteem. This postponement validates their inability to assume proper social roles. An inferiority complex can be internalized by a person with a disability after having many negative, unpleasant social experiences. Deviation from a normal body image receives little acceptance or tolerance in the mainstream media; as a consequence, frequent traumatizing rejections erode the ego. Some individuals with disabilities would rather stay single than date or marry another person with a disability for fear that the countertransference of a disabled image may be too painful.

Family

Children with congenital disabilities are more susceptible to health perils and social rejection. Parents have a tendency to shield these children, both emotionally and physically, from feeling vulnerable. Overprotection out of concern for the child's safety typically has an adverse influence on psychosexual development. Children or youth with congenital or acquired disabilities of early onset do not have the chance to experience the stages of growth in a "normal" way; immaturity is a common characteristic of the personality of persons with disabilities, both in casual social interaction and in more intimate relationships. Parents or guardians of children with disabilities must educate them on how to handle sexuality in an appropriate manner (Best, 1993; Robinault, 1978; Roland, 1999).

Culture

Reincarnation is the supreme belief of Buddhism and other non-Judeo-Christian religions in many parts of the non-Western world. In some Eastern cultures, disability is believed to be a punishment from God to an individual and his or her family for sins committed in this life or even in previous lives. The concept of karma in the Hindu culture attributes a life of suffering in the present to sins committed in a former life. One can imagine how a person with a disability feels serving a "sentence" for a crime which he or she, or someone in the family, had presumably committed hundreds or thousands of years ago. According to ancient Chinese folklore, there are 18 courts in purgatory to judge a person who passes on. An evil individual's spirit will be interrogated and tortured for bad deeds committed during his or her lifetime. A thief will be reincarnated without arms, a mute is paying the price for lying too much, and a bald person for ridiculing shaven-headed monks and nuns. The stigma attached to this kind of religious belief condemns interaction between able-bodied and disabled persons. Under no circumstance is a person with a disability an ideal candidate for marriage considering these religious beliefs (Arokiasamy, Rubin, & Roessler, 1995; M. G. Brodwin et al., 1992; Fine & Asch, 1988).

Early Abandonment

Attitudes of ancient civilizations were far from compassionate. In the early Greek and Roman eras, children born with disabilities were subject to infanticide; in Sparta, the immature, weak, and "damaged" were eliminated purposefully (Arokiasamy et al., 1995).

Child neglect and abuse occur with much greater frequency for children with all kinds of disabilities when compared to nondisabled children (Carter, 1999; Chubon, 1994). Growing up in an abandoned and unloving environment, children with disabilities may never have been exposed to nurturing and warm parents. It is very likely for them to think they will not be able to become good parents; as a result, they may choose not to marry. Fears of attachment and intimacy with other people are results of the continuing rejection and neglect they endure in an indifferent and cold atmosphere. Lutfiyya (1997) stated that if people with disabilities are to form friendships and be a part of society as adults, relationships must begin to develop during the early school years. Unfortunately, despite the mainstreaming and integration of children with disabilities at school, children with disabilities make few nondisabled friends. As long as children with disabilities are seen as having severe limitations and complex deficiencies, without provided support, they are vulnerable to a return to a more segregated and restricted environment (Walker & Shoultz, 1997). Aside from family members and care providers, individuals with disabilities may have no freely given and chosen relationships (Lutfiyya, 1997). Emotional barriers become difficult to remove; the passage and enactment of protective laws has lessened discrimination but may not ease the feeling of isolation and loneliness among many people with disabilities.

Heredity

Disabilities can be grouped into two major categories based on their cause: congenital and acquired. How disabled persons construct their schema or worldview can be determined in part by the nature of the disability. A person with a genetic defect (e.g., neuromuscular disease or deafness) will be aware of the danger of conceiving a similarly disabled child. Having gone through so much hardship in life, a person with a disability may have concerns about having children who may have to endure similar hardships. In comparison, a person who has lost a limb in an accident, for example, will more likely consider having children.

Other Factors

Both men and women appreciate physical attractiveness because individuals with beauty are assumed to possess admirable qualities such as intelligence, kindness, and honesty. "Image is everything" has become a way of life in American culture. This notion carries more weight than "beauty is in the eye of the beholder" or "beauty is only skin deep." People with altered body images thus can be left out of the process of mate selection. Similar to animals, human mate selection is programmed by one's preferences; only the supposedly fittest will survive the elimination process (S. K. Brodwin, Orange, & M. G. Brodwin, 1994; Kammerer-Quayle, 1993; Kerckhoff & Davis, 1962).

Institutional settings are not conducive to socialization among clients with disabilities, because privacy is often limited due to management and safety issues, as well as negative attitudes. The institutionalized population is therefore deprived of opportunities to make friends with the opposite sex because care providers can be overprotective and believe that people with disabilities are not capable of functioning independently and appropriately at a social level. Living in segregated settings, such as board and care facilities or convalescent hospitals, further decreases the opportunity to meet eligible partners (Webster, 1994). The chance of extending a relationship into a friendship with care providers is also minimal.

Transportation poses a problem for people with visual and ambulatory limitations who wish to date. Driving safety may prevent some people from possessing a driver's license. Not all public transit systems have wheelchair lifts; this certainly restricts freedom to travel. In addition, architectural barriers stand in the way; few places are designed for the participation of wheelchair users and other types of disabled people. If a person with a disability is confined to home or to a board and care facility, socialization is dramatically curtailed. Fortunately, with successful passage of the ADA in 1990, many of these architectural barriers are slowly but systematically being removed, allowing people with physical disabilities greater access to American society.

COPING SKILLS

Clinicians need familiarity with the coping skills that are used by individuals with disabilities in adjusting and adapting to their disabilities. The major skills were described by Moos and Schaeffer (1989) as follows:

1. *Logical Analysis and Mental Preparation.* This coping skill involves breaking down problems into manageable components, using mental testing for difficult problems, and drawing on prior experiences for resolving persistent problems.
2. *Cognitive Redefinition.* The individual alters his or her values and restructures the situation (e.g., "It could always be worse").
3. *Cognitive Avoidance or Denial.* These self-protective defense mechanisms are used as a temporary coping mechanism.
4. *Seeking Information and Support.* One learns about the condition and seeks help from family, friends, and community.
5. *Taking Problem-Solving Action.* The person learns specific skills to help in certain situations.
6. *Identifying Alternative Rewards.* This coping skill involves maintaining hope and controlling emotions.
7. *Emotional Discharge.* This includes the venting of anger and despair.
8. *Resigned Acceptance.* At this point, the person is able to accept "fate" and move on with life.

CONCLUSION

Through use of the information contained within this contribution, clinicians can develop greater knowledge of and sensitivity toward clients with disabilities, especially in the areas of intimacy and sexuality. With information in this area, mental health professionals can have a better understanding of their clients who express concerns in these areas. The clinician's psychological support, knowledge of information about sexuality and societal attitudes toward disability, and expressions of validation will enhance the client's sense of health and well being.

Martin G. Brodwin, PhD, CRC, is Professor and Coordinator of the Rehabilitation Education Programs at California State University, Los Angeles. He received his PhD in rehabilitation counseling from Michigan State University in East Lansing, Michigan, and became a certified rehabilitation counselor (CRC) in 1975. Currently, he serves on the Commission on Standards and Accreditation of the Council on Rehabilitation Education (CORE) and as a vocational expert for the Office of Hearings and Appeals of the Social Security Administration. His recent book, *Medical, Psychosocial, and Vocational Aspects of Disability,* is used in rehabilitation counseling graduate programs throughout the country. Dr. Brodwin may be contacted at California State University, Los Angeles, Division of Administration and Counseling, 5151 State University Drive, Los Angeles, CA 90032.

Roy K. Chen, MS, received his Master of Science degree in rehabilitation counseling from California State University, Los Angeles. Presently, he is a doctoral candidate in rehabilitation counseling at Michigan State University in East Lansing, Michigan. Mr. Chen also holds a Master of Business Administration (MBA) degree from Azusa Pacific University in Azusa, California. Areas that interest Mr. Chen include mental retardation, psychiatric disabilities, and cross-cultural issues. While a graduate student at California State University, Los Angeles, he was awarded the California State University Graduate Scholarship and the Barnes and Noble USA Academic Scholarship. Mr. Chen may be contacted at 10954 Ranchito Street, El Monte, CA 91731.

RESOURCES

Americans With Disabilities Act of 1990, 42 U.S.C. § 12101 *et seq.*

Antonak, R. F., & Livneh, H. (1995). Direct and indirect methods to measure attitudes toward persons with disabilities with an exegesis of the error-choice test method. *Rehabilitation Psychology, 40,* 3-24.

Arokiasamy, C. M. V., Rubin, S. E., & Roessler, R. T. (1995). Sociological aspects of disability. In S. E. Rubin & R. T. Roessler (Eds.), *Foundations of the Vocational Rehabilitation Process* (4th ed., pp. 123-155). Austin, TX: Pro-Ed.

Atkinson, D. R., & Hackett, G. (1998). *Counseling Diverse Populations* (2nd ed.). Boston: McGraw-Hill.

Bernstein, W., Stephenson, B., Snyder, M., & Wicklund, R. (1983). Casual ambiguity and heterosexual affiliation. *Journal of Experimental Social Psychology, 19,* 78-92.

Berscheid, E., & Walster, E. (1978). *Interpersonal Attraction.* Menlo Park, CA: Addison-Wesley.

Best, G. A. (1993). Sexuality and disability. In M. G. Brodwin, F. Tellez, & S. K. Brodwin (Eds.), *Medical, Psychosocial, and Vocational Aspects of Disability* (pp. 79-90). Athens, GA: Elliott and Fitzpatrick.

Boyle, P. S. (1998). Rehabilitation counselors as providers: The issue of sexuality. In D. R. Atkinson & G. Hackett, *Counseling Diverse Populations* (2nd ed., pp. 171-178). Boston: McGraw-Hill.

Brodwin, M. G., Hong, G. K., & Soriano, M. (1992). Discrimination, disability, and cultural considerations: Implications for counselors. *California Association for Counseling and Development Journal, 12,* 9-14.

Brodwin, M. G., Parker, R., & DeLaGarza, D. (1996). Disability and accommodation. In E. M. Symanski & R. M. Parker (Eds.), *Work and Disability: Issues and Strategies in Career Development and Job Placement* (pp. 165-207). Austin, TX: Pro-Ed.

Brodwin, S. K., Orange, L. M., & Brodwin, M. G. (1994). Disabled clients: What every therapist needs to know. In L. VandeCreek, S. Knapp, & T. L. Jackson (Eds.), *Innovations in Clinical Practice: A Source Book* (Vol. 13, pp. 419-430). Sarasota, FL: Professional Resource Press.

Burling, K., Tarvydas, V. M., & Maki, D. R. (1994). Human sexuality and disability: A holistic interpretation of rehabilitation counseling. *Journal of Applied Rehabilitation Counseling, 26*(3), 6-12.

Carter, B. (1999). Becoming parents: The family with young children. In B. Carter & M. McGoldrick (Eds.), *The Expanded Family Life Cycle: Individual, Family, and Social Perspectives* (3rd ed., pp. 249-273). Boston: Allyn and Bacon.

Chandani, A., McKenna, K., & Maas, F. (1989). Attitudes of university students toward physically disabled people. *British Journal of Occupational Therapy, 52*(6), 233-236.

Chubon, R. A. (1994). *Social and Psychological Foundations of Rehabilitation.* Springfield, IL: Charles C. Thomas.

Civil Rights Act of 1964, 42 U.S.C. § 2000 *et seq.*

Cobb, N. J. (1995). *Adolescence: Continuity, Change, and Diversity* (2nd ed.). Mountain View, CA: Mayfield.

Corey, G., & Corey, M. S. (1997). *I Never Knew I Had a Choice* (6th ed.). Pacific Grove, CA: Brooks/Cole.

Cromer, A., Enrile, B., McCoy, K., & Gerchardstein, M. J. (1990). Knowledge, attitudes and behavior related to sexuality in adolescents with chronic disability. *Developmental Medicine and Child Neurology, 32*(7), 602-610.

Danek, M. M. (1992). The status of women with disabilities revisited. *Journal of Applied Rehabilitation Counseling, 23,* 7-13.

Danek, M. M., Coyers, L. M., Enright, M. S., Munson, M., Brodwin, M., Hanley-Maxwell, C., & Gugerty, J. (1996). Legislation concerning career counseling and job placement for people with disabilities. In E. M. Szymanski & R. M. Parker (Eds.), *Work and Disability: Issues and Strategies in Career Development and Job Placement* (pp. 39-78). Austin, TX: Pro-Ed.

Dart, J., & West, J. (1995). Americans With Disabilities Act. In A. E. Dell Orto & R. P. Marinelli (Eds.), *Encyclopedia of Disability and Rehabilitation* (pp. 47-54). New York: Macmillan.

DeLoach, C. P. (1994). Attitudes toward disability: Impact on sexual development and forging intimate relationships. *Journal of Applied Rehabilitation Counseling, 25*(1), 18-25.

DeLoach, C. P., & Greer, B. G. (1981). *Adjustment to Severe Physical Disability: A Metamorphosis.* New York: McGraw-Hill.

Ducharme, S. H. (1993). Beyond the management of sexual problems: Creating a therapeutic environment for addressing sexuality issues. In C. J. Durgin, N. D. Schmidt, & L. J. Fryer (Eds.), *Staff Development and Clinical Intervention in Brain Injury Rehabilitation* (pp. 211-228). Gaithersburg, MD: Aspen.

Ducharme, S. H. (1995). Sexuality and disability. In A. E. Dell Orto & R. P. Marinelli (Eds.), *Encyclopedia of Disability and Rehabilitation* (pp. 668-673). New York: Macmillan.

Evans, J., & Conine, T. (1985). Sexual habilitation of youngsters with chronic illness or disabling conditions. *Journal of Allied Health, 14,* 79-87.

Fine, M., & Asch, A. (1988). Disability beyond stigma: Social interaction, discrimination, and activism. *Journal of Social Issues, 44,* 3-21.

Gething, L., LaCour, J., & Wheeler, B. (1994). Attitudes of nursing home administrators and nurses toward people with disabilities. *Journal of Rehabilitation, 60*(4), 66-70.

Goffman, E. (1963). *Stigma: Notes on the Management of Spoiled Identity.* Englewood, NJ: Prentice Hall.

Hahn, H. (1988). The politics of physical differences: Disability and discrimination. *Journal of Social Issues, 44,* 39-47.

Horenstein, S. (1974, June). *Sexuality and Multiple Sclerosis.* Report of the National Multiple Sclerosis Society Conference, St. Louis, MO.

Huston, T. (1973). Ambiguity of acceptance, social desirability, and dating choices. *Journal of Experimental Psychology, 9,* 32-42.

Jenkins, W., Patterson, J. B., & Szymanski, E. M. (1998). Philosophical, historical, and legislative aspects of the rehabilitation counseling profession. In R. M. Parker & E. M. Szymanski (Eds.), *Rehabilitation Counseling: Basics and Beyond* (3rd ed., pp. 1-40). Austin, TX: Pro-Ed.

Kammerer-Quayle, B. (1993). Image of people with visible disfigurement and disabilities. In M. G. Brodwin, F. Tellez, & S. K. Brodwin (Eds.), *Medical, Psychosocial, and Vocational Aspects of Disability* (pp. 139-150). Athens, GA: Elliott and Fitzpatrick.

Keller, M. C., & Young, R. K. (1996). Mate assortment in dating and married couples. *Personality and Individual Differences, 21*(2), 217-221.

Kelley, S. D., & Lambert, S. S. (1992). Family support in rehabilitation: A review of research 1980-1990. *Rehabilitation Counseling Bulletin, 36,* 98-119.

Kelly, G. F. (1996). *Sexuality Today: The Human Perspective* (5th ed.). Dubuque, IA: Brown and Benchmark.

Kerckhoff, A. C., & Davis, K. (1962). Value consigns and needs complementary in mate selection. *American Sociological Review, 27,* 295-303.

Kroll, K., & Klein, E. L. (1995). *Enabling Romance: A Guide to Love, Sex, and Relationships for the Disabled.* Bethesda, MD: First Woodbine House.

Lim-Kee, J. Y. (1994). Sexuality, marriage and disability. *International Journal of Adolescent Medicine and Health, 7*(3), 199-202.

Livneh, H. (1982). On the origins of negative attitudes toward people with disabilities. *Rehabilitation Literature, 43,* 338-347.

Livneh, H. (1991). On the origins of negative attitudes toward people with disabilities. In R. P. Marinelli & A. E. Dell Orto (Eds.), *The Psychological and Social Impact of Disability* (pp. 181-196). New York: Springer.

Lloyd, M. (1992). Does she boil eggs? Toward a feminist model of disability. *Disability, Handicap and Society, 7,* 207-221.

Lutfiyya, A. M. (1997, September-last update). The importance of friendship between people with and without mental retardation (Homepage of the ARC Organization) [On-line]. Available: http://www.thearc.org

Masters, W., Johnson, V., & Kolodny, R. (1995). *Human Sexuality* (5th ed.). New York: Harper Collins.

Moos, R. H., & Schaeffer, J. A. (1989). The crisis of physical illness: An overview and conceptual approach. In R. H. Moos (Ed.), *Coping With Physical Illness: New Perspectives* (Vol. 2, pp. 3-25). New York: Plenum.

Murstein, B. I. (1976). *Who Will Marry Whom?* New York: Springer.

Nosek, M. A., Fuhrer, M. J., & Potter, C. (1995). Life satisfaction of people with physical disabilities: Relationship to personal assistance, disability status, and handicap. *Rehabilitation Psychology, 40,* 191-202.

Robinault, I. P. (1978). *Sex, Society, and the Disabled: A Developmental Inquiry into Roles, Reactions, and Responsibilities.* Hagerstown, MD: Harper and Row.

Roland, J. S. (1999). Chronic illness and the family life cycle. In B. Carter & M. McGoldrick (Eds.), *The Expanded Family Life Cycle: Individual, Family, and Social Perspectives* (3rd ed., pp. 492-511). Boston: Allyn and Bacon.

Rubin, S. E., & Roessler, R. T. (1995). Rehabilitation clients and their needs. In S. Rubin & R. Roessler (Eds.), *Foundations of the Vocational Rehabilitation Process* (4th ed., pp. 175-208). Austin, TX: Pro-Ed.

Schilder, P. (1964). *Image and Appearance of the Human Body.* New York: Wiley.

Smith-Hanen, S. (1976). Socialization of the physically handicapped. *Journal of Applied Rehabilitation Counseling, 7*(3), 131-141.

Smith-Hughes Act of 1917, 20 U.S.C. § 11 *et seq.*

Soldier Rehabilitation Act of 1918, 40 Stat. 617.

Solomon, S. E. (1993). Women and physical distinction: A review of the literature and suggestions for intervention. *Women and Therapy, 14*(3/4), 91-103.

Sprecher, S., Sullivan, Q., & Hatfield, E. (1994). Mate selection preferences: Gender differences in a national sample. *Journal of Personality and Social Psychology, 66*(6), 1074-1080.

Steward, V. (1964). *Are They Qualified for Marriage?* Minneapolis, MN: T. S. Denison.

Vargo, J. W. (1987, August). *"And Sometimes I Wonder about Thee": A Misconception Hypothesis Approach to Viewing Attitudes Toward People With Disabilities.* Paper presented at the meeting of the Canadian Guidance and Counseling Association, Toronto, Ontario, Canada.

Vargo, J. W. (1989). "In the house of my friend": Dealing with disability. *International Journal for the Advancement of Counselling, 12,* 281-287.

Vash, C. (1981). *The Psychology of Disability.* New York: Springer.

Vash, C. (1994). *Personality and Adversity: Psychospiritual Aspects of Rehabilitation.* New York: Springer.

Walker, P., & Shoultz, B. (1997-copyright). Community Integration Report: Supporting children and youth with disabilities in integrated recreation and leisure activities (Homepage of the ARC Organization) [On-line]. Available: http://www.thearc.org

Walster, E., & Walster, G. (1976). Interpersonal attraction. In B. Seidenberg & A. Snadowsky (Eds.), *Social Psychology: An Introduction* (pp. 279-308). New York: Free Press.

Webster, S. K. (1994). A personal essay on sexuality and integration: Opportunity and challenge. *Journal of Applied Rehabilitation Counseling, 25*(1), 59-61.

Weinberg, A. N. (1984). Physically disabled people assess the quality of their lives. *Rehabilitation Literature, 45*(1-2), 12-15.

Wohlander, K., & Petal, M. (1985). People who are gay or lesbian and disabled. In H. Hildago, H. Peterson, & N. Woodman (Eds.), *Lesbian and Gay Issues: A Resource Manual for Social Workers* (pp. 59-73). Silver Spring, MD: National Association for Social Workers.

Yuker, H. E. (1992). Attitudes toward persons with disabilities: Conclusions from the data. *Rehabilitation Psychology News, 19*(2), 17-18.

Yuker, H. E. (1995). Attitudes. In A. E. Dell Orto & R. P. Marinelli (Eds.), *Encyclopedia of Disability and Rehabilitation* (pp. 94-99). New York: Macmillan.

Working With Marital Affairs: Learning From the Clinton Triangles

Emily M. Brown

We didn't really want to know all this! We could have clung to our fantasy that it wasn't so bad - even if we've known otherwise for a long time. Who wants to face the fact that he betrayed us?! How could he betray us so? Why would he take such foolhardy risks? Why was he willing to throw our interests over for her? What did he see in her that he doesn't see in us?

Our national obsession with Clinton's "inappropriate behavior" parallels the response of those spouses who discover their partner's been cheating. As soon as the shock wears off, the betrayed spouse begins obsessing: "I can't believe that you would do this to me!" "How could you do this?" "Why are you willing to risk our relationship?" "What does she have that I don't have?"

You were probably sick of hearing about Bill Clinton's affairs, Monica, Hillary, Ken Starr, Linda Tripp, and all the others a long time ago. But before we send them off for a long rest (or for intensive treatment?) let's look at what we as therapists can learn from this cast of characters and their audience (the general public, including us) about working with affairs.

Affairs are extremely difficult for everyone involved. They have little to do with rationality and a lot to do with intense emotions and strong beliefs. These emotions and beliefs incorporate aspects of religion, fantasy, family values, pain, repression, and personal history. If we have betrayed or been betrayed in some way (and what adult hasn't?), our reactions to Clinton's betrayal of us may be tinged with echoes from our personal past. Clinton's behavior and that of all the other players gives us an opportunity to reflect and address our own unfinished business about affairs and betrayal.

It might be helpful to recap your reactions:

- What aspect of Clinton's behavior drew your strongest response?
- Which emotions did you experience? How intense were they?
- Did your response to Clinton echo prior responses in your life? To what prior events?
- What judgments did you make?
- What did you feel like doing? Why was this what you wanted to do?
- Which of the other players did you have a strong response to? (Ask yourself the same questions listed above.)
- Was your experience in working with clients experiencing an affair any different while the Clinton scandal was constantly in the news?
- In what ways, if any, has the Clinton scandal changed your knowledge or your practice in working with affairs?

PRIVACY VERSUS SECRECY

Clinton's situation raises many questions at the national level. For our president and for other top officials, what is appropriate privacy, what should remain secret, and what is dishonest? Where are the boundaries? Is a sitting president entitled to have a secret sexual life outside of marriage that is undisclosed to the public? Is this privacy or dishonesty? What is the relevance of this information to the public? Does it matter who the third party is? Should the rules about affairs in the workplace with subordinates be any different for our president? What about the possibility of sexual harassment charges?

Many of us felt disgusted or outraged by Clinton's behavior once we knew about it. Should we have known? Maybe not. In the past we have had presidents who handled the responsibilities of their office in a presidential manner, despite having one or more affairs. Franklin Delano Roosevelt took us successfully through the Depression and World War II, although he had an ongoing affair with Lucy Mercer. John F. Kennedy brought hope and vitality to this country notwithstanding his affairs. These affairs were not trumpeted by the media and were not generally known to the public.

On the other hand, maybe we should know. Knowing raises questions about judgment (important for a president), concerns about blackmail (Kennedy's sexual ties with Judith Exner, Mafia girlfriend, were of concern), and doubts about whether subsequent decisions are being made to distract us (the Kosovo war). What we don't need to know is all the details. I doubt that Starr's crew or Congress needed them either.

OUR ROLE AS THERAPISTS

The questions about privacy versus secrecy raised about Clinton pertain equally to our clients. The major difference, and it is a significant one, is that our clients are talking about secrets in an intimate relationship, rather than between an elected president and his constituents. Thus the answers are somewhat different.

The national obsession with Clinton's affair has parallels to our work with clients as well. It seemed that everyone in the country was reading the paper, watching TV, analyzing, speculating on the outcome, and discussing the situation nonstop. Likewise, it's much easier for the betrayed spouse to obsess (a thinking process) about the partner's affair than to feel the pain and fear that lie inside. As therapists we need to keep an intensive focus on process as opposed to content when dealing with affairs, and especially with the issues of disclosure and obsession.

Secrecy and Disclosure

The issue of disclosure is one of the most difficult aspects for therapists in treating affairs. Some therapists question whether a client is entitled to hide an extramarital affair from the spouse when participating in marital therapy. Rationales include the belief that working on the marriage will solve the underlying problems and the affair doesn't have to be dealt with, that it will be too painful for the spouse to handle, that it is best to leave sleeping dogs lie, or that "everyone does it" and it is no big deal.

Other therapists believe that hidden affairs need to be brought into the open in marital therapy. I'm of this school. Yes, it will be painful for the marital partner to know, but it's impossible to work on a marriage when the big secrets remain hidden. The spouse who later finds out about his or her partner's affair feels hoodwinked or worse and views any work that was done as meaningless because it was done under false pretenses. The *marital* therapist who knows of the affair and colludes with the betraying spouse to hide it will be seen as a traitor. The therapist working *individually* with the spouse who is hiding an affair is in a somewhat different position. That therapist is not betraying one of his or her clients - the other spouse - as is the marital therapist. Even so, this therapist also needs to help the client confront the reality of his or her dishonesty and reach a decision on how to deal with it. Helping clients deal with the hard stuff is the nature of our work.

As therapists, the issue of honesty is central, both for our clients and for ourselves. Clinton's lies were much more problematic than the affair itself. Just as with our clients, his lies raise doubts about everything else he says. We want and need to be able to believe the president of our country. Marital partners need to be able to believe each other. We need to help our clients recognize that the price of hiding their betrayal is high and that it is paid by spouses, family, friends, and colleagues as well as by the betraying partner. The price is higher when the lying has continued over time. Moreover, lying seldom works. Someone, somehow lets the cat out of the bag. Although the betraying spouse doesn't want to believe that anyone knows of the affair, somebody else always knows (usually many somebodies know). Granted that Clinton's affair had many more tentacles and consequences than the average affair, the spillover provides a strong example of the reach of an affair.

What would you have done if Bill Clinton came to see you individually during the period he was hiding his affair with Monica? I would suggest individual treatment to help him face his childhood wounds, see his sexual addiction in the context of those wounds, and examine all the possible consequences of telling or not telling Hillary and the public. I would propose to Bill that we have a session with his top advisors to discuss telling and its consequences. Couple's sessions are out until Hillary knows of Bill's affair with Monica.

We can not *make* a client disclose a hidden affair, nor should we, but we too have decisions to make about how to maintain the integrity of our process and ourselves. Can we continue to work with a *couple*, when one partner is hiding an affair? Yes, if that spouse comes clean promptly. If not, what then? It's time to terminate couple's work and refer them to individual therapists. (For a more detailed discussion of disclosure, see Brown, 1991, 1999).

The Cost of Dishonesty

As is true with Clinton, it is not the sex, but the dishonesty that is the most destructive aspect of an affair for our clients. For the spouse, an affair means the person in whom they chose to place their utmost faith can no longer be trusted. Can the spouse believe it when the partner says the affair is over? What else is he or she lying about? Can the partner's word ever be trusted again? The longer the affair is hidden and the more lies told, the more questions there are about trust. We see this with Clinton. His lies continued until he was caught on tape. Prior to that, many of his close associates put themselves on the line for him. His betrayal was not just of Hillary (and Chelsea) but of his close associates, various others who inadvertently got caught up in this mess, and the public. Although the public stood behind Clinton during the crisis, questions are cropping up these days about his behavior: "The lawyers, flacks, hacks and good Democrats who assured us that it didn't really matter that the president was a pathologically dedicated liar - because, you will recall, he only lied about that which gentlemen should lie about - might now wish . . . to revisit their position" (Kelly, 1999).

Clinton has squandered the country's hope and trust - trust in him, and faith in government. An entire year in the life of Congress, and other branches of government has been wasted, not to mention the $40 million spent on Starr's inquisition. Questions arise as to whether the war in Yugoslavia was entered into precipitously without the necessary planning because Clinton felt he needed to prove himself. Even Clinton's strongest supporters feel betrayed.

Imagine the difference for our country if Clinton had volunteered the truth back in the beginning: "Yes, I have behaved inappropriately, and it's not right. I've ended it (even 'I'm going to end it') and I am starting on the work I need to do to get myself back on track." Every human being who is able to admit to having done something wrong could have identified with him and most would admire his courage in facing his failings and taking responsibility for making needed changes.

And so it goes with our clients. The betraying spouse has destroyed the partner's hope and trust and often used family resources as well in pursuit of the affair. Taking responsibility for doing so is a necessary first step.

Obsession and Rumination

The entire country was caught up in the Clinton soap opera. Defenses were offered, moral judgments proclaimed, courses of action prescribed, and outcomes predicted, while voyeurism ran rampant. The country behaved like the chorus of friends and relatives that surround the average couple that is struggling with an affair. As therapists, we can warn our clients about the kinds of "advice" they are likely to get and help them pay attention to their own inner truths instead.

More than anyone else, the betrayed spouse obsesses about the affair: "How could you do this to me? What did you see in him? Was he better in bed than me? What did you do together? Are you sure it's over? I don't know why I should believe you. I just don't understand how you could do this to me." Hillary's obsession wasn't obvious to the public. However the public made up for it with its own obsession about the latest news. Many of us were like kids looking for any sign about whether the sky was going to fall, while at the same time wanting to stay away from our own fears, our own issues, and our own experience with honesty or betrayal. Grace under pressure has paid off for Hillary.

The spillover nationally of this "mess" was extensive: Much of the work of Congress and various branches of government was on hold for a year. Again, this parallels what happens with families. The endless obsession and rumination are paralyzing. It's not just the marital partners who are affected. The spillover touches children, family members, friends, work colleagues, neighbors, school personnel, and babysitters. Even managed care gets into the act - denying an adequate number of sessions, of course. Parental functioning, relationships within the extended family, and work performance suffer.

One of the most important aspects of our work as therapists is to help the betrayed spouse move beyond obsession about the affair. Contrary to what most betrayed spouses think, it is not an expression of feeling, but a way of trying to make rational sense of the affair (however irrationally). Obsession's appropriate function is to soften the initial emotional impact of disclosure. Continuing obsession means it is being used to avoid the underlying emotions.

Although obsession about the affair may sound like justifiable anger, it's not. It's really rumination, which utilizes the rational mind and not the emotional self. The obsessive spouse is like a squirrel in a cage, going round and round over the same terrain without end. Ruminating offers the illusion that rational understanding is just one question away, that it will explain everything, and then the issue can be boxed up and put away. In reality, ruminating offers the betrayed spouse protection from experiencing the pain and the powerlessness that are part of betrayal.

When both spouses engage in this version of "Twenty Questions" (more like 2,000!), the situation escalates. In response to the barrage of accusatory questions, the betraying spouse offers another tidbit about the affair, trying to appease the partner without doing too much damage. Because you get more of what you reinforce, the questioning escalates with each tidbit, as does the sense of being out of control. Both spouses, in trying to avoid their painful emotions, are drawn deeper into the muck. Neither pursuing rational answers nor exacting punishment solves the emotional problem. Resolution of betrayal occurs at the emotional level.

For the betrayed spouse, obsessing obscures the fact that together the couple made enough room in their relationship for a third party. Obsessing is a way of saying, "I'm an innocent victim. My spouse is the bad guy." Yes, it was the betraying spouse who chose to have an affair. However both spouses colluded in not addressing the underlying issues in their relationship. As long as the situation is defined as one in which there is an innocent victim and a guilty party, work on the relationship cannot proceed. In keeping with systems thinking, we need to reframe the affair as a symptom of deeper problems in the relationship to which each spouse has contributed.

It is easy for us as therapists to get caught up in feeding the obsession. We may think that providing more details will be helpful, or that we should let our client vent. Or we may view the betrayed spouse as an innocent victim and the betraying spouse as the bad guy, or we may be reluctant to be present with our client's most difficult emotions. It is essential, however, for the therapist to help the betrayed spouse get to the emotions being blocked by the obsession. The step that allows betrayed spouses to make the transition from obsessing to working on their own issues is daring to feel their own deep-down genuine emotions: usually a combination of pain, fear, and helplessness. These emotions are real, and because they are real they are grounding. Getting to the emotions enables real work to begin.

We need to keep in mind that it takes considerable time to recover from betrayal. Urging the betrayed spouse to move on won't end the obsession. The emotional risk of paying attention to one's feelings is not learned in an instant nor is such a risk taken all at once. Rather it comes in small increments over time.

Thus, as therapists, we need to push from the beginning for the deep feelings, while allowing the person to enter this space at a pace that feels safe enough (no pace feels safe). Don't settle for a focus on anger - anger is a secondary feeling and the route to resolution is through the primary emotions: in this case pain, fear, and helplessness.

Affairs and Parenting

It is unclear what was happening with Chelsea after her father's behavior became the country's obsession. Bob Woodward reported that on August 18, 1998, the day after Bill admitted to his affair with Monica, Bill and Hillary weren't speaking and Chelsea looked incredibly sad (Woodward, 1999). It appears that the Clintons tried to protect Chelsea from direct contact with the media. However, no amount of protection would be enough to shelter Chelsea from the barrage of media exposure of her father's behavior.

The obsessive phase following disclosure of an affair is usually the hardest for kids. Obsessing leaves little time for parenting and poisons the air. The parental crisis often leads to poor decisions regarding what is said to the kids.

We need to check out what is happening to the children and troubleshoot the situation. Are the kids being triangled in? Do they need information about what is causing the craziness in their family? Are they getting too much information? What information do they need? Who can provide support to the kids while their parents are in crisis? What needs to happen in this family to calm the situation and prevent further damage?

Grieving

Part of the devastation of an affair is the loss of hopes, dreams, and trust. It is no wonder that the betrayed spouse is slow to put the pieces together and realize that it adds up to an affair. Acknowledging an affair means life as one has known it is over. Disclosure of an affair has similar meaning for the betraying partner. No longer is there an illusion of having a solid marriage or of being a "good husband" or a "doting wife." This betrayal means having to rework one's approach to life.

Grief for the losses sets in as the obsession begins to subside. If either spouse has a history of losses or abandonment issues, grieving will be particularly difficult. I would assume that Chelsea is grieving, but it appears that Bill and Hillary have turned to the work of politics rather than to personal work. Our clients are often tempted to do much the same: They work endless hours, they focus on the children, and they talk endlessly to friends about what their spouse has done to them - all as a way of avoiding the emotional issues bubbling inside. When they come for therapy, one of the most important things we can do is help them pay attention to their emotions and to be present as they experience them.

Rebuilding

One of the things we're not seeing with the Clintons is serious work on rebuilding their relationship. Nor do they seem to be looking at themselves and how they got to this point. The only identified source of help has been ministerial, and it seems to be more of a look good/feel good maneuver than truly therapeutic.

Many couples who experience an affair act similarly, staying busy with other matters, burying emotions, focusing on the children, maintaining distance from each other - anything but tackling the difficult and painful work of facing one's self. Some couples remain stuck in the obsessive phase for years, often telling themselves that they are staying together for the sake of the kids. These are the couples who don't get to therapy, or where one or both drop out after a few sessions. An affair is a wake-up call, but these couples have turned off the alarm. In so doing, they miss the opportunity to make changes for the better in their lives.

Of the individuals and couples who come to see us following an affair, many know they want the marriage to continue. Others are not sure, or want help with separating. As therapists, we need to look at the rebuilding process as one involving both spouses, in keeping with the fact that both spouses contributed to making enough room for an affair. Depending on the type of affair, the best treatment format may be individual therapy, couples therapy, or some combination of individual and couples work. (For a discussion of the five types of affairs see Brown, 1991, 1999).

For the Conflict Avoiders and Intimacy Avoiders, the two types of affairs where the spouses still care about each other, the work is much the same whether they do it together or separately. Doing the work together gives the marriage its best chance. Couples don't need to decide whether they want their marriage to continue in order to do couples work. In fact, that would be putting the cart before the horse. However, each partner needs to be committed to working on some aspect of themselves, as well as exploring and making changes in their relationship. Much of the couples work has to do with sharing the vulnerable self, talking about the hard stuff, and learning to live in the present. Once the work is underway, they are in a better position to *begin* considering whether their marriage has potential.

A great majority of the Conflict Avoiders and Intimacy Avoiders who seriously work on changing their relationship patterns will opt to stay in the marriage. Many of them comment that the work they have done has resulted in a much better marriage than ever before - some go so far as to be grateful that the affair woke them up before it was too late. For those who do the work of rebuilding, but decide to end the marriage, the increased self-awareness and ability to share one's real self will positively influence the choice of a subsequent partner and the quality of that relationship. It will also contribute to a sad but sane divorce.

With the Conflict Avoiders and the Intimacy Avoiders, affairs have more to do with the lack of emotional self-knowledge and communication skills. Here, couples work is the treatment of choice. In contrast, Sexual Addiction Affairs and Split Self Affairs reflect deep childhood wounds. Before marital therapy will be effective, these wounds need to be addressed in individual therapy. In the case of Exit Affairs, a decision has already been made to end the marriage, and the affair serves as the vehicle. Using a couples format to focus on the issues of ending can be helpful, followed by individual therapy, especially for the betrayed spouse. Often the betraying spouse in an Exit Affair is unaware of needing to do any work at this time - the hope is that the third party is the answer.

The Societal Context

Both the betrayed and the betraying spouse are getting an overload of advice from friends and relatives - not as much as Bill and Hillary got, but just as "helpful." Generally the advice they are getting is bad. The "advisors" are reacting from their own situation, whatever that may be. They react emotionally, and they have none of the consequences of what they advise.

We can help our clients by coaching them in how to cut off the advice, however well-intended, so that they have space to pay attention to their own ideas and feelings about how they might proceed. Getting the clutter out of the way provides room to get clarity about direction and goals.

Despite all the divorce talk of our betrayed and betraying clients and their friends and relatives, don't ever assume divorce unless the affair is an Exit Affair. Most affairs don't result in divorce. Bill and Hillary are a good illustration. They have been together for a long time, despite his history of womanizing. Hillary has her reasons for putting up with Bill's behavior. Whatever their personal agenda, their public agenda has been power. Being the president's wife has given Hillary access to pursue her own agenda in ways she could not otherwise. If Hillary eventually leaves Bill, it will likely be because she has acquired the power she wants and doesn't need Bill's help anymore. On the personal front, it may be that they have an arrangement, such as an open marriage. Although it didn't happen with the Clintons, such arrangements often include an agreement to be discreet, not to embarrass the other.

Our betrayed clients sometimes turn to attorneys to make everything alright. These clients usually have a frame of reference that says, naïvely, that our legal system and our judges are fair, or that the legal system will extract justice (read: punishment) from the betraying spouse, or will offer security. The legal system's frame of reference is adversarial, one against the other, win/lose. The lawyer's responsibility is to get the most for his or her client. This framework runs counter to the approach of therapists. When our clients get involved prematurely with the legal system, it can diminish the client's opportunity to sort out and resolve the emotional issues. At the national level, Ken Starr's handling of the Clinton situation is similar to the worst that divorce lawyers have to offer: sensationalism, lack of privacy, calling in every possible witness, and the emotional devastation of a public win/lose battle.

Professional Values/Personal Feelings

We each have our own personal responses to betrayal. These relate to our own life course: the times we have betrayed or been betrayed, our fears, our ways of interacting in our intimate relationships, and our family history regarding betrayals, family secrets, values, and beliefs.

When it comes to Clinton, we feel much like the betrayed spouse. Some of us are obsessing about the situation; others are disgusted; some said they knew from the beginning he couldn't be trusted; still others don't want to have to look at the situation; some want him punished. Many of us would like to make our sense of betrayal go away. Reactions to Hillary are important too. Many therapists, especially women, admire her "cool," her refusal to reveal all to the media, and her decision to run for the Senate. Although it's admirable that she has refrained from revealing all to the media, does this really make her a heroine?

What does our obsession save us from feeling? What feelings do we have about the power dynamics here? About sexual addiction? What is our personal history regarding trust in intimate relationships? To which of our own life experiences are we resonating? If anything, we need the opportunity to experience and to talk about our own pain, our disappointment and disillusionment, and our grief. We have been betrayed and we are upset about it. We need to give voice to our feelings. We need to be heard.

Do we need a public forum? In some ways the media provides us with that, but the media also tends to get preoccupied with sensational details or with judgmental concerns. We may need private forums of our own making. Our reactions to Clinton's betrayal of us may be tinged with echoes from our personal past. Clinton's behavior gives us an opportunity to reflect and address our own unfinished business about betrayal.

After all the disturbing aspects of Bill and Monica's affair, some positive consequences are emerging. For centuries, a hush-hush atmosphere combined with moral judgments have made affairs taboo to talk about seriously and harder to deal with. However, this hasn't dampened people's tendency to engage in affairs. A side benefit of Clinton's "inappropriate behavior" may be that our society learns to talk more openly and directly about affairs. We've been pretty irrational as a culture, focusing on blame and punishment while encouraging sexual acting out and enjoying the titillation. Therapists are in a prime position to contribute to serious discussion about the nature of affairs, so that the public is better informed about the reality as opposed to the fantasies and the gossip.

RESOLUTION AND FORGIVENESS

Our client's desire for a quick "I'm sorry" is understandable but unrealistic. We know that if Clinton told us now that he is sorry, we wouldn't be able to trust that he means it. Healing doesn't happen in a week or even two, even when you're working on it at Martha's Vineyard. Healing from betrayal is not just a matter of giving or getting more facts, or of asking or granting forgiveness. It is not a matter of the "bad guy" completing penance and the "innocent victim" bestowing forgiveness. Resolving betrayal requires changes in behavior and attitudes on the part of both spouses. It requires facing the inner demons that prompted the betrayal. At a minimum, the betrayer needs to learn to pay attention to the emotional self so that it informs behavior rather than driving it. The betrayed spouse, who likely has been the betrayer in some lesser events in the marriage (e.g., withholding information, lying, or violating agreements), will need to work on the emotional self as well. Along with that comes being honest, giving one's self a voice, owning one's responsibility, and developing realistic expectations. Real apologies can come only after listening to the partner's pain and fear and fully understanding and taking responsibility for one's own actions and for the pain those actions caused. Just like Clinton, our clients often want to skip these steps and move directly to forgiveness.

On August 17, 1998, Clinton wasn't ready to ask for forgiveness or to be forgiven. More than a year later he still isn't ready, despite some words of acknowledgment during the impeachment proceedings. It will be some time before he is ready, assuming he does the necessary work on himself. Although many of us want to see Clinton redeem himself, we need to take time to observe whether changes on Clinton's part are real or designed only to move this problem to the sidelines in a hurry. In the meantime, let's put Clinton's betrayal aside, so that we can pay attention to our own feelings about betrayal and work on resolving our own issues with betrayal. That is our part in moving beyond obsession to more important matters in our national life.

CONTRIBUTOR

Emily M. Brown, LCSW, is Director of the Key Bridge Therapy and Mediation Center in Arlington, Virginia. As a Clinical Social Worker and a Marriage and Family Therapist, she works with couples, individuals, and families regarding the underlying issues in marriage, divorce, and betrayal. She also trains mental health professionals throughout North America and in Europe on treating the issues associated with extramarital affairs and other relationship issues. She is the author of *Affairs: A Guide to Working Through the Repercussions of Infidelity* (1999), *Patterns of Infidelity and Their Treatment* (1991), and numerous articles on affairs, divorce, and divorce mediation. She encourages those who are struggling with an affair to face their chaotic feelings so that the affair becomes a catalyst for positive change rather than a tragedy. Ms. Brown has made appearances on *The Early Show, Oprah, Donahue,* the *Today Show,* CNBC's *Real Personal, The Shirley Show* (Canada), National Public Television, NPR's *Talk of the Nation,* and numerous other radio and television programs. Ms. Brown may be contacted at 1925 N. Lynn Street, Suite 700, Arlington, VA 22209.

RESOURCES

Cited Resources

Carnes, P. (1991). *Don't Call It Love*. New York: Bantam.

Fisher, H. (1992). *Anatomy of Love: The Natural History of Monogamy, Adultery and Divorce*. New York: Norton.

Gottman, J. (1994). *Why Marriages Succeed or Fail*. New York: Simon & Schuster.

Kasl, C. D. (1989). *Women, Sex, and Addiction*. New York: Ticknor & Fields.

Lawson, A. (1988). *Adultery: An Analysis of Love and Betrayal*. New York: Basic Books.

Lerner, H. G. (1993). *The Dance of Deception: Pretending and Truth-Telling in Women's Lives*. New York: HarperCollins.

Lusterman, D. (1998). *Infidelity: A Survival Guide*. Oakland, CA: New Harbinger.

Markman, H., Stanley, S., & Blumberg, S. L. (1994). *Fighting for Your Marriage*. San Francisco: Jossey-Bass.

Reibstein, J., & Richards, M. (1993). *Sexual Arrangements: Marriage and the Temptation of Infidelity*. New York: Scribners.

Smedes, L. B. (1996). *The Art of Forgiving*. New York: Ballantine.

Spring, J. A. (1996). *After the Affair*. New York: HarperCollins.

Vaughan, P. (1998). *The Monogamy Myth: A Personal Handbook for Recovering From Affairs* (rev. ed.). New York: Newmarket Press.

Additional Resources

Brown, E. M. (1991). *Patterns of Infidelity and Their Treatment*. New York: Brunner/Mazel.

Brown, E. M. (1999). *Affairs: A Guide to Working Through the Repercussions of Infidelity*. San Francisco: Jossey-Bass.

Kelly, M. (1999, May 26). The Clinton syndrome. *The Washington Post,* p. A29.

Woodward, B. (1999). *Shadow: Five Presidents and the Legacy of Watergate*. New York: Simon & Schuster.

Web Sites

www.affairs-help.com	Emily Brown's web site. Provides information and guidance for those involved in any part of the affair triangle, bulletin boards, and information about training for mental health professionals.
www.itstessie.com (Religious)	Provides information and guidance for those struggling with an affair.
www.pages.prodigy.com/divorceplus/div00.htm	Provides information about divorce-related issues.
www.vaughan-vaughan.com	Provides information and guidance for those involved in an affair, plus chat rooms and message boards.

Introduction to the Client Handouts

Two client handouts are included in this section of Volume 18. The handouts in each volume are designed so that they may be photocopied and distributed to your clients.

Both handouts are published by the American Psychological Association Practice Directorate. The first, entitled "Managing Traumatic Stress: Tips for Recovering From Disasters and Other Traumatic Events," is certainly timely in the context of multiple natural disasters.

The second handout is entitled "Breast Cancer: How Your Mind Can Help Your Body." The fact sheet tells patients how psychological treatment can help the body.

Managing Traumatic Stress: Tips for Recovering From Disasters And Other Traumatic Events*

Because you are reading this fact sheet, you probably are in the process of recovering from a natural disaster or other type of traumatic event. Perhaps you experienced a flood, hurricane, or earthquake. Or maybe you have been in a serious accident or the victim of a crime. Traumatic experiences such as these tend to be sudden and overwhelming. In some cases, there are no outwardly visible signs of physical injury, but there is nonetheless a serious emotional toll. It is common for people who have experienced traumatic situations to have very strong emotional reactions. Understanding normal responses to these abnormal events can aid you in coping effectively with your feelings, thoughts, and behaviors, and help you along the path to recovery.

What Happens to People After a Disaster or Other Traumatic Event?

Shock and denial are typical responses to disasters and other kinds of trauma, especially shortly after the event. Both shock and denial are normal protective reactions.

Shock is a sudden and often intense disturbance of your emotional state that may leave you feeling stunned or dazed. Denial involves your not acknowledging that something very stressful has happened, or not experiencing fully the intensity of the event. You may temporarily feel numb or disconnected from life.

As the initial shock subsides, reactions vary from one person to another. The following, however, are normal responses to a traumatic event:

- *Feelings become intense and sometimes are unpredictable.* You may become more irritable than usual, and your mood may change back and forth dramatically. You might be especially anxious or nervous, or even become depressed.
- *Thoughts and behavior patterns are affected by the trauma.* You might have repeated and vivid memories of the event. These flashbacks may occur for no apparent reason and may lead to physical reactions such as rapid heart beat or sweating.

  You may find it difficult to concentrate or make decisions, or become more easily confused. Sleep and eating patterns also may be disrupted.
- *Recurring emotional reactions are common.* Anniversaries of the event, such as at 1 month or 1 year, as well as reminders such as aftershocks from earthquakes or the sounds of sirens, can trigger upsetting memories of the traumatic experience. These "triggers" may be accompanied by fears that the stressful event will be repeated.
- *Interpersonal relationships often become strained.* Greater conflict, such as more frequent arguments with family members and coworkers, is common. On the other hand, you might become withdrawn and isolated and avoid your usual activities.
- *Physical symptoms may accompany the extreme stress.* For example, headaches, nausea, and chest pain may result and may require medical attention. Preexisting medical conditions may worsen due to the stress.

How Do People Respond Differently Over Time?

It is important for you to realize that there is not one "standard" pattern of reaction to the extreme stress of traumatic experiences. Some people respond immediately, while others have delayed reactions - sometimes months or even years later. Some have adverse effects for a long period of time, while others recover rather quickly.

And reactions can change over time. Some who have suffered from trauma are energized initially by the event to help them with the challenge of coping, only to later become discouraged or depressed.

A number of factors tend to affect the length of time required for recovery, including:

- *The degree of intensity and loss.* Events that last longer and pose a greater threat, and where loss of life or substantial loss of property is involved, often take longer to resolve.
- *A person's general ability to cope with emotionally challenging situations.* Individuals who have handled other difficult, stressful circumstances well may find it easier to cope with the trauma.
- *Other stressful events preceding the traumatic experience.* Individuals faced with other emotionally challenging situations, such as serious health problems or family-related difficulties, may have more intense reactions to the new stressful event and need more time to recover.

How Should I Help Myself and My Family?

There are a number of steps you can take to help restore emotional well-being and a sense of control following a disaster or other traumatic experience, including the following:

- *Give yourself time to heal.* Anticipate that this will be a difficult time in your life. Allow yourself to mourn the losses you have experienced. Try to be patient with changes in your emotional state.
- *Ask for support from people who care about you* and who will listen and empathize with your situation. But keep in mind that your typical support system may be weakened if those who are close to you also have experienced or witnessed the trauma.

  Communicate your experience in whatever ways feel comfortable to you - such as by talking with family or close friends, or keeping a diary.
- *Find out about local support groups* that often are available such as for those who have suffered from natural disasters, or for women who are victims of rape. These can be especially helpful for people with limited personal support systems.

  Try to find groups led by appropriately trained and experienced professionals. Group discussion can help people realize that other individuals in the same circumstances often have similar reactions and emotions.
- *Engage in healthy behaviors* to enhance your ability to cope with excessive stress. Eat well-balanced meals and get plenty of rest. If you experience ongoing difficulties with sleep, you may be able to find some relief through relaxation techniques. Avoid alcohol and drugs.
- *Establish or reestablish routines* such as eating meals at regular times and following an exercise program. Take some time off from the demands of daily life by pursuing hobbies or other enjoyable activities.
- *Avoid major life decisions* such as switching careers or jobs if possible because these activities tend to be highly stressful.
- *Become knowledgeable about what to expect* as a result of trauma. Some of the "Additional Resources" listed at the end of this fact sheet may help you with this learning process.

How Do I Take Care of Children's Special Needs?

The intense anxiety and fear that often follow a disaster or other traumatic event can be especially troubling for children. Some may regress and demonstrate younger behaviors such as thumb sucking or bed wetting. Children may be more prone to nightmares and fear of sleeping alone. Performance in school may suffer. Other changes in behavior patterns may include throwing tantrums more frequently, or withdrawing and becoming more solitary.

There are several things parents and others who care for children can do to help alleviate the emotional consequences of trauma, including the following:

- *Spend more time with children and let them be more dependent of you* during the months following the trauma - for example, allowing your child to cling to you more often than usual. Physical affection is very comforting to children who have experienced trauma.
- *Provide play experiences to help relieve tension.* Younger children in particular may find it easier to share their ideas and feelings about the event through nonverbal activities such as drawing.
- *Encourage older children to speak* with you, and with one another, about their thoughts and feelings. This helps reduce their confusion and anxiety related to the trauma. Respond to questions in terms they can comprehend. Reassure them repeatedly that you care about them and that you understand their fears and concerns.
- *Keep regular schedules* for activities such as eating, playing, and going to bed to help restore a sense of security and normalcy.

When Should I Seek Professional Help?

Some people are able to cope effectively with the emotional and physical demands brought about by a natural disaster or other traumatic experience by using their own support systems. It is not unusual, however, to find that serious problems persist and continue to interfere with daily living. For example, some may feel overwhelming nervousness or lingering sadness that adversely affects job performance and interpersonal relationships.

- *Individuals with prolonged reactions that disrupt their daily functioning should consult with a trained and experienced mental health professional.* Psychologists and other appropriate mental health providers help educate people about normal responses to extreme stress. These professionals work with individuals affected by trauma to help them find constructive ways of dealing with the emotional impact.
- *With children, continual and aggressive emotional outbursts, serious problems at school, preoccupation with the traumatic event, continued and extreme withdrawal, and other signs of intense anxiety or emotional difficulties all point to the need for professional assistance.* A qualified mental health professional can help such children and their parents understand and deal with thoughts, feelings, and behaviors that result from trauma.

How May I Use APA As a Resource?

"Talk to Someone Who Can Help," brochure about psychotherapy and choosing a psychologist from the American Psychological Association, can be ordered free of charge. Call 800-964-2000.

Contact the *APA Practice Directorate* at (202) 336-5800 for the name and telephone number of your *state psychological association.* These associations, along with *city* and *county psychological associations,* can refer you to psychologists in your area. They may also be able to put you in touch with *other local organizations and groups that help victims of disasters and other traumatic events.*

"Helping Children Cope," may be accessed via the *APA home page on the Internet,* at http://www.apa.org/kids.html

Additional Resources

Local chapters of the American Red Cross may be able to direct you to additional resources. Check your local telephone directory for the chapter nearest you.

National Organization for Victims' Assistance, 1757 Park Road, NW, Washington, DC 20010; toll-free, 800-TRY-NOVA; in DC metropolitan area, (202) 232-6682.

Two other materials available via the Internet offer additional information about coping with disaster:

- "After a Disaster: Steps You Can Take to Cope With a Stressful Situation," Los Angeles County Department of Mental Health, http://gladstone.uoregon.edu/~dvb/dissteps.htm
- "Emotional Reactions to Disasters," University of Illinois Cooperative Extension Service, http:www.ag.uiuc.edu/~disaster/facts/emotion.html

Breast Cancer: How Your Mind Can Help Your Body*

Each year 185,000 people in this country learn that they have breast cancer. Because less than a quarter of them have genetic or other known risk factors, the diagnosis often comes as a devastating surprise. The emotional turmoil that results can affect women's physical health as well as their psychological well-being. This question-and-answer fact sheet explains how psychological treatment can help these women harness the healing powers of their own minds.

What Impact Does a Breast Cancer Diagnosis Have on Psychological Well-Being?

Receiving a diagnosis of breast cancer can be one of the most distressing events women ever experience. And women may not know where to turn for help.

Distress typically continues even after the initial shock of diagnosis has passed. As women begin what is often a lengthy treatment process, they may find themselves faced with new problems. They may find their personal relationships in turmoil, for instance. They may feel tired all the time. They may be very worried about their symptoms, treatment, and mortality. They may face discrimination from employers or insurance companies. Factors like these can contribute to chronic stress, anxiety, and depression.

Why Is It Important to Seek Psychological Help?

Feeling overwhelmed is a perfectly normal response to a breast cancer diagnosis. But negative emotions can cause women to stop doing things that are good for them and start doing things that are bad for anyone but especially worrisome for those with a serious disease. Women with breast cancer may start eating poorly, for instance, eating fewer meals and choosing foods of lower nutritional value. They may cut back on their exercise. They may have trouble getting a good night's sleep. And they may withdraw from family and friends. At the same time, these women may use alcohol, cigarettes, caffeine, or other drugs in an attempt to soothe themselves.

A breast cancer diagnosis can also lead to more severe problems. Researchers estimate that anywhere from 20% to 60% of cancer patients experience depressive symptoms, which can make it more difficult for women to adjust, participate optimally in treatment activities, and take advantage of whatever sources of social support are available. Some women become so disheartened by the ordeal of having cancer that they refuse to undergo surgery or simply stop going to radiation or chemotherapy appointments. As a result, they may get even sicker. In fact, studies show that missing as few as 15% of chemotherapy appointments results in significantly poorer outcomes.

How Can Psychological Treatment Help Women Adjust?

Licensed psychologists and other mental health professionals with experience in breast cancer treatment can help a great deal. Their primary goal is to help women learn how to cope with the physical, emotional, and

---

* The American Psychological Association Practice Directorate gratefully acknowledges the assistance of Alice F. Chang, PhD, and Sandra B. Haber, PhD, in developing this fact sheet.

lifestyle changes associated with cancer as well as with medical treatments that can be painful and traumatic. For some women, the focus may be on how to explain their illness to their children or how to deal with a partner's response. For others, it may be on how to choose the right hospital or medical treatment. For still others, it may be on how to control stress, anxiety, or depression. By teaching patients problem-solving strategies in a supportive environment, psychologists help women work through their grief, fear, and other emotions. For many women, this life-threatening crisis eventually proves to be an opportunity for life-enhancing personal growth.

Breast cancer patients themselves aren't the only ones who can benefit from psychological treatment. Psychologists often help spouses who must offer both emotional and practical support while dealing with their own feelings, for instance. Children, parents, and friends involved in caretaking can also benefit from psychological interventions.

The need for psychological treatment may not end when medical treatment does. In fact, emotional recovery may take longer than physical recovery and is sometimes less predictable. Although societal pressure to get everything back to normal is intense, breast cancer survivors need time to create a new self-image that incorporates both the experience and their changed bodies. Psychologists can help women achieve that goal and learn to cope with such issues as fears about recurrence and impatience with life's more mundane problems.

Can Psychological Treatment Help the Body, Too?

Absolutely. Take the nausea and vomiting that often accompany chemotherapy, for example. For some women, these side effects can be severe enough to make them reject further treatment efforts. Psychologists can teach women relaxation exercises, meditation, self-hypnosis, imagery, or other skills that can effectively relieve nausea without the side effects of pharmaceutical approaches.

Psychological treatment has indirect effects on physical health as well. Researchers already know that stress suppresses the body's ability to protect itself. What they now suspect is that the coping skills that psychologists teach may actually boost the immune system's strength. In one well-known study, for example, patients with advanced breast cancer who underwent group therapy lived longer than those who did not.

Research also suggests that patients who ask questions and are assertive with their physicians have better health outcomes than patients who passively accept proposed treatment regimens. Psychologists can empower women to make more informed choices in the face of often-conflicting advice and can help them communicate more effectively with their health care providers. In short, psychologists can help women become more fully engaged in their own treatment. The result is an enhanced understanding of the disease and its treatment and a greater willingness to do what needs to be done to get well again.

What Type of Psychological Treatment Is Helpful?

A combination of individual and group treatment sometimes works best. Individual sessions with a licensed psychologist typically emphasize the understanding and modification of patterns of thinking and behavior. Group psychological treatment with others who have breast cancer gives women a chance to give and receive emotional support and learn from the experiences of others. To be most effective, groups should be made up of women at similar stages of the disease and led by psychologists or other mental health professionals with experience in breast cancer treatment.

Whether aimed at individuals or groups, psychological interventions strive to help women adjust to their diagnoses, cope with treatment, and come to terms with the disease's impact on their lives. These interventions offer psychologists an opportunity to help women better understand breast cancer and its treatment. Psychologists typically ask women open-ended questions about their assumptions, ideas for living life more fully, and other matters. Although negative thoughts and feelings are addressed, most psychological interventions focus on problem-solving as women meet each new challenge.

> A breast cancer diagnosis can severely impair women's psychological functioning, which in turn can jeopardize their physical health. It doesn't have to be that way. Women who seek help from licensed psychologists with experience in breast cancer treatment can actually use the mind-body connection to their advantage to enhance both mental and physical health.

Subject Index
To Volume 18

A cumulative index to all 18 volumes is available from the publisher. (To order the cumulative index, contact Professional Resource Press, P.O. Box 15560, Sarasota, FL 34277-1560. Include a $5.00 check or money order payable to Professional Resource Press.)

A

Abandonment, risk management issues regarding, 231-245
Acupuncture, 404-405
Adolescent sex offenders, psychoeducational groups for, 311-322
Adolescents,
 adventure therapy for, 335-347
 chronic headaches in, 121-134
  assessment of, 123-126
  classification of, 121-123
  cognitive-behavioral treatment program for, 127-129
  incidence of, 121
  intervention for, 126-129
  medication for, 127-129
Adventure therapy with adolescents, 335-347
Affairs, marital, 471-478
Aging (*see* Elderly)
Alternative medicine in mental health treatment, 401-416
 Acupuncture, 404-405
 Ayurvedic Medicine, 406-408
 Chinese Medicine, 403-405
 Homeopathy, 410-411
 Naturopathy, 408-410
Antisocial personality disorder, 78-79
Assertiveness skills and surgery patients, 330-331
Assessment of resistant children, strategy for, 455-458
Athletes, motivating, 349-367
Attributional styles in athletes, 349-367
Avoidant personality disorder, 80-81
Ayurvedic Medicine, 406-408

B

Borderline personality disorder, 79-80
 with mental retardation, 82
Breast Cancer: How Your Mind Can Help Your Body (Handout), 485-486
Brief psychotherapy, termination and, 233-234

C

Caregivers, compassion fatigue in, 441-453
Children
 effects of high interparental conflict on, 154-156
 resistant, 455-458
Chinese Medicine, Classical and Traditional, 403-405
Chronic headaches in adolescents, 121-134
Chronic medical conditions, 33-45
 elderly and, 33-34
Clinical supervision documentation, 301-307
Clinical Supervision Notes Record Form, 304-306
Clinton, Bill, 471-473, 475-478
Cognitive techniques for motor vehicle accident survivors, 145-148
Cognitive-behavioral therapy for,
 chronic headaches in adolescents, 127-129
 depression, 21
 frottage, 189-190
 surgical patients, 328-329
Cognitive-experiential model of dream interpretation for couples, 85-101
Collaborative Divorce, 169-184
Compassion fatigue, 441-453
Competence, with culturally diverse and elderly clients, 264-266
Complaints,
 ethics, 215
 legal, 216-217
 regulatory, 215-216

Computers, use of, in telehealth,
networked, 393-395
stand-alone, 392-393
Contract, psychotherapist-patient, 281-287
Couples, dream interpretation for, 85-101
Covert sensitization, as treatment for frottage, 189-190
Cultural competence in sex therapy, 68-69
Culturally diverse clients, competence and, 257-272

D

Deaf community, mental health services for, 369-381
Defensive strategies for dealing with ethic complaints, 218-228
Dementia, assessment of, 199-209
Dependent personality disorder, 81
Depression,
cognitive-behavioral therapy for, 21
Interpersonal Psychotherapy for, in late life, 21-31
interpersonal relationships and, 21-23
medication for, 21
in motor vehicle accident survivors, 149
Diaphragmatic Breathing, Sample Script, 131
Difficult patients, Time-Limited Dynamic Psychotherapy for, 5-19
Directed Family Therapy, 153-168
Disability, marital and sexual issues and, 459-470
Disasters, tips for recovering from (Handout), 481-483
Divorce,
Collaborative, 169-184
intimacy and, 289
Divorcing families in conflict, Directed Family Therapy for, 153-168
Dream interpretation for couples, 85-101
Dyslexia,
Information Sheets, 427-435
overview and treatment of, 417-440

E

Elderly,
chronic medical conditions in, 33
competence and, 257-272
dementia assessment in, 199-209
depression in, 21-31
maintaining professional competence with, 264-266
Emotion management techniques for motor vehicle accident survivors, 148-150
Emotional, Sexual, and Spiritual Intimacy Scale (ESSI), 289-296
Erection dysfunction, 57-71
future of, 69
sex therapy and, 64-65
treatment strategies for, 63-68
Ethical dilemmas in interactions with the media, 247-255
Ethics,
aging and culturally diverse clients and, 259-260
complaints, 213-229
issues regarding termination and abandonment, 231-245
and services to Deaf community, 371-374
Expert testimony, effect of legal complaints on, 217
Exposure therapy for motor vehicle accident survivors, 141-145

F

Facsimile machines, use of, in telehealth, 390-391
Family of Origin Therapy, 47-56
Family, role of, in chronic illness, 35-43
Family Therapy,
as part of adventure therapy, 339-340
Directed, for divorcing families, 153-168
Financial policy form, 298
Forms
Clinical Supervision Notes Record, 304-306
Dyslexia, Information Sheets, 427-435
Emotional, Sexual, and Spiritual Intimacy Scale (ESSI), 292-295
Informed Consent to Participate in Directed Family Therapy, 164-166
Nondeviant Sexual History, 194
Our Financial Policy, 298
Outpatient Services Contract, 283-286
Paraphilic History, 195
Pre-Authorized Health Care Form, 299
Termination Process, Sample Letters from Clinician to Patient for Use in, 242-243
Worksheet for Identifying Attributional Styles in Athletes, 359-362
Worksheet for Modifying Attributions in Athletes, 363-365
Frottage, evaluation and treatment of, 185-197
cognitive-behavioral therapy for, 189-190
covert sensitization for, 189-190
medication for, 190-191
obsessive-compulsive disorder and, 190
olfactory aversion treatment for, 190
relapse prevention therapy for, 191

G

Group therapy for adolescent sex offenders, 311-322

H

Handouts:
Breast Cancer: How Your Mind Can Help Your Body, 485-486
Managing Traumatic Stress: Tips for Recovering From Disasters and Other Traumatic Events, 481-483
Headaches, chronic, in adolescents, 121-134
Hill method for dream interpretation, 86-100
Histrionic personality disorder, 80
Homeopathy, 410-411

I

Illness, context of, in chronic medical conditions, 34-42
Informed Consent to Participate in Directed Family Therapy (Form), 164-166
Interaction Therapy for parents and children, 103-120
Interpersonal Psychotherapy for treating late life depression, 21-31
Intimacy,
disability and, 459-470
emotional, sexual, and spiritual, 289-291

L

Learning disabilities (*see* Dyslexia)
Legal complaints, 213-215, 216-217
Licensing complaints, 213-229

M

Malpractice, defensive strategies against, 213-229
Managing Traumatic Stress: Tips for Recovering From Disasters and Other Traumatic Events (Handout), 481-483
Marital affairs, 471-478
Marketing, quality of care indicators and, 273-278
Marriage,
  affairs and, 471-478
  disability and, 459-470
Media, ethical issues and, 247-255
Medication,
  for chronic headache in adolescents, 127-129
  for depression, 21
  for erection dysfunction, 64, 66-67
  for frottage, 190-191
  integrated with psychotherapy in treatment of severe personality disorders, 73-84
Mental retardation and severe personality disorders, 82
Motor vehicle accident survivors, PTSD in, 135-152

N

Narcissistic personality disorder, 80
Naturopathy, 408-410
Neurobiogenic factors in dyslexia, 420-422
Nondeviant Sexual History (Form), 194

O

Obsessive-compulsive personality disorder, 81
  and frottage, 190
Olfactory aversion treatment for frottage, 190
Our Financial Policy (Form), 298
Outpatient Services Contract (Form), 283-286

P

Pain control in surgical procedures, 327-328
Paranoid personality disorder, 77
Paraphilia: Frottage, 185-197
Paraphilic History (Form), 195
Parent-Child Interaction Therapy, 103-120
Personality disorders, severe, integration of psychotherapy and medication in treatment of, 73-84 (*see also* specific disorders)
Pre-authorization forms and policies for increasing fee collections, 297-300
Pre-Authorized Health Care Form, 299
Psychoeducational groups for adolescent sex offenders, 311-322
Psychopharmacology (*see* Medication)
Psychotherapist-patient contract, 281-287
Psychotherapy,
  brief, and termination, 233-234
  Interpersonal, for late life depression, 21-31
  Time-Limited Dynamic, for difficult patients, 5-19
PTSD in motor vehicle accident survivors, 135-152
  cognitive techniques for, 145-148
  emotion management techniques for, 148-150
  exposure therapy for, 141-145
  relaxation therapy for, 145

Q

Quality of care indicators as marketing tool, 273-278

R

Relapse prevention therapy for frottage, 191
Relaxation techniques for,
  chronic headaches in adolescents, 127-128
  motor vehicle accident survivors, 145
  surgery patients, 329-330
Resistant children, assessment strategy for, 455-458
Risk management,
  in ethics, legal, and regulatory complaints, 213-229
  and termination, 231-245

S

Schizoid personality disorder, 77
Schizotypal personality disorder, 77-78
Severe personality disorders, integration of medication with psychotherapy for, 73-84
  Antisocial, 78-79
  Avoidant, 80-81
  Borderline, 79-80
    with mental retardation, 82
  Dependent, 81
  Histrionic, 80
  Narcissistic, 80
  Obsessive-Compulsive, 81
  Paranoid, 77
  Schizoid, 77
  Schizotypal, 77-78
Sex offenders, adolescent, 311-322
Sex therapy for erection dysfunction, 64-65
Sexual disorders: frottage, 185-197
Sexual intimacy, 289-291
Sexuality and disability, 459-470
Solution Focused Family of Origin Therapy, 47-56
Spiritual intimacy, 289-291
Spiritual issues for surgery patients, 330
Stress, traumatic (Handout), 481-483
  in motor vehicle accident survivors, 135-152
Substance use, erection dysfunction and, 60-61, 64
Surgery patients, psychological interventions for, 323-334
  assertiveness skills for, 330-331
  cognitive-behavioral therapy for, 328-329
  pain control for, 327-328
  relaxation techniques for, 329-330
  spiritual issues and, 330

T

Telehealth in mental health care, 385-400
  computers, networked, 393-396
  computers, stand-alone, 392-393
  facsimile machines, 390-391
  telecommunications technology, 386-389

Telehealth in mental health care *(Continued)*
teleconferencing, 391-392
telephony, 389-390
virtual reality, 395
Termination,
premature or forced, 236-237
risk management issues of, 231-245
sample letters from clinician to patient for use in process of, 242-243
voluntary, 234-235
Time-Limited Dynamic Psychotherapy for difficult patients, 5-19
Traumatic events, tips for managing (Handout), 481-483

V

Vacuum constriction devices for erection dysfunction, 64, 65-66
Virtual reality, use of, in telehealth, 395

W

Wilderness therapy, 341-343
Worksheet for Identifying Attributional Styles in Athletes (Form), 359-362
Worksheet for Modifying Attributions in Athletes (Form), 363-365

Information for Contributors

The editors of *Innovations in Clinical Practice* welcome the opportunity to review manuscripts that are consistent with the goals of the series. Manuscripts will be reviewed only if they are not simultaneously under consideration elsewhere. While we will attempt to handle all manuscripts with care, it is important to note that we assume no responsibility for unsolicited manuscripts. Any obligations we make to contributors are specified by written agreement after manuscript acceptance, and we reserve the right to accept or reject manuscripts at our discretion. All submissions should be accompanied by the author's current vita or a brief letter outlining the author's professional experience and training relevant to the topic. Accepted manuscripts are subject to editing.

Manuscript Submission

Interested contributors should submit an original and one copy of double-spaced manuscripts with a vita or letter describing their relevant experience to: Leon VandeCreek, Senior Editor, School of Professional Psychology, 3640 Colonel Glenn Highway, Wright State University, Dayton, OH 45435. Receipt of all manuscripts will be acknowledged and authors will be contacted again and notified of our editorial decision following review. Contributions not accepted for publication can be returned only if authors include a large, self-addressed envelope with sufficient return postage. When manuscripts are accepted for publication, authors are asked to provide the entire contribution on IBM-compatible disks as well as printed copies.

Manuscript Preparation

Brief contributions are preferred, and unsolicited manuscripts should generally not exceed 25 double-spaced typed pages. Each manuscript should begin with a title page that includes the name(s), address(es), and telephone number(s) of the author(s). The second page should have the title of the contribution centered at the top, but should not contain the name(s) of the author(s). No abstract is required. Manuscripts should generally follow the style specified by the current *Publication Manual of the American Psychological Association.* There is, however, an exception in that each manuscript should include a "Resource" instead of a "Reference" section and "Reference Notes." The use of footnotes is discouraged. Contributors may refer to the contents of the present volume for a general sense of the style that should be followed. Three levels of headings should be used to facilitate the organization of contributions: (a) a centered main heading, (b) a flush side heading, and (c) an indented side heading. Manuscripts should be written in a concise, professional, but readable manner. Writing in the first person, for example, is quite acceptable. Sexist language should be avoided.

Assessment Instruments and Forms

The *Innovations* volumes contain informal clinical assessment instruments and checklists. We do not usually publish formal psychological tests. Assessment instruments are designed to help the clinician be more thorough in collecting information. Contributors of assessment instruments should contact the publisher to receive a copy of the special instructional guidelines that pertain to this type of material.

Continuing Education Available for Home Study

The most recent volumes of *Innovations in Clinical Practice: A Source Book* are available as formal home-study continuing education programs. This best-selling, comprehensive source of practical clinical information is complemented by examination modules which may be used to earn continuing education credits.

Credits may be obtained by successfully completing examinations based on those contributions in each volume which have been selected by the editorial advisory board. Each of these contributions explores a timely topic designed to enhance your clinical skills and provide the knowledge necessary for effective practice. After studying these selections, a 200-item multiple-choice examination is completed and returned to the Professional Resource Exchange for scoring. Upon passing the examination (80% of test items answered correctly), your credits will be recorded and you will receive a copy of your official transcript.

At the time of publication of this volume, continuing education modules are available for Volumes 15 through 18 of *Innovations in Clinical Practice*. Each module contains examination materials for 20 credits (equivalent to 20 hours of continuing education activity).

The *Innovations in Clinical Practice* Continuing Education (CE) Program is one of the most efficient ways to stay current on new clinical techniques and obtain formal credit for your study. If your professional associations and state boards do not currently require formal CE activities, you may still wish to consider this program as an excellent means of receiving feedback on your professional development. This self-study program is . . .

- ***Relevant*** - selections are packed with information pertinent to your practice.
- ***Inexpensive*** - typically less than half the cost of obtaining credits through workshops and these expenses may still be tax deductible as a professional expense.
- ***Convenient*** - study at your own pace in the comfort of your home or office.
- ***Useful*** - the volume will always be available as a practical reference and resource for day-to-day use in your professional practice.
- ***Effective*** - as a means of staying up to date and obtaining feedback on your knowledge acquisition and professional development. In most states with continuing education requirements, credits earned from American Psychological Association (APA) approved sponsors are automatically approved for licensure renewal. Consult your profession's state board for their policies regarding the status of programs offered by APA approved sponsors.

Specific learning objectives and faculty credentials are available upon request.

The Professional Resource Exchange, Inc. is approved by the American Psychological Association to offer continuing education for psychologists. The Professional Resource Exchange maintains responsibility for the program. The Professional Resource Exchange, Inc. is also recognized by the National Board for Certified Counselors to offer continuing education for National Certified Counselors. We adhere to NBCC Continuing Education Guidelines (Provider #5474). Florida provider #CM-069-Exp. 1/2001. Our programs also meet the qualifications for continuing education credit for MFCCs and/or LCSWs as required by the CA Board of Behavioral Sciences (PCE #816).

Professional Resource Exchange offers other CE programs as well. Please see next page ——▸

More Continuing Education Programs

Ethics Program - 6 Credits

Based on the book, *Keeping Up the Good Work: A Practitioner's Guide to Mental Health Ethics* and companion audiotape by Leonard J. Haas, PhD, and John L. Malouf, PhD, this program will increase your understanding of ethical standards and practices and expand your expertise in resolving ethical dilemmas. The authors teach you how to identify potential ethical problems, and offer practical guidelines for resolving those problems. Numerous examples are given of instances in professional practice where clinicians frequently misunderstand their ethical obligations, and a straightforward process is presented for reaching decisions that are ethically appropriate.

Credits are earned by self-paced home study of the book and tape, and successful completion of a 50 question multiple-choice examination. Six continuing education (CE) credits (equivalent to 6 contact hours) will be awarded if you correctly answer at least 80% of the test questions. To participate in this program you must purchase the CE module and purchase or have access to the book and tape.

Hardbound Book	1995	304pp.	ISBN: 1-56887-012-4
Audiocassette Tape		50 min.	ISBN: 0-943158-37-0

Continuing Education Packet contains book, tape, and CE module

Domestic Violence and Spouse Abuse Program - 3 Credits

A domestic violence and spouse abuse home-study continuing education (CE) course based on the book, *Spouse Abuse,* by Michele Harway, PhD, and Marsali Hansen, PhD. This program grants 3 CE credits to participants who correctly answer 80% of the 30 multiple-choice questions contained in the CE test module. To participate in this program, you must purchase or have access to the book, *Spouse Abuse.*

Paperbound Book	1994	118pp.	ISBN: 1-56887-005-1

Continuing Education Packet contains book and CE module

Child Sexual Abuse Program - 10 Credits

Based on the book *Assessing Allegations of Child Sexual Abuse* by Kathryn Kuehnle, PhD, this continuing education program will instruct you in navigating through the clinical, scientific, and ethical minefields you encounter when involved with child sexual abuse allegations. Credits are earned by self-paced home study of the book and successful completion of at least 80% of the 100 multiple-choice questions. To participate in this program, you must purchase the CE module and purchase or have access to the book.

Hardbound Book	1996	400pp.	ISBN: 1-56887-009-4

Continuing Education Packet contains book and CE module

Ethics Program - 3 Credits

Based on the book *Ethical Risk Management: Guidelines for Practice* by William F. Doverspike, PhD. The author offers a practical approach to integrating ethical principles into clinical practice, balancing scholarly analysis with the practical application of ethical principles. This book presents useful risk-management strategies based on a conceptual framework which can be applied to a variety of clinical situations. Also included are an ethics checklist and numerous office forms for putting ethics into practice. This program grants 3 CE credits to participants who correctly answer 80% of the 30 multiple-choice questions contained in the CE test module. To participate in this program, you must purchase or have access to the book, *Ethical Risk Management: Guidelines for Practice.*

Paperbound Book	1999	112pp.	ISBN: 1-56887-057-4

Continuing Education Packet contains book and CE module

Specific learning objectives and faculty credentials are available upon request.

For additional information, please photocopy and return the form on the next page ——————▶

Do You Want More Information?

Yes! Please Send Me . . .

❒ Information on the other volumes in the *Innovations in Clinical Practice: A Source Book* series (Tables of Contents for all 18 volumes and ordering information).

❒ Information on your Home-Study Continuing Education Programs.

❒ Your latest catalog.

Name:____

(Please Print)

Address:____

Address:____

City/State/Zip:_____________________________________

Telephone: (______)________________________________

My Primary Profession Is:_____________________________

For Fastest Response . . .

Fax to Our 24 Hour FAX Line at **1-941-343-9201**

OR

E-mail to **mail@prpress.com**

OR

Call **1-800-443-3364**

OR

Visit Our Website at **http://www.prpress.com**

Or Mail This Form To . . .

Professional Resource Press
PO Box 15560 • Sarasota FL 34277-1560